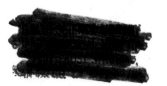

PLASTIC SURGERY

Indications, Operations, and Outcomes

Bruce M. Achauer, MD, FACS
Professor of Surgery,
Division of Plastic Surgery,
University of California Irvine,
California College of Medicine,
Orange, California

Elof Eriksson, MD, PhD, FACS
Joseph E. Murray Professor of Plastic and Reconstructive Surgery,
Harvard Medical School;
Chief, Division of Plastic Surgery,
Brigham and Women's Hospital;
Chief, Division of Plastic Surgery,
Children's Hospital,
Boston, Massachusetts

Bahman Guyuron, MD, FACS
Clinical Professor of Plastic Surgery,
Case Western Reserve University,
Cleveland, Ohio;
Medical Director,
Zeeba Medical Campus,
Lyndhurst, Ohio

John J. Coleman III, MD, FACS
Professor of Surgery;
Chief of Plastic Surgery;
Staff Physician,
Indiana University Medical Center;
Director, Pediatric Burn Unit;
Staff Physician,
Riley Children's Hospital;
Staff Physician,
Wishard Memorial Hospital,
Indianapolis, Indiana

Robert C. Russell, MD, FRACS, FACS
Clinical Professor of Surgery,
Division of Plastic Surgery,
Southern Illinois University School of Medicine,
Springfield, Illinois

Craig A. Vander Kolk, MD, FACS
Associate Professor of Plastic Surgery;
Director, Cleft and Craniofacial Center,
Johns Hopkins University School of Medicine,
Baltimore, Maryland

PLASTIC SURGERY

Indications, Operations, and Outcomes

Volume Two

Craniomaxillofacial, Cleft, and Pediatric Surgery

EDITOR
Craig A. Vander Kolk, MD, FACS
Associate Professor of Plastic Surgery;
Director, Cleft and Craniofacial Center,
Johns Hopkins University School of Medicine,
Baltimore, Maryland

OUTCOMES EDITOR
Edwin G. Wilkins, MD, MS
Associate Professor of Plastic Surgery,
University of Michigan Health Systems,
Ann Arbor, Michigan

MANAGING EDITOR
Victoria M. VanderKam, RN, BS, CPSN
Clinical Nurse, Division of Plastic Surgery,
University of California Irvine Medical Center,
Orange, California

ILLUSTRATIONS BY
Min Li, MD
Indiana University School of Medicine,
Department of Surgery, Section of Plastic Surgery,
Indianapolis, Indiana

with 6279 illustrations, including 963 in color, and 18 color plates

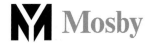

A Harcourt Health Sciences Company

St. Louis   London   Philadelphia   Sydney   Toronto

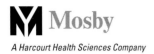

Mosby

A Harcourt Health Sciences Company

Acquisitions Editor: Richard Zorab
Developmental Editor: Dolores Meloni
Project Manager: Carol Sullivan Weis
Senior Production Editor: Rick Dudley
Designers: Dave Zielinski/Mark Oberkrom

NOTICE

Medicine is an ever-changing field. Standard safety precautions must be followed, but as new research and clinical experience broaden our knowledge, changes in treatment and drug therapy may become necessary or appropriate. Readers are advised to check the most current product information provided by the manufacturer of each drug to be administered to verify the recommended dose, the method and duration of administration, and contraindications. It is the responsibility of the treating physician, relying on experience and knowledge of the patient, to determine dosages and the best treatment for each individual patient. Neither the publisher nor the editor assumes any liability for any injury and/or damage to persons or property arising from this publication.

Mosby, Inc.
A Harcourt Health Sciences Company
11830 Westline Industrial Drive
St. Louis, Missouri 63146

Printed in the United States of America

Volume 2 ISBN 0-8151-1020-0
Set ISBN 0-8151-0984-9

00 01 02 03 04 GW/MVY 9 8 7 6 5 4 3 2 1

Contributors

BRUCE M. ACHAUER, MD, FACS
Professor of Surgery,
Division of Plastic Surgery,
University of California Irvine,
California College of Medicine,
Orange, California

GREGORY J. ADAMSON, MD
Clinical Instructor of Orthopedics,
University of Illinois College of Medicine at Peoria;
Staff, St. Francis Medical Center,
Peoria, Illinois

GHADA Y. AFIFI, MD
Clinical Assistant Professor,
Division of Plastic Surgery,
Department of Surgery,
Loma Linda University Medical Center and Children's
    Hospital;
Attending Surgeon, Plastic Surgery,
Jerry L. Pettis Memorial Veterans Affairs Medical Center,
Loma Linda, California;
Private Practice,
Newport Beach, California

RICHARD D. ANDERSON, MD
Plastic Surgery Staff,
Scottsdale Healthcare Hospitals;
Private Practice,
Scottsdale, Arizona

JAMES P. ANTHONY, MD
Associate Professor of Surgery,
Division of Plastic Surgery,
University of California–San Francisco,
San Francisco, California

HÉCTOR ARÁMBULA, MD
Professor of Plastic Surgery,
Postgraduate Division of Medicine,
Universidad Nacional Autonoma de Mexico;
Chairman, Plastic Surgery Service,
Hospital de Traumatologia Magdalena de las Salinas,
Instituto Mexicano del Seguro Social, IMSS,
Mexico City, Mexico

LOUIS C. ARGENTA, MD
Julius A. Howell Professor and Chairman,
Department of Plastic Surgery,
Wake Forest University School of Medicine;
Professor and Chairman,
Department of Plastic and Reconstructive Surgery,
North Carolina Baptist Hospital,
Winston-Salem, North Carolina

DUFFIELD ASHMEAD IV, MD
Assistant Clinical Professor of Plastic Surgery and
    Orthopedics,
University of Connecticut School of Medicine,
Farmington, Connecticut;
Director, Division of Hand Surgery,
Connecticut Children's Medical Center,
Hartford, Connecticut

CHRISTOPHER J. ASSAD, BS, MD, FRCSC
Plastic and Reconstructive Surgeon;
Associate Staff,
Halton Health Care Services Corporation,
Milton District Hospital,
Milton, Ontario, Canada

THOMAS J. BAKER, MD
Professor of Plastic Surgery–Voluntary,
University of Miami School of Medicine;
Senior Attending Physician,
Mercy Hospital,
Miami, Florida

TRACY M. BAKER, MD
Instructor in Plastic Surgery,
University of Miami School of Medicine,
Miami, Florida

JUAN P. BARRET, MD
Professor, Rijksuniversiteit Groningen;
Plastic and Reconstructive Surgeon,
University Hospital Groningen,
Groningen, The Netherlands

MUNISH K. BATRA, MD
Assistant Clinical Instructor–Voluntary,
Division of Plastic Surgery,
University of California–San Diego Medical Center,
San Diego, California;
Private Practice,
Del Mar, California

BRUCE S. BAUER, MD, FACS
Associate Professor of Surgery,
Northwestern University Medical School;
Head, Division of Plastic Surgery,
The Children's Memorial Hospital,
Chicago, Illinois

STEPHEN P. BEALS, MD, FACS, FAAP,
Assistant Professor of Plastic Surgery,
Mayo Medical School;
Adjunct Professor,
Department of Speech and Hearing Science,
Arizona State University;
Craniofacial Consultant,
Barrow Neurological Institute
Phoenix, Arizona

MICHAEL S. BEDNAR, MD
Associate Professor,
Department of Orthopedic Surgery and Rehabilitation,
Stritch School of Medicine,
Loyola University–Chicago,
Maywood, Illinois

RAMIN A. BEHMAND, MD
Chief Resident,
Division of Plastic and Reconstructive Surgery,
University of Michigan Hospitals,
Ann Arbor, Michigan

RUSSELL W. BESSETTE, DDS, MD
Clinical Professor of Plastic Surgery,
State University of New York–Buffalo,
School of Medicine;
Executive Director of Research,
Sisters Hospital,
Buffalo, New York

MARINA D. BIZZARRI-SCHMID, MD
Instructor in Anesthesia,
Harvard Medical School;
Anesthesiologist,
Brigham and Women's Hospital,
Boston, Massachusetts

GREG BORSCHEL, MD
Plastic Surgery Resident,
University of Michigan Hospitals,
Ann Arbor, Michigan

MARK T. BOSCHERT, MS, MD
Attending Physician,
St. Joseph Health Center;
Private Practice,
St. Charles, Missouri,
Attending Physician,
Barnes-St. Peters Hospital,
St. Peters, Missouri

JOHN BOSTWICK, MD, FACS
Professor and Chairman of Plastic Surgery,
Emory University School of Medicine;
Chief of Plastic Surgery,
Emory University Hospital,
Atlanta, Georgia

J. BRIAN BOYD, MB, ChB, MD, FRCSC, FACS
Professor of Surgery,
The Ohio State University College of Medicine,
Columbus, Ohio;
Chairman of Plastic Surgery,
Cleveland Clinic–Florida,
Fort Lauderdale, Florida

WILLIAM R. BOYDSTON, MD, PhD
Pediatric Neurosurgeon,
Children's Healthcare of Atlanta,
Scottish Rite Children's Hospital,
Atlanta, Georgia

KARL H. BREUING, MD
Instructor in Surgery,
Harvard Medical School;
Attending Physician, Plastic Surgery,
Brigham and Women's Hospital;
Attending Physician, Plastic Surgery,
Children's Hospital;
Attending Physician, Plastic Surgery,
Faulkner Hospital;
Attending Physician, Plastic Surgery,
Dana Farber Cancer Institute,
Boston, Massachusetts

FORST E. BROWN, MD
Emeritus Professor of Plastic Surgery,
Dartmouth Medical School,
Hanover, New Hampshire;
Consultant,
Veterans Administration Hospital,
White River Junction, Vermont

RICHARD E. BROWN, MD, FACS
Clinical Associate Professor;
Hand Fellowship Director,
Division of Plastic Surgery,
Southern Illinois University School of Medicine,
Springfield, Illinois

MARIE-CLAIRE BUCKLEY, MD
Plastic Surgery Fellow,
University of Minnesota Medical School,
Division of Plastic and Reconstructive Surgery,
Minneapolis, Minnesota

GREGORY M. BUNCKE, MD, FACS
Clinical Assistant Professor of Surgery,
University of California–San Francisco,
San Francisco, California;
Clinical Assistant Professor of Surgery,
Stanford University,
Stanford, California;
Co-Director, Division of Microsurgery,
California Pacific Medical Center,
San Francisco, California

HARRY J. BUNCKE, MD
Clinical Professor of Surgery,
University of California–San Francisco,
San Francisco, California;
Associate Clinical Professor of Surgery,
Stanford Medical School,
Stanford, California;
Director, Microsurgical Transplantation–Replantation
   Service,
California Pacific Medical Center–Davies,
San Francisco, California

RUDOLF BUNTIC, MD
Clinical Instructor,
Division of Plastic Surgery,
Stanford University,
Stanford, California;
Attending Microsurgeon,
California Pacific Medical Center,
San Francisco, California

ELISA A. BURGESS, MD
Resident in Plastic Surgery,
Oregon Health Sciences University,
Portland, Oregon

FERNANDO D. BURSTEIN, MD
Clinical Associate Professor,
Plastic and Reconstructive Surgery,
Emory University School of Medicine;
Chief, Plastic and Reconstructive Surgery;
Co-Director, Center for Craniofacial Disorders,
Scottish Rite Children's Medical Center,
Atlanta, Georgia

GRANT W. CARLSON, MD
Professor of Surgery,
Emory University School of Medicine;
Chief of Surgical Services,
Crawford Long Hospital;
Chief of Surgical Oncology,
Emory Clinic,
Atlanta, Georgia

JAMES CARRAWAY, MD, AB
Professor of Plastic Surgery;
Chairman, Division of Plastic Surgery,
Eastern Virginia Medical School,
Norfolk, Virginia

STANLEY A. CASTOR, MD
Plastic Surgery Staff Physician,
The Watson Clinic,
Lakeland, Florida

BERNARD CHANG, MD
Director, Plastic and Reconstructive Surgery,
Mercy Medical Center,
Baltimore, Maryland

YU-RAY CHEN, MD
Professor, Department of Plastic Surgery,
Chang Gung University Medical School
Tao-Yuan, Taiwan;
Superintendent and Attending Surgeon,
Department of Plastic Surgery,
Chang Gung Memorial Hospital,
Taipei, Taiwan

ANDREAS CHIMONIDES, BS, MD
Staff Physician,
Butler Memorial Hospital,
Butler, Pennsylvania;
Staff Physician,
St. Francis Medical Center;
Staff Physician,
University of Pennsylvania Medical Center–St. Margaret's
   Hospital,
Pittsburgh, Pennsylvania

MARK A. CODNER, MD
Clinical Assistant Professor,
Emory University School of Medicine;
Private Practice,
Atlanta, Georgia

I. KELMAN COHEN, MD
Professor of Surgery;
Director, Wound Healing Center,
Medical College of Virginia,
Virginia Commonwealth University,
Richmond, Virginia

MYLES J. COHEN, MD
Clinical Assistant Professor of Surgery,
University of Southern California School of Medicine;
Attending Physician,
Cedars Sinai Medical Center,
Los Angeles, California

STEVEN R. COHEN, MD
Associate Clinical Professor,
Division of Plastic and Reconstructive Surgery,
University of California Medical Center–San Diego;
Chief, Craniofacial Surgery,
Children's Hospital of San Diego,
San Diego, California

VICTOR COHEN, MD
Resident Physician,
McGill University Health Center,
McGill University School of Medicine,
Montreal, Quebec, Canada

JOHN J. COLEMAN III, MD, FACS
Professor of Surgery;
Chief of Plastic Surgery;
Staff Physician,
Indiana University Medical Center;
Director, Pediatric Burn Unit;
Staff Physician,
Riley Children's Hospital;
Staff Physician,
Wishard Memorial Hospital,
Indianapolis, Indiana

LAWRENCE B. COLEN, MD
Associate Professor of Plastic and Reconstructive Surgery,
Eastern Virginia Medical School,
Norfolk, Virginia

E. DALE COLLINS, MD, MS
Assistant Professor of Surgery,
Dartmouth Medical School,
Hanover, New Hampshire;
Medical Director, Comprehensive Breast Program,
Dartmouth-Hitchcock Medical Center,
Lebanon, New Hampshire

MATTHEW J. CONCANNON, MD, FACS
Assistant Professor;
Director of Hand and Microsurgery,
University of Missouri,
Columbia, Missouri

BRUCE F. CONNELL, MD
Clinical Professor of Surgery,
University of California Irvine,
California College of Medicine,
Orange, California

AISLING CONRAN, MD
Assistant Professor, Clinical Anesthesia,
University of Chicago,
Chicago, Illinois

PAUL C. COTTERILL, BS, MD, ABHRS,
Honorary Lecturer,
Sunnybrook Hospital,
Department of Dermatology,
University of Toronto,
Toronto, Ontario, Canada

KIMBALL MAURICE CROFTS, MD
Staff Physician,
Utah Valley Regional Medical Center,
Provo, Utah;
Staff Physician,
Timpanogos Regional Hospital,
Orem, Utah;
Staff Physician,
Mt. View Hospital,
Payson, Utah;
Staff Physician,
Sevier Valley Hospital,
Richfield, Utah

LISA R. DAVID, MD
Assistant Professor,
Department of Plastic and Reconstructive Surgery,
Wake Forest University School of Medicine;
Attending Physician,
North Carolina Baptist Hospital,
Winston-Salem, North Carolina

WILLIAM M. DAVIDSON, AB, DMD, PhD
Professor and Chairman,
Department of Orthodontics,
University of Maryland Dental School;
Associate Staff, Dentistry,
Johns Hopkins Hospital,
Baltimore, Maryland

MARK A. DEITCH, MD
Assistant Professor of Surgery,
Division of Orthopedic Surgery,
University of Maryland School of Medicine,
Baltimore, Maryland

MARK D. DeLACURE, MD, FACS
Chief, Division of Head and Neck Surgery and Oncology;
Associate Professor of Otolaryngology–Head and Neck
   Surgery,
Department of Otolaryngology;
Associate Professor of Reconstructive Plastic Surgery,
Institute of Reconstructive Plastic Surgery,
Department of Surgery,
New York University School of Medicine,
New York, New York

VALERIE BURKE DeLEON, MA,
Department of Cell Biology and Anatomy,
Johns Hopkins University School of Medicine,
Baltimore, Maryland

JOHN Di SAIA, MD
Assistant Clinical Professor,
Division of Plastic Surgery,
University of California Irvine,
California College of Medicine,
Orange, California

RICHARD V. DOWDEN, MD
Clinical Assistant Professor,
Case Western Reserve University,
Cleveland, Ohio

CRAIG R. DUFRESNE, MD, FACS
Clinical Professor of Plastic Surgery,
Georgetown University,
Washington, DC;
Plastic Surgery Section Chief;
Co-Director, Center for Facial Rehabilitation,
Fairfax Hospital,
Inova Hospital System,
Fairfax, Virginia

FELMONT F. EAVES III, MD, FACS
Assistant Clinical Professor,
University of North Carolina,
Chapel Hill, North Carolina;
Attending Physician,
Charlotte Plastic Surgery Center;
Attending Physician,
Carolinas Medical Center;
Attending Physician,
Presbyterian Hospital;
Attending Physician,
Mercy Hospital,
Charlotte, North Carolina

PHILIP EDELMAN, MD
Associate Professor of Medicine;
Director, Toxicology and Clinical Services,
Division of Occupational and Environmental Medicine,
George Washington University School of Medicine,
Washington, DC

ERIC T. EMERSON, MD
Private Practice,
Gastonia, North Carolina

TODD B. ENGEN, MD
Clinical Faculty,
University of Utah School of Medicine,
Salt Lake City, Utah;
Clinical Director,
Excel Cosmetic Surgery Center,
Orem, Utah

BARRY L. EPPLEY, MD, DMD
Assistant Professor of Plastic Surgery,
Indiana University School of Medicine,
Indianapolis, Indiana

ELOF ERIKSSON, MD, PhD, FACS
Joseph E. Murray Professor of Plastic and Reconstructive
  Surgery,
Harvard Medical School;
Chief, Division of Plastic Surgery,
Brigham and Women's Hospital;
Chief, Division of Plastic Surgery,
Children's Hospital,
Boston, Massachusetts

GREGORY R.D. EVANS, MD, FACS
Professor of Surgery;
Chair, Division of Plastic Surgery,
University of California Irvine,
California College of Medicine
Orange, California

JEFFREY A. FEARON, MD, FACS, FAAP
Director, The Craniofacial Center,
North Texas Hospital for Children at Medical City Dallas,
Dallas, Texas

LYNNE M. FEEHAN, MS, PT
Senior Hand Therapist,
Hand Program,
Workers' Compensation Board of British Columbia,
Richmond, British Columbia, Canada

RANDALL S. FEINGOLD, MD, FACS
Assistant Clinical Professor, Plastic and Reconstructive
  Surgery,
Albert Einstein College of Medicine,
Bronx, New York;
Attending Surgeon,
Long Island Jewish Medical Center,
New Hyde Park, New York;
Chief, Division of Plastic Surgery,
North Shore University Hospital at Forest Hills,
Forest Hills, New York

ROBERT D. FOSTER, MD
Assistant Professor in Residence,
Division of Plastic and Reconstructive Surgery,
University of California–San Francisco,
San Francisco, California

FRANK J. FRASSICA, MD
Professor of Orthopedic Surgery and Oncology,
Johns Hopkins University School of Medicine,
Baltimore, Maryland

ALAN E. FREELAND, MD
Professor, Department of Orthopedic Surgery;
Director, Hand Surgery Service,
The University of Mississippi Medical Center,
Jackson, Mississippi

MENNEN T. GALLAS, MD
Junior Faculty Associate,
University of Texas M.D. Anderson Cancer Center,
Houston, Texas

BING SIANG GAN, MD, PhD, FRCSC
Assistant Professor,
Departments of Surgery and Pharmacology-Toxicology,
University of Western Ontario;
Staff Surgeon,
Hand and Upper Limb Centre;
Staff Surgeon,
St. Joseph's Health Centre,
London, Ontario, Canada

WARREN L. GARNER, MD
Associate Professor of Surgery,
University of Southern California;
Associate Professor of Plastic Surgery;
Director, LAC & USC Burn Center,
Los Angeles, California

DAVID G. GENECOV, MD
Attending Surgeon,
International Craniofacial Institute,
Dallas, Texas

GEORGE K. GITTES, MD
Associate Professor,
Department of Surgery,
University of Missouri–Kansas City;
Holder and Ashcraft Chair of Pediatric Surgical Research,
Children's Mercy Hospital,
Kansas City, Missouri

JEFFREY A. GOLDSTEIN, MD
Associate Professor of Surgery,
Case Western Reserve University;
Medical Director, Craniofacial Center;
Chief of Plastic and Reconstructive Surgery,
Rainbow Babies and Children's Hospital,
Cleveland, Ohio

HECTOR GONZALEZ-MIRAMONTES, MD
Private Practice,
Guadalajara, Mexico

LAWRENCE J. GOTTLIEB, MD
Professor of Clinical Surgery,
University of Chicago,
Pritzker School of Medicine,
Chicago, Illinois

MARK S. GRANICK, MD
Professor of Surgery;
Chief of Plastic Surgery,
MCP-Hahnemann University,
Philadelphia, Pennsylvania

FREDERICK M. GRAZER, MD, FACS
Associate Clinical Professor,
Division of Plastic Surgery,
University of California Irvine,
California College of Medicine;
Staff Physician,
University of California Irvine Medical Center,
Orange, California;
Clinical Professor of Surgery,
The Pennsylvania State University Milton S. Hershey
    Medical Center College of Medicine,
Hershey, Pennsylvania;
Staff Physician,
Hoag Memorial Hospital Presbyterian,
Newport Beach, California

JON M. GRAZER, MD, MPH
Staff Physician,
Hoag Memorial Hospital Presbyterian,
Newport Beach, California;
Staff Physician,
Western Medical Center,
Santa Ana, California

JUDITH M. GURLEY, MD
Assistant Professor of Surgery,
Division of Plastic and Reconstructive Surgery,
Washington University School of Medicine;
Attending Physician,
St. Louis Children's Hospital;
Attending Physician,
Shriner's Hospital for Children,
St. Louis, Missouri

BAHMAN GUYURON, MD, FACS
Clinical Professor of Plastic Surgery,
Case Western Reserve University,
Cleveland, Ohio;
Medical Director,
Zeeba Medical Campus,
Lyndhurst, Ohio

HONGSHIK HAN, MD
Plastic Surgery Resident,
Division of Plastic Surgery,
Northwestern University Medical School,
Chicago, Illinois

ROBERT A. HARDESTY, MD
Professor,
Loma Linda University School of Medicine;
Medical Staff President;
Chief of Plastic Surgery,
Loma Linda University Medical Center,
Loma Linda, California

MAUREEN HARDY, PT, MS, CHT
Clinical Assistant Professor,
University of Mississippi Medical Center;
Director, Hand Management Center,
St. Dominic Hospital,
Jackson, Mississippi

ALAN SCOTT HARMATZ, BS, MD
Assistant Professor of Surgery,
University of Vermont College of Medicine,
Burlington, Vermont;
Attending Physician,
Maine Medical Center,
Portland, Maine

STEPHEN U. HARRIS, MD
Staff Physician,
Nassau County Medical Center,
East Meadow, New York;
Staff Physician,
North Shore Hospital,
Manhasset, New York;
Staff Physician,
Winthrop University Hospital,
Mineola, New York;
Plastic Surgeon,
Long Island Plastic Surgical Group,
Garden City, New York

ROBERT J. HAVLIK, MD
Associate Professor of Surgery,
Indiana University School of Medicine,
Indianapolis, Indiana

DETLEV HEBEBRAND, MD, PhD
Attending Physician,
Hand and Burn Center,
Bergmannsheil Clinic,
Ruhr University,
Bochum, Germany

MARC H. HEDRICK, MD
Assistant Professor of Surgery and Pediatrics,
Division of Plastic and Reconstructive Surgery,
University of California–Los Angeles School of Medicine,
Los Angeles, California

DOMINIC F. HEFFEL, MD
Resident, General Surgery,
University of California–Los Angeles Center for Health
    Sciences,
Los Angeles, California

CHRIS S. HELMSTEDTER, MD
Director of Orthopedic Oncology–Southern California,
Kaiser Permanente,
Baldwin Park, California;
Assistant Clinical Professor, Orthopedics and Surgery,
University of Southern California School of Medicine,
Los Angeles, California

VINCENT R. HENTZ, MD
Professor of Functional Restoration (Hand Surgery),
Stanford University School of Medicine,
Stanford, California

JEFFREY HOLLINGER, DDS, PhD
Professor, Biology and Biomedical Health Engineering;
Director, Center for Bone Tissue Engineering,
Carnegie Mellon University,
Pittsburgh, Pennsylvania

HEINZ-HERBERT HOMANN, MD
Attending Physician,
Hand and Burn Center,
Bergmannsheil Clinic,
Ruhr University,
Bochum, Germany

CHARLES E. HORTON, MD, FACS, FRCSC
Professor of Plastic Surgery,
Eastern Virginia Medical School,
Norfolk, Virginia;
Clinical Professor of Surgery,
Medical College of Virginia,
Richmond, Virginia

CHARLES E. HORTON, Jr., MD
Assistant Professor of Urology,
Eastern Virginia Medical School;
Chief, Department of Urology,
Children's Hospital of the King's Daughters,
Norfolk, Virginia

ERIC H. HUBLI, MD, FACS, FAAP
Craniomaxillofacial Surgeon,
International Craniofacial Institute,
Dallas, Texas

ROGER J. HUDGINS, MD
Assistant Professor,
Morehouse University School of Medicine;
Chief of Pediatric Neurosurgery,
Children's Healthcare of Atlanta,
Scottish Rite Children's Hospital,
Atlanta, Georgia

LAWRENCE N. HURST, MD, FRCSC
Professor and Chairman,
Division of Plastic Surgery,
The University of Western Ontario;
Chief, Division of Plastic Surgery
London Health Sciences Centre, University Campus,
London, Ontario, Canada

ETHYLIN WANG JABS, MD
Dr. Frank V. Sutland Professor of Pediatric Genetics;
Professor of Pediatrics, Medicine, and Plastic Surgery,
John Hopkins University School of Medicine,
Baltimore, Maryland

MOULTON K. JOHNSON, MD
Associate Professor of Orthopedic Surgery,
University of California–Los Angeles,
Los Angeles, California

GLYN JONES, MD, FRCS, FCS
Associate Professor of Plastic Surgery;
Chief of Plastic Surgery,
Crawford Long Hospital,
Emory Clinic,
Atlanta, Georgia

NEIL F. JONES, MD
Professor, Division of Plastic and Reconstructive Surgery,
Department of Orthopedic Surgery,
University of California–Los Angeles;
Chief of Hand Surgery,
University of California–Los Angeles Medical Center,
Los Angeles, California

JESSE B. JUPITER, MD
Professor of Orthopedic Surgery,
Harvard Medical School;
Head, Orthopedic Hand Service,
Massachusetts General Hospital,
Boston, Massachusetts

M.J. JURKIEWICZ, MD, DDS
Professor of Surgery, Emeritus,
Emory University School of Medicine,
Atlanta, Georgia

MADELYN D. KAHANA, MD
Associate Professor of Anesthesiology and Pediatrics,
The University of Chicago Hospital,
Chicago, Illinois

CHIA CHI KAO, MD
Fellow, Department of Reconstructive and Plastic Surgery,
University of Southern California,
Los Angeles, California

AJAYA KASHYAP, MD
Assistant Professor,
University of Massachusetts Medical Center,
Worcester, Massachusetts;
Attending Plastic Surgeon,
Metrowest Medical Center,
Framingham, Massachusetts

JULIA A. KATARINCIC, MD
Consultant, Department of Orthopedic Surgery,
Mayo Clinic,
Rochester, Minnesota

DANIEL J. KELLEY, MD
Assistant Professor;
Director, Head and Neck Oncology/Skull Base Surgery,
Department of Otolaryngology and Bronchoesophagology,
Temple University School of Medicine,
Philadelphia, Pennsylvania

KEVIN J. KELLY, DDS, MD
Associate Professor,
Department of Plastic Surgery,
Vanderbilt University School of Medicine;
Director, Craniofacial Surgery,
Department of Plastic Surgery,
Vanderbilt Medical Center,
Nashville, Tennessee

PRASAD G. KILARU, MD
Clinical Assistant Professor of Surgery,
University of Southern California–Los Angeles,
Los Angeles, California;
Staff Physician,
City of Hope National Medical Center,
Duarte, California

GABRIEL M. KIND, MD
Assistant Clinical Professor,
Department of Surgery,
Division of Plastic and Reconstructive Surgery,
University of California–San Francisco;
Assistant Director of Research;
Assistant Fellowship Director,
The Buncke Clinic,
San Francisco, California

BRIAN M. KINNEY, MD, FACS, MSME
Clinical Assistant Professor of Plastic Surgery,
University of Southern California–Los Angeles;
Former Chief,
Century City Hospital,
Los Angeles, California

ELIZABETH M. KIRALY, MD
Fellow, Hand and Microvascular Surgery,
University of Nevada School of Medicine,
Department of Surgery,
Division of Plastic Surgery,
Las Vegas, Nevada

JOHN O. KUCAN, MD
Professor of Surgery,
Institute of Plastic Surgery,
Southern Illinois University School of Medicine,
Springfield, Illinois

M. ABRAHAM KURIAKOSE, MD, DDS, FACS
Assistant Professor of Otolaryngology,
Division of Head and Neck Surgery,
Department of Otolaryngology,
New York University School of Medicine;
Attending Surgeon,
New York University Medical Center,
New York, New York

AMY L. LADD, MD
Associate Professor,
Division of Hand and Upper Extremity,
Department of Functional Restoration,
Stanford University;
Chief, Hand and Upper Extremity Clinic,
Lucile Salter Packard Children's Hospital,
Stanford, California

PATRICK W. LAPPERT, MD
Assistant Professor of Surgery,
Uniformed Services University of the Health Sciences,
Bethesda, Maryland;
Chief, Department of Plastic Surgery,
Naval Medical Center,
Portsmouth, Virginia

DON LaROSSA, MD
Professor of Plastic Surgery,
The University of Pennsylvania School of Medicine;
Staff Physician,
Hospital of The University of Pennsylvania;
Senior Surgeon,
Children's Hospital of Philadelphia,
Philadelphia, Pennsylvania

DAVID L. LARSON, MD
Professor and Chair of Plastic and Reconstructive Surgery,
Medical College of Wisconsin,
Milwaukee, Wisconsin

DONALD R. LAUB, Jr., MS, MD
Assistant Professor,
Departments of Surgery and Orthopedics,
University of Vermont;
Attending Plastic and Hand Surgeon,
Fletcher Allen Health Care,
Burlington, Vermont

MICHAEL LAW, MD
Fellow, Microsurgery,
University of Southern California–Los Angeles,
Division of Plastic Surgery,
Los Angeles, California

W. THOMAS LAWRENCE, MPH, MD
Professor and Chief,
Section of Plastic Surgery,
University of Kansas Medical Center,
Kansas City, Kansas

W.P. ANDREW LEE, MD, FACS
Assistant Professor of Surgery,
Harvard Medical School;
Chief of Hand Service,
Department of Surgery,
Massachusetts General Hospital,
Boston, Massachusetts

SALVATORE LETTIERI, MD
Senior Associate Consultant,
Mayo Clinic,
Division of Plastic and Reconstructive Surgery,
Rochester, Minnesota

JAN S. LEWIN, PhD
Assistant Professor and Director,
Speech Pathology and Audiology Section,
University of Texas M.D. Anderson Cancer Center,
Houston, Texas

TERRY R. LIGHT, MD
Dr. William M. Scholl Professor;
Chairman, Department of Orthopedic Surgery and
  Rehabilitation,
Stritch School of Medicine,
Loyola University–Chicago,
Maywood, Illinois

SEAN LILLE, MD
Research Professor,
Department of Chemistry and Biochemistry,
Arizona State University,
Tempe, Arizona;
Research Scientist,
Mayo Clinic–Scottsdale,
Scottsdale, Arizona;
Private Practice,
Phoenix, Arizona

TED LOCKWOOD, MD
Associate Clinical Professor,
University of Kansas Medical School;
Assistant Clinical Professor,
University of Missouri–Kansas City Medical School,
Kansas City, Missouri

MICHAEL T. LONGAKER, MD, FACS
John Marquis Converse Professor of Plastic Surgery Research;
Director of Surgical Research,
New York University School of Medicine;
Attending Plastic Surgeon,
New York University Medical Center,
New York, New York

H. PETER LORENZ, MD
Assistant Professor of Plastic Surgery,
University of California–Los Angeles School of Medicine,
Los Angeles, California

GEORGE L. LUCAS, MD
Professor and Chairman,
Orthopedic Surgery;
Program Director,
University of Kansas–Wichita;
Orthopedic Surgeon,
Via Christi Hospital;
Orthopedic Surgeon,
Wesley Medical Center,
Wichita, Kansas

PETER J. LUND, BS, MD
Orthopedic/Hand Surgery,
Methodist Volunteer General Hospital,
Martin, Tennessee

STEVEN D. MACHT, MD, DDS
Clinical Professor of Plastic Surgery,
George Washington University,
Washington, DC

JOHN S. MANCOLL, MD
Private Practice,
Fort Wayne, Indiana

GREGORY A. MANTOOTH, MD
Chief Resident,
Division of Plastic and Reconstructive Surgery,
Indiana University,
Indianapolis, Indiana

BENJAMIN M. MASER, MD
Community Physician,
Department of Functional Restoration,
Stanford University,
Stanford, California

BRUCE A. MAST, MD
Assistant Professor,
Department of Surgery,
Division of Plastic and Reconstructive Surgery,
University of Florida;
Chief, Section of Plastic Surgery,
Malcolm Randall Gainesville Veterans Administration
  Medical Center,
Gainesville, Florida

ALAN MATARASSO, MD
Clinical Associate Professor of Plastic Surgery,
Albert Einstein College of Medicine;
Surgeon,
Manhattan Eye, Ear, Throat Hospital,
New York, New York

G. PATRICK MAXWELL, MD
Assistant Professor of Plastic Surgery,
Vanderbilt University;
Director, Institute for Aesthetic Surgery,
Baptist Hospital,
Nashville, Tennessee

MICHAEL H. MAYER, MD
Physician and Surgeon,
Plastic and Reconstructive Surgery,
Portland, Oregon

TRACY E. McCALL, MD
Chief Plastic Surgery Resident,
State University of New York,
Health Science Center at Brooklyn,
Brooklyn, New York

ROBERT L. McCAULEY, MD
Chief, Plastic and Reconstructive Surgery,
Shriners Burns Hospital Galveston;
Professor of Surgery and Pediatrics,
University of Texas Medical Branch,
Galveston, Texas

LAWRENCE R. MENENDEZ, MD
Associate Professor, Clinical Orthopedics;
Associate Professor, Department of Surgery,
Division of Tumor and Endocrine,
University of Southern California;
Chief of Orthopedics,
Kenneth Norris Jr. Cancer Hospital,
Los Angeles, California

FREDERICK J. MENICK, MD
Private Practice,
Tucson, Arizona

WYNDELL H. MERRITT, MD, FACS
Clinical Assistant Professor of Surgery,
Medical College of Virginia,
Richmond, Virginia

BRYAN J. MICHELOW, MBBCh, FRCS
Clinical Assistant Professor,
Case Western Reserve University,
Cleveland, Ohio

SCOTT R. MILLER, MD
Clinical Instructor of Plastic Surgery,
University of California–San Diego,
San Diego, California;
Attending Surgeon,
Scripps Memorial Hospital,
La Jolla, California

TIMOTHY A. MILLER, MD
Professor,
University of California–Los Angeles;
Chief, Plastic Surgery,
Wadsworth Veterans Administration Medical Center,
Los Angeles, California

FERNANDO MOLINA, MD
Professor, Plastic, Aesthetic, and Reconstructive Surgery;
Head, Division of Plastic and Reconstructive Surgery,
Hospital General Dr. Manual Gea Gonzalez,
Mexico City, Mexico

ROBERT E. MONTROY, MD
Associate Clinical Professor,
Division of Plastic Surgery,
University of California Irvine,
California College of Medicine,
Orange, California;
Chief, Plastic Surgery Section;
Assistant Chief, Spinal Cord Injury/Disease Health Care
    Group,
Department of Veterans Affairs Medical Center,
Long Beach, California

THOMAS S. MOORE, MD
Clinical Professor of Plastic Surgery,
Indiana University School of Medicine;
Chairman, Department of Plastic Surgery,
St. Vincent Hospital,
Indianapolis, Indiana

FARAMARZ MOVAGHARNIA, DO
Plastic Surgeon;
Staff Physician,
Emory Northlake Regional Medical Center,
Atlanta, Georgia

ARIAN MOWLAVI, MD
Plastic Surgery Resident,
Southern Illinois University School of Medicine,
Springfield, Illinois

JOSEPH E. MURRAY, MD
Emeritus Professor of Surgery,
Harvard Medical School,
Boston, Massachusetts

THOMAS A. MUSTOE, MD
Professor and Chief, Division of Plastic Surgery,
Northwestern University Medical School,
Chicago, Illinois

ARSHAD R. MUZAFFAR, MD
Chief Resident,
Department of Plastic Surgery,
University of Texas Southwestern Medical Center,
Parkland Memorial Hospital,
Dallas, Texas

NASH H. NAAM, MD, FACS
Clinical Professor,
Department of Plastic and Reconstructive Surgery,
Southern Illinois University School of Medicine,
Springfield, Illinois;
Director, Southern Illinois Hand Center,
Effingham, Illinois

SATORU NAGATA, MD, PhD
Visiting Professor,
Division of Plastic Surgery,
University of California Irvine,
California College of Medicine,
Orange, California;
Department Director,
Reconstructive Plastic Surgery,
Chiba Tokushukai Hospital,
Narashinodai, Funabashi, Chiba, Japan

DANIEL J. NAGLE, MD
Associate Clinical Professor of Orthopedic Surgery,
Northwestern University Medical School;
Attending Hand and Microsurgeon,
Northwestern Memorial Hospital,
Chicago, Illinois

FOAD NAHAI, MD, FACS
Private Practice,
Atlanta, Georgia

DAVID T. NETSCHER, MD, FACS
Associate Professor,
Division of Plastic Surgery,
Baylor College of Medicine;
Chief, Plastic Surgery,
Veterans Affairs Medical Center,
Houston, Texas

MICHAEL W. NEUMEISTER, MD
Assistant Professor;
Plastic Surgery Program Director;
Chief, Microsurgery and Research,
Southern Illinois University School of Medicine;
Director, Hyperbaric Oxygen Unit,
Co-Director, Regional Burn Unit,
Memorial Medical Center,
Springfield, Illinois

RONALD E. PALMER, MD
Clinical Assistant Professor,
University of Illinois College of Medicine at Peoria,
Peoria, Illinois

FRANK A. PAPAY, MS, MD, FACS, FAAP
Assistant Clinical Professor,
The Ohio State University College of Medicine,
Columbus, Ohio;
Staff Surgeon;
Head, Section of Craniofacial and Pediatric Plastic Surgery,
The Cleveland Clinic Foundation,
Department of Plastic and Reconstructive Surgery,
Cleveland, Ohio

ROBERT W. PARSONS, MD
Professor Emeritus in Plastic Surgery and Pediatrics,
University of Chicago,
Pritzker School of Medicine,
Chicago, Illinois

WILLIAM C. PEDERSON, MD, FACS
Clinical Associate Professor,
Department of Surgery and Orthopedic Surgery,
University of Texas Health Science Center–San Antonio,
San Antonio, Texas

LINDA G. PHILLIPS, MD
Professor of Plastic Surgery;
Chief, Division of Plastic Surgery,
University of Texas Medical Branch,
Galveston, Texas

GEORGE J. PICHA, MD, PhD, FACS
Clinical Assistant Professor,
Division of Plastic Surgery,
Case Western Reserve University,
Cleveland, Ohio;
Private Practice,
Lyndhurst, Ohio

JEFFREY C. POSNICK, DMD, MD, FRCSC, FACS
Clinical Professor, Plastic Surgery, Pediatrics, Oral and
    Maxillofacial Surgery, and Otolaryngology/Head and Neck
    Surgery,
Georgetown University,
Washington, DC;
Director, Posnick Center for Facial Plastic Surgery,
Chevy Chase, Maryland

JASON N. POZNER, MD
Private Practice,
Boca Raton, Florida

STEFAN PREUSS, MD
Fellow, Plastic and Reconstructive Surgery,
Harvard Medical School;
Staff Physician,
Brigham and Women's Hospital;
Staff Physician,
Children's Hospital,
Boston, Massachusetts

JULIAN J. PRIBAZ, MD
Associate Professor of Surgery;
Program Director,
Harvard Plastic Surgery Residency Training Program,
Harvard Medical School;
Associate Surgeon,
Brigham and Women's Hospital;
Associate Surgeon,
Children's Hospital,
Boston, Massachusetts

C. LIN PUCKETT, MD, FACS
Professor and Head, Division of Plastic Surgery,
University of Missouri,
Columbia, Missouri

OSCAR M. RAMIREZ, MD
Clinical Assistant Professor,
Johns Hopkins University School of Medicine;
Clinical Assistant Professor,
University of Maryland,
Baltimore, Maryland;
Director,
Esthétique International,
Plastic Surgical Center,
Timonium, Maryland

GERALD V. RAYMOND, MD
Assistant Professor,
John Hopkins University School of Medicine;
Neurologist,
Kennedy Krieger Institute,
Baltimore, Maryland

RILEY REES, MD
Professor of Plastic and Reconstructive Surgery,
University of Michigan Medical Center;
Chief, Plastic Surgeon Section,
Veterans Administration Medical Center,
Ann Arbor, Michigan,
Associate,
Chelsea Community Hospital,
Chelsea, Michigan

DANIEL REICHNER, MD
Plastic Surgery Resident,
University of California Irvine,
California College of Medicine,
Orange, California

JOAN RICHTSMEIER, MA, PhD
Professor, Department of Cell Biology and Anatomy,
Department of Plastic Surgery,
Johns Hopkins University School of Medicine,
Baltimore, Maryland

DAVID RING, MD
Fellow, Orthopedic Hand Service,
Massachusetts General Hospital,
Boston, Massachusetts

THOMAS L. ROBERTS III, MD
Associate Clinical Professor of Surgery,
Medical University of South Carolina at Spartanburg,
Spartanburg, South Carolina

ROD J. ROHRICH, MD, FACS
Professor and Chairman,
Department of Plastic Surgery,
University of Texas Medical Center at Dallas,
Dallas, Texas

LORNE E. ROTSTEIN, MD, FRCSC, FACS
Associate Professor,
Department of Surgery,
University of Toronto;
Staff Surgeon,
Princess Margaret Hospital,
The Toronto General Hospital University Health Network,
Toronto, Ontario, Canada

J. PETER RUBIN, MD
Fellow in Plastic Surgery,
Harvard Medical School,
Boston, Massachusetts

ROBERT C. RUSSELL, MD, FRACS, FACS
Clinical Professor of Surgery,
Division of Plastic Surgery,
Southern Illinois University School of Medicine,
Springfield, Illinois

A. MICHAEL SADOVE, MD
Professor of Surgery (Plastics),
Indiana University School of Medicine;
Chief, Plastic Surgery,
James Whitcomb Riley Hospital for Children,
Indianapolis, Indiana

KENNETH E. SALYER, MD
Adjunct Professor, Department of Orthodontics,
Baylor College of Dentistry,
Baylor University,
Dallas, Texas;
Clinical Professor, Department of Surgery,
Division of Plastic and Reconstructive Surgery,
University of Texas Health Science Center at San Antonio,
San Antonio, Texas;
Founding Director,
International Craniofacial Institute,
Cleft Lip and Palate Treatment Center,
Dallas, Texas

NICOLAS SASTRE, MD
Professor of Plastic Surgery,
Postgraduate Division of Medical Faculty,
Universidad Nacional Autonoma de Mexico;
Chairman, Plastic Surgery Department,
Hospital General de Mexico,
Mexico City, Mexico

STEPHEN A. SCHENDEL, MD, DDS
Professor and Head, Division of Plastic and Reconstructive
   Surgery;
Chairman, Department of Functional Restoration,
Stanford University,
Stanford, California

STEPHEN B. SCHNALL, MD
Associate Professor of Clinical Orthopedics,
University of Southern California School of Medicine,
Los Angeles, California

ALAN E. SEYFER, MD
Chief, Plastic Surgery,
Professor of Surgery, Anatomy, and Cell Developmental
   Biology,
Oregon Health Sciences University;
Chief, Plastic Surgery,
Doernbecher Childrens Hospital;
Staff Surgeon,
Shriners' Hospital for Crippled Children;
Portland Veterans Administration Medical Center,
Portland, Oregon

JATIN P. SHAH, MD, FACS, FRCS, FDSRCS
Professor of Surgery,
Weill Medical College,
Cornell University;
E.W. Strong Chair in Head and Neck Oncology;
Chief, Head and Neck Service,
Memorial Sloan-Kettering Cancer Center,
New York, New York

ARTHUR SHEKTMAN, MD
Attending Surgeon,
Newton-Wellesley Hospital,
Newton, Massachusetts;
Attending Surgeon,
St. Elizabeth's Medical Center,
Boston, Massachusetts

RANDY SHERMAN, MD
Professor and Chief,
Division of Plastic and Reconstructive Surgery,
University of Southern California–Los Angeles;
Chief, Plastic Surgery,
University of Southern California University Hospital;
Chief, Plastic Surgery,
Los Angeles County Hospital,
Los Angeles, California

PETER P. SIKO, MD
Research Manager,
The Buncke Clinic,
San Francisco, California

CARL E. SILVER, MD
Professor of Surgery,
Albert Einstein College of Medicine;
Chief, Head and Neck Surgery,
Montefiore Medical Center,
Bronx, New York

JEFFREY D. SMITH, MD
Clinical Fellow in Surgery,
Harvard Medical School;
Chief Resident, Plastic Surgery,
Brigham and Women's Hospital;
Chief Resident, Plastic Surgery,
Children's Hospital,
Boston, Massachusetts

NICOLE ZOOK SOMMER, MD
Plastic Surgery Resident,
Southern Illinois University School of Medicine,
Springfield, Illinois

RAJIV SOOD, MD
Associate Professor of Plastic Surgery,
Indiana University Medical Center;
Chief, Plastic Surgery Section,
Wishard Memorial Hospital,
Indianapolis, Indiana

CAROL L. SORENSEN, PsyD
Adjunct Professor of Psychology,
Concordia University,
Irvine, California

PANAYOTIS N. SOUCACOS, MD, FACS
Professor and Chairman,
Department of Orthopedics,
University of Ioannina School of Medicine,
Ioannina, Greece

MYRON SPECTOR, BS, MS, PhD
Professor of Orthopedic Surgery (Biomaterials),
Harvard Medical School;
Director of Orthopedic Research,
Department of Orthopedic Surgery,
Brigham and Women's Hospital,
Boston, Massachusetts

MELVIN SPIRA, MD, DDS
Professor of Surgery,
Division of Plastic Surgery,
Baylor College of Medicine,
Houston, Texas

HANS U. STEINAU, MD
Professor, Department of Plastic Surgery,
Director, Clinic for Plastic Surgery,
Hand and Burn Center,
Bergmannsheil Clinic,
Ruhr University,
Bochum, Germany

PETER J. STERN, MD
Professor and Chairman,
Department of Orthopedic Surgery,
University of Cincinnati College of Medicine,
Cincinnati, Ohio

BERISH STRAUCH, MD
Professor and Chairman,
Department of Plastic Surgery,
Albert Einstein College of Medicine,
Montefiore Medical Center,
Bronx, New York

JAMES M. STUZIN, MD
Clinical Assistant Professor of Plastic Surgery–Voluntary,
University of Miami School of Medicine;
Senior Attending Physician,
Mercy Hospital,
Miami, Florida

MARK R. SULTAN, MD
Associate Clinical Professor of Surgery,
Columbia University;
Chief, Division of Plastic Surgery,
Beth Israel Medical Center,
New York, New York

WILLIAM M. SWARTZ, MD, FACS
Clinical Associate Professor,
Department of Surgery,
University of Pittsburgh,
Pittsburgh, Pennsylvania

JULIA K. TERZIS, MD, PhD, FRCSC
Professor, Department of Surgery,
Division of Plastic and Reconstructive Surgery;
Director, Microsurgery Program,
Eastern Virginia Medical School,
Microsurgical Research Center,
Norfolk, Virginia

VIVIAN TING, MD
Resident in General Surgery,
University of Rochester Medical Center,
Strong Memorial Hospital,
Rochester, New York

BRYANT A. TOTH, MD, FACS
Assistant Clinical Professor of Surgery,
Department of Surgery,
University of California–San Francisco;
Attending Surgeon,
California Pacific Medical Center,
San Francisco, California;
Chief, Division of Plastic Surgery,
Children's Hospital of Northern California,
Oakland, California

LAWRENCE C. TSEN, MD
Assistant Professor of Anesthesia,
Harvard Medical School;
Attending Anesthesiologist,
Department of Anesthesiology,
Perioperative and Pain Medicine,
Brigham and Women's Hospital,
Boston, Massachusetts

MARTIN G. UNGER, MD, FRCSC, ABCS, ABHRS
Clinical Teacher and Lecturer,
University of Toronto;
Chief of Plastic Surgery,
One Medical Place Hospital,
Toronto, Ontario, Canada

ALLEN L. VAN BEEK, BS, MD
Clinical Associate Professor,
University of Minnesota,
Department of Surgery,
Minneapolis, Minnesota

VICTORIA M. VANDERKAM, RN, BS, CPSN
Clinical Nurse, Division of Plastic Surgery,
University of California Irvine Medical Center,
Orange, California

CRAIG A. VANDER KOLK, MD, FACS
Associate Professor of Plastic Surgery,
Director, Cleft and Craniofacial Center,
Johns Hopkins University School of Medicine,
Baltimore, Maryland

NICHOLAS VEDDER, MD
Associate Professor,
University of Washington,
Seattle, Washington

MARIOS D. VEKRIS, MD
Orthopedic Attending Surgeon,
Ioannina University Hospital,
Ioannina Medical School,
Ioannina, Greece

PETER M. VOGT, MD, PhD
Associate Professor;
Attending Physician,
Hand and Burn Center,
Bergmannsheil Clinic,
Ruhr University,
Bochum, Germany

JEFFREY D. WAGNER, MD
Associate Professor of Surgery,
Department of Surgery,
Division of Plastic and Reconstructive Surgery,
Indiana University School of Medicine,
Indianapolis, Indiana

ROBERT L. WALTON, MD, FACS
Professor of Surgery,
University of Chicago School of Medicine;
Chief, Section of Plastic Surgery,
University of Chicago Hospitals,
Chicago, Illinois

BERNADETTE WANG, MD
Fellow, Hand and Microsurgery,
Curtis National Hand Center,
Union Memorial Hospital,
Baltimore, Maryland

H. KIRK WATSON, MD
Director, Connecticut Combined Hand Surgery Fellowship;
Assistant Clinical Professor of Orthopedics, Rehabilitation,
    and Plastic Surgery,
Yale University School of Medicine,
New Haven, Connecticut;
Clinical Professor, Department of Orthopedics,
University of Connecticut School of Medicine,
Farmington, Connecticut;
Senior Staff,
Hartford Hospital;
Connecticut Children's Medical Center,
Hartford, Connecticut

M. SHARON WEBB, MD, PhD, JD
Attorney-at-Law,
Boston, Massachusetts

DENTON D. WEISS, LCDR, MC, USNR
Department of Plastic Surgery,
Naval Medical Center Portsmouth,
Portsmouth, Virginia

KATHLEEN J. WELCH, MD, MPH
Instructor in Anesthesia,
Harvard Medical School;
Director of Plastic Surgical Anesthesia,
Brigham and Women's Hospital,
Boston, Massachusetts

DEBORAH J. WHITE, MD
Staff Physician,
Scottsdale Healthcare,
Scottsdale, Arizona

GORDON H. WILKES, BS, MD, FRCSC
Clinical Professor of Surgery,
University of Alberta;
Chief of Surgery,
Misericordia Hospital,
Edmonton, Alberta, Canada

J. KERWIN WILLIAMS, MD
Clinical Associate Professor,
Division of Plastic Surgery,
Emory University School of Medicine;
Attending Physician,
Pediatric and Craniofacial Associates,
Atlanta Plastic Surgery,
Atlanta, Georgia

TODD WILLIAMS, MD
Chief Plastic Surgery Fellow,
Southern Illinois University School of Medicine,
Institute for Plastic and Reconstructive Surgery,
Springfield, Illinois

PETER D. WITT, MD, FACS
Associate Professor of Plastic Surgery;
Director, Pediatric Plastic Surgery,
Sutherland Institute,
University of Kansas School of Medicine,
Kansas City, Kansas

JOHN F. WOLFAARDT, BDS, MDent, PhD
Professor,
Faculty of Medicine and Dentistry,
University of Alberta;
Director, Craniofacial Osseointegration and Maxillofacial
    Prosthetic Rehabilitation Unit,
Misericordia Hospital,
Edmonton, Alberta, Canada

WILLIAM A. ZAMBONI, MD
Professor and Chief,
Division of Plastic Surgery,
University of Nevada School of Medicine,
Las Vegas, Nevada

JAMES E. ZINS, MD
Chairman, Department of Plastic Surgery,
The Cleveland Clinic Foundation,
Cleveland, Ohio

ELVIN G. ZOOK, MD
Professor of Plastic Surgery,
Southern Illinois University School of Medicine;
Chairman, Department of Plastic Surgery,
Memorial Medical Center,
Springfield, Illinois

**RONALD M. ZUKER, MD, FRCSC,
  FACS, FAAP**
Professor of Surgery,
University of Toronto;
Head, Division of Plastic Surgery,
The Hospital for Sick Children,
Toronto, Ontario, Canada

*To the families and loved ones of the authors, who are owed
a great deal for the time that we have missed with them while caring
for our patients and writing chapters for this book.
To quote a popular song, they are the "wind beneath our wings."
Thank you for helping us soar to new heights in the practice of plastic surgery.*

General Preface

This large project is dedicated to our colleagues who have contributed individual chapters to this textbook. Those who write chapters for books know that they are the unsung heroes of the medical publishing business. The chapter authors are recognized experts in their fields who have given their time in an effort to communicate their knowledge to the rest of the world. This unselfish work involves a long time commitment and a multistaged process. We would not have plastic surgery textbooks if it were not for the many people who give so freely of their time and expertise. We thank each of our chapter authors; this project is by you and for you, and we hope that you are proud of the finished product.

Plastic Surgery: Indications, Operations, and Outcomes was envisioned as a comprehensive overview of the entire discipline of plastic surgery. The concept was to create a practical book that would be useful for plastic surgeons in practice and for those in training. Each clinical chapter follows a standard format as closely as possible; the chapters first describe the indications for surgery, then discuss the operation of choice, including procedural details, and finally present outcomes information when available.

A project such as this has a history of its own. Bruce Achauer started the process in 1992 by talking to publishers and potential coeditors. He has provided leadership throughout the project. Working together, Achauer, Elof Eriksson, and Bahman Guyuron determined the title, focus, outline, and editors. In the fall of 1995, Achauer, Eriksson, and Guyuron signed a contract with Mosby, agreeing that they would edit the textbook. Jack Coleman, Bob Russell, and Craig Vander Kolk agreed to serve as volume editors.

Early on it was decided that the authors would focus on outcomes as much as possible, although we knew full well that there was little information on outcomes in plastic surgery. The goal was to increase awareness of this need and guide readers to begin thinking toward measuring outcomes. Ed Wilkins accepted the challenge of serving as outcomes editor.

The actual writing of the text began in 1996. The entire process of writing and editing took several years and involved a long-term commitment. The publishing business, like many others, has undergone tremendous change, including consolidation and the creation of larger firms from several companies. There was also an inevitable change of personnel during the process. Although Mosby started the project, Harcourt Health Sciences completed it. Throughout the years, our editorial staff has been extremely helpful.

Many individuals have been involved with this project. We extend our gratitude to the following people: John DeCarville and Bob Hurley, who captured our vision from the start and fully embraced it; Richard Zorab, Senior Editor, and Dolores Meloni, Senior Developmental Editor, of Harcourt Health Sciences, who saw the project through to its fruition; our tireless production staff of Carol Weis, Project Manager, and Florence Achenbach, Rick Dudley, Karen Rehwinkel, Christine Schwepker, and David Stein, Production Editors; and finally, Victoria VanderKam, who was willing to do anything necessary to see this project through.

It has been a fabulous experience, and we are grateful for the opportunity to participate. We thank everybody (authors, illustrators, and editors) for their commitment, hard work, and friendship and for creating this excellent textbook for plastic surgery.

BRUCE M. ACHAUER
ELOF ERIKSSON
BAHMAN GUYURON
JOHN J. COLEMAN
ROBERT C. RUSSELL
CRAIG A. VANDER KOLK

Preface to the Second Volume

As this volume of *Plastic Surgery: Indications, Operations, and Outcomes* goes to press, it seems appropriate to reflect on where the specialty of plastic surgery is at the beginning of the new millennium. It is easy to get lost in paperwork, insurance forms, or the most recent media release regarding problems in the health care industry and forget what a privilege it is to practice plastic surgery. As plastic surgeons, we have an opportunity to change people's lives at a time when they may feel that not much help can be offered to them or that not much about them can be improved upon. What greater honor could we possibly have than to take a young child with a cleft lip and reposition the tissue in such a way to make that child complete? Ideally, we would accomplish this task in such a way that the child would no longer be asked about the deformity or even have to remember the name of his or her plastic surgeon.

I am reminded of a time in the early 1980s when, as a young plastic surgery resident, I sat down with Reed Dingman after a day of surgery. I told him that I found it difficult to read everything necessary to learn about a particular problem because I was being exposed to a new deformity or surgical technique every day. He wisely advised me to concentrate on the principles because they never change, that techniques will come and go, and that there would be many advances throughout my lifetime. He explained that understanding the principles and then keeping up with the latest advances through reading and research would allow me to find the necessary information for each problem that I encountered. His advice has served many other plastic surgeons and myself well over the years.

Two of the hallmarks of plastic surgery are innovation and creativity. Innovation and creativity are easier for some than for others; however, when each of us critically evaluates our results, we can advance our understanding of plastic surgery. As a colleague of Paul Manson, I have been fortunate to witness both the innovation and creativity that come from this approach. The extensive advancements in facial trauma that he has published over the past 15 years have been based on a thorough understanding of what occurs with facial fractures and analysis of the results of treatment. Each of Paul Manson's cases is critically analyzed in an attempt to find "a better way to do it." This analysis can involve talking with the patient, comparing results based on preoperative and postoperative photographs, and evaluating the position of the reconstructed underlying structures via CT examination. Each of us has this information at our fingertips. To be innovative and creative, all we need to do is ask ourselves how to "do it better."

Paul Tessier became one of the greatest plastic surgeons of the twentieth century by practicing outcome studies of craniofacial problems and procedures. He analyzed the results of the old reconstructive techniques for complex facial anomalies, took this analysis to the laboratory to develop new techniques, critically reviewed these improvements, submitted them to peer review, and then advanced these techniques throughout the world. Essentially, Tessier stands for what this textbook is all about, which is understanding a problem, determining the best way to treat it, and then analyzing the results. Essentially, I have tried to accomplish these three goals in this volume on Craniofacial and Pediatric Plastic Surgery.

Therefore, as we enter this new century, I hope that this textbook will serve many readers in a variety of ways. I believe that it will teach indications and principles to residents, assist practicing surgeons in refining their techniques, and encourage all of us to begin to analyze our results. All of these things will serve to improve the care of our patients, which is what plastic surgery is all about.

CRAIG A. VANDER KOLK

Outcomes Preface

At the dawn of a new millennium, we are witnessing the most dramatic overhaul of the American health care system in more than a century. Health care reform is well underway, driven by economic and political forces within both the public and private sectors. The watchwords of this not-so-quiet revolution, terms such as *efficiency, cost-effectiveness,* and *value,* reflect the new demand by payers that health care interventions deliver measurable benefit at reasonable costs. Contrary to long-standing traditions in the United States, exactly what constitutes a "reasonable" cost is determined not by those who provide health care but rather by those who foot the bill. The growing emphasis on cost-effectiveness, or "value" for every dollar spent, is forcing providers to fundamentally rethink traditional patterns of care. In this brave new world, medical decisions are made only after the perceived benefits have been weighed against the risks *and* costs of treatment.

Recent reforms also reflect changes in the traditional standards by which we have assessed the effectiveness of care. Treatment options are no longer being judged simply in terms of morbidity and mortality. Instead, interventions are evaluated by studying their impacts on long-term functioning, well-being, and quality of life. This new emphasis on measurement of outcomes from the "patient's viewpoint" is of particular interest to plastic surgeons. Unlike cardiac or transplant surgeries, aesthetic and reconstructive procedures usually do not produce life-saving results. Instead, plastic surgeons endeavor to bestow more subtle benefits on their clientele, improving their body image, psychosocial well-being, and physical functioning. Lest plastic surgeons downplay the significance of their work, it is important to note that health services researchers and payers now evaluate the value of health care interventions in terms of quality-adjusted life years (QALYs) contributed. Interventions that substantially improve quality of life may be viewed as comparable (or superior) to treatment options that increase longevity.

Clearly, assessment of patient-centered outcomes is of critical importance not only to plastic surgeons but to all health care providers. Outcomes data are playing increasingly important roles in determining which treatment modalities are supported by payers and managed care providers. Research assessing the results and costs of care also may determine where and by whom that care is delivered. Outcomes studies also provide key information to patients and providers to assist in medical decision-making. In managing health care delivery systems, outcomes data (such as patient satisfaction) identify potential targets for quality improvement efforts and provide meaningful yardsticks with which to assess progress.

Given the growing importance of assessing and reporting patient-centered results of care, the chapter authors of this textbook have included "Outcomes" sections where appropriate. Available data on a diverse array of outcomes parameters are referenced. However, as the reader will note, considerable gaps still exist in our knowledge of surgical outcomes, particularly in the areas of quality of life and cost analyses. While we attempt to summarize existing outcomes data in each chapter, we also have endeavored to highlight some areas in which more research is needed. For many aesthetic and reconstructive problems and procedures, the quantity of unanswered research questions dwarfs our current body of knowledge. It is the hope of the volume authors and editors that some of the issues raised in these chapters will stimulate new outcomes studies to answer these questions.

EDWIN G. WILKINS

Contents

VOLUME TWO CRANIOMAXILLOFACIAL, CLEFT, AND PEDIATRIC SURGERY
Craig A. Vander Kolk, Editor

VOLUME THREE   HEAD AND NECK SURGERY
John J. Coleman III, Editor

VOLUME FOUR HAND SURGERY
Robert C. Russell, Editor

PART I

BASIC PRINCIPLES OF CRANIOMAXILLOFACIAL SURGERY

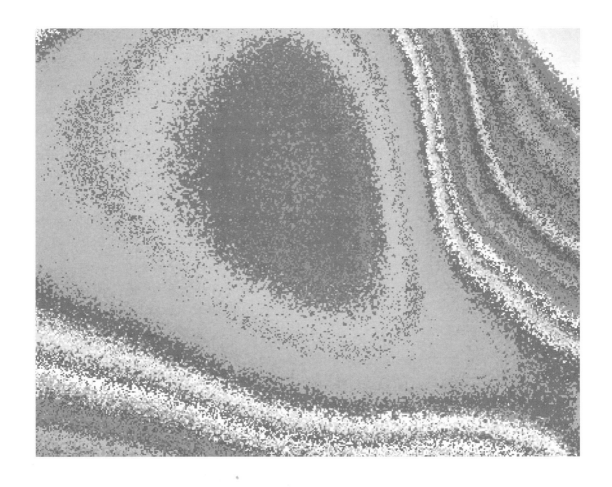

Concepts in Pediatric and Craniomaxillofacial Plastic Surgery

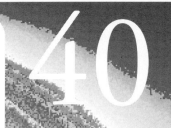

40

Craig A. Vander Kolk

INTRODUCTION

This volume of *Plastic Surgery: Indications, Operations, and Outcomes* concentrates on craniomaxillofacial surgery. It covers all aspects of this specialty, and the chapters are divided in such a way to cover the majority of topics pertinent to this field. The first section covers general topics that are important conceptually to treatment of the diverse groups of patients encountered. The subsequent chapters cover the field in depth. The underlying theme within the entire volume is the treatment of children. Therefore this chapter seeks to lay the groundwork for understanding the unique strategies and issues that need to be kept in mind in treating the patient with a complex craniofacial problem. Furthermore, we attempt to review the important considerations in indications, operations, and outcomes in the pediatric patient population that is constantly changing and needs to be followed for an extended period of time.

INDICATIONS

Plastic surgeons must consider a multitude of factors when determining the appropriate time for surgical intervention. With each particular diagnosis, the timing of treatment may be well established, but depending on their presentation, each individual patient's needs must be considered. Obviously, when there are functional limitations, early surgery is usually indicated. This can be seen in situations in which airway compromise can occur, such as in Pierre Robin sequence, Treacher-Collins syndrome, Nager syndrome, Apert and Crouzon syndromes, and the other craniofacial dysostoses. Although a tracheostomy occasionally needs to be considered, this should be done only as a last resort. The technique of

distraction osteogenesis is improving our treatment for complex airway problems because it not only repositions the bone, particularly the mandible or maxilla, but it also carries the soft tissues with the bone advancement. Distraction osteogenesis decreases the incidence and amount of relapse. This increases the success of preserving the airway and limiting the need for a tracheostomy. Fortunately, this technique is being performed at an earlier and earlier age, improving outcomes for complex problems.

Distraction osteogenesis not only revolutionizes the outcome but also allows definitive surgical intervention to be performed at an earlier age. This is particularly true in early maxillary surgery for cleft midface hypoplasia. Rather than waiting until full maxillary and mandibular growth has occurred, treatment can be instituted in late childhood. This improves not only the functional deformity that can be seen but also the appearance of the child. This is especially advantageous for patients as they go through or endure adolescence.

Cleft palate surgery is another functional correction in which the timing has been shown to be important in the overall outcome of speech. Although cleft palate surgery is not necessary for nutrition, it is important to reconstruct the anatomic deformity, reposition the muscles, and lengthen the palate to allow for subsequent speech and language development with the best chance for a normal outcome.

In craniosynostosis, long-term neuropsychologic outcomes are still being debated. However, there are specific times in which release of the sutures is necessary. When this is combined with frontal-orbital advancement, the growth restriction of the brain, skull, and potentially even the midface may be unlocked by early surgery.

One of the advantages of plastic surgery in the new millennium is that anesthesia and critical care patient management have allowed the safe performance of procedures at an earlier age. In addition, more complex procedures can be safely accomplished with improvement in both outcomes and limitation in morbidity and mortality. In the past the consideration of doing lip repair based on 10 weeks, 10 g of hemoglobin, and 10 lb was important. This no longer needs to be the overwhelming consideration for the timing of surgery. There may be other advantages to waiting, such as increased size, that improve the overall outcome in cleft lip repair and are more important than an arbitrary age based on old criteria.

Advancements in outpatient surgery have changed a whole host of surgical procedures, which have all been beneficial in outcomes for both cost and ease for the patient and family.

Early surgery is thought to be advantageous for healing. Although extensive work has been done to understand fetal wound healing, to date we are not yet at the point of controlling scar formation in a fashion that allows scarless wound healing. On the other hand, scarring needs to be kept in mind in determining a time for surgery. Generally it is believed that scarring becomes more prominent throughout the first few years of life, and I generally recommend that final cleft lip surgery for shape and symmetry be accomplished within the first year of life. In a similar fashion, thicker, redder scars seem to be prominent during the active growth phases of the child. Often this is thought to occur between the ages of 4 and 14.

Psychologic concerns as an indication for surgery is a difficult issue to pursue. There is, however, no doubt that there are various phases in development that predispose to psychologic trauma. Although is it often thought that surgery should be accomplished before a child goes to school, now with preschool being very common, this issue may need to be reconsidered. It appears that a more consistent presence with peers from one year to the next may bring about psychologic issues and teasing at an earlier age. However, generally speaking, it is not until the end of first grade, or around 6 to 7 years of age, that children finally understand the difference between themselves and others in their peer group, resulting in questions about deformities or congenital anomalies. The next, and perhaps most major, time for psychologic concerns is in the adolescent years. There is no doubt that children with facial deformities have a difficult time in this period of growth, and this should always be kept in mind as part of the indications for treatment.

Unfortunately, although there are numerous articles establishing the psychologic issues with such problems as cleft lip and cleft palate, insurance companies and health maintenance organizations have certainly limited the availability of psychologic care when this is the major indication for treatment. United efforts among a host of organizations may change this in the future, spearheaded by groups such as the Coalition for Craniofacial Anomalies Treatment, supported by the American Society of Plastic Surgeons, the American Cleft Palate-Craniofacial Association, the American Society of Craniofacial Surgery, the American Society of Pediatric Neurosurgeons, the American Medical Association, and numerous other organizations that advocate for children and the treatment of birth deformities.

OPERATIONS

Whereas indications for procedures are gradually refined and oftentimes performed at earlier and earlier ages, perhaps the greatest advancements in plastic surgery have been in the innovative and creative thought processes that have taken place in developing new operations along with significant advancements in technology. Although we rarely see advancements, such as those operations that were created and established by Paul Tessier, many new and innovative techniques have been built upon principles established by this pioneer and continue to be a hallmark of the field of plastic surgery.

Although the indications for removal of congenital nevus continue to be debated as to potential for malignant degeneration, techniques of serial excision and, more importantly, tissue expansion have allowed the removal of large congenital nevi before puberty. This is important because puberty is the time that there appears to be the greatest potential for malignant change. Recently this technique has been extended to expansion of donor sites for free-tissue transfer and expansion of the skin overlying an area where a full-thickness skin graft can be harvested to lessen the scarring.

Advances in technology have allowed the greatest advances in surgical operations. Not only can procedures be done at an earlier date because of the advances in anesthesia and critical care, but also we can now more safely advance or modify bone segments to achieve the desired result. Previously, complex osteotomies needed to be performed to stabilize a segment that was advanced beyond the previous boundary of the deformed facial skeleton. Wires typically provided stabilization of a segment in only one plane. Therefore solid surrounding bone needed to be available to stabilize the segment in more than one degree of rotation. Complex tongue-and-groove and Z-plasty techniques helped the field move forward, but there were limitations with each of these techniques. With the advent of plate-and-screw fixation, stable fixation could be accomplished and the boundaries of movement of bone expanded. Not only did it allow for more creative operations, but results also improved with this expansion of the craniofacial skeleton. Earlier healing occurred, and this improved the outcomes.

More recently, the use of absorbable plates and screws has further extended the use of fixation into younger patients and decreased the incidence of less ideal outcomes when plates and screws became loose or irritated, requiring removal.

Nothing probably has advanced cranial facial and pediatric construction as much as distraction osteogenesis. Beginning in the late 1980s, McCarthy established this technique based on principles pioneered by Ilizarov. Following the tradition of Le Fort and Tessier of first taking the concepts to the laboratory and then performing them in clinical cases allowed the field to gradually and safely expand to a wide variety of cases and deformities. The utility and advantages of this technique have resulted in a rapid succession of advancements.

OUTCOMES

The field of pediatric and craniofacial surgery is fortunate to have a rich history in the outcome analysis of treatment plans and surgical procedures. Often outcomes are weighed as to the type of surgical procedure and the timing of that procedure. All of this has been tempered by a general understanding that changes always occur in the growth and development of the child. In addition, outcomes must be evaluated according to appearance and function.

This is well highlighted in our understanding of the timing and procedures for cleft lip and cleft palate surgery. Early surgery is felt to give a superior result, both in the esthetics of the lip and the function of the palate. However, it is always kept in mind that the extensive undermining necessary to do a lip repair can have detrimental effects on the subsequent growth of the midfacial skeleton. This concept needs to be considered for both lip repair and palate repair. Improved results occur with palate repair when it is accomplished at an earlier age and with advances and changes in the technique used.

The craniofacial literature has attempted to extensively study rigid fixation on its outcome and potential deleterious effect on cranial growth. Animal studies have shown that, although there can be a local effect, this is minimal and does not outweigh the advantages of more accurate positioning of the segments and more stabilization of the reconstructed skeletal construct.

Although distraction osteogenesis is known to allow earlier surgical reconstruction of complex facial skeleton anomalies, the long-term outcomes of this technique are currently being evaluated. These studies will evaluate the new bone formed and the potential for relapse. They will also study the responses of the soft tissues. Both of these results appear to be favorable and in the patient's best interest.

Perhaps the key to all of plastic surgery is the understanding of the indications, operations, and outcomes in the treatment of complex congenital problems and the pediatric population. Fortunately, plastic surgeons have been dedicated not only to utilizing all of the available technology to improve the timing of treatment but also to utilizing advances in technology to analyze these outcomes. This is best exemplified by the use of three-dimensional computed tomography scans to categorize the deformity; determine the indications for treatment; plan the surgery; and analyze the reconstruction, outcome, and even the growth of the patient undergoing the procedure. This and other examples reported and illustrated in this volume have been the hallmark of plastic surgery.

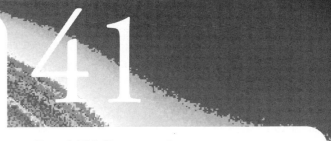

CHAPTER 41

Craniofacial Genetics and Dysmorphology

Gerald V. Raymond

INTRODUCTION

The role of genes in congenital abnormalities of the head and neck is presently an area of intense investigation. It is readily apparent that certain conditions are genetic, and there has been a striking increase in knowledge of the developmental genes that control cranial and facial development. As a clinician, the dilemma is often how to incorporate this expanding information into useful knowledge.

This chapter attempts to present information on common malformations of the face and head and their recurrence risks, as well as introducing new genetic understanding. For the surgeon who is seeing a patient with a congenital abnormality of the head or face, it is important to recognize that there may be implications beyond the operating room, for the patient and for the family. Whether this will have implications in treatment remains to be seen. The proper identification of certain conditions may also allow one to predict associated problems, reduce morbidity, and place results in proper context.

The chapter outlines some of what is known about particular craniofacial syndromes and their genetics. I use some specific examples, but it is not possible nor is it my intention to be exhaustive. It is always appropriate to seek the assistance of a clinical geneticist in evaluating a patient with multiple congenital anomalies. It is important to emphasize that there are limits to both clinical and laboratory identification. Although it is often frustrating to all involved when a child with multiple congenital anomalies cannot be assigned a diagnosis, it serves no purpose to force a label on the child, and appropriate caution should be exercised in counseling.

OROFACIAL CLEFTS

The genetics of the orofacial clefts, cleft lip and palate (CL/P), and cleft palate (CP) are one of the most important areas of study in craniofacial genetics. Although there are over 200 syndromes with clefts, both chromosomal and mendelian, an orofacial cleft is an isolated birth defect in most situations. It is

the complex genetics of this isolated cleft that have provoked intense interest.

Genetics of Isolated Clefts

Early studies focused on the recurrence risk of either having a second affected child or for someone affected with a cleft to have a similarly affected child. It was shown that cleft lip with or without a cleft palate was a distinct entity from isolated cleft palate. Families who have had one child with CL/P or CP have a higher risk than the general population of having a similarly affected child. For CL/P, this is generally reported as being 4% if one child has a cleft, 4% if one parent has it, 17% if one parent and one child have it, and 9% if two children have it.[7] This recurrence risk varies with the gender of the individual and ethnic origin. For CP, Curtis et al[7] estimated that the risk of recurrence in subsequently born children is about 2% if one child has it, 6% if one parent has it, and 15% if one parent and one child have it. These empiric recurrence risks have been variously interpreted as evidence of a multifactorial threshold model, a single major gene with decreased penetrance, or a single gene with environmental influence.

Genetic Models

The multifactorial model was advanced to explain a variety of birth defects that recurred in families but did not fit classic mendelian inheritance. The hypothesis is based on an individual carrying genes that raise the chance of having a cleft. Inherent in this model is a threshold above which one expresses the phenotype. Either genetic or environmental factors can carry one beyond the threshold.

In cleft lip and palate, Carter et al[4] stated that the most consistent explanation was that a single gene was unlikely and believed that the multifactorial threshold model best fit the data. Chung et al[6] analyzed several previous epidemiologic studies in the Danish and the Japanese. They concluded that the Danish data were explained best by a combination of a single gene and multifactorial inheritance and the Japanese data could only be explained by a multifactorial model. Finally, other analyses have shown that dominant or codominant inheritance of a major locus was the closest fit.[16]

In a study of 561 Danish probands with nonsyndromic isolated cleft palate, Shields et al[25] determined that neither a multifactorial-threshold model nor a single major locus model was completely compatible with the distribution of cases. They proposed two forms of nonsyndromic cleft palate: (1) familial CP, which has an autosomal dominant component, and (2) nonfamilial CP, which appears to be related to environmental factors. Christensen and Mitchell[5] estimated the prevalence of nonsyndromic CP in Denmark, obtained estimates of the risks to first-, second-, and third-degree relatives, and analyzed the data for mode of inheritance. A total of 2301 CP cases were born in Denmark during 1936-1987. The majority, 1952 (84.8%), were nonsyndromic. The recurrence risks for the three classes of relatives of the nonsyndromic CP probands was 2.74%, 0.28%, and 0.00%, respectively. Analyses of these data were considered consistent with CP being determined by several interacting loci.

OROFACIAL CLEFT SYNDROMES

Whereas the genetics of isolated clefts remain a matter for continued study, there is an equally important role for understanding the common syndromes that can result in orofacial clefts, both in clinical diagnosis and also in the understanding of the etiology of all clefts (Table 41-1).

Deletion of 22q11.2 —DiGeorge Sequence/Velocardiofacial Syndrome

The DiGeorge sequence (DGS) is composed of coarctation of the aorta, thymic aplasia, and parathyroid abnormalities with resultant hypocalcemia. The DiGeorge sequence is generally a sporadic condition. A cytogenetic deletion of the long arm of chromosome 22 was first noted by de la Chapelle et al[8] and has

subsequently been found in over 90% of cases to have a specific deletion of 22q11.2. Velocardiofacial syndrome (VCFS), or Shprintzen's syndrome, is manifested by velopharyngeal insufficiency, cleft palate, cardiac anomalies, unusual facies, and learning difficulties (Figure 41-1). Although (as with the

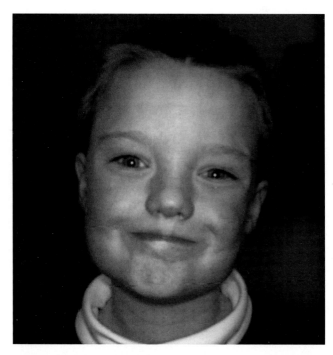

Figure 41-1. Velocardiofacial syndrome. An affected boy with congenital heart disease (atrium septal defect and right-sided aortic arch), learning disabilities with language delays, early feeding difficulties, nasal speech, and deletion of velocardiofacial region on chromosome 22 detected by FISH. Note the facies with upslanting palpebral fissures; broad, square nasal root; and thin upper lip.

Table 41-1.
List of Other Conditions Associated with Orofacial Clefts

SYNDROME	FEATURES	INHERITANCE
Cerebrocostomandibular	CP, abnormal ribs, small mandible	Reports of both recessive and dominant inheritance
Ectrodactyly-ectodermal dysplasia-clefting (EEC)	CL/P, sparse hair, defects in mid-hands and feet (ectrodactyly)	Autosomal dominant
Roberts'-SC phocomelia	Phocomelia, CL/P, sparse hair, genitourinary anomalies	Autosomal recessive, premature separation of centromeres
Oral-facial-digital (OFD) type I	CP, multilobulated tongue, abnormal digits, mild mental retardation	X-linked dominant
Mohr (OFD type II)	Midline cleft of the upper lip, polysyndactyly, cleft tongue	Autosomal recessive
Oto-palatal-digital type I	CP, short stature, bone dysplasia	X-linked recessive

DiGeorge sequence) most cases were sporadic, there were cases that were transmitted vertically from one generation to the next. It was determined that 83% of individuals with this condition are deleted for the same specific region on the long arm of chromosome 22q11.2.[11,20,22]

The specific genes that result in DGS/VCFS are not yet known. There are several lost, including the putative transcription factor TUPLE-1 (Tup-like enhancer of split gene 1)[15]; CDCREL-1, which in mice is expressed during skeletal embryogenesis[3]; and the Goosecoid-like gene (GSCL),[14] which contains a homeobox region. Any proposed candidates will have to be shown to produce their effect when only one copy (hemizygosity) is present.

The diagnosis of this condition and certain other chromosomal deletions has been greatly aided by the use of molecular genetic techniques, especially fluorescent in situ hybridization (FISH). The technique uses fluorescently tagged deoxyribonucleic acid (DNA) probes and can be performed in conjunction with routine cytogenetic examination. In the case of examination for deletions, the normal situation will demonstrate two signals visible with a fluorescent microscope, one on each chromosomal segment. When there is deletion of the targeted sequence, there will be only one signal visible rather than the expected two.

This is an extremely powerful tool and may be used to search for deletions and other chromosomal abnormalities. Given its speed and relative ease, it continues to find uses in cytogenetics and will play an increasing role in clinical diagnosis in the future.

Stickler Syndrome

Stickler syndrome is one of the most commonly reported syndromes resulting in cleft palate[19] (Figure 41-2). Characterized by myopia, retinal detachment, clefts, and arthropathy, at least one form is due to a defect in the collagen type II gene. This form of Stickler is allelic with the defect in Kneist dysplasia and spondyloepiphyseal dysplasia. It is, like many of the collagen disorders, autosomal dominant. Individuals who are suspected of having Stickler syndrome should be periodically screened for vision and retinal abnormalities.

Robin Sequence

The triad of cleft palate, micrognathia, and glossoptosis comprises this field defect or association. It has heterogeneous etiology, but it has been stated that one of the most common causes is Stickler syndrome.[13]

Van der Woude Syndrome

This autosomal dominant syndrome is associated with either cleft lip and palate or cleft palate. Lower lip pits that are accessory salivary glands are the specific feature of this condition. In many series, this condition represents one of the most common causes of cleft palate. The gene for this condition has been localized to the long arm of chromosome 1. It has been suggested that at least in some families there may be a submicroscopic deletion in the area of 1q32-q41.[2,24]

CRANIOSYNOSTOSIS

Premature fusion of the cranial sutures may result alone or occur with other anomalies. Craniosynostosis may result from single-gene mutations, from chromosomal abnormalities, and in association with certain teratogens. The incidence of craniosynostosis is 0.4/1000 in the general population.[13] The most commonly involved suture is the sagittal, accounting for one half of the cases. The other involved sutures are the coronal (18% to 29%) and a small percentage of metopic or lambdoidal. When craniosynostosis is part of a syndrome, it is most often associated with malformations of the limbs, ears, and heart. The common craniosynostosis syndromes include

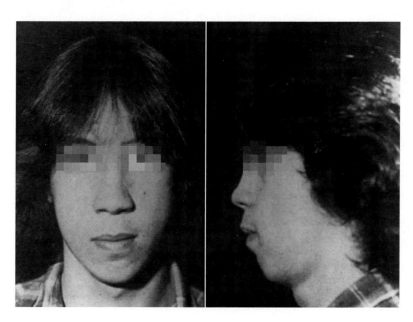

Figure 41-2. Stickler syndrome. Young man with myopia and retinal detachments, arachnodactyly, repaired cleft palate, and hearing loss. His facial features demonstrate depressed bridge of nose, maxillary hypoplasia, and small chin. (From Liberfarb RM, Hirose T, Holmes LB: *J Pediatr* 99:394-399, 1981.)

Apert syndrome, Crouzon syndrome, Saethre-Chotzen syndrome, Pfeiffer syndrome, and others[13] (Table 41-2).

Apert Syndrome

Apert syndrome is a constellation of craniosynostosis, midface malformations, and symmetric syndactyly of the hands and feet.[13,18] The skull in infancy is characterized by fusion of the coronal suture and a complete, wide-gaping, midline bony defect extending from the root of the nose to the posterior fontanelle. After the first year of life, bony islands form within the defect, grow, and fuse until the gap is completely covered. In this defect, proper sutures do not form. Only the lambdoidal forms a true suture with interdigitation of bone. In spite of the craniosynostosis, the head circumference is normal at birth.

The face in Apert syndrome is characteristic. There is a steep forehead and a horizontal groove above the supraorbital ridge. The children have shallow orbits with proptosis, hypertelorism, and downslanting of the palpebral fissures. There is occasionally subluxation of the orbits. The cranial base is malformed and asymmetric. The middle third of the face is hypoplastic, with an apparently normal mandible giving the appearance of prognathism. The nasal bridge is depressed, and the nose is beaked and humped. There is a high frequency of cleft palate or bifid uvula (30%). Even when intact, the palate is highly arched, is constricted, and has a deep median furrow giving the appearance of a Byzantine cross. With the combination of reduced nasopharyngeal dimensions and decreased patency of the posterior nasal choanae, there may be obstructive apnea.

Mental retardation is seen in a significant percentage of individuals. The mean intelligence quotient (IQ) has been reported in one series to be 74, with a range of 52 to 89.[21] Individuals with normal intelligence have been reported.[13] There are a variety of malformations of the brain, especially of the corpus callosum and limbic structures, and defects of neuronal migration. Later intelligence does not clearly correlate with early surgical correction. The altered cranial base and incidence of clefts often result in hearing loss, which affects testing of cognition and language.

Individuals with this condition have syndactyly of fingers 2, 3, and 4. The thumb and digit 5 may also be involved in the fused hand mass. When the thumb is free, it is broad and deviated radially. All of the bones of the hand are shortened. The feet are similarly involved. The joints may become stiff with age.

Crouzon Syndrome

Crouzon syndrome is the other common craniosynostosis syndrome. It is characterized by variable craniosynostosis, maxillary hypoplasia, and ocular proptosis.[13,18] Brachycephaly is commonly observed. Craniosynostosis may not be evident at birth, but it usually becomes apparent during the first year of life and complete by age 2 or 3. Ocular proptosis is a defining feature. Shallow orbits are the skeletal cause of the proptosis and result in involvement of the eye with exposure keratitis, poor vision, and rarely optic atrophy and blindness. The rest of the face is characterized by abnormality of the maxillas, shortening of the dental arch, and a beaked nose. Conductive hearing loss is present in over 50% of cases. There may be atresia of the external auditory canals.

The presence of limb anomalies has been a controversial point. There have been reports of skeletal anomalies, especially when determined by radiographs; however, significant abnormalities of the limbs are not seen on physical examination. This lack of abnormality separates it from Apert syndrome and many of the other craniosynostosis syndromes.

Genetics

Most cases of Apert syndrome are sporadic. There have been a few cases that document autosomal dominant inheritance with complete penetrance, and there has been at least one episode of germinal mosaicism.[13] Approximately two thirds of cases of Crouzon are familial, and the remainder are sporadic. Both conditions demonstrate a paternal age effect, indicating that most are the result of paternal mutation in spermatogenesis.

An understanding of the genetic basis has come with the demonstration that both Crouzon and Apert syndromes

Table 41-2.
Features of Craniosynostosis Syndromes

SYNDROME	ASSOCIATED CLINICAL FEATURE	FGF RECEPTOR
Apert	Syndactyly of fingers, mental retardation	FGFR2
Crouzon	Shallow orbits proptosis, beaked nose	FGFR2
Jackson-Weiss	Midface hypoplasia, foot abnormalities	FGFR2
Pfeiffer	Broad thumbs and toes, polysyndactyly	FGFR2
Crouzon with acanthosis nigricans	Acanthosis nigricans	FGFR3
Beare-Stevenson cutis gyrata	Cloverleaf skull, thick scalp folds, acanthosis nigricans	FGFR2

result from mutations in the fibroblast growth factor receptor 2 (FGFR2).[9,12,26,27] FGFR2 has been localized to chromosome 10. The fibroblast growth factor receptors comprise a family of tyrosine kinase receptors sharing a common protein structure. They have three immunoglobulin-like domains in the extracellular regions, a transmembrane region, and the internal tyrosine kinase. Binding of fibroblast growth factor to the receptor results in activation of the tyrosine kinase signaling the transduction pathways for cell replication and differentiation.

Reardon et al[23] showed in 9 out of 20 patients with Crouzon syndrome mutations in the FGFR2 gene. Jabs et al[17] found mutations in FGFR2 in Crouzon and in individuals with Jackson-Weiss syndrome. In Apert syndrome, Wilkie et al[28] found mutations in FGFR2. In all 40 cases, they identified specific missense mutations involving the adjacent amino acids ser252-to-trp and pro253-to-arg. This is the linker region between the second and third extracellular immunoglobulin domain. The mutation has been shown in all cases identified to date to be a change from cytosine to guanine at base pair position 934 or the same change at base pair position 937. How different mutations in this single molecule result in different phenotypes is not yet known.

CONDITIONS AFFECTING THE EXTERNAL EARS AND FACE

Mandibulofacial Dysostosis (Treacher Collins Syndrome)

Malformation of structures derived from the first and second pharyngeal arches and pouch characterize this condition. It is autosomal dominant with variability of expression from one generation to another. As demonstrated by several cases associated with chromosomal translocations, there appears to be some degree of genetic heterogeneity.[1]

The facial abnormalities are symmetric and bilateral. There is hypoplasia of the supraorbital area and the zygoma. The resultant face is narrow, with downward-sloping palpebral fissures; depressed cheekbones; malformed pinnae; a receding chin; and a large, downturned mouth. Coloboma of the outer third of the lower lid is present. The ear lobe is malformed, with microtia in 60% of affected individuals. The bridge of the nose is raised. The nares are narrow, and the alar cartilage may be absent. A cleft palate is seen in about 35%. In an additional 30% to 40%, palatopharyngeal incompetence is present.[13]

The genetic defect of one form has been localized to the long arm of chromosome 5 (5q32-q33.1), and the gene has been labeled TCOF1. It codes for a low-complexity protein called treacle, which shares characteristics with nucleolar trafficking proteins. It is hypothesized that this protein has an important role in early human facial development.[10,29]

Hemifacial Microsomia and Goldenhar's Syndrome

Affecting the ears, mouth, and mandible, this condition is predominantly unilateral but does occur bilaterally.

Goldenhar's syndrome, most likely a variant, also involves vertebral anomalies and epibulbar dermoids. This heterogeneous group of disorders has been referred to under various labels, and minimum criteria appears to include microtia or other ear abnormality.

Most cases are sporadic, and there is evidence to suggest that a vascular disruption is the cause. Even so, there appears to be etiologic heterogeneity with both rare reports of affected families and affected siblings. The empiric recurrence risk is in the range of 2% to 3%. It has been suggested that other first-degree relatives be evaluated.[13]

Abnormalities of the ear range from complete absence to anotia to an ill-defined mass of tissue that is displaced anteriorly and inferiorly to a mildly unusual ear. Preauricular tags and sinuses are common. Tags may occur anywhere from the tragus to the angle of the mouth. The affected auditory canal may be narrow to atretic, and conductive and sensorineural hearing loss is frequently seen.

Ocular abnormalities include blepharoptosis, anophthalmia, or microphthalmia. Epibulbar tumors are found in about one third and appear as solid yellowish or pinkish-white ovoid masses. These are seen at the inferotemporal portion of the eye and are usually asymmetric. Other eye abnormalities include leukoma, vision impairment, microcornea, and eyelid abnormalities.

Facial asymmetry is marked in about 20%. This is due to the abnormal ear and changes in the bones of the face, especially of the mandible. Approximately one third have bilateral involvement, but it is nearly always asymmetric in involvement.

A wide range of central nervous system (CNS) and vertebral anomalies have been described. Cranial nerve involvement, especially of the trigeminal (V) and facial (VII) nerves, is seen and results in facial anesthesia and weakness, respectively. Cervical spine and cranial base anomalies occur with increased frequency and include vertebral fusions, platybasia, Klippel-Feil anomaly, scoliosis, and anomalous ribs.

A variety of other abnormalities have been described. Cleft lip and palate may be present. Radial ray defects have been noted in about 10%. Other anomalies include defects of the lung, renal disease, and congenital heart disease. Affected infants are often small for their gestational age.

REFERENCES

1. Arn PH, Mankinen C, Jabs EW: Mild mandibulofacial dysostosis in a child with a deletion of 3p, *Am J Med Genet* 46:534-536, 1993.
2. Bocian M, Walker AP: Lip pits and deletion 1q32-41, *Am J Med Genet* 26:437-443, 1987.
3. Botta A, Lindsay EA, Jurecic V, et al: A member of the septin gene family is deleted in DiGeorge Syndrome and its mouse homolog is highly expressed during embryogenesis in the nervous system and skeletal primordia, *Am J Hum Genet* 61:A174, 1997.

4. Carter CO, Evans K, Coffery R, et al: A three generation family study of cleft lip with or without cleft palate, *J Med Genet* 19:246-261, 1982.

5. Christensen K, Mitchell LE: Familial recurrence-pattern analysis of nonsyndromic isolated cleft palate—a Danish Registry study, *Am J Hum Genet* 58:182-190, 1996.

6. Chung CS, Bixler D, Watanabe T, et al: Segregation analysis of cleft lip with or without cleft palate: a comparison of Danish and Japanese data, *Am J Hum Genet* 39:603-611, 1986.

7. Curtis EJ, Fraser FC, Warburton D: Congenital cleft lip and palate, *American Journal of Diseases in Children* 102:853-857, 1961.

8. de la Chapelle A, Herva R, Koivisto M, et al: A deletion in chromosome 22 can cause DiGeorge syndrome, *Hum Genet* 57:253-256, 1981.

9. De Moerlooze L, Dickson C: Skeletal disorders associated with fibroblast growth factor receptor mutations (review), *Curr Opin Genet Dev* 7:378-385, 1997.

10. Dixon MJ: Treacher Collins syndrome, *Hum Mol Genet* 5:1391-1396, 1996.

11. Driscoll DA: Genetic basis of DiGeorge and velocardiofacial syndromes, *Curr Opin Pediatr* 6:702-706, 1994.

12. Gorlin RJ: Fibroblast growth factors, their receptors and receptor disorders, *J Craniomaxillofac Surg* 25:69-79, 1997.

13. Gorlin RJ, Cohen MM, Levin LS: *Syndromes of the head and neck,* New York, 1990, Oxford University Press.

14. Gottlieb S, Emmanuel BS, Driscoll DA, et al: The DiGeorge syndrome minimal critical region contains a goosecoid-like (GSCL) homeobox that is expressed early in human development, *Am J Hum Genet* 60:1194-1201, 1997.

15. Halford S, Wadey R, Roberts C, et al: Isolation of a putative transcriptional regulator from the region of 22q11 deleted in DiGeorge syndrome, Shprintzen syndrome and familial congenital heart disease, *Hum Mol Genet* 2:2099-2107, 1993.

16. Hecht JT, Yang P, Michels VV, et al: Complex segregation analysis of nonsyndromic cleft lip and palate, *Am J Hum Genet* 49:674-681, 1991.

17. Jabs EW, Li X, Scott AF, et al: Jackson-Weiss and Crouzon syndromes are allelic with mutations in fibroblast growth factor receptor 2, *Nature Genetics* 8:275-279, 1994.

18. Jones KL: *Smith's recognizable patterns of malformation,* Philadelphia, 1982, WB Saunders.

19. Jones MC: Facial clefting: etiology and developmental pathogenesis, *Clin Plast Surg* 20:599-606, 1993.

20. Leana-Cox J, Pangkanon S, Eanet KR, et al: Familial DiGeorge/velocardiofacial syndrome with deletions of chromosome 22q11.2: report of five families with a review of the literature, *Am J Med Genet* 65:309-316, 1996.

21. Lefebvre A, Travis F, Arndt EM, et al: A psychiatric profile before and after reconstructive surgery in children with Apert's syndrome, *Br J Plast Surg* 39:510-513, 1986.

22. Morrow BE, Edelman L, Ferreira J, et al: A duplication on chromosome 22q11 is the basis for the common deletion that occurs in velo-cardio-facial syndrome patients, *Am J Hum Genet* 61:A25, 1997.

23. Reardon W, Winter RM, Rutland P, et al: Mutations in the fibroblast growth factor receptor 2 gene cause Crouzon syndrome, *Nature Genetics* 8:98-103, 1994.

24. Sander A, Schmelzle R, Murray J: Evidence for a microdeletion in 1q32-41 involving the gene responsible for Van der Woude syndrome, *Hum Mol Genet* 3:575-578, 1994.

25. Shields ED, Bixler D, Fogh-Andersen P: Facial clefts in Danish twins, *Cleft Palate J* 16:1-6, 1979.

26. Webster MK, Donoghue DJ: FGFR activation in skeletal disorders: too much of a good thing, *Trends Genet* 13:178-182, 1997.

27. Wilkie AO: Craniosynostosis: genes and mechanisms, *Hum Mol Genet* 6:1647-1656, 1997.

28. Wilkie AO, Slaney SF, Oldridge M, et al: Apert Syndrome results from localized mutations of FGFR3 and is allelic with Crouzon syndrome, *Nature Genetics* 9:165-172, 1995.

29. Wise CA, Chiang LC, Paznekas WA, et al: TCOF1 gene encodes a putative nucleolar phosphoprotein that exhibits mutations in Treacher Collins Syndrome throughout its coding region, *Proc Natl Acad Sci USA* 94:3110-3115, 1997.

CHAPTER

Craniofacial Growth: Genetic Basis and Morphogenetic Process in Craniosynostosis

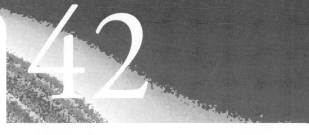

Valerie Burke DeLeon
Ethylin Wang Jabs
Joan Richtsmeier

INDICATIONS

Craniosynostosis is defined as the premature fusion of the neurocranial bones and is thought to be etiologically and pathogenetically heterogeneous. The occurrence of craniosynostosis is estimated as 3 to 5 per 10,000 births,[9] and the lack of a functional suture produces morphologic effects ranging from mild to severe. Recent research has focused on two areas that represent separate ends of an etiologic continuum: the study of cranial morphology, development, and suture biology, and the study of molecular genetics in individuals exhibiting premature synostoses. As we expand our knowledge of the physiologic processes evident in normal and abnormal suture morphogenesis and of the genetic mutations that result in craniosynostosis, the extent of uncertainty in the causal progression is narrowed. Eventually, science will bridge the gap between these areas of study with a full understanding of the mechanisms responsible for craniosynostosis. We believe that insights into the etiology of the individual presentation of synostosis can be valuable in planning surgical approaches and in anticipating postoperative results.

CRANIOSYNOSTOSIS: A SHORT SURVEY

Craniosynostosis may result from a number of different factors, some of which have been classified by Cohen[9] as malformational, metabolic, monogenic, or chromosomal in character. Different causes produce different mechanisms that result in craniosynostosis. In malformational cases, such as

microcephaly, Cohen[8] proposed the absence of brain growth and tensile stresses across sutures as the pathogenesis of synostosis. On the other hand, metabolic disorders, such as hyperthyroidism, may result in accelerated osseous maturation and premature fusion of the cranial bones, whereas monogenetic and chromosomal causes may interfere with the normal function of the osteogenic fronts and mesenchymal blastema in suture formation or maintenance.[8]

Craniosynostosis can occur as an isolated birth defect, in association with other anomalies, or as one of a set of anomalies that define a syndrome. Ninety syndromes involving craniosynostosis had been delineated by 1991, almost half of which are monogenic.[8] By the end of 1998, there were 81 entries involving craniosynostosis included in the Online Mendelian Inheritance in Man (OMIM) database.[64]

Syndromic characterization is subject to continuous reevaluation as clinical descriptions are revised in light of genetic information. Some of the more commonly recognized syndromes that involve craniosynostosis include Apert, Crouzon, Jackson-Weiss, Pfeiffer, and Saethre-Chotzen syndromes, all of which are associated with gene mutations as discussed below. Apert syndrome is characterized by craniosynostosis and bony syndactyly of the hands and feet (Figure 42-1). The distinctions between Crouzon, Jackson-Weiss, and Pfeiffer syndromes are blurred. These three produce a range of clinical manifestations from craniosynostosis with involvement primarily in the cranium in Crouzon syndrome (Figure 42-2), through inclusion of broad great toes and bony fusion in the feet in Jackson-Weiss syndrome patients, to the inclusion of broad thumbs and toes in Pfeiffer syndrome patients. However, radiology of Crouzon syndrome patients has

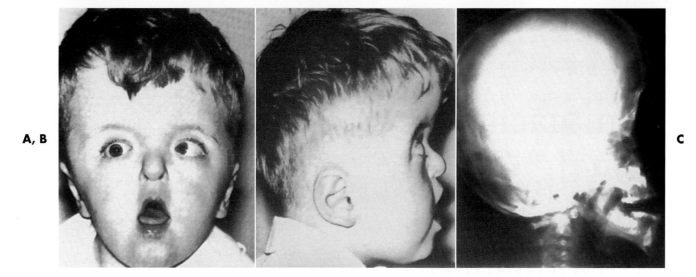

Figure 42-1. **A** and **B,** Apert syndrome patient. Note turribrachycephaly, ocular hypotelorism, proptosis, down-slanting palpebral fissures, strabismus, midface deficiency, and beaked nose. **C,** Radiograph showing Apert skull. (**A** and **B** from Cohen MMJ: *Birth Defects* 11:137-189, 1975; **C** modified from Cohen MM Jr: *Craniosynostosis: diagnosis, evaluation, and management,* New York, 1986, Raven Press.)

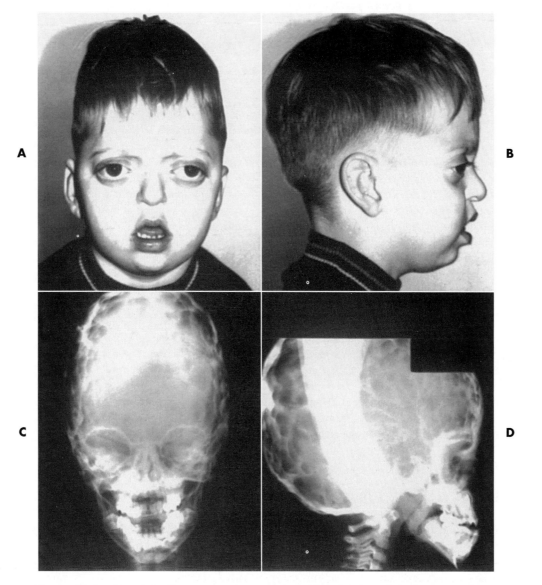

Figure 42-2. **A** and **B,** Crouzon syndrome patient. Note brachycephaly, ocular proptosis, maxillary hypoplasia, and beaked nose. **C** and **D,** Radiographs of a different individual showing Crouzon cranial morphology. (Modified from Jones K: *Smith's recognizable patterns of human malformation,* ed 5, Philadelphia, 1997, WB Saunders.)

revealed subtle limb abnormalities, obscuring the clinical distinction between Jackson-Weiss and Crouzon syndromes.[3] The distinction between Jackson-Weiss and Pfeiffer syndromes is disputed, as well.[99] Saethre-Chotzen syndrome is characterized predominantly by coronal synostosis, facial dysmorphology, brachydactyly, and cutaneous syndactyly (Figure 42-3) but can be confused with Crouzon syndrome when a patient with Saethre-Chotzen syndrome presents with no limb abnormalities.[28]

Syndromes that share craniosynostosis as a characteristic phenotype, as well as mutations on the same gene as a common cause, may still involve different pathogenetic mechanisms. For example, mutations associated with Apert and Crouzon syndromes are located on the same gene but are mutually

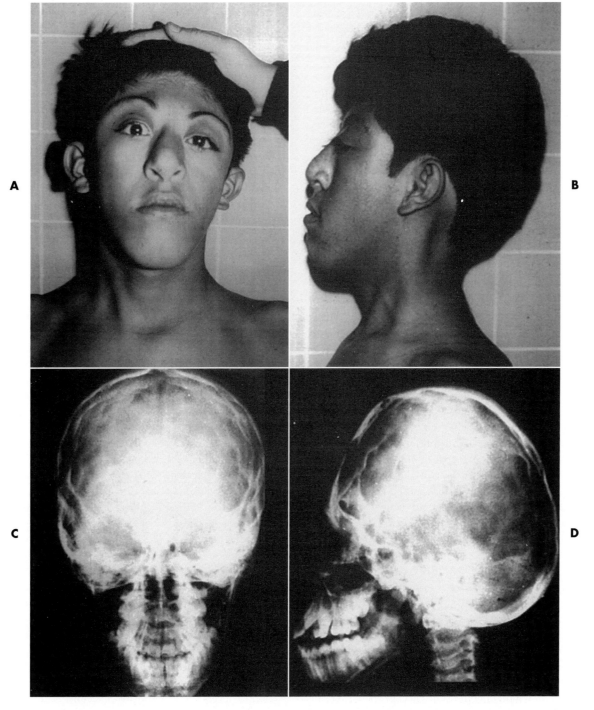

Figure 42-3. **A** and **B,** Saethre-Chotzen syndrome patient. Note the high forehead, decreased anteroposterior diameter, asymmetry of the face and ears, ptosis, and maxillary hypoplasia. **C** and **D,** Radiographs of the same individual. (Modified from Howard TD, et al: *Nat Genet* 15:36-41, 1997.)

exclusive of one another. These two subgroups of mutations may result in different pathogenetic mechanisms. Mathijssen et al[52] have demonstrated a displacement of the frontal and parietal ossification centers (tubers) *toward* the coronal suture in cases of Apert syndrome and isolated coronal synostosis. They also noted an apparent caudal dispositioning of the bony tubers in Apert dry skulls. However, these displacements were not found in Crouzon syndrome patients, indicating a distinction in the pathogenesis of suture closure in these two syndromes.[52] Richtsmeier et al[81] found an inferior displacement of the parietal tubers in a sample of patients with isolated sagittal synostosis, suggesting a possible link in pathogenesis (but not necessarily etiology) between Apert syndrome and certain types of isolated synostosis.

The idea that craniosynostosis sometimes results from the failure of sutures to form has also been proposed.[20,36] If the suture never forms, agenesis rather than synostosis is a more appropriate term for the condition,[52] and the presumptive location of the unformed suture may be termed the *sutural default zone*.[10] The concept of a "window of opportunity" for suture induction has been noted in the literature.[9,66] Cohen and Kreiborg[10] suggested that the agenesis of sagittal and metopic sutures in Apert syndrome patients results from the widening of the formative suture areas caused by primary cranial base synostosis. The approximation of the approaching bone fronts is delayed, and the window of opportunity for suture induction is missed, resulting in fusion when the bones meet rather than suture formation.

Isolated craniosynostosis involves the premature fusion of one or more cranial sutures without any other primary abnormalities. In most cases, only one suture is involved, and the phenotype is often described solely on the basis of cranial morphology. Isolated sagittal synostosis results in dolichocephaly, metopic synostosis in trigonocephaly, and unicoronal and bicoronal synostosis in asymmetric and symmetric brachycephaly, respectively. The face may also appear to be affected in isolated synostosis, especially metopic and unicoronal synostosis, although these are by definition secondary effects. The shape of the cranium can appear similar in syndromic and nonsyndromic cases, based on shared patterns of suture fusion. However, comparable cranial morphology does not necessarily indicate a shared etiology and pathogenesis of the craniosynostosis.

CRANIAL VAULT DEVELOPMENT AND SUTURE FORMATION

Two important processes are involved in normal development of the cranial vault. First, embryonic intercellular interactions trigger the differentiation of osteogenic cells, followed by the formation of bone. Second, bone is continually remodeled through resorption and deposition of new bone. Therefore craniofacial form is a product of the original morphogenesis of the bony precursors and the subsequent growth pattern of the bone in concert with surrounding soft tissue.

Up until the 1980s, most quantitative research focusing on postnatal craniofacial development in isolated and syndromic craniosynostosis used two-dimensional roentgenographic cephalograms as data and superimposition of tracings as the method of analysis.[38-40] Analysis of global craniofacial shape and change in shape through time using three-dimensional data from computed tomography scans and magnetic resonance imaging has recently become more common.[50,81,85] The objectives of studying growth patterns of craniosynostosis patients are manifold, sometimes involving the prediction or evaluation of postoperative results. More commonly, however, such studies target proximate goals that might help to understand the pathogenesis of craniosynostosis. These goals include local and global quantitative measures of the difference between normal craniofacial morphology and the morphology associated with craniosynostosis, tabulation of the age specificity of these differences, and quantification of the geometric relationship of cranial bones to one another as the skull grows. This information can provide a better understanding of abnormal morphogenesis when joined with information pertaining to the molecular mechanisms and cellular processes that ultimately produce cranial form.

The cranial vault is formed by five bones that develop in an osteogenic membrane around the brain: a pair of frontal bones, a pair of parietal bones, and a squamous occipital bone. The osteogenic membrane is the outermost layer of the developing meninges. It is generally understood that epithelial-mesenchymal interactions result in osteogenic condensations around the developing brain.[101] The condensations are a result of chemotaxis and proliferation. In intermembranous bone, differentiation of mesenchyme into preosteoblasts may occur before condensation and as a direct result of epithelial-mesenchymal interactions.[17] A wave of osteodifferentiation radiates outward from ossification centers in each of these condensations. As osteoblasts are formed, they secrete an extracellular matrix, osteoid, which is then mineralized through the deposition of hydroxyapatite crystals. Bone growth occurs through a combination of bone deposition at the margins of the bony plate and bone deposition and resorption from the ectocranial and endocranial surfaces. Sutures are induced when the osteoinductive fronts of adjacent bones either abut or overlap each other, and a fibrous matrix is formed and incorporated between the bones.

Cranial sutures are fibrous articulations between contiguous bones of the cranium that permit some movement at compression during parturition and allow localized growth of the bone to accommodate the developing brain. The precise mechanisms of suture formation, maintenance, and fusion are not well understood despite significant investigation.[36,65-67,87] At a histologic level, sutures are formed when approaching wedge-shaped osteogenic fronts meet. The suture initially consists of five layers, a central vascular area surrounded by two cellular cambrial layers and two fibrous periosteal layers. The cambrial layers merge to form the cellular blastema, leaving continuous periosteum ectocranially and continuous dura endocranially around the functioning suture. Osteogenic cells at the sutural margins produce new bone, resulting in appositional growth at the sutures. The metopic suture begins ossification in the second year, but the other cranial sutures usually do not begin to fuse until the third decade of life, well after the brain has reached its full volume.[36]

Moss[56] proposed a biomechanical model for suture formation, maintenance, and premature fusion, which posited fiber tracts running through the dura between sites of dural attachment on the cranial base and the sutural edges of the calvarial bones. According to this model, tensile forces produced by the dural fiber tracts induce the compensatory deposition of new bone along the margins of the bone while maintaining suture patency.[56] This model also posits that abnormalities in the cranial base result in transmission of abnormal stresses to the vault, inducing premature fusion.[56]

More recent research has given support to a biochemical model for suture biology. As with the biomechanical model, the dura plays a critical role in suture formation, maintenance, and fusion. However, the biochemical model appears to have a molecular component instead of, or in addition to, a mechanical effect. Implantation of presumptive coronal sutures with underlying fetal dura into an adult rat model resulted in normal development and patency of the suture.[67] This study demonstrated that physical connection to the cranial base via dural fiber tracts was not required for the formation and maintenance of the suture. Transplantation of the presumptive suture without underlying fetal dura also resulted in the expected suture morphogenesis, but fusion inevitably followed, suggesting that the dura plays a role in maintaining suture patency but is not required for suture formation.[67] Fetal dura is able to regenerate calvarial bone and sutures in proper anatomic position, indicating some kind of signaling mechanism in the dural tissue.[15,48] Opperman et al[67] suggested that morphogenesis of the suture is initiated by the meeting of osteogenic fronts, and that an interaction between the osteogenic fronts and the blastema imprints the dura in such a way that it causes the dura to maintain suture patency and, in fact, recreate the suture in the event of removal and regrowth of the calvarial bone.

The signaling mechanism in the dura apparently involves soluble chemical factors rather than cell-cell or cell-matrix interactions, because the interposition of a permeable membrane between the fetal dura and the presumptive suture did not produce premature bony fusion.[66] However, neonatal calvarial sutures cultured without underlying dura in vitro remained patent, suggesting that these sutures had achieved some sort of internal stabilization to maintain patency. When the neonatal suture was transplanted into an adult in vivo model with underlying adult parietal dura, the suture fused. These latter results indicate that an osteogenic signal in the adult dura was able to override the internal patency of the neonatal calvarial suture and produce bony fusion.[66] Opperman et al[66] reiterated the suggestion that formation of the suture marks the dura and proposed further that the dura then sends an osteoinhibitory signal to the suture. This osteoinhibitory signal is necessary to suture patency for a period of time, but at some point the suture becomes internally

stabilized. After stabilization the signaling mechanism beneath the suture then functions to limit the normal osteoinductive signal of the majority of the dura. Therefore, if the dura is not properly imprinted with the osteoinhibitory signal, or if the suture does not become stabilized during this critical time period, then premature fusion of the suture may ensue.[66]

Additionally, development of the calvarial bones in the absence of dura resulted in a decreased level of calcium deposition, suggesting that the dura also plays a role in normal mineralization.[66] The soluble factor that influences mineralization may be bound to the cells of the dura because interposition of the permeable membrane also resulted in reduced mineralization compared with bone with intact dura but still more mineralization than when the dura was entirely removed.[66] Interposition of the membrane only partially limited the influence of the dura on the mineralization of the bone. This may implicate a transmembrane molecule that is attached to an individual cell but has an extracellular component. One such molecule is the protein product of a gene, FGFR2, that has been associated with craniosynostosis and is discussed below.

Many extracellular signaling molecules have been implicated in the regulation of bone cell proliferation and differentiation, including fibroblast growth factors (FGFs), transforming growth factors β (TGF-βs), bone morphogenetic proteins (BMPs), platelet-derived growth factors (PDGFs), insulin-like growth factors (IGFs), and interleukins. Generally, these factors act by binding receptors at a target cell and triggering a signal transduction cascade that influences the nature of the gene products of the target cell and may affect its differentiation potential. TGF-βs are among the most abundant of the growth factors and are produced by bone cells and by the cells of the dura.[65] TGF-β molecules are produced by osteoblasts, which also possess high-affinity receptors for TGF-βs, suggesting an autocrine regulatory mechanism.[22] The differential expression of TGF-β1, TGF-β2, and TGF-β3 in patent and fusing sutures suggests a role for these molecules in suture formation, maintenance, and/or fusion.[65,87] During normal suture development in a rat model, TGF-β1, TGF-β2, and TGF-β3 were all expressed.[65] TGF-β1 and TGF-β2 remained active in the fusing frontonasal suture but declined concurrent with an increase in TGF-β3 during maintenance of the patent coronal suture.[65] Exogenous application of TGF-β2 induced early fusion of the posterior frontal suture in a rat model.[87] These experimental results suggest a loose connection between TGF-β2 and suture fusion and between TGF-β3 and suture patency and lead one to conclude that a disruption in the timing or production of these factors may result in premature synostosis or sutural agenesis.

Winograd et al[103,104] have conducted recent research into the cellular enzymatic changes that occur in vivo and ex vivo during programmed suture fusion in a rat model. In particular, they have found that levels of alkaline phosphatase, a marker of osteoblastic activity, and tartrate-resistant acid phosphatase, a marker of osteoclastic activity, increase significantly within the fusing suture, indicating regulatory control of bone synthesis and resorption in the fusion process.[103,104]

We note that the molecular mechanisms involved in suture fusion may differ depending on the suture involved. For example, the signaling process that induces the bluntly opposed, midline sagittal suture may not be the same as the induction mechanism of the overlapping, transversely oriented coronal suture. These distinct mechanisms could relate to the fact that the coronal suture marks the junction of two different bones (frontal and parietal), whereas the sagittal suture joins two of the same bone (parietal). Perhaps differential timing of formation and rates of growth of the parietal and frontal bones require that suture formation be induced in the coronal suture in some way different from the sagittal suture, where the abutting parietal bones are expected to grow symmetrically in terms of morphology and rate. Any distinction in mechanisms could also be a product of differential molecular patterning on the anterior-posterior and axial planes, as seen in *Drosophila* (e.g., sonic hedgehog and anterior-posterior patterning). These types of molecular issues, in addition to morphologic and genetic issues relating to craniosynostosis, remain open to further investigation.

GENETIC COMPONENT OF CRANIOSYNOSTOSIS

In the early 1990s, Cohen[8] and Lewanda et al[42] discussed the genetic heterogeneity of syndromic craniosynostosis. Since then, the genetic basis of several autosomal dominant craniosynostosis syndromes, primarily involving the coronal sutures, have been elucidated for Boston-type craniosynostosis,[32] Crouzon syndrome,[79] Jackson-Weiss syndrome,[31] Pfeiffer syndrome,[58] Apert syndrome,[100] Crouzon syndrome with acanthosis nigricans,[54] Beare-Stevenson cutis gyrata syndrome,[75] and Saethre-Chotzen syndrome[19,28] (Table 42-1). Several of these mutations associated with craniosynostosis suggest that in

some cases craniosynostosis may result from changes in the genes that regulate ontogeny.[32] Genetic studies have identified at least five genes that, when mutated, lead to craniosynostosis (MSX2, FGFR1, FGFR2, FGFR3, TWIST). These genetic correlations provide clues to the molecular pathways of human craniofacial development and the mechanisms of craniofacial malformations, such as craniosynostosis.

The first mutant gene implicated was MSX2.[31] The MSX family of transcription factors, of which MSX2 is a member, are homeobox genes that code for proteins that regulate the expression of unknown gene targets. MSX2 was mapped to chromosome 5, where the locus responsible for Boston-type craniosynostosis, an autosomal dominant condition, had also been mapped. A single, common nucleotide change causing an amino acid substitution in a highly conserved region of the MSX2 homeodomain was found in all affected members of a large New England family (Table 42-2). These individuals displayed a range of phenotypes, including variable involvement of sutures and cranial morphology (ranging from frontal orbital recession to cloverleaf skull anomaly), cleft of the soft palate, triphalangeal thumb, and shortened first metatarsals.

In the mouse, Msx2 is expressed in premigratory and migratory cephalic neural crest, neural crest-derived mesenchyme of the first through fourth branchial arches, osteogenic tissue of the mandible and maxilla, developing teeth, apical ectodermal ridge and underlying mesenchyme of the limb bud, and endocardial cushion of the developing heart.[26,49] Moreover, it was found to be expressed at calvarial sutures.[32] Many of these locations are sites of epithelial-mesenchymal interactions, and tissue recombination experiments have shown that, in at least some of these sites, the expression of the Msx2 gene depends on such interactions.[97] Another mouse study showed that Msx2 was intensely expressed in sutural mesenchyme and

Table 42-1.
Craniosynostosis Syndromes: Chromosome Loci and Genes

SYNDROME	CHROMOSOME	GENE
Craniosynostosis, Boston type	5q34-q35	MSX2[32]
Crouzon	10q25.3-q26	FGFR2[31,79]
	4p16.3	FGFR3[4,55]
Crouzon with acanthosis nigricans	4p16.3	FGFR3[54]
Jackson-Weiss	10q25.3-q26	FGFR2[31]
Pfeiffer	8p11	FGFR1[58]
	10q25.3-q26	FGFR2[88]
	4p16.3	FGFR3[4]
Apert	10q25.3-q26	FGFR2[70,100]
Beare-Stevenson cutis gyrata	10q25.3-q26	FGFR2[75]
Saethre-Chotzen	7p22-p21.3	TWIST[19,28]

Table 42-2.
Mutations in Craniosynostosis

MUTATION	SYNDROME	MUTATION	SYNDROME
MSX2		**IgIII-like Domain—cont'd**	
P147H	Craniosynostosis, Boston type[32]	D321A	Pfeiffer[41]
FGFR1		Y328C	Crouzon[31]
IgII-IgIII Linker		N331I	Crouzon[93]
P252R	Pfeiffer[58]	A337P	Crouzon[72]
FGFR2		DA337-338ins	Crouzon[93]
IgII-like Domain		G338R	Crouzon[23]
Y105C	Crouzon[76]	G338E	Crouzon[76]
IgII-IgIII Linker		Y340H	Crouzon[31,79]
S252W	Apert,[a] Pfeiffer[b; 70,71,100]	Y340C	Pfeiffer[13]
S252L	Crouzon[c; 61]	T341P	Pfeiffer[88]
S252F	Apert[d; 61]	C342R	Pfeiffer, Crouzon, Jackson-Weiss[69,79,88]
SP252-253FS	Pfeiffer[61]	C342S[f]	Pfeiffer, Crouzon, Jackson-Weiss[23,53,79]
P253R	Apert[a; 70,100]		
S267P	Pfeiffer, Crouzon[13,62]	C342Y	Pfeiffer, Crouzon[79,88]
G268-269ins	Crouzon[53]	C342W	Crouzon, Pfeiffer[69,94]
VV269-270del	Saethre-Chotzen[74]	C342F	Crouzon[62]
F276V	Pfeiffer, Crouzon[96]	C342G	Pfeiffer[13]
C278F	Pfeiffer, Crouzon, Jackson-Weiss[53,62]	**IgIII-Transmembrane Linker**	
Y281C	Crouzon[e]	A344A(G→A)[g]	Crouzon, Unclassified syndrome[31,69,79,95]
IgIII-like Domain			
HIQ287-289del	Crouzon[62]	A344P	Pfeiffer[53]
Q289P	Crouzon, Jackson-Weiss[23,62]	A344G	Crouzon, Jackson-Weiss[23,31]
W290G	Crouzon[69]	G-P345-361del	Pfeiffer[53]
W290R	Crouzon[62]	S347C	Crouzon[31]
W290C[f]	Pfeiffer, Antley-Bixler?[89,98]	I220-1221insAlu	Apert[d; 63]
K292E	Crouzon[92]	S351C	Pfeiffer, Crouzon, Antley-Bixler?, Unclassified syndrome[7,24,51,60,76]
Y301C	Crouzon[96]		
I119-3-4insAlu[g]	Apert[d; 63]		
I119-3T→G[g]	Pfeiffer[90]	S354C	Crouzon[79]
I119-2A→G[g]	Pfeiffer, Apert[d; 41,73]	WLT356-358del	Crouzon[93]
I119-2A→T[g]	Pfeiffer[2]	L357S	Crouzon[25]
I119-1G→C[g]	Pfeiffer[27]	V359F	Pfeiffer[53]
I119-1G→A[g]	Pfeiffer[13]	S372C	Beare-Stevenson[75]
I119+3A→G[g]	Pfeiffer[13]		
A314S[g]	Pfeiffer, Unclassified syndrome[90,96]		

Continued

Table 42-2.
Mutations in Craniosynostosis—cont'd

MUTATION	SYNDROME	MUTATION	SYNDROME
FGFR—cont'd		**DNA-Binding Domain—cont'd**	
Transmembrane		A129R[j]	Saethre-Chotzen[74]
Y375C	Beare-Stevenson[75]	L131P	Saethre-Chotzen[19]
G384R	Unclassified syndrome[76]	R132P	Saethre-Chotzen[74]
FGFR3		I134M	Saethre-Chotzen[86]
IgII-IgIII Linker		AALRKI1135-136ins	Saethre-Chotzen[28]
P250R[h]	Syndromic and nonsyndromic coronal craniosynostosis[4,55,74]	P136L	Saethre-Chotzen[33]
Transmembrane		**Loop**	
A391E	Crouzon with acanthosis nigricans[a; 54]	P139S	Saethre-Chotzen[74]
TWIST		KIIPTLP139-140ins[f]	Saethre-Chotzen[19,28,74,86]
Prior to DNA Binding		S140X	Saethre-Chotzen[86]
G61X	Saethre-Chotzen[86]	IIPTLPS140-141ins	Saethre-Chotzen[86]
E65X	Saethre-Chotzen[86]	D141Y	Saethre-Chotzen[74]
L77S[i]	Saethre-Chotzen[33,86]	D141G	Saethre-Chotzen[86]
Y103X[f]	Saethre-Chotzen[19,28,74]	K145G[j]	Saethre-Chotzen[28]
E104X	Saethre-Chotzen[18]	K145E	Saethre-Chotzen[18]
DNA-Binding Domain		K145N	Saethre-Chotzen[86]
R116W	Saethre-Chotzen[74]	T148N	Saethre-Chotzen[77]
R118Q	Saethre-Chotzen[18]	L149F	Saethre-Chotzen[74]
R118H	Saethre-Chotzen[86]	A152V	Saethre-Chotzen[74]
Q119P	Saethre-Chotzen[28]	**Helix II**	
Helix I		R154G	Saethre-Chotzen[86]
Q122X	Saethre-Chotzen[74]	L159F	Saethre-Chotzen[18]
S123W	Saethre-Chotzen[33]	Q161X	Saethre-Chotzen[18]
S123X	Saethre-Chotzen[19]		
E126X	Saethre-Chotzen[19,86]		

Numbering of FGFR2 nucleotides was based on the complimentary DNA (cDNA) sequence reported by Dionne et al.[14] Table represents mutations implicated in craniosynostosis identified through 1998.

[a]Recurrent mutations with consistent spectrum of clinical features.
[b]Only one of more than 200 patients with this mutation displays the Pfeiffer syndrome phenotype.
[c]This mutation is also found in normal phenotype.
[d]Apert-like phenotype observed in one case.
[e]Jabs EW: Unpublished data; and Wilkie AOM: Personal communication.
[f]Different nucleotide mutations have been shown to cause this amino acid mutation.
[g]Presumed or proven to affect ribonucleic acid (RNA) splicing.
[h]High degree of phenotypic variation associated with this mutation. Syndromic phenotypes have included Crouzon, Pfeiffer, and Saethre-Chotzen. "Muenke craniosynostosis" is sometimes used to refer to all phenotypes with this mutation.
[i]Rose et al[86] referred to this mutation as S78P, which has been corrected by Johnson et al.[33]
[j]Mutation causes frameshift so that all subsequent amino acids are altered.

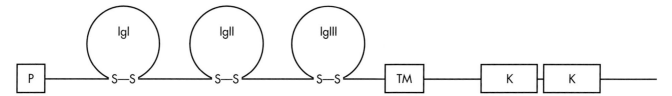

Figure 42-4. Schematic structure of fibroblast growth factor receptors (FGFRs). *P,* Signal peptide; *Ig,* immunoglobulin-like domains (I, II, and III); *TM,* transmembrane region; *K,* split tyrosine kinase domain; *S-S,* disulfide bond created between cysteine residues. Note that the cysteine residues serve an important function in protein structure and that mutations affecting one of these amino acids can leave the corresponding cysteine available to bond with and activate other receptors without the presence of growth factors. (Modified from Jabs EW, et al: *Nat Genet* 8:275-279, 1994.)

dura mater during embryonic stages.[35] However, after birth, the expression of Msx2 was dramatically reduced in the mesenchyme and completely disappeared from the dura mater.[35] Expression of Msx2 in fetal dura only may relate to the unique ability of fetal dura to maintain suture locations.

The mutation identified in the MSX2 homeodomain has been shown to result in enhanced affinity of the MSX2 protein for binding to downstream target deoxyribonucleic acid (DNA) sequence but has little or no effect on the site specificity of MSX2 binding.[47,91] These findings suggest that the mutation may exert its pathophysiologic effects on craniofacial development by a gain of function rather than either a loss of function or dominant-negative mechanism. Transgenic mice experiments in which either a wild-type or mutant mouse Msx2 was expressed from a heterologous promoter support the role for MSX2 in Boston-type craniosynostosis because the mutant mice displayed closely opposed sutures and ectopic bone formation.[44] Transgenic mice carrying a 34-kb DNA fragment encompassing a human MSX2 gene encoding either the wild-type or mutant MSX2 and its regulatory flanking regions were created. The mutant mice exhibited variable phenotypes with multiple craniofacial malformations of varying severity, including aplasia of the interparietal bone, decreased ossification of the hyoid, mandibular hypoplasia, cleft secondary palate, exencephaly, and median facial cleft.[102]

Fibroblast growth factor receptors are a family of four genes for which three members (FGFR1, FGFR2, and FGFR3) have been found to have mutations in individuals diagnosed with one of more than six different craniosynostosis syndromes, including Apert, Crouzon, Jackson-Weiss, Pfeiffer, Beare-Stevenson cutis gyrata, and Crouzon with acanthosis nigricans syndromes.[43,57,68] Affected individuals exhibit additional craniofacial features of hypertelorism, ocular proptosis, midface hypoplasia, high-arched palate, dental malocclusion, and conductive hearing loss. Two of these craniosynostosis syndromes are also associated with skin disorders, Beare-Stevenson cutis gyrata (furrowing of the skin) syndrome[75] and Crouzon syndrome with acanthosis nigricans (hyperkeratosis and hyperpigmentation of the skin).[54] The FGFR genes encode highly related glycoproteins with a common structure: an extracellular domain with a signal peptide and three immunoglobulin-

like (IgI, IgII, and IgIII) domains containing characteristic cysteine residues, a single transmembrane domain, and an intracellular split tyrosine kinase domain (Figure 42-4). At least seventeen ligands, called fibroblast growth factors, have been identified that bind to the IgII-IgIII-like domains of FGFRs. FGFs act in concert with heparan sulfate proteoglycans to bind these receptors, forming dimers and leading to transphosphorylation of the kinase domains. The activated receptors can then phosphorylate intracellular proteins that transmit biological signals into the nucleus and mediate an array of biologic processes, including cell growth, differentiation, mitogenesis, migration, angiogenesis, and wound healing.[21] FGFRs have distinct spatial and temporal expression patterns and are all expressed in bone primordia, suggesting a specialized role or roles in bone development. FGFR1, FGFR2, and FGFR3 are all expressed in the developing suture.[29,35]

Interestingly, similar craniosynostosis syndromes have been mapped to point mutations or inframe small deletions or insertions in all three of these receptors (see Table 42-2). For instance, a proline-to-arginine substitution in the linker region between the IgII and IgIII loops has been identified in each of the three receptors, resulting in Pfeiffer syndrome when present in FGFR1, Apert syndrome when present in FGFR2, and a highly variable form of craniosynostosis when present in FGFR3.[57] The latter mutation in FGFR3 can be associated with a broad range of phenotypes; individuals with this mutation can resemble Crouzon syndrome, Saethre-Chotzen syndrome, or isolated coronal synostosis patients. It has also been shown that mutations in this IgII-IgIII linker region of each of the three receptors can result in apparently the same phenotype (e.g., Pfeiffer syndrome). A variety of mutations in the extracellular domain of FGFR2 cause Pfeiffer, Crouzon, and Jackson-Weiss syndromes, and often the identical mutation can result in two or more of these disorders.

In contrast, virtually all cases of Apert syndrome in which a mutation has been identified are associated with one of only two mutations in FGFR2 (see Table 42-2). Apert syndrome is a clinically distinct condition with a consistent suite of associated clinical features, although the craniofacial phenotype has been described as variable. The two craniosynostosis conditions associated with skin disorders, Beare-Stevenson cutis gyrata and Crouzon syndrome with acanthosis nigricans, result from mutations at the juxtamembrane and transmembrane domains of FGFR2 and FGFR3, respectively.

The FGFR2 mutations that have been found in Crouzon and Pfeiffer syndromes result in receptors that are constitutively activated, suggesting that these conditions result from a gain-of-function mechanism.[21,59] In other words, the mutant receptor turns on the signal transduction cascade, even when the appropriate trigger, the FGF ligand, is not present. In contrast, the FGFR2 mutations that result in Apert syndrome modify the receptor in a way that reduces the dissociation of the FGF2 ligand, resulting in prolonged activation of the receptor.[1] However, it is unclear whether these modifications to FGFR activity produce similar or different responses by the receptor cell. The extent of abnormal activation of the FGFR signal transduction cascade may differ from one syndrome to the next. Clearly, these findings suggest modifying genes, perhaps upstream or downstream of FGFRs, that modulate the phenotype. Factors such as genetic background, epistasis, environment (maternal and postnatal), and other stochastic processes can not be ignored in proposing any mechanism for the pathogenesis of Pfeiffer syndrome, Crouzon, Jackson-Weiss, Apert, or any other FGFR-related syndrome.

The TWIST gene codes for a transcription factor with a basic helix-loop-helix motif. The protein contains a loop domain that maintains the tertiary structure between the helical elements that dimerize before binding DNA. Mutations in TWIST result in Saethre-Chotzen syndrome (see Table 42-2), a common autosomal dominant disorder of craniosynostosis, usually affecting the coronal suture. Facial asymmetry, ptosis, prominent ear crus, low-set posteriorly rotated small ears, conductive deafness, deviated nasal septum, cleft palate, and malocclusion are additional craniofacial features of this condition. The limb anomalies include brachydactyly and syndactyly. The locus for Saethre-Chotzen syndrome was mapped to the chromosome 7p21-p22 region by linkage analysis. Case reports with the phenotype and apparently balanced translocations and deletions involving 7p21-p22 support the localization of the disease locus to this region.[33,37,78,80] Many different mutations in TWIST, including missense, nonsense, duplications, and deletions, have been identified and are presumed to cause loss of function. Interestingly, mice who have lost one copy of Twist (heterozygous null) have a phenotype that resembles Saethre-Chotzen syndrome.[19] Twist expression in mouse embryos occurs along a dorsoventral gradient until the headfold stage, then it is observed along the rostrocaudal axis in the mesoderm and in neural crest cell derivatives. Specifically, it is expressed during the embryonic mesodermal development of the head and limbs. Later Twist message is predominantly found in the somites, head mesenchyme, first aortic arches, second and fourth branchial arches, limb buds, and mesenchyme underneath the epidermis. Twist transcripts have also been detected in primary osteoblastic cells from newborn mouse calvaria.

Our understanding of the genetic causes of craniosynostosis is generally limited to the syndromic forms discussed above. When occurring as one of several features of a syndrome such as Apert, Crouzon, Jackson-Weiss, Pfeiffer, or Saethre-Chotzen syndromes, craniosynostosis is seen predominantly in the coronal suture. If there are distinct mechanisms of suture fusion for each of the different sutures of the cranium, then different molecular pathways may be involved. Pathogenetic studies of these syndromes should include histochemical analyses of each of the involved sutures because comparisons between multiple sutures from one individual may provide clues regarding the differential nature of premature fusion.

It is remarkable that so little is known about the pathogenesis of isolated forms of craniosynostosis. Although a FGFR3 Pro250Arg mutation has been shown to result in nonsyndromic coronal synostosis,[4] there are no known mutations associated with isolated sagittal, lambdoid, or metopic synostosis. This prompts us to ask, why not? Are these isolated forms of craniosynostosis not caused by genetic conditions, or have they simply not yet been discovered? We believe that isolated craniosynostosis has various causes, some of which are genetic in nature and some of which are not. We suggest that mutations in gene products other than MSX2, FGFRs, and TWIST produce some forms of craniosynostosis, of the sagittal or metopic suture at least, and remain undiscovered.

HYPOTHETICAL MECHANISMS

It has been shown that MSX2, FGFRs, and TWIST are each expressed at some point in the development of the cranial vault and that mutations in these genes are associated with syndromes that include craniosynostosis as a feature. Note that MSX2 and TWIST are transcription factors and the FGFRs are transmembranic receptors for extracellular factors. We have seen that certain growth factors (e.g., TGF-βs) also play an important role in the maintenance and premature fusion of cranial sutures. At the morphologic level, craniofacial growth patterns of children with syndromic and nonsyndromic craniosynostosis have been shown to follow craniofacial growth trajectories that are different from normal.[38,39,83,84] Our goal is to understand the regulatory mechanisms that might connect the gene products, the growth factors, the growth pattern, and the morphology. Gene interactions, including epistasis and the effects of a variable genetic background, may obscure our understanding of these mechanisms, and for the time being we can only speculate on these possible connections.

It has been postulated, based on tissue culture experiments, that Msx2 is involved in craniofacial development by functioning as a transcriptional repressor.[91] The MSX2 gain-of-function mutation, then, may result in a reduced expression of the unknown target protein. Overexpression of Msx2 in a transgenic mouse model, simulating the effect of a gain-of-function mutation, resulted in a higher number of proliferating, preosteoblastic cells in the postnatal sagittal suture and enhanced growth of the parietal bones into the sutural space.[45] This suggests that the target protein for MSX2 is involved with the final stages of osteoblast differentiation. Data from this study also indicated that Msx2 in the cranium was expressed primarily along the margins of the parietal and interparietal bones.[45]

A study of Apert syndrome infant and fetal sutures showed that the Apert FGFR2 mutations lead to an increase in the number of mesenchymal cells that enter the osteogenic pathway and an increase in the rate of osteoblast maturation.[46] This suggests that the normal function of FGFR2 may relate to the recruitment of uncommitted cells as preosteoblasts, in addition to or instead of the proliferation of preosteoblast cells. Given that the FGFR2 mutations result in a gain of function, it is also interesting to note that synostosed coronal sutures from Crouzon syndrome patients contain fewer cells with active FGFR2 than nonsynostosed sutures from the same individuals.[6] In addition, patients with Crouzon syndrome showed less FGFR2 activity in both synostosed and nonsynostosed sutures compared with either synostosed or nonsynostosed sutures in children with nonsyndromic, isolated coronal synostosis.[6] These results may demonstrate a balance between abnormal gain of function, correlated with proliferative osteogenic stem cells, and an eventual, compensating down-regulation of FGFR2 at the cellular level, correlated with cell differentiation, bone formation, and suture fusion.[99]

In a study involving Fgfr2 expression in a fetal mouse model, Iseki et al[30] described Fgfr2 down-regulation as an autocrine response to FGF ligand binding. Fgfr2 is most strongly transcribed in the proliferating cells along the margins of the developing calvarial bones.[30] Its activity is adjacent to and mutually exclusive of the transcription of osteopontin, a marker for cell differentiation.[30] Ectopic application of FGF2, intended to simulate the overexpression of Fgfr2, induced strong osteopontin expression in the immediate area of FGF2 application. Fgfr2 expression was absent from the osteopontin region but encircled it.[30] These results led Iseki et al[30] to propose the following model for calvarial growth. Fgfr2 is expressed in the proliferating cells at the margins of the developing bone, and trace amounts of FGF2 are available in the local extracellular environment. The osteoid matrix of the developing bone binds FGF2, making it available to adjacent undifferentiated cells. High levels of activated Fgfr2 in these cells result in the down-regulation of Fgfr2, the expression of osteopontin, and differentiation into preosteoblasts. These preosteoblasts become osteoblasts, secreting osteoid and binding more FGF2 from the environment. Thus a paracrine loop is created that results in the continually expanding proliferation and differentiation of bone cells.[30] Further research by Iseki and Morriss-Kay[29] indicates that Fgfr1 is expressed in the differentiating cells along with osteopontin. They suggest that Fgfr1 signaling plays a key role in the regulation of osteogenic cell differentiation.[29] Note the temporal and functional differences in the expression of FGFR1 and FGFR2 and the apparent association of FGFR2 with cell proliferation and of FGFR1 with cell differentiation.

Gain of function at the molecular level associated with mutations in FGFR2 may result in overactive cell proliferation, followed by a down-regulation of the FGFR2 protein and differentiation of bone cells, as discussed above. The expression of FGFR1 and other markers of differentiation may be triggered by high levels of FGFR2 or merely associated with its

down-regulation. The FGF-FGFR pathways likely involve many other gene products, as well. For example, there is evidence to suggest that TGF-βs potentiate the proliferative effect of FGFs.[22] If TGF-β2 is loosely associated with suture fusion,[65,87] we might expect to see that TGF-β2 in particular produces an increase in osteogenic cell proliferation.

It is also possible that the FGFRs and MSX2 genes are involved in the same regulatory cascade but that the mutations in these genes affect the mechanism in different ways. For example, assuming that MSX2 is upstream of FGFR2 in this hypothetic cascade, the MSX2 mutation may result in an *underexpression* of FGFR2 and decreased functionality of the FGFR2 protein, whereas the FGFR2 mutation may cause an increased functionality of the FGFR2 protein and a corresponding down-regulation of FGFR2 protein at the tissue level. Although the ultimate result is the same histochemically (reduced FGFR2 activity at the cellular level), the heterogenous mechanisms involved and variable effects on parallel regulatory cascades may yield potentially diverse developmental programs susceptible to various insults, and ultimately different phenotypes.

Alternatively, MSX2 may be a downstream target of FGFR2. The gain-of-function mutation of FGFR2 may activate MSX2 in excess of normal levels, or the MSX2 mutation itself may cause an MSX2 gain of function. Increased MSX2 function would repress the normal expression of its target gene, possibly delaying osteoblast differentiation. Under this mechanism, both the FGFR2 mutation and the MSX2 mutation would result in excessive cell proliferation along the edges of calvarial bone, and the delayed differentiation of osteoblasts may adversely affect the induction of one or more sutures.

Mutations in TWIST, on the other hand, result in a loss of function. It has been suggested that the TWIST gene product may be a prerequisite for FGFR signaling during mesoderm formation.[19,28] Given the expression of TWIST in the osteoblast cells of the developing calvaria, we speculate that a loss-of-function mutation in the TWIST gene may also affect cell proliferation at the periphery of the calvarial bones. If this is the case, craniosynostosis in Saethre-Chotzen syndrome may result from the failure of the bones to approximate each other within the time frame required for suture morphogenesis, as discussed above. This error in timing may produce an immediate fusion of the bone rather than normal suture formation. If we assume that TWIST is included in the same molecular cascade as MSX2 and FGFR2, it is possible that MSX2 has the effect of repressing TWIST.

Speculations such as these are helpful primarily in identifying issues for further research. Additional data on the differential expression of growth factors in normal and abnormal cranial sutures in individuals with syndromic and nonsyndromic synostosis would help us to better understand the potentially complex regulatory cascade involved in suture morphogenesis and cranial growth. It is possible that MSX2, the FGFRs, and TWIST are all involved in a single, probably complex regulatory cascade for cranial bone and suture formation. They may also each play a role in multiple developmental processes throughout the body, as suggested by their expression patterns in tissues both in and outside of the craniofacial region. If there is a genetic basis for the sagittal and metopic forms of isolated synostosis, then that gene product may also be involved in this cascade. However, whereas a mutation in this unidentified gene produces an isolated form of craniosynostosis, a mutation in FGFR2 or TWIST produces a syndromic form of craniosynostosis. Further research of both syndromic and nonsyndromic synostosis may elucidate the morphogenetic processes involved in normal and synostotic suture formation.

OPERATIONS

Currently, molecular mechanisms are not considered in planning surgical correction of the deformities associated with craniosynostosis. The phenotype (i.e., the dysmorphic skull) continues to be the most obvious and accessible indication of treatment requirements and goals. However, it is our contention that if the cause and progression of the dysmorphology were understood, this information could be of great use in surgical reconstruction. Different forms of craniosynostosis have been shown to have variable causes, and even where the specific genetic cause is known (i.e., in certain syndromic forms), the pathogenesis is unclear. The dynamic nature of the craniofacial complex and variable growth trajectories make reliable prediction of outcomes problematic.

Surgical treatment of syndromic dysmorphology is complicated by the likelihood of multiple abnormal elements in the dynamic craniofacial system and the need to repair those of functional significance first. In comparison, isolated synostosis of a cranial suture appears as a less complex deformity, especially for midline sutures, but the genetic and developmental basis for the majority of cases of nonsyndromic synostosis remains unknown and may be more complex than anticipated. Different causes of craniosynostosis may produce similar cranial morphologies, but whether they result in different growth patterns and deserve differential surgical treatment is a subject of speculation.

Surgical procedures are designed to address the specific, dysmorphic aspects of the synostosed skull. These range from simple, neurocranial strip craniectomies to more complex, multiple-operation reconstructions. Surgeons rely on previous experiences but generally cannot control for all factors so as to ensure prediction of the best procedure at the best time for a given patient. Previous experience is often a good guide to postoperative success, but the ideal situation would enable us to link etiology and phenotype (including growth pattern) in an algorithm of reliable predictive value.

Techniques based on a strip craniectomy involve release of the fused suture with variable extensions of the craniectomy but usually without additional reconstructive measures. In isolated sagittal synostosis, a simple release of the suture coupled with minimal cranial excavation can sometimes result in immediate improvement in overall form of the calotte (Figure 42-5). However, immediate postoperative correction may not always occur, depending on the age of the child and the severity of the dysmorphology. More extensive techniques, often including the removal and modification of bone elements, involve more reconstruction and carry a higher risk of complications, but they can provide a more immediate improvement in overall morphology. A predictive algorithm based on pathogenetic mechanisms would assist in the identification of patients requiring more extensive surgery and those who do not.

OUTCOMES

The aesthetic goal of surgical intervention for craniosynostosis is to modify an abnormal cranial morphology and produce a cranial form that is within the normal range. This can sometimes be accomplished through the release of the synostosed suture but may require reconstruction to correct any abnormal morphology secondary to the synostosis. In most cases it is assumed that the skull will continue to develop in a normal fashion once the fused suture is released. However, if there is an inherent abnormality in the craniofacial growth pattern, then an intervention that brings cranial morphology to a form deemed normal for that stage of development may not be adequate.[12,16] Although normal for that developmental stage, the morphology will continue to develop along an abnormal trajectory, eventually moving outside the range deemed normal (Figure 42-6). The dynamic nature of the craniofacial complex must be taken into account, and the possibility of further growth along an abnormal trajectory should be understood by the medical team and the patient's family. Definition of these growth trajectories is a goal of our laboratory.

Resynostosis is also possible. In a follow-up study to surgical correction of sagittal synostosis, poor results were reported in three out of 85 cases involving the pi procedure, all three of which were performed on children under 3 months of age.[5] The propensity for resynostosis is probably correlated with the cause or mechanism that produced the original fusion of the suture. If a genetic mutation results in abnormal proliferation of osteogenic cells at the presumptive suture, then cell proliferation after suture release is possible, although by no means ensured. The postoperative suture area, which is no longer either a fused suture or a functional suture, may display a bone deposition mechanism and a growth pattern that are different from the fused or functional sutures.

Awareness of the possibility of abnormal postintervention growth is extremely important, both in planning an intervention and in maintaining realistic expectations for postintervention results. The craniofacial complex is a dynamic system, and surgical intervention that impacts the neurocranium may affect

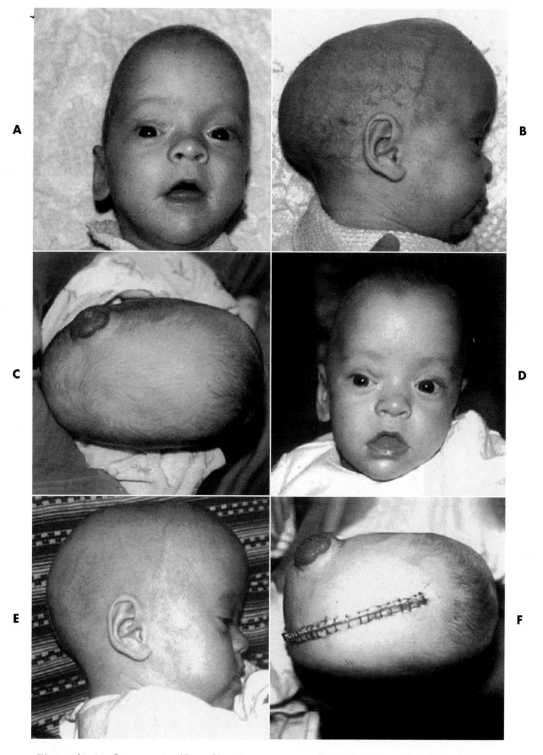

Figure 42-5. Preoperative (**A** to **C**) and postoperative (**D** to **F**) photographs of an infant with sagittal synostosis who underwent a sagittal strip craniectomy and strip craniectomies of pseudolambdoid sutures. Note marked improvement of overall head shape. The preoperative photographs were taken 1 week before surgery. The postoperative photographs were taken 5 days after surgery. The patient has a large hemangioma on her left superior parietal area. The patient was a premature infant born at 24 weeks. At the time of surgery, the patient was approximately 7 months old by calendar dates, 3 months old corrected for her premature birth.

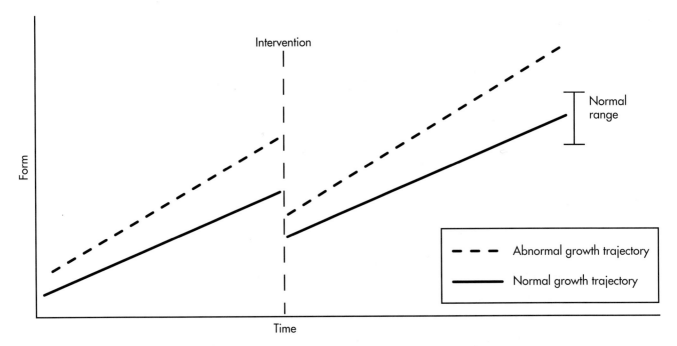

Figure 42-6. Schematic graph comparing form and growth trajectory. Following surgical intervention, the skull with a normal growth pattern continues to develop with a morphology in the "normal" range. However, the skull with an abnormal growth pattern continues to develop abnormally after intervention, and the morphologic form ultimately falls outside of the normal range. (Modified from Cole TM III, Krovitz GE, Richtsmeier JT: Paper presented at American Cleft Palate-Craniofacial Annual Meeting, New Orleans, 1997.)

other regions of the head or face. In addition, particularly for syndromic craniosynostosis cases, the underlying pathogenetic mechanisms may result in an abnormal growth trajectory that cannot be normalized by a single reconstructive procedure. Insights into the molecular processes involved with suture formation and maintenance may help to elucidate the pathogenetic mechanisms involved with craniosynostosis and suggest preventative treatments at the molecular level. Further, predictive algorithms based on an understanding of pathogenesis will assist in the timing and design of surgical intervention and produce an outcome that is more likely to be acceptable to the patient's family and medical team.

Our future research goals include acquisition of genetic information on patients who have undergone surgical correction of isolated sagittal synostosis. If the patients fall into two discernible subgroups based on postoperative results, these groups might correlate with the presence or absence of specific gene mutations. If these expectations are supported by subsequent research, then we suggest an open discussion on the possible incorporation of genetic testing in intervention planning. The incidence of a mutation does not enable us to definitively predict phenotype, however. As with any clinical problem, other variables will confound relationships, making it difficult to match cause with effect and to differentiate correlation from causation. These covariates include the nature of the synostosis (i.e., total versus partial synostosis), the genetic "background" of the patient, the type of intervention used, and the age at surgery. However, if we know something about the nature of the growth process that results in the osseous defect, the craniofacial team can anticipate the postoperative growth trajectory and predict postoperative morphology.[82] For example, if molecular information prompts the anticipation of resynostosis, the timing and nature of the intervention, as well as preventative measures taken, might be different than when resynostosis is not anticipated. Knowledge of the incidence and genetic basis for postoperative refusion might lead to research into the application of exogenous growth factors for prevention of resynostosis. Awareness of a genetic basis for the synostosis and the mode of bone formation that results in the synostosis can only improve realistic expectations of the intervention for the craniofacial team and for the family.

We hope that this chapter will serve as an overview of molecular research into the etiology and pathogenesis of craniosynostosis and its relation to intervention outcomes. We would like to encourage a continuing discourse among surgeons, geneticists, and molecular biologists with the goal of integrating knowledge, hypotheses, data, and conclusions from multiple fields of study. Specifically, we hope that plastic surgeons will maintain an awareness of the molecular and genetic context of their patients. Further, we would like to prompt geneticists to report more detailed, even quantitative, phenotypic information about their patients and animal models. A multilevel assessment of craniosynostosis patients, including genetic, molecular, and morphologic characters, will eventually allow us to bridge the existing gap between genotype and phenotype, leading to a full understanding of the genetic basis and morphogenetic process of craniosynostosis.

ACKNOWLEDGEMENTS

We would like to thank the editors for inviting us to contribute to this volume. We thank Gregg Semenza for helpful comments on the manuscript and Craig Vander Kolk in particular for editorial comments and for access to patient data. This work was supported in part by PHS awards P50DE11131 (Project IV: EWJ; Project II: JTR) and F33 DE05706-02 (JTR).

REFERENCES

1. Anderson J, Burns H, Enriquez-Harris P, et al: Apert syndrome mutations in fibroblast growth factor receptor 2 exhibit increased affinity for FGF ligand, *Hum Mol Genet* 7:1475-1483, 1998.

2. Anderson P, Hall C, Evans R, et al: The feet in Pfeiffer syndrome, *J Craniofac Surg* 9:83-87, 1998.

3. Anderson PJ, Hall CM, Evans RD, et al: Hand anomalies in Crouzon syndrome, *Skeletal Radiol* 26:113-115, 1997.

4. Bellus GA, Gaudenz K, Zackai EH, et al: Identical mutations in three different fibroblast growth factor receptor genes in autosomal dominant craniosynostosis syndrome, *Nat Genet* 14:174-176, 1996.

5. Boop FA, Chadduck WM, Shewmake K, et al: Outcome analysis of 85 patients undergoing the pi procedure for correction of sagittal synostosis, *J Neurosurg* 85:50-55, 1996.

6. Bresnick S, Schendel S: Crouzon disease correlates with low fibroblastic growth factor receptor activity in stenosed cranial sutures, *J Craniofac Surg* 6:245-248, 1995.

7. Chun K, Siegerl-Bartelt J, Chitayat D, et al: FGFR2 mutation associated with clinical manifestations consistent with Antley-Bixler syndrome, *Am J Med Genet* 77:219-224, 1998.

8. Cohen MM Jr: Sutural biology and the correlates of craniosynostosis, *Am J Med Genet* 47:581-618, 1993.

9. Cohen MM Jr: *Craniosynostosis: diagnosis, evaluation, and management*, New York, 1986, Raven Press.

10. Cohen MM Jr, Kreiborg S: Suture formation, premature sutural fusion, and suture default zones in Apert syndrome, *Am J Med Genet* 62:339-344, 1996.

11. Cohen MMJ: An etiologic and nosologic overview of craniosynostosis syndromes, *Birth Defects* 11:137-189, 1975.

12. Cole TM III, Krovitz GE, Richtsmeier JT: Patterns of calvarial growth in unilateral lambdoid synostosis and posterior plagiocephaly without synostosis. Paper presented at American Cleft Palate-Craniofacial Annual Meeting, New Orleans, 1997.

13. Cornejo L, Gaudenz K, Gripp K, et al: Mutational analysis in 79 patients with Pfeiffer syndrome in FGFR2 reveals variable phenotype with one exception: Ser351Cys, *Am J Hum Genet* 63(suppl):A33, 1998.

14. Dionne C, Crumley G, Bellot F, et al: Cloning and expression of two distinct high-affinity receptors cross-reacting with acidic and basic fibroblast growth factors, *EMBO J* 9:2685-2692, 1990.

15. Drake D, Persing JA, Berman DE, et al: Calvarial deformity regeneration following subtotal calvariectomy for craniosynostosis: a case report and theoretical implications, *J Craniofac Surg* 4:85-89, 1993.

16. Dufresne C, Richtsmeier JT: Interaction of craniofacial dysmorphology, growth, and prediction of surgical outcome, *J Craniofac Surg* 6:270-281, 1995.

17. Dunlop LL, Hall BK: Relationships between cellular condensation, preosteoblast formation, and epithelial-mesenchymal interactions in initiation of osteogenesis, *Int J Dev Biol* 39:357-371, 1995.

18. El Ghouzzi V, Lajeunie E, Le Merrer M, et al: TWIST mutations disrupting the b-HLH domain are specific to Saethre-Chotzen syndrome, *Am J Hum Genet* 61(suppl):A332, 1997a.

19. El Ghouzzi V, Le Merrer M, Perrin-Schmitt F, et al: Mutations of the TWIST gene in Saethre-Chotzen syndrome, *Nat Genet* 15:42-46, 1997b.

20. Furtwangler JA, Hall SH, Koskinen-Moffett LK: Sutural morphogenesis in the mouse calvaria: the role of apoptosis, *Acta Anat (Basel)* 124:78-80, 1985.

21. Galvin BD, Hart KC, Meyer AN, et al: Constitutive receptor activation by Crouzon syndrome mutations in fibroblast growth-factor receptor (FGFR)-2 and FGFR2/neu chimeras, *Proc Natl Acad Sci USA* 93:7894-7899, 1996.

22. Globus RK, Patterson-Buckendahl P, Gospodarowicz D: Regulation of bovine bone cell proliferation by fibroblast growth factor and transforming growth factor "b," *Endocrinology* 123:98-105, 1988.

23. Gorry MC, Preston R, White G, et al: Crouzon syndrome: mutations in two spliceoforms of FGFR2 and a common point of mutation shared with Jackson-Weiss syndrome, *Hum Mol Genet* 4:1387-1390, 1995.

24. Gripp K, Stolle C, McDonald-McGinn D, et al: Phenotype of the fibroblast growth factor receptor 2 Ser351Cys mutation: Pfeiffer syndrome type III, *Am J Med Genet* 78:356-360, 1998.

25. Hertz JM, Juncker I, Molhave B, et al: Mutations in the FGFR2-gene in Crouzon syndrome, *Eur J Hum Genet* 5(suppl):155-156, 1997.

26. Hill RE, Jones PF, Rees AR, et al: A new family of mouse homeobox-containing genes: molecular structure chromosomal location, and developmental expression of Hox7.1, *Genes Dev* 3:26-37, 1989.

27. Hollway G, Suthers G, Haan E, et al: Mutation detection in FGFR2 craniosynostosis syndromes, *Hum Genet* 99:251-255, 1997.

28. Howard TD, Paznekas WA, Green ED, et al: Mutations in TWIST, a basic helix-loop-helix transcription factor in Saethre-Chotzen syndrome, *Nat Genet* 15:36-41, 1997.

29. Iseki S, Wilkie AOM, Morriss-Kay GM: Fgfr1 and Fgfr2 have distinct differentiation- and proliferation-related roles in the developing mouse skull vault, *Development* 126:5611-5620, 1999.

30. Iseki S, Wilkie AOM, Heath JK, et al: Fgfr2 and osteopontin domains in the developing skull vault are mutually exclusive and can be altered by locally applied FGF2, *Development* 124:3375-3384, 1997.

31. Jabs EW, Li X, Scott AF, et al: Jackson-Weiss and Crouzon syndromes are allelic with mutations in fibroblast growth factor receptor 2, *Nat Genet* 8:275-279, 1994.

32. Jabs EW, Muller U, Li X, et al: A mutation in the homeodomain of the human MSX2 gene in a family affected with autosomal dominant craniosynostosis, *Cell* 75:443-450, 1993.

33. Johnson D, Horsley S, Moloney D, et al: A comprehensive screen for TWIST mutations in patients with craniosynostosis identifies a new microdeletion syndrome of chromosome band 7p21.1, *Am J Hum Genet* 63:1282-1293, 1998.

34. Jones K: *Smith's recognizable patterns of human malformation,* ed 5, Philadelphia, 1997, WB Saunders.

35. Kim H, Rice DPC, Kettunen PJ, et al: FGF-, BMP- and Shh-mediated signalling pathways in the regulation of cranial suture morphogenesis and calvarial bone development, *Development* 125:1241-1251, 1998.

36. Kokich VG: The biology of sutures. In Cohen MM Jr (ed): *Craniosynostosis: diagnosis, evaluation, and management,* New York, 1986, Raven Press.

37. Krebs I, Weis I, Hudler M, et al: Translocation breakpoint maps to 5 kb 3' from TWIST in a patient affected with Saethre-Chotzen syndrome, *Hum Mol Genet* 6:1079-1086, 1997.

38. Kreiborg S: Postnatal growth and development of the craniofacial complex in premature craniosynostosis. In Cohen MM Jr (ed): *Craniosynostosis: diagnosis, evaluation, and management,* New York, 1986, Raven Press.

39. Kreiborg S: *Crouzon syndrome: a clinical and roentgencephalometric study,* Copenhagen, 1981, The Royal Dental College.

40. Kreiborg S, Pruzansky S: Craniofacial growth in premature craniofacial synostosis, *Scand J Plast Reconstr Surg* 15:171-186, 1981.

41. Lajeunie E, Ma HW, Bonaventure J, et al: FGFR2 mutations in Pfeiffer syndrome, *Nat Genet* 9:108, 1995.

42. Lewanda AF, Cohen MM Jr, Jackson CE, et al: Genetic heterogeneity among craniosynostosis syndromes: mapping the Saethre-Chotzen locus between D7S513 and D7S516 and exclusion of Jackson-Weiss and Crouzon syndrome loci from 7p, *Genomics* 19:115-119, 1994.

43. Lewanda AF, Meyers GA, Jabs EW: Craniosynostosis and skeletal dysplasia: fibroblast growth factor receptor defects, *Proc Assoc Am Physicians* 108:19-24, 1996.

44. Liu YH, Ma L, Wu L-Y, et al: Premature suture closure and ectopic cranial bone in mice expressing Msx2 transgenes in the developing skull, *Proc Natl Acad Sci USA* 92:6137-6141, 1995.

45. Liu Y-H, Tang Z, Kundu RK, et al: *Msx2* gene dosage influences the number of proliferative osteogenic cells in growth centers of the developing murine skull: a possible mechanism for *MSX2*-mediated craniosynostosis in humans, *Dev Biol* 205: 260-274, 1999.

46. Lomri A, Lemonnier J, Hott M, et al: Increased calvaria cell differentiation and bone matrix formation induced by fibroblast growth factor receptor 2 mutations in Apert syndrome, *J Clin Invest* 101:1310-1317, 1998.

47. Ma L, Golden S, Wu L, et al: The molecular basis of Boston-type craniosynostosis: the Pro1486His mutation in the N-terminal arm of the MSX2 homeodomain stabilizes DNA binding without altering nucleotide sequence preferences, *Hum Mol Genet* 5:1915-1920, 1996.

48. Mabbutt LW, Kokich VG: Calvarial and suture development following craniectomy in neonatal rabbit, *J Anat* 129:413-422, 1979.

49. MacKenzie A, Ferguson MWJ, Sharpe PT: Expression patterns of the homeobox gene, Hox8, in the mouse embryo suggest a role in specifying tooth initiation and shape, *Development* 115:403-420, 1992.

50. Marsh JL, Vannier MW: Cranial base changes following surgical treatment of craniosynostosis, *Cleft Palate J* 23:9-18, 1986.

51. Mathijssen I, Vaandrager J, Hoogeboom A, et al: Pfeiffer syndrome resulting from an S351C mutation in the fibroblast growth factor receptor-2 gene, *J Craniofac Surg* 9:207-209, 1998.

52. Mathijssen IMJ, Vaandrager JM, van der Meulen JC, et al: The role of bone centers in the pathogenesis of craniosynostosis: an embryologic approach using CT measurements in isolated craniosynostosis, Apert and Crouzon syndrome, *Plastic Reconst Surg* 98:7-25, 1996.

53. Meyers GA, Day D, Goldberg R, et al: FGFR2 exon IIIa and IIIc mutations in Crouzon, Jackson-Weiss, and Pfeiffer syndromes: evidence for missense changes, insertions, and a deletion due to alternative RNA splicing, *Am J Hum Genet* 58:491-498, 1996.

54. Meyers GA, Orlow SJ, Munro IR, et al: Fibroblast growth factor receptor 3 (FGFR3) transmembrane mutation in Crouzon syndrome with acanthosis nigricans, *Nat Genet* 11: 482-484, 1995.

55. Moloney DM, Wall SA, Ashworth GJ, et al: Prevalence of Pro250Arg mutation of fibroblast growth factor receptor 3 in coronal craniosynostosis, *Lancet* 349:1059-1062, 1997.

56. Moss ML: The pathogenesis of premature cranial synostosis in man, *Acta Anat* 37:351-370, 1959.

57. Muenke M, Francomano C, Cohen M Jr, et al: Fibroblast growth factor receptor related skeletal disorders: craniosynostosis and dwarfism syndromes. In Jameson L (ed): *Principles of molecular medicine,* Totowa, NJ, 1998, Humana Press.

58. Muenke M, Schell U, Hehr A, et al: A common mutation in the fibroblast growth factor receptor 1 gene in Pfeiffer syndrome, *Nat Genet* 8:269-274, 1994.

59. Neilson KM, Friesel RE: Constitutive activation of fibroblast growth factor receptor 2 by a point mutation associated with Crouzon syndrome, *J Biol Chem* 270:26037-26040, 1995.

60. Okajima K, Robinson L, Mart M, et al: Ocular anterior chamber dysgenesis in craniosynostosis syndromes with a fibroblast growth factor receptor 2 mutation, *Am J Hum Genet* 85:160-170, 1999.

61. Oldridge M, Lunt PW, Zackai EH, et al: Genotype-phenotype correlation for nucleotide substitutions in the IgII-IgIII linker of FGFR2, *Hum Mol Genet* 6:137-143, 1997.

62. Oldridge M, Wilkie AOM, Slaney SF, et al: Mutations in the third immunoglobulin domain of the fibroblast growth factor receptor-2 gene in Crouzon syndrome, *Hum Mol Genet* 4:1077-1082, 1995.

63. Oldridge M, Zackai E, McDonald-McGinn D, et al: *De novo Alu* element insertions in FGFR2 identify a distinct pathological basis for Apert syndrome, *Am J Hum Genet* 64:446-461, 1999.

64. Online Mendelian Inheritance in Man, OMIM. Baltimore, Institute of Genetic Medicine, Johns Hopkins University; and Bethesda, Md, National Center for Biotechnology Information, National Library of Medicine, World Wide Web URL: http://www.ncbi.nlm.nih.gov/omim, 1998.

65. Opperman LA, Nolen AA, Ogle RC: TGF-β1, TGF-β2, and TGF-β3 exhibit distinct patterns of expression during cranial suture formation and obliteration in vivo and in vitro, *J Bone Miner Res* 12:301-310, 1997.

66. Opperman LA, Passarelli RW, Morgan EP, et al: Cranial sutures require tissue interactions with dura mater to resist osseous obliteration in vitro, *J Bone Miner Res* 10:1978-1987, 1995.

67. Opperman LA, Sweeney TM, Redmon J, et al: Tissue interactions with underlying dura mater inhibit osseous obliteration of developing cranial sutures, *Dev Dyn* 198:312-322, 1993.

68. Park WJ, Bellus GA, Jabs EW: Mutations in fibroblast growth factor receptors: phenotypic consequences during eukaryotic development, *Am J Hum Genet* 57:748-754, 1995a.

69. Park WJ, Meyers GA, Li X, et al: Novel FGFR2 mutations in Crouzon and Jackson-Weiss syndromes show allelic heterogeneity and phenotypic variability, *Hum Mol Genet* 4:1229-1233, 1995b.

70. Park WJ, Theda C, Maestri NE, et al: Analysis of phenotypic features and FGFR2 mutations in Apert syndrome, *Am J Hum Genet* 57:321-328, 1995c.

71. Passos-Bueno M, Richieri-Costa A, Sertie AL, et al: Presence of the Apert canonical S252W FGFR2 mutation in a patient without severe syndactyly, *J Med Genet* 35:677-679, 1998.

72. Passos-Bueno M, Sertie A, Richieri-Costa A, et al: Description of a new mutation and characterization of FGFR1, FGFR2, and FGFR3 mutations among Brazilian patients with syndromic craniosynostosis, *Am J Med Genet* 78:237-241, 1998.

73. Passos-Bueno MR, Sertie AL, Zatz M, et al: Pfeiffer mutation in an Apert patient: how wide is the spectrum of variability due to mutations in the FGFR2 gene? *Am J Med Genet* 71:243-245, 1997.

74. Paznekas W, Cunningham M, Howard T, et al: Genetic heterogeneity of Saethre-Chotzen syndrome, due to TWIST and FGFR mutations, *Am J Hum Genet* 62:1370-1380, 1998.

75. Przylepa KA, Paznekas W, Zhang M, et al: Fibroblast growth factor receptor 2 mutations in Beare-Stevenson cutis gyrata syndrome, *Nat Genet* 13:492-494, 1996.

76. Pulleyn LJ, Reardon W, Wilkes D, et al: Spectrum of craniosynostosis phenotypes associated with novel mutations at the fibroblast growth factor receptor 2 locus, *Eur J Hum Genet* 4:283-291, 1996.

77. Ray P, Siegel-Bartelt J, Chun K: A unique mutation in TWIST causes Saethre-Chotzen syndrome, *Am J Hum Genet* 61(suppl):A344, 1997.

78. Reardon W, McManus SP, Summers D, et al: Cytogenetic evidence that the Saethre-Chotzen syndrome gene maps to 7p21.2, *Am J Med Genet* 47:633-636, 1993.

79. Reardon W, Winter RM, Rutland P, et al: Mutations in the fibroblast growth factor receptor 2 gene cause Crouzon syndrome, *Nat Genet* 8:98-193, 1994.

80. Reid CS, McMorrow L, McDonald-McGinn D, et al: Saethre-Chotzen syndrome with familial translocation at chromosome 7p22, *Am J Med Genet* 47:637-639, 1993.

81. Richtsmeier JT, Cole TM, Krovitz G, et al: Preoperative morphology and development in sagittal synostosis, *J Craniofac Gen Dev Biol* 18:64-78, 1998.

82. Richtsmeier JT, Fang S, Raghavan R: Volumetric morphing, the study of craniofacial growth and the prediction of surgical outcome. Paper presented at American Cleft-Palate and Craniofacial Association Annual Meeting, Baltimore, 1998.

83. Richtsmeier JT, Grausz HM, Morris GR, et al: Growth of the cranial base in craniosynostosis, *Cleft Palate Craniofac J* 28:55-67, 1991.

84. Richtsmeier JT, Lele S: Analysis of craniofacial growth in Crouzon syndrome using landmark data, *J Craniofac Genet Dev Biol* 10:39-62, 1990.

85. Richtsmeier JT, Marsh JL, Vannier ML: Three-dimensional analysis of craniofacial morphology and growth in craniosynostosis. Paper presented at American Cleft-Palate Craniofacial Association Annual Meeting, Williamsburg, Va, 1988.

86. Rose C, Patel P, Reardon W, et al: The TWIST gene, although not disrupted in Saethre-Chotzen patients with apparently balanced translocations of 7p21, is mutated in familial and sporadic cases, *Hum Mol Genet* 6:1369-1373, 1997.

87. Roth DA, Longaker MT, McCarthy JG, et al: Studies in cranial suture biology: Part I. Increased immunoreactivity for TGF-β isoforms (β1, β2, and β3) during rat cranial suture fusion, *J Bone Miner Res* 12:311-321, 1997.

88. Rutland P, Pulleyn LJ, Reardon W, et al: Identical mutations in the FGFR2 gene cause both Pfeiffer and Crouzon syndrome phenotypes, *Nat Genet* 9:173-176, 1995.

89. Schaefer F, Anderson C, Can B, et al: Novel mutation in the FGFR2 gene at the same codon as the Crouzon syndrome mutations in a severe Pfeiffer syndrome type 2 cases, *Am J Med Genet* 75:252-255, 1998.

90. Schell U, Hehr A, Feldman G, et al: Mutations in FGFR1 and FGFR2 cause familial and sporadic Pfeiffer syndrome, *Hum Mol Genet* 4:323-328, 1995.

91. Semenza GL, Wang GL, Kundu R: DNA binding and transcriptional properties of wild-type and mutant forms of the homeodomain protein MSX2, *Biochem Biophys Res Commun* 209:257-262, 1995.

92. Steinberger D, Collamn H, Schmalenberger B, et al: A novel mutation (a886g) in exon 5 of FGFR2 in members of a family with Crouzon phenotype and plagiocephaly, *J Med Genet* 34:420-422, 1997.

93. Steinberger D, Mulliken J, Muller U: Crouzon syndrome: previously unrecognized deletion, duplication, and point mutation within FGFR2 gene, *Hum Mutat* 8:386-390, 1996a.

94. Steinberger D, Mulliken JB, Muller U: Predisposition for cysteine substitutions in the immunoglobulin-like chain of FGFR2 in Crouzon syndrome, *Hum Genet* 96:113-115, 1995.

95. Steinberger D, Reinhartz T, Unsoeld R, et al: FGFR2 mutation in clinically nonclassifiable autosomal dominant craniosynostosis with pronounced phenotypic variation, *Am J Med Genet* 66:81-86, 1996b.

96. Steinberger D, Vriend G, Mulliken J, et al: The mutations in FGFR2-associated craniosynostosis are clustered in five structural elements of immunoglobin-like domain III of the receptor, *Hum Genet* 102:145-150, 1998.

97. Takahashi Y, Bontoux M, Le Douarin NM: Epithelio-mesenchymal interaction are critical for Quox 7 expression and membrane bone differentiation in the neural crest derived mandibular mesenchyme, *EMBO J* 10:2387-2393, 1991.

98. Tartaglia M, Valeri S, Velardi F, et al: Trp290Cys mutation in exon IIIa of the fibroblast growth factor receptor 2 (FGFR2) gene is associated with Pfeiffer syndrome, *Hum Genet* 99:602-606, 1997.

99. Wilkie AOM: Craniosynostosis: genes and mechanisms, *Hum Mol Genet* 6:1647-1656, 1997.

100. Wilkie AOM, Slaney SF, Oldridge M, et al: Apert syndrome results from localized mutations of FGFR2 and is allelic with Crouzon syndrome, *Nat Genet* 9:165-172, 1995.

101. Williams PL: *Gray's anatomy,* ed 38, New York, 1995, Churchill Livingstone.

102. Winograd J, Reilly MP, Roe R, et al: Perinatal lethality and multiple craniofacial malformations in MSX2 transgenic mice, *Hum Mol Genet* 6:369-379, 1997.

103. Winograd JM, Im MJ, Vander Kolk CA: Enzymatic activation associated with programmed fusion of the posterior interfrontal sutures in rats (submitted).

104. Winograd JM, Im MJ, Vander Kolk CA: Osteoblastic and osteoclastic activation in coronal sutures undergoing fusion *ex vivo, Plast Reconstr Surg* 100:1103-1112, 1997.

Anthropometrics, Cephalometrics, and Orthodontics

43

William M. Davidson

INTRODUCTION

The purpose of this chapter is to provide the reader with a working knowledge of the role orthodontics may play in treatment of patients with craniofacial deformity and the interaction the surgeon should expect with the orthodontist. The diagnosis and treatment plan for a patient with maxillary hypoplasia and mandibular prognathism illustrate the relationships among facial form, dental harmony and function, facial balance, and facial aesthetics. The steps taken in physical assessment of the patient are outlined and include patient assessment, data collection and evaluation, formulation and prediction of results of alternative treatment plans, and evaluation of chosen treatment plans.

INDICATIONS

Orthodontic patients are self-referred or referred by other dentists or patients. The dental problems are usually obvious to the layperson and appear as chief complaints of "crooked teeth," "gaps," "teeth sticking out," etc. Underlying skeletal problems may be described as "top teeth stick out," "chin too small or big," etc., or may not be obvious to the patient.

The patient who will serve as an example of the interrelationships between orthodontics and surgery is a female, 15-year-2-month-old, 5-foot 7-inch Caucasian high school student who was referred by her mother with a chief complaint of "lower teeth sticking out." She presented with a Class III malocclusion with the clinical appearance of both maxillary insufficiency and mandibular prognathism.

Subsequent to completion of a routine medical history, which in her case provided no events relevant to her problem, a dental clinical examination was performed. The lateral profile and dental relationship are shown in Figures 43-1 and 43-2.

OPERATIONS

CLINICAL EVALUATION

A clinical examination can be performed in a few minutes and is supplemented with a more detailed examination of specific problem areas, if necessary. All adult patients are referred to their dentist or periodontist before the start of orthodontics for correction of dental problems. New crowns are generally not placed until after orthognathic surgical treatment is complete, so they may be made to fit the new occlusion. All dental caries and active periodontal disease must be arrested before initiation of orthodontic treatment.

A significant amount of data may be derived during the initial patient visit with a simple yet sophisticated facial form analysis. Although this information must be supplemented with models, radiographs and radiographic quantitation through cephalometric analysis of facial proportions relative to approximated facial reference lines, the facial form analysis has clinical value and often provides important clues to further treatment.

Assessment of lower and upper facial height is demonstrated in Figure 43-3 and illustrates a normal 1-to-1 ratio of upper to lower facial height. Lower facial height may be subdivided into thirds; one third from base of the nose to corner of the mouth, and two thirds from the corner of the mouth to base of the chin.

Further assessment of facial height is seen in Figure 43-4 by measurement of the interlabial gap at rest. This gap should be 1 to 2 mm with the upper lip covering most of the crown of the maxillary central incisor. Exposure of 1 to 3 mm is considered normal and aesthetic. An approximation of the mandibular plane gives an estimate of the direction of facial growth, with a steep plane suggesting vertical and a horizontally oriented plane suggesting a forward direction of growth. The relative protrusion of the upper lip may be estimated by the nasolabial angle, which may be either acute (protrusive) or obtuse (retrusive).

An approximation of anteroposterior relationships of the middle and lower face can be made by establishing

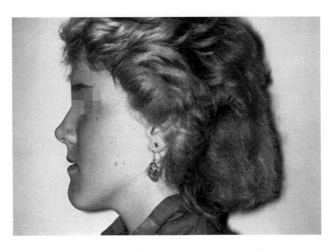

Figure 43-1. Pretreatment lateral profile.

a perpendicular line dropped from the supraorbital ridge in the midline. This can serve as a guide to evaluate the relative protrusion of the maxilla and mandible to each other or to upper facial structures. This is shown in Figure 43-5.

Symmetry of the frontal profile may be evaluated relative to a midline constructed from forehead, tip of nose, center of upper lip, dental midlines, center of lower lip, and midpoint of chin (Figure 43-6). Vertical perpendiculars from the inner and outer canthi of the eyes should divide the face into fifths and may also serve as guides to width of the nose and mouth and interocular distance (Figure 43-7).

There are many more complex measurement systems, but these quickly gathered observed relationships provide a useful beginning to the database that will result in the appropriate diagnosis and treatment plan.

Comprehensive, useful discussions of facial form analyses

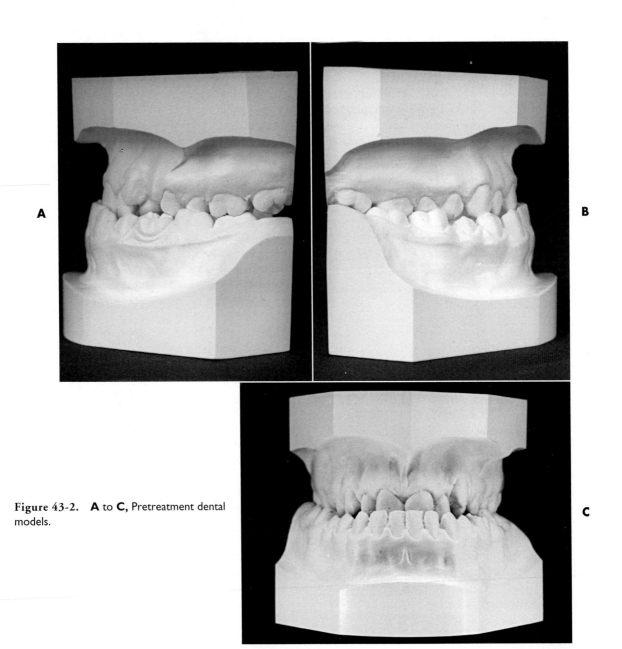

Figure 43-2. **A** to **C,** Pretreatment dental models.

may be found in the Proffit text *Contemporary Orthodontics,* pp. 143-150, and the chapter Soft Tissue Evaluation, by Alexander Jacobson and Christos Vlachros.[21]

The evaluation shown in Figure 43-8 is routinely performed for all patients.

EXPLANATION OF CLINICAL EXAMINATION

The *profile* is assessed as convex, straight, or concave. *Show of maxillary incisors* at rest should be 2 or 3 mm[11] beneath the upper lip. When the patient smiles, most or all of the maxillary incisor teeth crowns should be seen. If more than 2 or 3 mm of upper gum is visible at rest in a patient with deep bite, treatment may require intrusion of maxillary teeth either with orthodontics alone if anterior facial height is acceptable, or with surgery and orthodontics if the maxilla is displaced downward, resulting in increased facial height and lip incompetence. This observation is an important part of treatment planning for assessment and correction of vertical

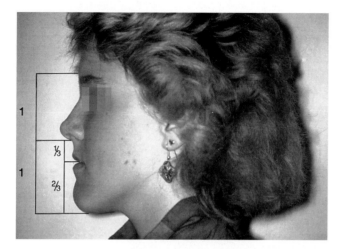

Figure 43-3. Estimation of anterior facial height.

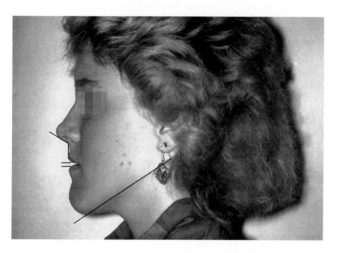

Figure 43-4. Estimation of interlabial gap and direction of facial growth.

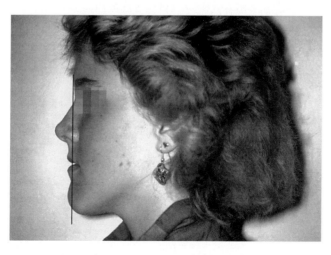

Figure 43-5. Estimation of facial protrusion.

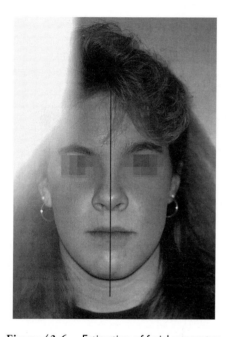

Figure 43-6. Estimation of facial symmetry.

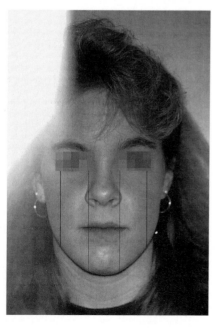

Figure 43-7. Estimation of frontal proportions.

Name _____ Age _15 yr 2 mo_ BD _02/07/70_ Sex _F_ Date _04/05/85_

Address/City/Zip Code _____

Chief Complaint _Lower teeth stick out._

Special Problems _No contributory medical history, no family history of Class 3 malocclusion._

CLINICAL EVALUATION

AESTHETICS/PROFILE		**TRANSVERSE**	_Crossbite anterior and posterior bilateral_
Profile	_Convex_	**ANTERIOR-POSTERIOR**	
Show of teeth	_Within normal limits_	Angle Class:	_RM 3 RC 3 LC 3 LM 3 OJ −3 mm_
Facial Symmetry	_Chin deviates to right 2 mm_	Nas Lab L	_Obtuse_
ALIGNMENT		**VERTICAL**	
Midline	_1 mm discrepancy_	Overbite	_50%_
Max dent/Max	_1 mm to left_	Openbite	
Mand dent/Mand	_No deviation_	Lower facial hgt	_Increased_
Max dent/Mand dent	_1 mm crowding_	Lip comp	_Slight strain on closure_
Maxillary:		Cleft	_None_
Crowding or space	_2 mm crowding_	Repaired	_None_
Arch form	_Constricted_	Procumbance	_Flat_
Symmetry	_Symmetric_	Length	_Adequate_
Mandibular:		Shifts	_No_
Crowding or space	_None—crowding_	Oral Hygiene:	G ☐ F ☒ P ☐
Arch form	_Due to retained primary molar_	TMJ	_No symptoms—normal excursions_
Symmetry	_Arch skewed to left_	Growth potential	_Little growth remaining_
		Habits	_No_
		Caries	_No_
		Roots	_No_
		Supernumerary	_No_
		Speech	_Good_

```
                e d c b a  a b c d e
      R  8 7 6 5 4 3 2 1  1 2 3 4 5 6 7 8  L
         8 7 6 5 4 3 2 1  1 2 3 4 5 6 7 8
                e d c b a  a b c d e
```

Unerupted

CONSULTS REQUIRED

√ Hygiene	__ Restorative
√ Oral Surgery	__ Perio
__ ENT	__ Hearing
√ Plastic	__ Speech
__ Other _____	

RECORDS REQUIRED

√ Study Cast   √ Photo   √ X-rays

CONSULTATION NOTES: Self-referred patient. Nongrowing female with Class 3 malocclusion, appears both maxillary retrusive and mandibular protrusive. _____

PROBLEM LIST	**TREATMENT PLAN**
Class 3 skeletal malocclusion	_Evaluate for 1 or 2 jaw surgery following 1 year ortho_
Midface hypoplasia	_6 months of orthodontics postsurgery_
Long lower face	_3rd molars to be extracted 6 months before surgery_

Est. Fee	**Funding Source**	**Initial**	**/month**	**Retention**
_$3600_	_Parents_	_$700_	_$120/24 mo_	_Hawley retainers_

Figure 43-8. Sample facial form analysis.

dysplasia and other supplements, particularly cephalometric diagnostic data.[11]

Facial and dental symmetry are determined by observation of a line from the center of the forehead through the nose, dental midline, lip midline, and chin midline. _Dental midline deviations_ are recorded and a preliminary judgment is made whether the cause of a midline deviation is dental or skeletal. Dental midline deviations can usually be corrected with orthodontics. Severe discrepancies may require removing teeth to make space for midline correction, or a surgical solution may be required, especially in the nongrowing patient.

Crowding, spacing, dental arch form, and *symmetry* are best evaluated on the dental models, as are crossbite discrepancies (transverse), *Angle's classification* (a dental classification of sagittal occlusal relationships between maxilla and mandible), *overjet, overbite,* and *open bite.* Refined details of tooth position, arch symmetry, and dental arch relationships are best evaluated on models.

The *nasolabial angle,*[5] the angle between the lower border of the nose and the upper lip, is an important aesthetic factor. Lip position is dependent on the position of the maxillary central incisors and has a significant effect on the treatment of malocclusion. An obtuse nasolabial angle may contraindicate retraction of maxillary incisors during an orthodontic treatment plan unless the maxilla were to be advanced surgically.[2]

Lower facial height is affected by orthodontic treatment. Intrusion or extrusion of molars has a significant effect on lower facial height and lip competence. Vertical development of the lower face may be desirable in brachycephalic patients. Dental eruption, except in the extreme brachycephalic patient, is easy to produce during treatment because orthodontic tooth movement tends to extrude teeth unless specific mechanics, often complex, are used to prevent extrusion. Thus dolichocephalic patients require careful planning to avoid dental extrusion and further dolichocephalic development.

Mandibular shifts when the teeth contact are indicative of poor transverse or anteroposterior intercuspation between maxillary and mandibular teeth. Mandibular shifts must be eliminated not only to avoid dental trauma and possible masticatory muscle spasm but also to ensure correct diagnosis of maxillomandibular relationships. The origin of these transverse discrepancies may be either dental or skeletal.

Oral hygiene must be excellent before beginning any orthodontic treatment. Orthodontic appliances may potentiate plaque accumulation, leading to gingivitis, periodontitis, and caries.[14,35] No orthodontic care should be started with poor oral hygiene, and a rigorous hygiene program should be followed during treatment. Dental prophylaxis every 3 months for adults may be necessary to maintain dental health. Fluoride rinses are also recommended to strengthen enamel and for an antimicrobial effect.[4]

Temporomandibular function must be normal. Mouth opening is measured from the edge of the maxillary incisor to the incisal edge of the mandibular incisor in the midline. Wide opening should be ±52 mm. Lateral excursions, right and left, should be 12 mm and protrusive excursion 10 mm in brachycephalic patients. Excursions of the jaws in patients with mesocephalic facial form are 43, 10, and 8 mm. Excursions in dolichocephalic patients are 42, 8, and 6 mm, respectively.[15] Occasional jaw clicking is not of concern, but locking or pain in the temporomandibular joint or masticatory muscles requires more detailed examination or referral. It is usual orthodontic practice to defer orthodontic treatment until temporomandibular joint symptoms have subsided. Because poor dental occlusion may cause functional maxilla-mandible malrelationships with resultant masticatory muscle spasm, an occlusal splint may be required to establish normal jaw

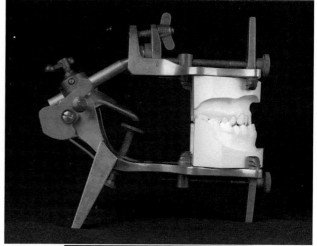

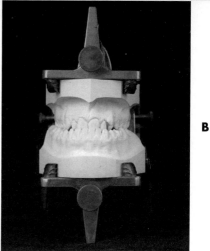

Figure 43-9. A and **B,** Pretreatment models mounted in plasterless articulator.

relationships before orthodontic or surgical treatment. Successful treatment is dependent on an accurate diagnosis made with the mandibular condyles in this normal position in the glenoid fossa. Records taken in an eccentric, abnormal position dictated by a poor occlusion may result in a faulty diagnosis and treatment plan.

Study models (Figs. 43-2, 43-9, 43-10, and 43-20) are prepared from alginate impressions of maxillary and mandibular dental arches. An interocclusal record is made by having the patient bite on a heat-softened wax wafer. It is recommended that the impressions be disinfected, kept moist, and sent as soon as possible to a commercial orthodontic laboratory for fabrication of quality study models. Alternatively, it is recommended that models be obtained from the patient's orthodontist.

Quality study models are necessary to analyze the occlusion and to evaluate details that may not be seen easily in the patient's mouth during the clinical examination. Normal occlusion[1] is described in all orthodontic texts and is demonstrated on models of this patient at the completion of her orthognathic surgical treatment (see Figure 43-20). The important relationships to note are 10% to 20% overbite, no crossbites, rotations corrected, good dental interdigitation, and minimal overjet. Models are also useful to simulate surgery[32] and to identify orthodontic corrections that must be accomplished before surgery in order that the teeth have the best possible ideal fit when surgery is performed. Ideal fit at this stage in treatment creates the most secure interdigitation between maxillary and mandibular teeth, thus the most reliable indexing for the surgeon as he or she locates the jaws relative to each using teeth as a guide. The orthodontist is expected to remove malocclusion in each dental arch and coordinate arch shape and size to allow excellent interdigitation between the maxillary and mandibular dental arches when the jaws are moved to their corrected positions.

Models may be sectioned if segmental surgery is anticipated and are mounted in an articulator (see Figures 43-9 and 43-10) to allow trial manipulations.[10] As can be seen in Figure 43-10, when sagittal relationships are corrected in this patient, expansion of the maxillary dental arch is needed to provide correct transverse dental relationships. Figures 43-3 and 43-4 show models mounted in a simple plasterless articulator. More complex mounting, a facebow transfer, and more complex articulators* may be necessary, especially if multijaw surgery is anticipated. Communication between surgeon and orthodontist is essential to decide what movements are possible dentally and which are best addressed surgically.

CEPHALOMETRIC EVALUATION

Cephalometric analysis aids in diagnosis by highlighting significant skeletal and dental deviations from normal values. Cephalometrics provides a method not only for identification of problems but also for formulation of a problem list, development of treatment plan, prediction of outcome, and prognosis of stability. This chapter presents a brief description of cephalometric principles. For a more comprehensive reference, two recent texts[3,16] or relevant sections in a contemporary orthodontic textbook[31] are recommended.

CEPHALOMETRIC TECHNIQUE

Just as it is necessary to establish a stable, reproducible reference position for the mandibular condyles in the glenoid fossa to assess the occlusion, it is necessary to orient the patient's head in a standardized position when taking clinical photographs or aligning the patient in the cephalometer. The patient's head is placed in a holder (cephalostat), the midsagittal plane of which is 60 inches from the anode of the x-ray source. A tightly collimated x-ray beam passes through the head and exposes the intensifying screen-equipped film cassette, which is fixed at a standard distance from the center of the fixation. All cephalometric machines in common

*Great Lakes Orthodontics, LTD, 199 Fire Tower Drive, Tonawanda NY 14150; and WhipMix Corporation, 361 Farmington Ave., Louisville KY 40217.

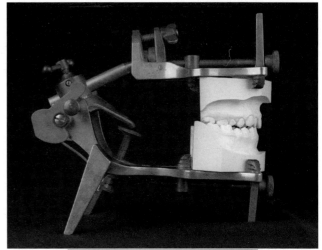

A

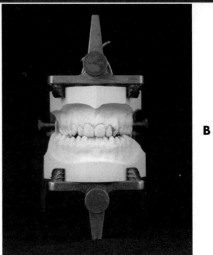

B

Figure 43-10. **A** and **B,** Models repositioned to correct buccal interdigitation.

orthodontic use feature a 60-inch x-ray tube anode to midline of fixator distance. The distance from the fixator to the film can be varied by the operator but should be set at a standard distance so that x-ray magnification is the same from patient to patient and from film to film. Standardization of tube, subject, and film distance allows for superimposition of serial films, sharing data with other clinicians, monitoring growth, and analyzing treatment results without fear of unknown magnification errors.

Typically, the patient's head is oriented by ear rods in the outer ear canal and by an orbital indicator, which provides a reproducible position of the head. This method may be neither possible nor accurate in patients presenting with aberrant positions and size of ear canals, absent ear canals, or marked skeletal asymmetries. In these instances, the operator should align one ear rod with the most normal ear canal, providing the patient with a tactile sense of position, and then place the patient in "natural head position." Natural head position,[34] in which the subject looks into his or her eyes in a mirror set several feet away, has been found to be highly reproducible[8,9] and should be used rather than the orbital pointer fitted to the

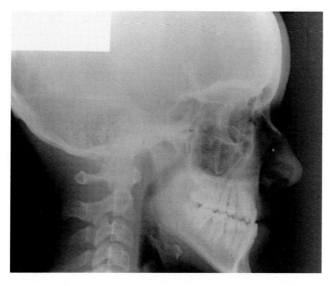

Figure 43-11. Pretreatment cephalometric radiograph.

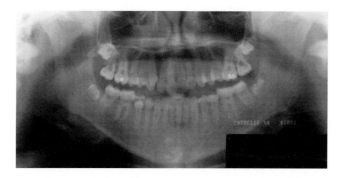

Figure 43-12. Pretreatment panoramic radiograph.

Measurement	Value		Mean	Diff	SD	
N – A – Pg	− 8.7	deg	(2.6)	−11.3	5.1	**
N – A (FH)	− 3.5	mm	(−2.0)	−1.5	3.7	
N – B (FH)	− 1.3	mm	(−6.9)	5.6	4.3	*
N – Pg (FH)	2.3	mm	(−6.5)	8.8	5.1	*
N – ANS (PFH)	56.7	mm	(50.0)	6.7	2.4	**
ANS – Gn (PFH)	72.0	mm	(61.3)	10.7	3.3	***
Face Ht Ratio	78.7	%	(81.0)	−2.3	6.0	
MP to HP	30.7	deg	(24.2)	6.5	5.0	*
U1 tip to NF	29.8	mm	(27.5)	2.3	1.7	*
L1 tip to MP	40.4	mm	(40.8)	−0.4	1.8	
U6 tip to NF	24.0	mm	(23.0)	1.0	1.3	
L6 tip to MP	32.0	mm	(32.1)	−0.1	1.9	
Wits: A – B (OP)	−11.9	mm	(−0.4)	−11.5	2.5	***
U1 to NF	105.9	deg	(112.5)	−6.6	5.3	*
L1 to MP	75.9	deg	(95.9)	−20.0	5.7	***

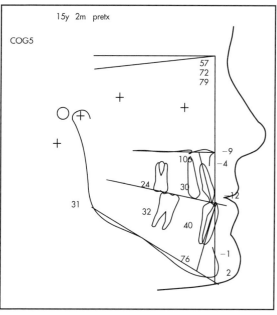

Figure 43-13. COGS analysis—pretreatment cephalometric film.

headholder. This method provides a postural position that leads to a good diagnosis of profile type, with neither the chin pushed up, appearing prognathic, nor tipped down into the neck, appearing retrognathic, nonrotated, or tipped resulting from asymmetry. The patient's lips are relaxed to allow radiographic assessment of interlabial gap and lip-tooth relationship. Frontal films (posteroanterior [PA]) are usually obtained, especially if a transverse problem exists. Once films are obtained (see Figure 43-5), cephalometric analysis allows quantitation of the size and position of cranial, facial, and dental structures. Many analyses are available.[3,10] All identify hard tissue relationships, and some identify soft tissue landmarks. Some analyses[17,19,22,23] simply use a template placed over the film to provide a "normal cephalometric tracing" with which the patient's film or tracing of the film can be compared. Cephalometric radiographs, lateral (Figure 43-11) and frontal (not shown here), are accompanied by panoramic films (Figure 43-12), which allow good visualization of interosseous dental anatomy. Panoramic films must be considered survey films because they will not reveal the details of subtle carious or periodontal lesions. They are useful in

establishing the position and development of unerupted teeth. Identify osseous lesions in the jaws. Suspected joint pathology may require more sophisticated imaging, usually laminography, bone scan, or MRI.[7]

The primary cephalometric analyses that are demonstrated for patients requiring orthognathic surgery are the Cephalometrics for Orthognathic Surgery (COGS) analysis[6] and Legan analysis.[29] The tables included in Figures 43-13 to 43-18 show the patient's measurements in the first column, normal (mean) measurement in the second column, difference between patient and normal standard in the third column, standard deviation of the normal values in the fourth column, and number of standard deviations of the patient's value from the normal standard in the fifth column. I may supplement these analyses with the McNamara[25,33] or Jarabak analysis.[21,26] The COGS analysis is shown (see Figures 43-13, 43-15, and 43-17) in tabular and graphic form on a computer-generated pretreatment tracing of the digitized pretreatment cephalomet-

Measurement	Value	Mean	Diff	SD	
G – Sn – Pg'	2.8 deg	(12.0)	−9.2	4.0	**
Sn – G (FH)	4.2 mm	(6.0)	−1.8	3.0	
Pg' – G (FH)	4.6 mm	(0.0)	4.6	4.0	*
G – Sn (PFH)	76.7 mm	(70.7)	6.0	3.5	*
Sn – Me' (PFH)	73.7 mm	(69.7)	4.0	3.3	*
G – Sn/Sn – Me'	104.1 %	(102.0)	2.1	8.0	
Chin – Throat Ang	84.4 deg	(100.0)	−15.6	7.0	**
Nasolabial	115.2 deg	(102.0)	13.2	8.0	*
UL to Sn – Pg'	−0.9 mm	(3.0)	−3.9	1.0	***
LL to Sn – Pg'	−1.2 mm	(2.0)	−3.2	1.0	***
Mentolabial Sul	5.2 mm	(4.0)	1.2	2.0	
Upper 1 Expos	3.2 mm	(2.0)	1.2	2.0	
Interlabial Gap	0.0 mm	(2.0)	−2.0	2.0	*

Measurement	Value	Mean	Diff	SD	
N – A – Pg	−8.7 deg	(2.6)	−11.3	5.1	**
N – A (FH)	−3.5 mm	(−2.0)	−1.5	3.7	
N – B (FH)	−1.3 mm	(−6.9)	5.6	4.3	*
N – Pg (FH)	2.3 mm	(−6.5)	8.8	5.1	*
N – ANS (PFH)	56.7 mm	(50.0)	6.7	2.4	**
ANS – Gn (PFH)	72.0 mm	(61.3)	10.7	3.3	***
Face Ht Ratio	78.7 %	(81.0)	−2.3	6.0	
MP to HP	30.7 deg	(24.2)	6.5	5.0	*
U1 tip to NF	29.8 mm	(27.5)	2.3	1.7	*
L1 tip to MP	38.8 mm	(40.8)	−2.0	1.8	*
U6 tip to NF	24.9 mm	(23.0)	1.9	1.3	*
L6 tip to MP	32.0 mm	(32.1)	−0.1	1.9	
Wits: A – B (OP)	−11.9 mm	(−0.4)	−11.5	2.5	***
U1 to NF	105.9 deg	(112.5)	−6.6	5.3	*
L1 to MP	64.5 deg	(95.9)	−31.4	5.7	***

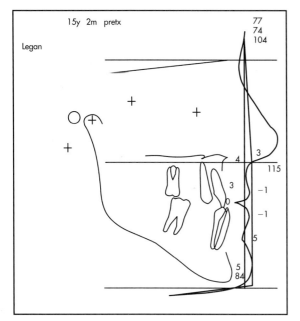

Figure 43-14. Legan soft tissue analysis—pretreatment cephalometric film.

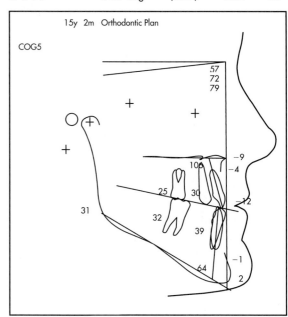

Figure 43-15. COGS analysis—orthodontic plan: no surgery.

ric film. Facial convexity and relationship of anterior projection of maxilla, mandible, and chin button to facial plane are measured. Upper and lower anterior facial height is measured, followed by a useful measurement of vertical dental development of both molars and incisors (palatal plane to occlusal plane and mandibular plane to occlusal plane). The sagittal relationships of maxilla and mandible are measured with the Wits analysis,[18,20] which is included in the COGS analysis. Angulation of maxillary and mandibular incisors are measured, providing an assessment of dental protrusion and procumbance. The COGS analysis was developed specifically for orthognathic surgery. Its reference line (SN) is corrected to a horizontal reference plane, and most measurements are in millimeters. The COGS analysis is an easy-to-use tool that provides surgically relevant direct measurements in a clinically useful context and is complemented by the Legan soft tissue analysis (see Figures 43-14, 43-16, and 43-18), which provides analogous soft tissue relationships quantifying mid and lower

face projection, lip position, interlabial gap, and chin-throat angle. These two analyses work well as a package and provide a comprehensive evaluation of hard and soft tissue relationships.

The McNamara analysis[25] is less complex but provides an estimate of the length of the mandible and maxilla measured from the condyle and assesses the relative relationship between these bones. This may be useful in some patients with whom a posterior rather than anterior reference point for mandibulomaxillary relationships is preferred. The Jarabak analysis[21] is also useful, providing direct measurements of anterior and posterior facial height and direct measurements of length of ramus and body of the mandible.

COMPUTERIZED DATA COLLECTION

Although these data can be collected by manually tracing and measuring films and predictions made by cutting out

Measurement	Value		Mean	Diff	SD	
G – Sn – Pg'	2.6	deg	(12.0)	–9.4	4.0	**
Sn – G (FH)	4.1	mm	(6.0)	–1.9	3.0	
Pg' – G (FH)	4.6	mm	(0.0)	4.6	4.0	*
G – Sn (PFH)	76.8	mm	(70.7)	6.1	3.5	*
Sn – Me' (PFH)	73.6	mm	(69.7)	3.9	3.3	*
G – Sn/Sn – Me'	104.3	%	(102.0)	2.3	8.0	
Chin – Throat Ang	84.5	deg	(100.0)	–15.5	7.0	**
Nasolabial	116.5	deg	(102.0)	14.5	8.0	*
UL to Sn – Pg'	–1.2	mm	(3.0)	–4.2	1.0	***
LL to Sn – Pg'	–2.6	mm	(2.0)	–4.6	1.0	***
Mentolabial Sul	4.4	mm	(4.0)	0.4	2.0	
Upper 1 Expos	3.3	mm	(2.0)	1.3	2.0	
Interlabial Gap	0.7	mm	(2.0)	–1.3	2.0	

Measurement	Value		Mean	Diff	SD	
N – A – Pg	5.0	deg	(2.6)	2.4	5.1	
N – A (FH)	1.8	mm	(–2.0)	3.8	3.7	*
N – B (FH)	–1.3	mm	(–6.9)	5.6	4.3	*
N – Pg (FH)	–1.5	mm	(–6.5)	5.0	5.1	
N – ANS (PFH)	58.2	mm	(50.0)	8.2	2.4	***
ANS – Gn (PFH)	68.2	mm	(61.3)	6.9	3.3	**
Face Ht Ratio	85.3	%	(81.0)	4.3	6.0	
MP to HP	30.6	deg	(24.2)	6.4	5.0	*
U1 tip to NF	29.8	mm	(27.5)	2.3	1.7	*
L1 tip to MP	40.4	mm	(40.8)	–0.4	1.8	
U6 tip to NF	24.0	mm	(23.0)	1.0	1.3	
L6 tip to MP	32.0	mm	(32.1)	–0.1	1.9	
Wits: A – B (OP)	–6.5	mm	(–0.4)	–6.1	2.5	**
U1 to NF	105.9	deg	(112.5)	–6.6	5.3	*
L1 to MP	76.0	deg	(95.9)	–19.9	5.7	***

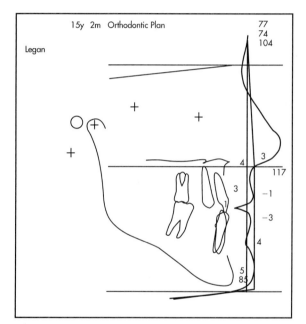

Figure 43-16. Legan analysis—orthodontic treatment: no surgery.

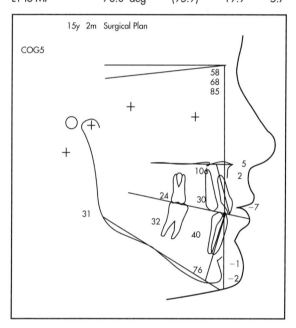

Figure 43-17. Orthodontics/orthognathic surgery. Le Fort I, genioplasty.

templates, it is recommended that a computerized method be used.[13] Having ready access to a number of analyses and ability to move dental and facial structures at will with built-in soft tissue adjustments is mandatory for a complete understanding of options in analysis or treatment. The leading systems are either Macintosh-or PC-based. These data were developed using Dentofacial Planner* PC-based software. Current versions provide a more elaborate display of output, better interface with word processing programs, and integrated video imaging and morphing. Integrated dental, skeletal, and facial morphing is possible without the investment in computerized cephalometrics, but data collection and presentation will be severely limited.

INTERPRETATION OF PRETREATMENT CEPHALOMETRIC FILMS

The patient presents with a concave profile (N-A-Pg) with retrusive maxilla and protrusive mandible. Both upper and lower facial height are increased. The mandibular plane is steep, and there is a significant Class III relationship (Wits) between maxilla and mandible. The mandibular incisor is tipped lingually, a characteristic of Class III malocclusions.

In summary, the COGS analysis demonstrates that the patient has a Class III malocclusion contributed to by both a retropositioned, or small, maxilla and a prognathic mandible. The McNamara analysis provides similar results, and the Jarabak analysis confirms these observations and shows an obtuse gonial angle and long body of the mandible. This is consistent with increased lower facial height, as in an increased S-Me.

---

*Dentofacial Software, Inc., 100 Simcoe Street, Suite 303, Toronto, Ontario, Canada M5H 3G2.

Measurement	Value		Mean	Diff	SD	
G – Sn – Pg'	8.7	deg	(12.0)	−3.3	4.0	
Sn – G (FH)	5.8	mm	(6.0)	−0.2	3.0	
Pg' – G (FH)	1.2	mm	(0.0)	1.2	4.0	
G – Sn (PFH)	76.7	mm	(70.7)	6.0	3.5	*
Sn – Me' (PFH)	71.4	mm	(69.7)	1.7	3.3	
G – Sn/Sn – Me'	107.4	%	(102.0)	5.4	8.0	
Chin – Throat Ang	75.4	deg	(100.0)	−24.6	7.0	***
Nasolabial	107.5	deg	(102.0)	5.5	8.0	
UL to Sn – Pg'	2.9	mm	(3.0)	−0.1	1.0	
LL to Sn – Pg'	1.6	mm	(2.0)	−0.4	1.0	
Mentolabial Sul	7.5	mm	(4.0)	3.5	2.0	*
Upper 1 Expos	4.5	mm	(2.0)	2.5	2.0	*
Interlabial Gap	0.0	mm	(2.0)	−2.0	2.0	*

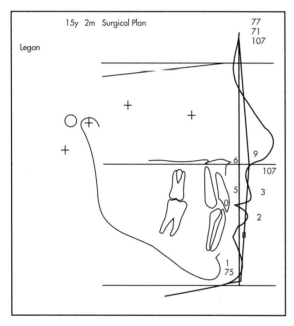

Figure 43-18. Orthodontics/orthognathic surgery. Le Fort I, genioplasty.

The Legan soft tissue analysis shows an obtuse nasolabial angle and retrusive upper lip. The lower lip is also retrusive.

OUTCOMES

A variety of treatment options may be explored and demonstrated using computerized cephalometrics. These may be presented to and discussed with the patient, who may then choose the program suitable to his or her needs from a good information base. Choice of treatment plan may depend on economic, aesthetic, and clinical criteria and estimates of risk/reward.

TREATMENT OPTIONS

No Treatment

No treatment is a viable option. This patient has a pleasant appearance and good self-image. However, the patient is dissatisfied with his or her appearance and seeks care with facial and dental aesthetic concerns as the chief complaints. The patient is asymptomatic, and there are no well-documented health reasons to correct his or her malocclusion, although it is generally assumed that a functional occlusion will result in healthier dental supporting tissues and better muscular balance.

Orthodontics with No Surgery

Orthodontic treatment without surgery may be considered. In cases in which surgery is refused or if the skeleton shows reasonable balance, treatment with orthodontics alone may be the only option available or acceptable to the patient because of finances, fear, or other reasons. A simulated example of treatment of this Class III patient with orthodontics is shown in Figures 43-15 and 43-16. If teeth are moved without orthognathic surgery, it is possible to effect modest profile changes. Protracting the maxillary dentition by tooth movement will provide support to the upper lip. Skeletal malocclusions often exhibit dental compensation to skeletal imbalance. In the Class III patient, this is usually manifest by maxillary incisors proclined labially and mandibular anterior teeth retroclined to the lingual. Orthodontic treatment of skeletal imbalance when surgery is unobtainable accentuates dental compensation. In a Class III patient, this results in accentuating the preexisting labial proclination of maxillary incisors and lingual inclination of mandibular incisors. In the Class II patient, it might mean retracting maxillary incisors to correspond to a retruded mandible or flaring mandibular incisors to reduce the overjet caused by maxillary protrusion. Thus an orthodontic treatment without surgery attempts to camouflage the underlying skeletal defect. Sometimes this is acceptable,[30] sometimes it is not. Small skeletal imbalances with minor preexisting dental compensations may be masked in this way. Results of this compromise are usually unacceptable if a severe skeletal imbalance exists. Patients may be pleased because dental aspects of their appearance may appear greatly improved, but the profile may not be improved and may even be made worse. This is a common sequela when a patient with a Class II malocclusion with deficient mandible has maxillary first bicuspids extracted and maxillary anterior teeth retracted to meet the deficient mandible. This treatment leads to a less aesthetic nasolabial angle than existed before treatment.[24] Conversely, a patient with maxillary protrusion may be greatly improved by the same orthodontic treatment that was contraindicated when the mandible is retrusive. Because many patients present with relatively minor skeletal deformities of both jaws rather than severe deformities of one jaw, orthodontic treatment alone may give acceptable, if not ideal, results. If severe skeletal imbalance is present, increased dental compensation in an orthodontic or nonsurgical treatment plan may provide not only poor dental and facial aesthetics but also decreased periodontal support and stability.

Surgery with No Orthodontics

Surgery without orthodontic alignment may be desirable in some patients. In this patient, surgery would provide the skeletal cephalometric values seen in Figures 43-17 and 43-18 and the dental results shown in Figure 43-10 in which pretreatment study models are articulated and moved into Class I buccal alignment. Because this patient does not have deep overbite or other dental interferences, it would be possible to protract the maxilla or retract the mandible with surgery to a position providing good facial balance without changing the vertical dimension. Good dental relationships would not be obtained. Many patients have dental relationships that would prevent surgical correction unless orthodontics were done before surgery. This is almost always the desirable sequence of treatment, although the reverse is sometimes indicated when a patient may present with jaws so far out of alignment that dental relationship correction is impossible unless preceded by surgery.

Combined Orthodontic-Orthognathic Surgical Treatment

This approach addresses dental, skeletal, and soft tissue problems. The orthodontist has specific responsibility for adjusting arch form and width and for alignment of the teeth within each dental arch so that all teeth are supported optimally by periodontal structures. Before initiation of any treatment, a mutually agreed upon comprehensive plan is necessary.[12] Prediction tracings and model analyses must be completed, and both the orthodontist and surgeon must agree on the surgeries that will be performed. The orthodontics treatment necessary in the presurgical phase of treatment depends on the surgical plan. For example, if vertical osteotomies are necessary, tooth roots must be moved away from the osteotomy sites to avoid surgical injury to the teeth. If the mandible of a brachycephalic patient is advanced, deep incisor overbite is usually corrected postsurgically by bicuspid extrusion. In contrast, a dolichocephalic patient usually requires deep overbite correction before surgery by orthodontic intrusion of anterior teeth. If maxillary dental expansion is indicated, as is often the case, a choice must be made between buccal tipping of the posterior teeth with orthodontic appliances or uprighting them over basal bone with subsequent surgical expansion or surgically assisted rapid palatal expansion.

This patient presented with a mildly retruded maxilla, normal show of teeth, mildly prognathic mandible, large chin button, and increased vertical facial height. The Dentofacial Planner cephalometric analysis program allowed these problems to be simulated and quantitated and tooth movement and trial surgeries to be performed on the computer (see Figures 43-17 and 43-18). Dental models were articulated and analyzed for optimum interdigitation when corrected to proper anteroposterior orientation. It was evident that correction of dental malposition was indicated and that maxillary dental expansion would be necessary to accommodate the

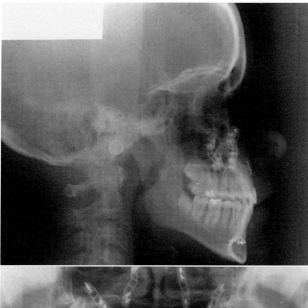

A

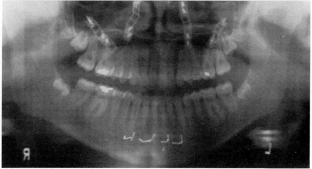

B

Figure 43-19. A and **B,** Posttreatment radiographs.

anticipated position of the mandible when the dentition was corrected to an ideal dental relationship.

The following possible treatment plans were considered:
1. Le Fort I osteotomy of maxilla with anterior movement to Class I dental occlusion
2. Bilateral sagittal split osteotomy with setback of mandible to Class I occlusion
3. Le Fort I osteotomy with reduction genioplasty

After careful explanation to the patient so that she would understand all benefits and risks, maxillary advancement was chosen rather than mandibular setback to provide improved aesthetics. Setback of the mandible would have resulted in poor chin-throat angle and retained the appearance of midface insufficiency. Maxillary advancement would result in improved nasolabial angle and midface fullness. The patient's increased lower facial vertical dimension was corrected with reduction genioplasty, which also reduced chin prominence while retaining good lip competence and dental display (see Figure 43-14). Although impaction of the maxilla during Le Fort osteotomy is a common way of reducing excess lower facial height, it reduces show of the maxillary anterior teeth and interlabial gap. Those effects may be desirable in many dolichocephalic patients with excessive gingival display but were not desirable for this patient.

The outcome was good. Posttreatment radiographs are shown in Figure 43-19. Good occlusion and facial balance are evident (Figures 43-20 and 43-21). The mother noted

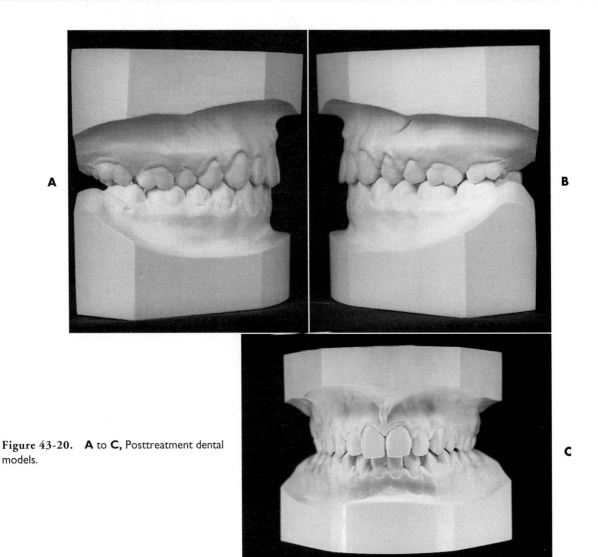

Figure 43-20. **A** to **C,** Posttreatment dental models.

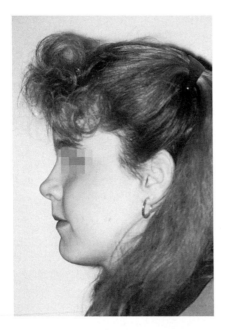

Figure 43-21. Posttreatment lateral profile.

broadening of the alar base of the nose secondary to the maxillary advancement. This might have been prevented with a tighter alar cinch.

SUMMARY

Cephalometrics, anthropometry, model analysis, and artistic perception provide the basis for good outcomes in orthognathic surgical cases. Use of computerized cephalometrics provides for trial manipulations to aid in treatment planning. Joint diagnosis and treatment planning and frequent consultation will result in the most consistent outcomes. The orthodontist must align the dentition optimally within each arch and set the stage for surgery to provide the best possible interarch occlusion. Subsequent to surgery, orthodontic details are completed, resulting in a well-finished case with excellent function and aesthetics.

ROTOCOL FOR ORTHODONTICS FOR THE PATIENT WITH CLEFT LIP AND PALATE

Cleft palate presents a unique challenge to orthodontists. Treatment may begin shortly after birth and be completed in the late teens or even the early twenties. Thus it is necessary to ration care so as to perform efficiently only the care absolutely necessary at the time it is needed.

Care may start with presurgical orthopedics to facilitate lip closure and alveolar alignment when the patient is a few days old.[28,38] A discussion of retraction devices to reduce procumbent premaxillas[16,31] and molding plates[28] to guide dental arch form are not further addressed in this chapter except to note that long-term results from use of these devices remains controversial.[39]

Dental development is usually slower than normal[6,7,36] and in the primary dentition is usually characterized by relatively normal arch form and tooth eruption sequence. It is important to recognize that the cleft deformity is superimposed on the underlying genetically predetermined and environmentally modified occlusion the child would have had if a cleft had not occurred. Teeth in the maxillary arch will always be affected by alveolar clefting but may not be affected if the alveolus (dental arch) is not involved. Maxillary molar width is often normal, but segment rotation medially in the cuspid region usually results in crossbite on the cleft side. The severity of crossbite is greater with larger clefts and heavily scarred repairs. Bilateral clefts will often present with bilateral posterior crossbites.

Anterior crossbite may also be present in the primary dentition and, if the dental overlap is severe, will require orthodontic correction. Posterior crossbites in the primary dentition do not seem to cause significant problems. We usually choose to correct posterior crossbites in the late mixed dentition by dental arch expansion before alveolar bone grafting. Severe anterior crossbites may have the potential to restrict mandibular growth and encourage anterior positioning of the mandible. Anterior crossbites should be corrected by orthodontics if poor aesthetics or interference with function is observed.

Maxillary lateral incisors are often missing on the side of the cleft. When present, they may be in normal or abnormal positions and are often found located in the palatal cleft. Teeth in the cleft are not extracted in the child patient before definitive orthodontic treatment unless they are causing problems (irritation or caries). Extraction results in alveolar shrinkage at the site and may contribute to a palatal fistula. It is important to remember that orthodontics corrections done at this time will probably require orthodontic retainers and add significantly to the number of patient visits and demands on patient and parent. Because much orthodontic care will be needed later, treatment at this age should be avoided unless absolutely necessary.

Orthodontic care is always needed in the mixed dentition during the eruption of permanent teeth. Because most children with cleft palate have delayed dental eruption,[6,7,36] it is necessary to evaluate dental eruption and set treatment intervals by the patient's individual biologic age rather than by reliance on chronologic age. Maxillary central incisors are usually severely rotated, especially adjacent to the cleft. Assessment of aesthetic and functional liability is required, and orthodontic correction of severe rotations may be performed if adequate bone is present adjacent to the cleft. Anterior crossbites may be present at this time and mandate correction to minimize potentially negative effects on growth and jaw position.

Eruption must be monitored on radiographs. Supernumerary teeth are removed if they have no future use. The development of the root of the permanent cuspid tooth is evaluated. Palatal expansion is performed with an orthodontic appliance when the root is one-half to two-thirds formed[5,13] before eruption of that tooth and the alveolar bone graft is placed by the surgeon in the void between major and minor segments.[40] Eruption of the cuspid tooth through the graft results in formation of normal periodontal structures and an intact bony alveolus. An orthodontic retainer is necessary to maintain the corrected arch width.

Definitive orthodontic treatment is completed in the permanent dentition. The lateral incisor on the cleft side is often absent and is replaced either by a prosthetic tooth or during orthodontic treatment by moving other teeth into that position. As the patient grows during puberty, maxillary retrusion may become evident and require orthognathic correction when facial growth is complete.

Orthodontic treatment of the cleft palate patient has an excellent prognosis. A synopsis of orthodontic treatment planning for cleft lip and palate patients is discussed by Proffit[37] (pp. 256-262). Treatment requires careful assessment of objectives at each stage of dental development. The goals of treatment should be to enable normal function of mastication, growth, and speech. Because treatment may be needed at a number of stages of development, one must be conservative and treat only what is absolutely necessary at that time to avoid the negative sequelae of excessively prolonged orthodontic care.

REFERENCES

1. Andrews LF: The six keys to normal occlusion, *Am J Orthod* 62:296-309, 1972.
2. Arnett GW, Bergman R: Facial keys to orthodontic diagnosis and treatment planning, Part II, *Am J Orthod* 103:395-411, 1993.
3. Athanasiou A: *Orthodontic cephalometry,* St Louis, 1995, Mosby.
4. Bader RL: Two-year longitudinal study of a peroxide-fluoride rinse on decalcification in adolescent orthodontic patients, *J Clin Dent* 3:83-87, 1992.
5. Bergland O, Semb G, Abyholm F: Elimination of the residual alveolar cleft by secondary bone grafting and subsequent orthodontic treatment, *Cleft Palate J* 23:175-205, 1986.

6. Bohn A: *Dental anomalies in harelip and cleft palate,* Oslo, 1963, Universitets-forloget, Scandinavian University Books.
7. Brouwers HJ, Kuijpers-Jagtman AM: Development of permanent tooth length in patients with unilateral cleft lip and palate, *Am J Orthod* 99:543-549, 1991.
8. Brown JB, McDowell F: *Plastic surgery of the nose,* St Louis, 1951, Mosby.
9. Burstone CJ, James RB, Legan H, et al: Cephalometrics for orthognathic surgery, *J Oral Surg* 36:269-277, 1978.
10. Christiansen EL, Thompson JR: *Temporomandibular joint imaging,* St Louis, 1990, Mosby.
11. Cooke MS: Five year reproducibility of natural head posture: a methodological study, *Am J Orthod Dentofacial Orthop* 97:489-494, 1990.
12. Cooke MS, Wei SHY: The reproducibility of natural head posture: a methodological study, *Am J Orthod Dentofacial Orthop* 93:280-288, 1988.
13. El Deeb M, Messer LB, Lehnert MW, et al: Canine eruption into grafted bone in maxillary cleft defects, *Cleft Palate J* 19:9-16, 1982.
14. Epker BN, Fish LC: Integrated orthodontic and surgical correction. In *Dentofacial deformities,* St Louis, 1986, Mosby.
15. Fields HW, Proffit WR, Nixon WL, et al: Facial pattern differences in long faced children and adults, *Am J Orthod* 85:217-223, 1984.
16. Figueroa AA, Reisberg DJ, Polley JW, et al: Intraoral-appliance modification to retract the premaxilla in patients with bilateral cleft lip, *Cleft Palate J* 33:497-500, 1996.
17. Fridrich KL, Tompach PC, Wheeler JJ, et al: Coordination of the orthosurgical treatment program, *Int J Adult Orthod Orthognath Surg* 9:195-199, 1994.
18. Gorelick L, Geiger A, Gwinnert AJ: Incidence of white spot formation after banding and bonding, *Am J Orthod* 81:93-98, 1981.
19. Graber TM, Vanarsdall RL: *Orthodontics: current principles and techniques,* St Louis, 1994, Mosby.
20. Grummons D: *Orthodontics for the TMJ-TMD patient,* Scottsdale, Ariz, 1994, Wright and Co.
21. Jacobson A: *Radiographic cephalometry, from basics to videoimaging,* Chicago, 1995, Quintessence Publishing.
22. Jacobson A: Orthognathic diagnosis using the proportional template, *Oral Surg* 28:820, 1980.
23. Jacobson A: The proportionate template as a diagnostic aid, *Am J Orthod* 75:156-172, 1979.
24. Jacobson A: Application of the "Wits" appraisal, *Am J Orthod* 70:179-189, 1976.
25. Jacobson A: The "Wits" appraisal of jaw disharmony, *Am J Orthod* 67:125-138, 1975.
26. Jarabak JR, Fizzell JA: *Technique and treatment with lightwire edgewise appliance,* St Louis, 1972, Mosby.
27. Johnston LE Jr: Template analysis, *J Clin Orthod* 21:484-590, 1987.
28. Kernahan DA, Rosenstein SW. *Cleft lip and palate, a system of management,* Philadelphia, 1990, Williams & Wilkins.
29. Legan H, Burston CJ: Soft tissue cephalometric analysis for orthognathic surgery, *J Oral Surg* 38:744-751, 1980.
30. Lo FD, Hunter WS: Changes in nasolabial angle related to maxillary incisor retraction, *Am J Orthod* 82:384-391, 1982.
31. Mason RM: A retraction headgear for bilateral cleft lip, *J Clin Orthod* 25:576, 1991.
32. McNamara JA Jr: A method of cephalometric evaluation, *Am J Orthod* 86:449-469, 1984.
33. McNamara JA Jr, Brudon WL: *Orthodontic and orthopedic treatment in the mixed dentition,* Ann Arbor, Mich, 1993, Needham Press.
34. Moorrees CF: Natural head position—a revival, *Am J Orthod Dentofac Orthop* 512-513, 1994 (guest editorial).
35. Ogaard B, Rola G, Arends J, et al: Orthodontic appliances and enamel demineralization. Part 1—lesion development, *Am J Dentofac Orthop* 93:68-73, 1988.
36. Peterka M, Peterkova R, Likovsky Z: Timing of exchange of the maxillary deciduous and permanent teeth in boys with three types of orofacial clefts, *Cleft Palate J* 33:318-323, 1996.
37. Proffit WR: *Contemporary orthodontics,* ed 2, St Louis, 1993, Mosby.
38. Rosenstein SW: Early habilitation of the cleft lip and palate child. In Johnston LE, editor: *New vistas in orthodontics,* Philadelphia, 1985, Lea & Febiger.
39. Ross B: Treatment variables affecting facial growth in unilateral cleft lip and palate, *Cleft Palate J* 24:24-32, 1987.
40. Stoelinga PJ, Haaers PEJJ, Leenen RJ, et al: Late management of secondarily grafted clefts, *Int J Oral Maxillofac Surg* 19:97-102, 1990.

Fixation Principles

Jeffrey A. Goldstein

INTRODUCTION

The purpose of this chapter is to discuss the theory, indications, operations, and outcomes surrounding the use of fixation in the craniomaxillofacial skeleton. Over the past 20 years, the importance of fixation in this area has been recognized and evolved from the use of wire fixation to more rigid forms of fixation. This chapter addresses this evolution, as well as the advantages and disadvantages of fixation.

INDICATIONS

PRINCIPLES OF BONE HEALING

To best understand the indications and principles of fixation, one must first understand the principles of bone healing. Bone is mesenchymally derived through the process of intramembranous ossification, endochrondal ossification, or a combination of both.[1,4,10,14,15] Endochrondal ossification requires the initial development of a cartilaginous anlage followed by resorption and replacement with bone. Membranous bone does not require an intermediate cartilaginous stage, with mesenchymal cells differentiating into osteoblasts that directly form mineralized bone. The majority of the craniomaxillofacial skeleton is membranous bone in origin, with the base of the skull and portions of the mandible and temporal and occipital bones endochrondal in nature. Until recently, fracture repair in the midface and cranial vault was thought to occur by fibrous healing, leading to a fibrous union. In the early 1990s, animal and human clinical studies demonstrated that the facial bones undergo true osseous union, albeit sometimes with a cartilaginous precursor similar to the endochrondal model.[21,23] It was postulated that the cartilage production may be related to motion between the two bony segments or to the presence of a gap between the segments. Interestingly, radiographic evaluation of membranous bone fracture healing is characterized by a persistent lucency at the fracture site despite a well-developed bony union demonstrated histologically. This may be explained by the presence of less dense reparative membranous bone or a difference in crystalline structure.[3,14]

The basic functions of bone are to support and protect other vital structures, as well as to carry load. Its function is therefore highly dependent on its characteristics of strength and rigidity. Fracturing destroys the continuity of the bone, resulting in a loss of rigidity and diminishment of strength. External dynamic forces will then displace the fracture ends, resulting in angular and rotational deformities and/or shortening. Such deformity can impair bony function, including its ability to carry load and to support and protect nearby vital structures. It is the aim of any form of fracture treatment to obtain function equal to the prefracture situation.

External dynamic forces applied across a fracture, usually by the differential pull of muscles attached to the involved bone, lead to deformation at the fracture site. Disruption of vessels in the surrounding soft tissue and bone lead to initial hematoma formation, which may actually assist in stabilizing the fracture. This stability is obtained in exchange for possible impediment of the bone at the fracture site as a result of vascular disruption. Fibrous tissue then replaces the initial hematoma, resulting in increased stiffness. The increased stiffness decreases the amount of mobility at the fracture site, allowing for a decrease in strain condition, which then allows for cartilage formation. Perren[16] and Phillips and Rahn[17-19] discussed the importance of strain effects on bony healing. Elongation, or strain tolerance, is defined as the capacity of any tissue to tolerate a certain amount of deformation before rupturing. Bone will rupture when elongated only 2%, whereas granulation tissue can tolerate 100% elongation and cartilage 10%. Consequently, the initial response of tissue deformation is fibrous tissue, which is replaced by cartilage, whose formation occurs only after the fibrous tissue results in decreased motion at the fracture site and a decrease in the strain condition. In spontaneously healing bone or in bony fractures placed in a situation of relative movement (e.g., cast fixation), resorption leading to fragment-end shortening is common. It has been postulated by Phillips and Rahn that the progression of fibrous tissue to cartilage to bone formation and fracture healing is driven by a diminishment of intrafragmentary strain. Therefore fragment-end resorption would appear to be an adaptive mechanism to reduce intrafragmentary strain for a given amount of motion because it is dependent on both motion and gap width. The second mechanism used to decrease intrafragmentary strain in this type of healing fracture is that of an increase in cross-sectional diameter at the fracture site caused by callus formation. Tissue rigidity increases to the fourth power as related to the radius from the center of rotation or bending. Consequently, endosteal callus is less efficient than the bony edges, which are less efficient than periosteal callus.

Based on this model, tissue can be formed in a fracture gap only if the tissue formed can tolerate the deformational strength present. Once a fragment site is filled by a given tissue, the properties of that tissue will increase the rigidity of the fracture site and thereby diminish the strain, allowing for the next stage of tissue differentiation. This accounts for the transition from fibrous tissue to cartilage formation to bone formation. This process of bony healing, which includes resorption, callus formation, and eventual bony healing, is defined as *indirect bone healing*. If the external dynamic load is greater than the biologic stabilization that is able to be achieved, delayed union or nonunion will result.

Although immobilization through casting will allow for indirect, or secondary, bone healing, it cannot hold the fractured bony ends in strict immobilization and contact. If one can achieve absolute immobilization with bony contact, bone union can theoretically proceed without requiring resorption of fragment ends or a cartilaginous intermediate stage. Fractures that can be stabilized and immobilized will then heal via the process of direct, or primary, bone healing. If such rigid fixation of the fracture is deemed appropriate, the most reliable means to achieve this is the use of plate and screw fixation. The bony union of the fracture ends occur by remodeling of the haversian canals by cutting cones.[19] Cutting cones are composed of osteoclasts and the conical surface of osteoblasts. In any fracture with adequate fixation and bone-to-bone contact, not all of the bony surface of the fracture line will be in contact. The gap areas will also be under a little strain, allowing bone to be deposited directly, originally randomly, followed by remodeling along the axis of the bone through haversian remodeling.[19] Direct bone healing does not require a cartilaginous intermediate and is not associated with resorption. It will result in a more efficient and reliable means of bony union when used in the correct situations.

PRINCIPLES OF OSTEOSYNTHESIS

To achieve fixation with adequate immobilization, two major fixation systems and principles exist: monocortical miniplate osteosynthesis and compression osteosynthesis. The principles behind compression osteosynthesis in the craniomaxillofacial skeleton are extrapolated from the Association of Osteosynthesis (AO) principles developed for long bone fractures and used only in the mandible, where the greatest deforming forces of the head and neck are present. The basis for fixation in both of these models is the clamping of the plate to the bone via the screws. The strength of the screw (limited by stripping of the bone thread or screw fracture) is the key determinant establishing functional load while still preserving the needed

rigid fixation. The strength of this relationship is then dependent on screw design, the screw-bone interface at the time of insertion and thereafter, and the reaction of the bone to the metallic screw and to any bony resorption and/or remodeling. Most craniofacial screws are now self-tapping in variety. Self-tapping screws, however, may result in a mild diminishment in holding power and require more torque for insertion, which can lead to screw failure and increased stress to the surrounding bones, leading to microfractures and possibly screw loosening.[19] Some authors have advocated the use of compression for stabilization of bone fractures. Without any form of compression, the stability of the fracture reduction is dependent on the plate rigidity and any friction between bony fragment ends. If a small gap exists, especially in conjunction with external muscle pull, the plate may bend, resulting in movement and high strain. Compression can be achieved with the use of compression plates or the lag screw technique. Compression results in absolute stability with a theoretic gap strain of zero. It also allows for friction, which diminishes the possibility of micromotion. The force of compression over time quantitatively decreases slowly. The surfaces under compression do not appear to develop fragment-end shortening because of resorption. The compression plates are best placed for fractures at the point nearest the center of the fracture plane. In mandibular fractures, these plates cannot be placed over the center of the fracture plane because of the presence of teeth roots. Placed in the lower border of the mandible, displacement may occur at the alveolar occlusal border when compression is applied. To overcome this, a tension band needs to be placed. In the areas in which teeth are present, a tension band can take the form of an arch bar. In the rest of the mandible, a second plate can be applied at the alveolar border. In general, a minimum of two screws should be placed on either side of a fracture for sufficient stability of the craniomaxillofacial skeleton. A second form of compression osteosynthesis is the use of the lag screw technique, which is addressed in this chapter.

The second form of rigid stabilization, in which interfragmentary compression does not play a role, is called *fixation osteosynthesis*. In most areas of the midface, upper face, and cranial vault where compression is not possible or desired, rigid stabilization can be provided by fixation osteosynthesis. The above-mentioned areas are composed of extremely thin bone. Fixation osteosynthesis can also be used quite successfully in the mandible. These systems come in a variety of sizes, including microsystems (1.0 mm), miniplate systems (1.3 to 2.0 mm), and mandibular systems (2.4 to 2.7 mm). In general, they are designed to be placed monocortically, especially in the bony structures of the midface and upper face that have no significant functional load. Experimental work has demonstrated that with either monocortical or bicortical placement of the screws, this form of fixation osteosynthesis is strong enough to withstand the masticatory forces in the mandible.[2] Mandibular bone will heal adequately without compression, perhaps, however, at a slower rate.[12] Although some groups advocate the use of miniplates in the mandible,[2] my preference is to use the larger mandibular (2.7 mm) plates. If dynamic compression at the fracture site is chosen, one must be aware that the bony segments can shift. If this shift is not realized or controlled, it can be transmitted to the alveolar occlusal plane or the condylar head, resulting in malocclusion or condylar torque. Gruss[12] warns that to use compression safely, good bone-to-bone contact of the fracture ends must be obtained, enabling the fracture ends to "lock together during compression without sliding or torquing." It should not therefore be used with oblique fractures, sagittal splitting fractures, comminuted fractures, segmental fractures, or fractures with bone loss. He further advocates the use of a longer plate with more screws based on a neutral and noncompressive mode to achieve the same goals.[12]

CHOICE OF FIXATION MATERIALS

Wire fixation in the craniomaxillofacial skeleton has historically been used for bone-to-bone orientation. However, because of its inability to control micromotion or rotational deformities, it does not provide the adequate immobilization necessary for primary bone healing. Originally, plates and screws were composed of stainless steel. The use of stainless steel was hampered by disadvantages, including corrosion, which potentially could lead to severe foreign body reactions and implant failure.[13] This has been a well-documented problem with orthopedic devices, but instances of this in maxillofacial utilization is unknown. Stainless steel also causes significant scatter on computed tomography (CT) scans and is extremely rigid to handle. Its rigidity may preexpose it to rebound after bending and subsequent screw instability. Most rigid fixation systems today are made of either titanium or Vitallium. These materials have excellent tissue compatibility, are corrosion resistant, and remain chemically inert. These current products allow for adequate malleability yet provide sufficient rigidity to resist deformation. Although Vitallium is somewhat stronger than titanium, it does have increased scatter on radiographic scanning. The titanium and Vitallium systems are produced in a variety of sizes. The 2.7-mm system is best used in the mandible. The 2.0-mm miniplates are frequently used along the structural pillars of the maxilla. The smaller microsystems (which are also the lowest profile) are best used in the periorbital regions, nasal dorsum, and frontal bone.

Although internal metallic bone fixation has becoming increasing popular over the past decade, several potential problems exist, including palpability, loosening of the hardware, sinusitis, long-term exposure or infection, scattering difficulties in both imaging and radiation therapy, intracranial migration when applied to the infant craniofacial skeleton, and concerns of growth restriction in the young.[5-7] In 1996 the U.S. Food and Drug Administration (FDA) approved the first resorbable fixation system for the craniomaxillofacial skeleton: the LactoSorb Craniomaxillofacial Fixation System. It is composed of a copolymer of L-polylactic acids and glycolic acids at a ratio of 82 to 18. For this polymeric material to be clinically valuable, it must meet the criteria of absolute biocompatibility, sufficient biomechanical strength over time to permit bone healing, complete resorption, and elimination of polymeric residues and by-products.[7] Lastly, upon total resorption, the body should "forget" the implant was ever present.[5-7,11,20] LactoSorb resorbs in two phases, with hydrolysis cleaving the chemical bonds that hold the polymer together. Second, as the polymer loses form and consistency, it will form particular debris, which will be metabolized by macrophages, with final oxidation products being carbon dioxide and water. Upon implantation of any foreign body, including the LactoSorb polymer, there may be an initial inflammatory response by the body, followed by encapsulation of the implant with a thin membrane, followed by resorption of the material with some small residuals of fibrous membrane remaining. LactoSorb, with its low molecular weight (approximately 60,000) and amorphous composition, has intermediate absorption characteristics, which allow it to be slow enough to not overwhelm the ability to clear degradation products yet fast enough to allow total clearance within 1 year. Its properties are that of a copolymer and are significantly different from those of the homopolymers L-lactic acid and pure polyglycolic acid, which are both of high degree of crystallinity and often a very high molecular weight. With appropriate design, a polymeric implant can be made to have strength comparable with a metal implant. The LactoSorb plate strength exceeds that of a 1.5-mm titanium plate for as long as 8 weeks after saline immersion in vitro.[20] Clinically, the palpability and profile of these resorbable plates significantly diminish as soon as 3 months after application. The LactoSorb fixation system appears to have strong indications for usage in cranial-orbital reconstruction, nasal-orbital ethmoidal reconstruction, and the midface. Its greatest applications appear to be in the pediatric population, where problems associated with permanent implants, including intracranial migration and growth restriction, appear to be avoided.

OPERATIONS

Surgical indications for the use of rigid fixation in the maxillofacial skeleton include facial trauma, posttraumatic deformities, elective osteotomies, congenital craniofacial reconstructions, bony tumor reconstruction, and onlay bone grafting. The technical details of these indications are far beyond the scope of this chapter and are well covered in Chapters 45, 47 to 51, and 63.

OUTCOMES

When assessing and discussing outcomes data in regards to fixation principles, a number of issues need to be addressed, including complications, aesthetic results, physical functioning, cost of care, patient satisfaction, and quality of life.

Although parameters such as quality of life are difficult to quantitatively measure, the use of rigid fixation often obviates the need for intermaxillary fixation after elective osteotomies or traumatic deformity repairs, making these procedures more tolerable to the patient without sacrificing stability and reliability of results. To fully discuss outcomes, one would need to address each indication for rigid fixation, including facial trauma, posttraumatic deformities, elective osteotomies, congenital craniofacial reconstruction, tumor reconstruction, and onlay grafting. This is again beyond the scope of this chapter. The reader is invited to explore each of these in their appropriate chapters listed above. In general, however, rigid fixation is preferable over nonrigid fixation (i.e., wires or sutures), which is preferable over no fixation for many craniomaxillofacial applications, including displaced fractures of the craniomaxillofacial skeleton (especially when comminuted); osteotomies from posttraumatic deformities; orthognathic surgery of the midface and/or mandible; pediatric craniorbital reconstruction for craniofacial deformities; bony tumor reconstruction of the orbits, midface, and mandible; and onlay bone grafting. In a number of studies there appears to be improved stability in both the short and long term with diminished relapse.[22] In addition, diminishment of intrafragmentary movement most likely diminishes postoperative infection to an extent that overcomes the risk of infection from implantation of foreign material.[8,9] Lastly, when infection does develop, especially in the repair of acute trauma, rigid fixation may in fact promote bony union even in the presence of infection. A number of studies, primarily retrospective in nature, describe the advantages of rigid fixation in all of the above-mentioned settings. These are detailed in their appropriate chapters.

With the advent of metallic bone plates and screws for internal fracture fixation, a reliable technique for achieving undisturbed fracture healing became available. However, disadvantages and complications of these systems must also be considered. Bony atrophy, or osteopenia, may occur as a result of stress shielding and corrosion by the rigid bone plates and screws, necessitating a second operation for removal. Metallic products may still carry a low carcinogenic risk. Metallic implant fixation devices may also interfere with imaging technology because resultant scattering on the desired image may obscure important details. In addition, the use of permanent metallic fixation in the pediatric patient may affect continued growth of the cranial bone. In the periorbital and nasal regions, conventional metallic plates and screws may be palpable or visible or may even get exposed. In the same pediatric population, intracranial migration of these plates and screws has also been described. Many of these complications could be avoided by the use of a resorbable fixation system, although the efficacy of this has only been proven in the non–weight-bearing regions of the craniofacial skeleton.

With the use of any fixation system, cost must also be considered. The resorbable and nonresorbable plate and screwing systems are clearly more expensive than wires and/or sutures. The advantages of rigid fixation must demonstrate a benefit that justifies the added expense. It is my experience that this benefit does exist, and this appears to be well documented in the literature.[22] Again the range of each indication and the relative costs are beyond the scope of this chapter and are dealt with in the previously referenced chapters of this book.

SUMMARY

The future advances in fixation principles and concepts are multifaceted. The use of glues and adhesives rather than plates is already being explored. A fixation implant may not necessarily be inert and may also act as a carrier to bring growth factors or other manipulators into the local wound-healing environment. Less invasive techniques of fixation implantation are also being explored with the hopes of minimizing devascularization of surrounding tissues. Lastly, the interface between an alloplastic implant and native bone is being explored to better understand and influence the interactions between the two. It is the hope of this author that plastic surgeons will stay in the forefront of these advances.

REFERENCES

1. Bassett C, Andrew L: Clinical implications of cell functioning and bone grafting, *Clin Orthop* 87:49-59, 1972.
2. Blez P, Khan JL: Principles of monocortical miniplate osteosynthesis. In Yaremchuk MJ, Gruss JS, Manson PN, editors: *Rigid fixation of the craniomaxillofacial skeleton,* Boston, 1992, Butterworth-Heinemann.
3. Craft PD, Sargent LA: Membranous bone healing and techniques in calvarial bone grafting, *Clin Plast Surg* 16:11-20, 1989.
4. Enlow PH: *Handbook of facial growth,* Philadelphia, 1982, WB Saunders.
5. Eppley B: Resorbable biotechnology for craniomaxillofacial surgery, *J Craniofac Surg* 8:85-86, 1997.
6. Eppley B, Prevel C: Non-metallic fixation in trauma midfacial fractures, *J Craniofac Surg* 8:103-109, 1997.
7. Eppley B, Sadove AM: A comparison of resorbable and metallic fixation of calvarial bone grafts, *Plast Reconstr Surg* 96:316-322, 1995.
8. Fialkov JA, Phillips JH, Walmsley SL: The effect of infection and lagscrew fixation on the union of membranous bone grafts in a rabbit model, *Plast Reconstr Surg* 93:574-581, 1994.
9. Fialkov JA, Phillips JH, Walmsley SL, et al: The effect of infection and lagscrew fixation on revascularization and new bone deposition in membranous bone grafts in a rabbit model, *Plast Reconstr Surg* 98:338-345, 1996.
10. Friedlaender GE: Current concepts review: bone grafts, *J Bone Joint Surg* 69a:786-799, 1987.
11. Goldstein JA, Quereshy FA, Cohen AR: Early experience with biodegradable fixation for congenital pediatric craniofacial surgery, *J Craniofac Surg* 8:110-115, 1997.

12. Gruss JS: Complications of rigid internal fixation of the mandible. In Yaremchuk MJ, Gruss JS, Manson PN, editors: *Rigid fixation of the craniomaxillofacial skeleton,* Boston, 1992, Butterworth-Heinemann.

13. Hobar PC: Methods of rigid fixation, *Clin Plast Surg* 19:31-40, 1992.

14. Manson PN: Facial bonehealing in bone grafts, *Clin Plast Surg* 21:331-348, 1994.

15. Mulliken JB, Kaban LB, Glowacki J: Induced osteogenesis: the biological principle and clinical applications, *J Surg Res* 37:487-496, 1984.

16. Perren SM: Physical and biological aspects of fracture healing with special reference to internal fixation, *Clin Orthop* 138:175-184, 1979.

17. Phillips JH, Rahn BA: Fixation effects on membranous and endochondral onlay bone graft resorption, *Plast Reconstr Surg* 82:872-877, 1988.

18. Phillips JH, Rahn BA: Fixation effects on membranous and endochondral onlay bone graft revascularization and bone deposition, *Plast Reconstr Surg* 85:891-897, 1990.

19. Phillips JH, Rahn D: Bone healing. In Yaremchuk MJ, Gruss JS, Manson PN, editors: *Rigid fixation of the craniomaxillofacial skeleton,* Boston, 1992, Butterworth-Heinemann.

20. Pietrzak WS, Sarver DR, Verstynen ML: Bioabsorbable polymer science for the practicing surgeon, *J Craniofac Surg* 8:87-91, 1997.

21. Rever LJ, Manson PN, Randolph MA, et al: The healing of facial bone fractures by the process of secondary union, *Plast Reconstr Surg* 87:451-458, 1991.

22. Rohrich RJ, Watumull D: Comparison of rigid plates versus wire fixation of the management of zygoma fractures: a long-term follow up clinical study, *Plast Reconstr Surg* 96:570-575, 1995.

23. Thaller SR, Kawamoto HK: A histologic evaluation of fracture repair in the midface, *Plast Reconstr Surg* 85:196-201, 1990.

Bone Grafting and Substitutes

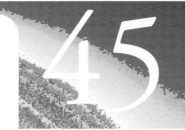

Elisa A. Burgess
Michael H. Mayer
Jeffrey Hollinger

INTRODUCTION

Reconstructive osseous surgery of the craniofacial skeleton is complex and extremely challenging. In attempting to restore the anatomic framework, the goals of aesthetically pleasing form and normal function are paramount. Obvious factors contributing to the challenge include the unique bony anatomy, a rich neurovasculature, and an extensive sensory motor consortium. Not uncommonly, soft tissue deformities are present, either from lack of bony support or from partial or complete absence resulting from congenital or traumatic causes. In addition, developmental influences may direct positional relationships among anatomic components of the craniofacial complex and thus replenishing deficient osseous tissue must not mitigate against synchronous growth of soft and hard tissues.

Osseous reconstruction of the craniofacial complex should be based on a rational progression of therapeutic intervention integrated with a fundamental respect for and appreciation of anatomy, embryology, biochemistry, and aesthetics. For example, the *anatomy* and *embryology* of the defect may dictate the origin and format of the donor bone graft. From a *biochemical* perspective, the autogenous bone graft, as the preeminent treatment to restore deficient form and function, is composed of a viable cell pool (which expresses *biochemical modulators*) and signaling factors (the *biochemical modulators*) prompting maximal bone regeneration. In contrast, allogeneic bank bone does not contain living cells; its effectiveness depends on intrinsic signaling molecules and the capacity to provide a foundation for bone regeneration. From an *aesthetic* perspective, restoring subtle nuances in deficient contour of craniofacial bone with either an autograft or allogeneic preparation demands a sculptor's prowess. Therefore to restore an aesthetically enduring and functional shape, a clinically convenient bone substitute that can be easily adapted and contoured may be used.

In keeping with the organizational framework of this textbook, under the heading of Indications, the anatomy of the craniofacial skeleton is discussed, along with the embryology of bone and the various biochemical regulators influencing bone formation. Under Operations, the various reconstructive materials and techniques are reviewed. Finally, in Outcomes, the options for the future are discussed.

INDICATIONS

The indications for bone grafting in the craniofacial skeleton are multifactorial. A bony defect requires the restoration of tissue that is functional, physiologic, and aesthetic. Fortunately, bone has the capacity to regenerate; however, beyond a certain level, this capacity must be augmented surgically, for example, with a bone graft.

In selecting a surgical procedure, the clinician and the patient must realize what is to be expected and consider the potential outcome. In making these decisions, the timing of the surgical intervention and the need for further surgery are important. Consideration must be given to the questions of whether a window of opportunity will be missed if surgery is delayed, if further bone or soft tissue growth will be inhibited, if soft tissue scarring and contraction will ensue, and if further grafting will be required. One option may involve early grafting, with the surgeon and the patient cognizant that supplemental surgical procedures still may be required. For example, patients with craniosynostosis syndromes may undergo early surgical intervention to promote appropriate brain development but may later require further bony revision.

The embryogenesis of the bone graft and the format of the graft may be considerations in the selection of donor and recipient sites. The clinician must consider the vascularity of the recipient site, the status of the overlying soft tissues, the bony volume requirements, and the need for load-bearing capability to achieve superior long-term results. As a result, when autogenous grafts are used, the best outcome for a specific site may involve a different donor site from one patient to the next. One must also consider the problems of donor supply and donor site morbidity. These considerations apply for calvaria, midface, mandible, and other sites in the craniofacial skeleton. Knowledge of the anatomy, embryology, and biochemistry of the craniofacial skeleton is essential to select the best therapeutic modality.

PREOPERATIVE PLANNING FOR CRANIOFACIAL DEFECTS

Clear surgical goals and recognition of associated comorbidities for each craniofacial category of congenital, traumatic, and oncologic defects should be well formulated before entering the operating room. For example, congenital defects, such as craniosynostosis or premature fusion of one or more cranial sutures in utero, require an extensive evaluation before surgical intervention. Evaluation commences in a multidisciplinary fashion with a craniofacial team. In addition, parental and patient expectations must be recognized and sometimes several preoperative clinic appointments are necessary. Based on these multiple interactions, the osseous pathology is identified and a reconstructive method encompassing ostectomy, bone graft, rigid fixation, and adjuvant therapies is generated. For example, the surgical goal for craniosynostosis surgery is to promote age-appropriate calvarial size and shape, which would allow for normal brain growth and improve intellectual development. Similar surgical goals would be generated for the other craniofacial conditions.

Preoperative planning is initiated with the history and physical examination in combination with photos documenting the current defect. Dental impressions and models should be made, along with a bite registration if dental reconstruction is an issue. Cephalometric radiographs and measurements assist with the two-dimensional analysis.[27] Computed tomography (CT) with three-dimensional reconstruction can support the initial evaluation and aid future follow-up examinations. CT software has advanced the technology of computer-generated models to assist in complex craniofacial reconstruction.[2,27,89] For example, Denta-Scan software (General Electric Tomography, Milwaukee) can generate CT scan data to provide unique three-dimensional views and allow accurate measurements for assessing fixation devices and implants. This allows for preoperative modifications and contouring while decreasing operative time and increasing accuracy. The technology is currently available to surgeons and provides assistance when using reconstructive materials and techniques.

ANATOMY

Anatomic Partitions of the Craniofacial Complex

The craniofacial complex may be partitioned anatomically into the neurocranium, midface, and mandible. The unique features (i.e., contour and function) of each anatomic partition can dictate selection of a particular type of graft or bone substitute. Bones under passive load, such as the parietal, occipital, and frontal bones, are broad, gently curved, and composed of an inner and outer cortex (i.e., table) with interposed marrow (i.e., diploë). Therefore a pastelike bone substitute that will harden in situ may be applicable for an outer table restoration. In contrast, the U-shaped mandible sustains challenging functional loading by providing origin and insertion for masticatory and suprahyoid muscles and may require supportive fixation in addition to a cortical graft or substitute.

EMBRYOGENESIS AND BIOCHEMICAL REGULATORS

Intramembranous Pathway

During embryogenesis, bones develop by two distinct pathways. The mandible (except for a segment of the coronoid process and the midsymphyseal region), vault of the cranium (i.e., from the supraorbital ridge posteriorly to the external occipital protuberance), parietal bones, squamous portion of the occipital and temporal bones, squama frontalis, part of the greater wing of the sphenoid, ilium, scapula, and clavicle[110] form directly from osteoblasts, whose pedigree can be traced to mesenchymal cell precursors.[10,77]

It is not certain what factors direct bone embryogenesis. Purportedly, adhesion molecules (e.g., fibronectin), soluble signals putatively identified as members of the *transforming growth factor-β family*,[72] and mesenchymal cells in the embryo coalesce, form *cell condensations,* and cells within this condensation differentiate into bone-forming cells, or *osteoblasts.*[40] This process is described as an intramembranous pathway and does not involve an intervening cartilage stage.

The *bone morphogenetic protein* (BMP) family (part of the transforming growth factor-β clan) probably plays key roles during bone embryogenesis.[98,101] Postnatally, BMPs promote osteoblast differentiation from pluripotential cells,[52] and the effect on cell phenotype expression depends on the concentration of BMP.[90] Perhaps a concentration gradient of BMPs in the developing embryo in the areas of the clavicle and craniofacial complex favors *intramembranous bone formation.* Moreover, antiangiogenic and angiogenic biochemical regulators modulating local vascularity will affect cell phenotype, determining whether undifferentiated cells become either osteoblasts or chondrocytes.

Endochondral Pathway

In the appendicular and axial regions, cells within primordial mesenchymal cell condensations develop into cartilage, which is replaced by bone. Cues to promote cell navigation through a *chondrogenic* rather than an *osteogenic* lineage pathway are unknown; however, as noted above, differential concentrations of BMPs and angiogenic or antiangiogenic factors could modulate phenotype.

A logical hypothesis is that concentration gradients of basic fibroblast growth factor (bFGF), BMP-related molecules, and BMPs in the embryo may favor site-specific functional activity and cell differentiation. Prompts for the appearance of these signaling cues have been a mystery. However, recent compelling evidence suggests signals from the zone of polarizing activity, the apical ectodermal ridge, and a network of regulatory genes (part of the Hox/Homeobox network and Wnt and sonic hedgehog genes) modulate BMP and FGF expression, thereby promoting cell and tissue differentiation and pattern formation.[24,33,58,87]

In vitro validation of the concentration gradient hypothesis for BMP regulation of cell differentiation has been proven with a mesenchymal stem cell line (C3H10T1/2).[107] C3H10T1/2 cells exposed to different concentrations of recombinant human (rh) BMP-2 differentiated into either adipocytes, chondrocytes, or osteoblasts—the phenotype observed was dose-dependent.[107] The highest concentration of rhBMP-2 promoted osteoblast formation.

BMP has angiogenic properties:[111] the capacity to cause endothelial cell differentiation and vessel formation.[31] Type IV collagen and matrix components of blood vessels bind to BMP-3, BMP-4, and BMP-7.[45] Moreover, FGF binds to vascular endothelium.[32] Therefore the more intense vascularity of the mandible and midfacial region compared with the appendicular region may favor sequestering of bFGF and BMPs by selective binding to type IV collagen of vascular basement membrane,[81] thus optimizing concentration gradients in favor of osteoblast phenotype.[15] Localization of bFGF could sustain the intensity of blood vessel formation, whereas undifferentiated cells populating the *condensations* could have an opportunity to interact with BMPs to pursue an osteogenic (i.e., *intramembranous*) rather than chondrogenic (i.e., *endochondral*) passage.[45]

Chondrolysis and concomitant osteogenesis can be correlated with angiogenesis.[86] Protamine is an antiangiogenic factor associated with cartilage,[99] and this biochemical regulator and others, such as angiostatin and endostatin, may thwart vascularization.[76] The mechanism by which these antiangiogenic factors operate is as yet undetermined. Perhaps at embryonic *endochondral* bone sites, either down-regulating bFGF synthesis or its receptor expression—or both—diminishes angiogenesis and the likelihood for direct, *intramembranous* bone formation.

Another mechanism that may modulate bone embryogenesis is *factor antagonism,* such as whether or not an *osteogenic inhibitory factor* is secreted.[11] An osteogenic inhibitory molecule could counteract the effect of osteogenic molecules (i.e., BMPs), thereby sustaining chondrogenesis.

A clinically relevant issue is whether bone embryogenesis influences the treatment outcome. It is noteworthy that, irrespective of its developmental pathway, there is no compelling evidence that biochemical, morphologic, and physiologic differences exist between endochondral and intramembranous bone. Moreover, during repair in the adult skeleton, the sequence of endochondral and intramembranous bone regeneration may not proceed through pathways recapitulating embryogenesis. Furthermore, the same cells, as well as soluble (i.e., growth factors) and insoluble (i.e., collagen) factors, are found in both types of bone.

Therefore it is unlikely that embryogenesis influences clinical performance.

However, differences in biofunctional loading and vascularity do exist between intramembranous and endochondral bones and merit therapy customization. For example, the intramembranous bones of the head and neck have a significantly more robust vascular supply than do bones in the extremities. Moreover, biofunctional loading of the calvaria is significantly less than for bone in the extremities. Consequently, release kinetics of BMPs from a delivery system for bone regeneration in the calvaria probably will be different than the long bone, blood supply being the determinant for localizing released BMP.

Thus the *format* of the bone graft may be of considerable importance. Format refers to the properties of the transplanted bone. The format may be cortical; cancellous; corticocancellous; vascularized; or contain a muscle pedicle and be transplanted as a cortical block, corticocancellous block, or as a various size range of particles. The format selected for the transplanted bone depends on the requirements at the recipient bed. The requirements may be for load bearing, maximal bony volume retention, or to allow for tooth eruption, as in alveolar clefts. For example, the requirement to onlay a deficient area of the zygoma may be fulfilled with a block of cortical bone. A segmental deficit in the body of the mandible may be treated with a vascularized fibula graft. Deficient alveolar bone in a cleft patient may be augmented with osseous coagulum (i.e., a composite of bone particles and marrow cells).

OPERATIONS

CRANIOFACIAL RECONSTRUCTIVE MATERIALS AND TECHNIQUES

Autogenous bone grafts are used in the vast number of craniofacial bone grafting procedures. As mentioned previously, the donor site is largely dependent on the requirements at the recipient site and the availability of donor graft. Specific procedures and bone graft formats are discussed in individual chapters devoted to a single subject and are not reviewed here. Rather, various bone graft options, along with the state-of-the-art technology either available or under investigation at the time of this writing, are presented.

Bone Transplants
AUTOGENOUS TRANSPLANTATION. The donor and recipient are the same for an autogenous graft and this therapy is the preeminent treatment to augment and regenerate deficient osseous form. Autogenous grafts are favored by surgeons for several reasons: outcome is predictable and the infectious, inflammatory, and immunologic reactions at the recipient bed are minimal. Despite benefits of autogenous grafts, there are liabilities, including blood loss, infection, pain, paresthesia, limited donor material, and contour mismatch between donor and recipient sites.

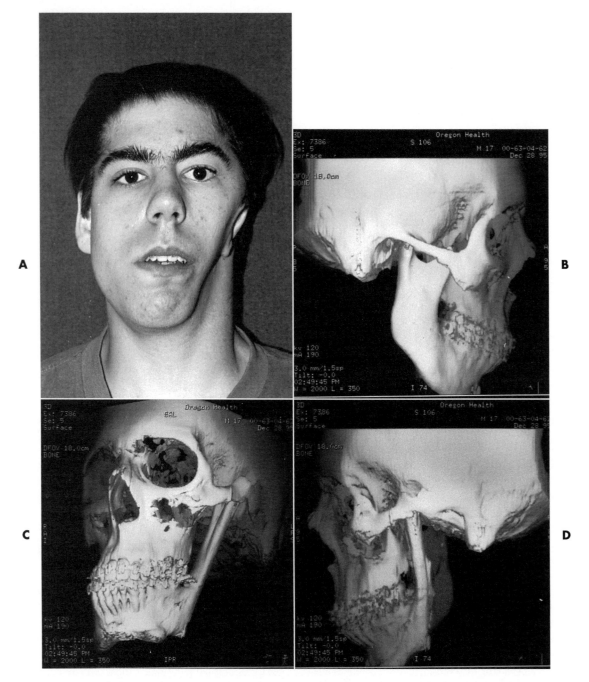

Figure 45-1. A, Preoperative photo of a patient with hemifacial microsomia. **B,** Three-dimensional postoperative CT scan showing normal right mandible of the patient with hemifacial microsomia. **C** and **D,** Three-dimensional postoperative CT scan showing the reconstructed left mandible using fibula autograft in the patient with hemifacial microsomia.   *Continued*

Bone regeneration superiority of autogenous grafts is due to sustained viability of bulk transplanted bone supported by its endogenous contingent of cells and soluble signaling factors. Transplanted cells consist of osteoblasts, osteoblast lineage cells, pluripotent cells that may become osteoblasts, and various phenotypes found in marrow and contiguous connective tissue stroma (e.g., periosteum). Soluble signaling factors within the autogenous bone, such as BMPs, enhance angiogenesis and promote osteoblast development from osteoblast lineage cells and pluripotent cells. BMPs have attracted

considerable attention for their bone regeneration prowess and therefore merit discussion in a section of this chapter.

An important selection criterion for a bone graft is whether viable osteoblast progenitor cells are included. Clearly, therefore, cancellous bone would be an optimal choice.[62] Cortical bone, which is relatively acellular, offers a nominal quantity of progenitor cells (from the cellular layer of the periosteum and endosteum). The clinical advantage offered by a combination of particulate corticocancellous graft material is the *bulk* provided by the cortical component, mitigating against tissue

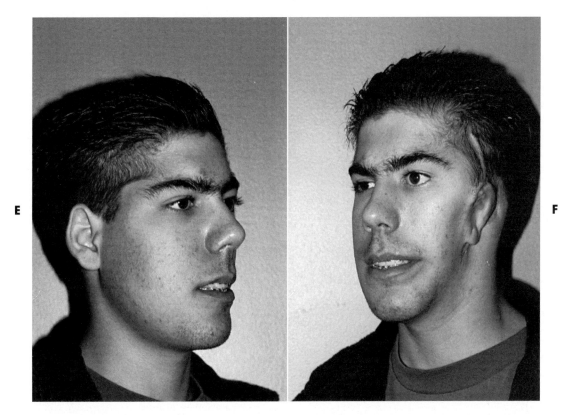

Figure 45-1, cont'd. E and **F,** Reconstructed postoperative photos of the patient with hemifacial microsomia.

prolapse, and the *cellularity* provided by the cancellous component. There seems to be a better rate of incorporation with corticomembranous bone, such as calvaria.[42] Cortico-membranous grafts are more rapidly vascularized than endochondral bone and thus will have better incorporation and less resorption.[56,95,119] In contrast, cancellous bone may migrate because of its spongy nature and will not be able to withstand stress. Other favorable factors influencing incorporation and limiting resorption of bone grafts include retained periosteum, adequate soft tissue coverage, and rigid fixation.[42]

From a surgical perspective, a graft can be divided into two broad categories: nonvascularized and vascularized bone transplantation. Nonvascularized bone grafting is performed with free transfer of donor material, such as rib, iliac crest, tibia, or fibula (Figure 45-1). In addition, the calvaria can serve as a source of nonvascularized bone by separation of the inner and outer tables. The tissue then may be used as inlay or onlay grafts. In brief, inlay grafts are placed within the defect and onlay grafts can be placed on other bony surfaces to improve contour. One example of an inlay is the use of an osseous coagulum (i.e., a composite of bone particles and marrow cells) to augment deficient alveolar bone circumscribing a dental prosthesis. In contrast, a zygoma deficit may be restored with an onlay of cortical bone that has been positionally stabilized with fixation to improve contour. However, with nonvascularized onlay grafts, the unfavorable long-term results caused by resorption merit alternative considerations.

Vascularized bone grafting occurs when an osteotomy is performed and bone is repositioned while maintaining

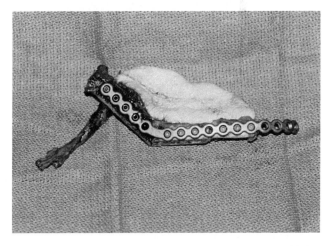

Figure 45-2. An example of a vascularized free fibular osteocutaneous autogenous bone graft.

periosteal blood supply. Vascularized bone grafting can also be performed by using microvascular free tissue transfer, which can be associated with donor site complications and technical difficulty. For example, a segmental deficit in the body of the mandible may be treated with a vascularized fibula graft (Figure 45-2).

Craniofacial surgery typically has involved a combination of techniques and materials for complex deformities. The traditional combination has involved an osteotomy segment with a bone graft and plate for internal fixation. Bone grafting has been important to promote healing of a fracture nonunion, in the replacement of bone at initial injury, and in stabilization of osteotomy segments during reconstructive surgery. In summary, a few principles of bone grafting are recommended: (1) harvest bone from familiar sites, (2) contour the bone, (3) perform tension-free placement of the bone with adequate immobilization, (4) avoid contaminated sites, and (5) ensure adequate graft coverage with blood supply.[39]

ALLOGENEIC TRANSPLANTATION. Transplantation of bone between non-genetically related individuals is referred to as *allogeneic transplantation,* and the term *syngeneic* is reserved for genetically related siblings. Stringent bone bank preparation protocols kill cells present in the transplant. Consequently, the correct nomenclature to describe the transplanted bone is an allogeneic implant and not an allograft. The latter therapy is not used, owing to the strident immunologic sequelae elicited by viable donor cells. Allogeneic implants are immunologic challenges to recipients as a consequence of transplanted cell debris and proteins.[34,102] Moreover, predictability for success with allogeneic preparations is significantly less than with autografts. The reasons for the inferiority include delayed vascularization, resorption, poor osteogenic capacity, potential for disease transmission, infection, morbidity, and mortality.

XENOGENEIC TRANSPLANTATION. The first report of unprocessed bone of nonhuman origin applied to human patients was in 1668 when the Dutch surgeon Job Van Meek'ren transplanted an unprocessed piece of dog calvaria to restore a segment of the calvaria of a Russian soldier who had been wounded in battle.[67] The Russian soldier survived with the transplant for 2 years. However, at the *suggestion* of the Russian church under threat of excommunication, the soldier requested removal of the graft, which led to his death. A Christian burial was provided!

Unprocessed xenogeneic bone is an unacceptable therapy. A limited number of bovine-derived products are available in Europe and the United States. A commercial product sold in the United States is Bio-Oss; it is deorganified cow bone prepared as particles (150-500 μm-sized chips) and blocks (2 cm) for alveolar ridge augmentation and mandibular reconstruction.

RIGID FIXATION FOR BONE GRAFTS

Significant documentation has validated that internal fixation provides graft stability and allows osseous integration with neovascularization.[115] Titanium or Vitallium metallic plates and cortical screws prevent movement of the grafts during the healing stage. In microplating systems, 0.8-mm to 1.2-mm diameter screws for children and 1.5-mm to 2.0-mm diameter screws for adults provide immobilization.[113] Larger-diameter screws of 2.4 mm to 2.7 mm are available for use in the mandible. Alternatively, a single lag screw can be effective with consideration of load requirements. Controversy lies in the

timing of bone grafting with rigid fixation in children because growth restriction can occur, especially across cranial sutures. Yaremchuk et al[114] demonstrated growth restriction with rigid fixation in a rhesus *(Macaca mulatta)* model. *M. mulatta* infants with ostectomized calvarial sites were fixated using wire or microplates with screws and were allowed to grow to near-adult size. Local shape changes were probably in part due to the ostectomy, but increasing degrees of rigid fixation led to an increased growth restriction. A surgeon may interpret this study as a recommendation to perform the minimum fixation to provide adequate stability. Mayer et al,[63] in a nonhuman primate model *(Macaca fascicularis)*, compared plate and screw fixation to stainless steel wire fixation for supraorbital bar and frontal bone advancement. They demonstrated specific alterations of the facial and orbital component of the zygomatic bone and skull. The changes were more pronounced in the wire fixation groups, suggesting the ability of rigid fixation in frontoorbital advancement to overcome the limitations of the surgical technique. Consideration may also be given to the later removal of rigid fixation to improve growth parameters or the use of biodegradable fixation, thus eliminating the need for hardware removal.

Although autogenous bone grafting with rigid fixation remains the gold standard therapy for craniofacial surgeons, there is a growing number of alternative techniques for bone regeneration. Distraction osteogenesis and guided bone regeneration are currently under clinical scrutiny in the craniofacial community.

DISTRACTION OSTEOGENESIS

In 1951, Ilizarov[48-50] introduced distraction osteogenesis after a patient reversed the compression rods of a primitive ring fixator used for compressive fracture management during World War II. The technique was applied to lengthen axial skeleton bone,[26,80] and eventually a group of Italian orthopedists began to study distraction osteogenesis.[4,7] The technique involves the regeneration of bone between vascularized bone surfaces that are separated by gradual distraction.[3] An osteotomy or corticotomy is performed and external fixation is applied followed by a 1-mm daily rate of distraction in extremities after a latency period (Figure 45-3, *A*). Failure of distraction osteogenesis can occur by (1) fibrocartilage nonunion, (2) failure of mineralization resulting from ischemia, (3) cystic degeneration, and (4) bending of the regenerated bone.[3]

After sufficient animal experimentation, clinical applications were undertaken in the axial skeleton of tibias, femurs, humeri, and other areas in over 100 human patients.[3] Indications were for lengthenings, deformity corrections, arthrodiastases, nonunions, acute fractures, and bone transportations. Greater than 90% of the patients healed by primary bone formation resulting from the distraction procedure. Complications presented were pain and soft tissue infection caused by the pins, and approximately 10% required supplemental autogenous bone grafts. The technique was applied to the craniofacial skeleton for jaw lengthening in the canine

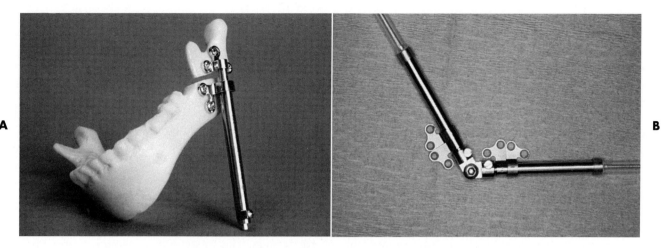

Figure 45-3. **A,** An example of a univectoral distraction osteogenesis device. **B,** An example of a multivectoral distraction osteogenesis device. (**A** and **B** courtesy Synthes, Paoli, Penn.)

mandible model.[51,69,96] McCarthy et al[66] applied this technology to cases requiring mandibular reconstruction. In a case report of four pediatric patients, three had unilateral craniofacial microsomia and one had Nager's syndrome (bilateral microsomia). All four patients underwent 18 to 24 mm of mandibular expansion with initial follow-up of 11 to 20 months. Only one patient had a 5-mm relapse. Complications from the expansion device included one inflammatory pin site and skin scars resulting from active expansion. Only one patient underwent revision of his scar. It is speculated that the slow expansion of the mandible also allows for lengthening of the supporting muscle and nerves, especially in the pediatric population.

Internal distraction devices minimize scar formation from the percutaneous pins. One series showed feasibility of internal distraction devices in five patients with craniofacial abnormalities.[18] Three patients underwent mandibular expansion, one patient underwent bilateral Le Fort III advancement, and one patient had segmental alveolar reconstruction through a transoral approach. All patients were able to obtain clinical lengthening, although one individual had mandibular relapse and two others had premature consolidation. Skin scarring was eliminated. Several issues surfaced in this series, including questions about the duration of the latency period before distraction commences and the rate of distraction in respect to the ages of patients. In the craniofacial skeleton, the latency period before distraction commences may be short in comparison with the extremities and the rate of distraction may be greater because of the increased vascularity of the head and neck.

Characteristics of a rich blood supply and a thin bony skeleton make the craniofacial region favorable to distraction osteogenesis. McCarthy[65] notes that no distraction cases in the craniofacial skeleton have required supplemental bone grafts. Multidimensional distraction with vector changes[64] (Figure 45-3, *B*) are currently available, and soon bidirectional and multidirectional internal devices will also be available. Applications have been applied to the cranium, midface, and mandible for traumatic and postoncologic reconstruction. Current research endeavors may investigate the endoscopic application of fixation devices. Many of these sites may alternatively be treated with other techniques, such as guided bone regeneration.

GUIDED BONE REGENERATION

An alternative technique for bone repair is guided bone regeneration (GBR). This can be defined as a controlled stimulation of new bone formation in a bony defect by osteoinduction, osteoconduction, or osteogenesis.[8] It is known that preservation of the periosteum over an osseous defect improves restoration of the lost bone. The proposed hypothesis assumes that the periosteum provides a source of osteoprogenitor cells and a blood supply. The osteopromoting cells from the bone populate the blood clot,[68] and the intact periosteum or barrier may inhibit the ingrowth of fibrous connective tissue.[6,74] This notion has been offered to justify resorbable and nonresorbable membranes in lieu of periosteum.

The application of membrane barrier-guided bone regeneration has garnered some attention in the periodontal literature with recent representation of other applications in the craniofacial literature. Five criteria for the design of an ideal barrier material have been described: spacemaking, cell occlusivity, tissue integration, ease of application, and biocompatibility.[91] The first and most common commercially available nonresorbable membrane barrier is polytetrafluoroethylene (Gore-Tex Periodontal Material, W.L. Gore & Associates, Flagstaff, Ariz.). The efficacy and safety have been examined,[13] and although polytetrafluoroethylene is relatively biocompatible, long-term studies are lacking.

Nyman et al[38] regenerated new bone in periodontal disease by using a barrier technique. Dahlin et al[25] also demonstrated bone regeneration in a rat mandible model using a standardized 5-mm trephine burr osseous defect. In this bilateral model, one side was treated with double membranes of polytetrafluoroethylene at the buccal and lingual margins and the contralateral defect site was left untreated as the control.

The mucoperiosteal flaps were repositioned, but the periosteum was not allowed to contact the bone. The animals were sacrificed at 3, 6, and 9 weeks, and histologic analysis revealed significant bone healing at the membrane-treated sites in all time frames, with little to no sign of healing at the control sites. The control sites displayed ingrowth of connective tissue.

Guided bone regeneration has been applied to experimental calvarial defects in rats, in which bilateral 5-mm parietal skull defects were made.[8] One cohort received a single polytetrafluoroethylene membrane over the extracranial defect with the contralateral defect left untreated as the control. The other cohort received a double membrane treatment (i.e., two membranes, with each positioned at the intracranial or extracranial margin) over the defect and the contralateral defect left untreated as the control. The animals were sacrificed at 30 days and evaluated for histologic bone regeneration. A significant amount of bone healing was found in the double membrane group when compared with the untreated control and to the single membrane. The authors postulate two theories of guided bone regeneration from this study: the soft tissue is excluded from the defect by the membrane, or the two membranes acted as a scaffold because new periosteum spread beneath the membrane and the original periosteum was not allowed contact with the defect.

Other rat studies have examined the effect of bone grafting with the membrane barrier technique.[1] Membranous and endochondral bone inlay were placed in mandibular critical size defects[93] with membrane barriers and membranous bone onlays were placed on the calvarial roof with membrane barriers. Controls were at contralateral sites and also were treated with the appropriate bone graft but without the membrane barrier. After 12 weeks, the sites were inspected and evaluated using light microscopy. The membranous bone inlay cohort with membrane barrier showed complete incorporation, in contrast to the controls. The endochondral bone inlays were not integrated with the surrounding bone even with a membrane barrier. The onlay grafts with or without membranes showed considerable resorption. Findings are consistent with our knowledge that inlay membranous autogenous bone grafts incorporate better than endochondral grafts, and this study implies that a membrane barrier enhances graft incorporation relative to controls.

Guided bone regeneration has now been performed in human patients for mandibular restoration and the placement of dental implants. In one study, 12 patients were selected for mandibular ridge enlargement or bony defect regeneration.[12] Mucoperiosteal flaps were raised and the cortical bone was perforated to create a bleeding surface. Polytetrafluoroethylene was placed over the surgical site to promote a space for bone regeneration and periosteum at the margins was removed. Digital subtraction radiographs, caliper measurements, and histology were used to evaluate patients after healing periods of 6 to 10 months. Three patients had acute infections that required early removal of the membranes, and two of these patients had foreign body materials from previous root canal fillings. Nine patients with 12 potential sites had sufficient bone for dental implants, and histology was consistent with

bone regeneration tissue. After adequate bone has been regenerated, the nonresorbable membrane is removed through an additional surgical procedure. In summary, the polytetrafluoroethylene membrane appears to be a fairly predictable way of obtaining new bone regeneration in several craniofacial sites.

Resorbable barriers, such as polylactic acid, polyglycolic acid, and collagen, are being evaluated in animal models of guided bone regeneration.[83] Resorbable barriers would have the benefit of not requiring surgical removal. The ideal resorbable barrier should allow the presence of osteopromoting cells, exclude connective tissue, and resorb without adverse effects on regeneration. Currently, some researchers are focusing on the period of time necessary for adequate bone regeneration. This information would assist in the development of a barrier undergoing a timely resorption. Testing in animal models continues, but two barriers have been approved for human periodontal applications in the United States. Guidor (John O. Butler Co., Chicago) and Resolut (W.L. Gore & Associates) have been approved by the U.S. Food and Drug Administration (FDA).[83] Guidor (a matrix of polylactic acid and a citric acid ester) has undergone primate studies[36,37] and human studies,[59] in which data appear to indicate an improvement in certain types of periodontal defects. Resolut (a matrix of lactide and glycolide homopolymers) has undergone primate studies,[46,84] as well as human clinical trial by Quinones et al. Clinical trial results have not been published, but the authors report that Resolut is comparable with the gold standard nonresorbable barrier in periodontal defects. Both versions of the resorbable barriers seem to be effective; however, additional craniofacial assessments are warranted.

BONE SUBSTITUTES

Polymethylmethacrylate

Polymethylmethacrylate (PMMA) is a polymer commonly seen in dentistry, orthopedics, neurosurgery, and craniofacial surgery. In dentistry, PMMA is used for dental prostheses. In orthopedics, PMMA cement secures a bone-prosthesis "bond." In craniofacial areas, PMMA has been used for cranioplasties.

There a number of attractive properties of PMMA. In its polymerized, hardened form, it is suitable for denture construction. Moreover, as a bone substitute, before setting as a hard polymer, PMMA can be manipulated relatively easily by the surgeon to conform to the bony recipient dimensions. Furthermore, PMMA is inexpensive. However, PMMA has significant liabilities. Shortcomings of PMMA include the inability to biodegrade and become replaced by functional bone; it is associated with chronic inflammation, including giant cells and macrophages that jeopardize longevity of cemented orthopedic prostheses; and infection and exfoliation of PMMA cranioplasties have been problematic. Therefore alternatives to PMMA should be sought. This consensus opinion has energized research and development to engineer cementless orthopedic prostheses that osseointegrate. Moreover, therapies that can be mortised and shaped to the irregular, sweeping contours of the craniofacial complex are available, especially as ceramic formulations that offer significant advantages over PMMA. These are presented in a subsequent section.

Polytetrafluoroethylene

Example products of polytetrafluoroethylene (PTFE) include Proplast, Gore-Tex, Teflon, and Medpor. Proplast is a nonbiodegradable, compressive, porous material with a pore size range of 50 to 400 μm and a void volume of 70% to 90%. Proplast HA contains hydroxyapatite. It is marketed for selected onlay procedures that do not involve biofunctional loading. The porous architecture of the PTFE construct combined with HA support fibrovascular ingrowth to sustain localization of the onlay device.

Gore markets a PTFE called Gore-Tex, produced as sheets, ranging from 0.4 mm to 2.0 mm in thickness. Gore-Tex has been used for guided bone regeneration around dental prostheses, for nasal augmentation, and for orbital floor reconstruction.[4,78] Another bone substitute product from Gore is known as SAM and consists of a combination of PTFE and fluorinated ethylene propylene manufactured as a bulk material suitable for carving and customized shaping to augment deficient facial contour.

Medpor is produced by Porex Medical for facial augmentation. It is porous, almost noncompressible, readily carvable, and nonbiodegradable with pores greater than 100 μm in diameter, permitting fibrovascular and bone ingrowth. Zygoma and chin augmentations may be accomplished with Medpor.

Polymethylmethacrylate/Polyhydroxy Ethylmethacrylate (PMMA/PHEMA)

This material is produced by W. Lorenz, manufactured under the name HTR, which stands for hard tissue replacement. A more recent version has been designated HTR-MFI.

HTR-MFI can be manufactured as blocks suitable for carving into shapes to augment anatomic sites, such as the zygomatic buttress and arch, pyriform aperture, chin, and ramus of the mandible. The product is a nonbiodegradable polymer with a porosity range of 250 to 350 μm. Porosity can support bone ingrowth and contour can be sustained because the polymer does not biodegrade. However, a potential liability is the resorption of the bone underneath the implant. A particulate version has been used by dentists to promote bone regeneration of deficient alveolar bone. To date, HTR has been received with muted enthusiasm from the dental community, but as an onlay for aesthetic facial augmentation, there appears to be controlled excitement.[28,29]

Biological Glasses

Two companies produce a therapeutic categorized as a "glass": Bioglass (USBiomaterials, Gainesville, Fla.) and Biogran (Orthovita, Malvern, Penn.). Biologically active glasses have enjoyed limited applications in the craniofacial complex. In a particulate format, they are used predominantly for alveolar bone augmentation associated with dental implants.[30] A recent report mentioned favorable results with biologically active glass in a preclinical orthopedic model.[75] Additional work is warranted in the craniofacial complex with this interesting class of therapeutics.

Collagen

The demineralization of bone by hydrochloric acid yields a product that is predominantly type I collagen and noncollagenous factors. The noncollagenous component containing BMP was studied extensively in the laboratories of Urist and Reddi because of its *osteoinductive* capacity: the ability to promote bone formation at a nonskeletal site (reviewed by Hollinger[45]). Several demineralized bone preparations are available for bone grafting procedures.

Grafton (Osteotech, Eatontown, NJ) is a formulation consisting of particles of demineralized human cortical bone matrix and glycerin that can be expressed through a syringe and placed into deficient alveolar bone around teeth.[61] Periodontal bone regeneration with this formulation has been claimed but poorly verified. Grafton has been used in patients for orbitocranial reconstruction for congenital deformities, orbital fracture repair, and orbital repair after tumor resection.[70] According to the authors, there were no complications and they concluded that properly prepared demineralized bone is safe for orbital reconstruction.[70] Long-term follow-up (5 years or greater) and conclusive objective assessment of the graft sites must be made to validate effectiveness of bone regenerative therapeutics.

There are many tissue banks throughout the United States that supply surgeons with demineralized human cortical bone in particulate formats and as blocks. However, the dental profession has been in the vanguard of clinicians using demineralized bone therapies. Many dentists prefer demineralized bone over substitutes, such as the biologically active glasses and the calcium phosphates (see below). Recent evidence from the dental literature suggests that particles of demineralized bone are poorly suited for periodontal bone regenerative procedures.[5]

Calcium Sulfate

This composition is identified by the familiar name of plaster of Paris. Favorable handling properties of calcium sulfate make it an attractive therapeutic candidate to restore contour to irregularly shaped bone deficiencies.[82] However, a number of significant liabilities with calcium sulfate mitigate against widespread clinical appeal, including an unpredictable biodegradation profile, concerns about biocompatibility, and toxicity. A contemporary generation of calcium-based products will be highlighted; it possesses the favorable handling features of plaster of Paris (i.e., moldability) without its negative features.

Calcium Phosphates

TRICALCIUM PHOSPHATE. This composition of calcium and phosphate presents many attractive possibilities for bone regeneration. Therefore it is curious why it has not become more commonly used. Favorable reports about biocompatibility, biodegradability, and usefulness as an autograft expander emphasize the significant benefits of tricalcium phosphate (TCP).[44] Hapset (Lifecore Biomedical, Chaska, Minn.) is a combination of tricalcium phosphate and calcium sulfate. Its suggested application is in dental extraction sockets; however, bone wounds in the alveolus (i.e., dental extraction sites) regenerate spontaneously and uneventfully without introduction of a foreign material.

Hydroxyapatites

Regarding the hydroxyapatites (HAs), they either do not biodegrade or biodegrade extremely slowly (a duration measured in years). This dogma is being dispelled by clever chemists. Contemporary HA formulations can biodegrade. This represents an unprecedented accomplishment having extensive, beneficial clinical ramifications in light of the fact that HA is probably the most biocompatible calcium-phosphate stoichiometry.

Several companies manufacture granular and block formats of HA consisting of either *laboratory-modified* HA, *bone-derived* HA, or *laboratory produced* HA.

LABORATORY-MODIFIED HA. Products by Interpore Cross International (Irvine, Calif.) are derived from calcium carbonate skeleton coral that are exposed to a sophisticated processing regimen, and through hydrothermal exchange after phosphoric acid processing, the carbonate is replaced with a "bone-like" HA framework endowed with interconnecting pores suitable for bone ingrowth.

Interpore offers a commercial product known as ProOsteon 500 that has FDA approval for repairing metaphyseal defects and ProOsteon 200 granules and blocks for periodontal, preprosthetic, and orthognathic surgery.[109] Persuasive clinical results from these products have prompted preclinical applications for anterior cervical discectomy and fusion[117] and calvaria repair.[88]

BONE-DERIVED HA. Two companies market an HA product derived from bovine-deorganified bone: CeraMed (Lakewood, Colo.) distributes the product OsteoGraf/N, and Osteohealth (Shirley, NY) distributes the product Bio-Oss (Figure 45-4). CeraMed products are prepared from U.S. cow bone, whereas those from Osteohealth are prepared from European cows. A third company, Sulzer (Winterthur, Switzerland), has begun to produce an anorganic bovine derivative. Bovine HA has found a niche in the dental marketplace for augmenting the alveolar ridge and maxillary sinus.[14,94] Craniofacial reconstruction with BioOss has been reported in a limited number of preclinical studies, and observations seem to indicate favorable responses.[54,100] A preclinical study with Bio-Oss recently reported positive results for long bone regeneration.[92]

LABORATORY-PRODUCED HA. CeraMed distributes two variations of particulate HA produced through laboratory chemistry, designated OsteoGraf/LD (for low density) and OsteoGraf/D (identifying this variation as dense). The latter

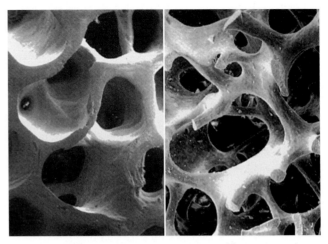

Autogenous   Natural bone mineral
bone mineral   low heat

Figure 45-4. Appearance of autogenous bone and natural bone mineral (BioOss) under scanning electron microscopy. (×50.) (Courtesy Osteohealth Company, Shirley, NY.)

iteration purportedly biodegrades less rapidly than the former. There were no quantitative, dynamic studies available at the time this chapter was prepared detailing the temporal degradation of the OsteoGraf products. Information regarding degradation profiles is clinically important and should be explored.

There has been remarkable progress in the field of calcium phosphate chemistry that will revolutionize prevailing treatment philosophies about the calcium phosphates. Three leading ceramic companies, Leibinger (a division of Stryker Howmedica, Kalamazoo, Mich.), Norian (Cupertino, Calif.), and Etex (Cambridge, Mass.), have independently developed compelling therapeutics that will benefit a wide spectrum of patients.

Leibinger has FDA approval for its product, BoneSource, as a craniofacial therapeutic touted for sinus obturation and cranioplasties with a surface area no larger than 25 cm^2 per defect. A number of excellent, compelling studies have supported the effectiveness of BoneSource.[19,20,57] The clinical appeal for Bone Source is based on its biocompatibility and ease of use in the operating room. Under aseptic conditions in the operating room, the appropriate quantity of water is combined with a known mass of BoneSource powder. A puttylike consistency is developed, and the surgeon has about 15 minutes of working time before the BoneSource (considered an HA *cement*) becomes hard. Another 4 to 6 hours in the host recipient bed is required for the HA to complete its reactive process. BoneSource is actually a composition of tetracalcium-phosphate plus dicalcium phosphate dihydrate[44] that, after curing within the recipient bed, may take a protracted period of time for resorption and subsequent replacement with bone.

Norian is another company marketing an HA cement called NorianSRS (which stands for skeletal replacement system).[21] The product consists of monocalcium phosphate monohydrate, alpha tricalcium phosphate, calcium carbonate, and sodium phosphate[44] and has similar handling properties to BoneSource. NorianSRS is likely to become a popular therapeutic for bone repair; however, it does not resorb, which can be a liability.

Etex is a third company producing HA cements; their product is referred to as alpha BSM (which stands for bone substitute material). In addition to the virtues of BoneSource and NorianSRS, such as biocompatibility and ease of handling, alpha BSM can be tailored to biodegrade. This feature significantly sets this bone cement apart from others. Moreover, an isothermic setting reaction (i.e., heat is not produced) underscores potential clinical superiority of alpha BSM. (Exothermic reactions plaguing certain calcium phosphates and calcium sulfates produce heat, which is deleterious to cells and tissues.) In addition, the spectral profile of alpha BSM is virtually indistinguishable from the HA component of bone.

Collagen-Calcium Phosphate Combination

COLLAGRAFT. Zimmer (Warsaw, Ind.) markets a product (Collagraft Bone Matrix) containing fibrillar collagens and HA/TCP. The collagens are bovine type I dermal collagen (95%) and type III collagen (5%). Collagraft has FDA approval for acute long bone fractures and traumatic osseous defects. Zimmer recommends Collagraft is mixed with bone marrow from the patient. The company clearly advises surgeons to take the appropriate precautions before administering Collagraft, noting potential immunologic problems that may arise in a very small percentage of patients.

Compelling results have been reported with Collagraft in long bone applications[22,23,55,116] and in a preclinical spinal fusion dog model.[118] At the time of preparing this chapter, there have not been any reports in the craniofacial literature with Collagraft.

Bone Morphogenetic Proteins

Spontaneous bone formation, that is, heterotopic osteogenesis at nonosseous sites, was noted by Neuhof[71] in 1917 and by Huggins[47] in 1930, and prompted Levander[60] in 1938 to state: "bone regeneration takes place as a result of some *specific bone formation substance* (emphasis added) activating the nonspecific mesenchymal tissue." In 1965, Urist[104] proposed the concept of *autoinduction* and derived the term *osteoinduction* in 1971: bone formation induced at a nonskeletal site caused by a diffusible protein, which he and Strates[105] called *bone morphogenetic protein*. Nearly 17 years after this seminal work, Wozney et al[108] cloned BMP genes and successfully expressed BMP gene products (Figure 45-5). It is now apparent that multiple BMPs exist; they are responsible for bone regeneration and the direction of embryologic development of cells, tissues, and organs, in addition to performing crucial roles in post fetal physiology.[52,53]

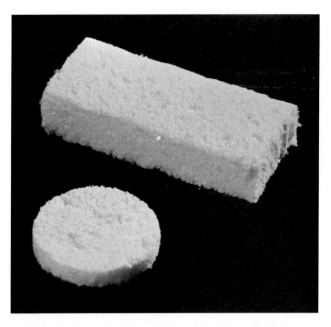

Figure 45-5. Osteoinductive proteins, such as rhBMP, may be imbedded on a d,d-l,l polylactic acid carrier (shown here) and placed into the osseous defect. (Courtesy THM Biomedical, Duluth, Minn.)

MULTIPLE BMPs, CLANS, AND FUNCTIONS. Contemporary literature has identified 15 BMPs, designated BMP-1 through BMP-13 (reviewed by Hollinger et al[45]). Except for BMP-1, the rest belong to the transforming growth factor-beta (TGF-β) family.[16,17,79,112] TGF-β is categorized as a superfamily that includes TGF-β-5, 15 BMPs (excluding BMP-1), the growth-differentiating factors (GDF-1 to GDF-10),[73] the inhibins, activins, Vg-related genes, nodal-related genes, Drosophila genes (e.g., dpp, 60A), and glial-derived neurotropic factor.[43,52,85]

It is becoming clear that BMPs are involved with a spectrum of functional activities, spanning embryogenesis to postnatal tissue repair. Apparently, groups of BMPs work synchronously in an organizational hierarchy that determines dorsal ventral orientation, the location of limbs, the number of bones in a limb, and their sizes.[98,101] Moreover, BMPs are associated with nonskeletal tissues and organs, including liver, brain, kidney, muscle, and spleen; however, details on the functional significance at these sites remains to be determined.[97,103,106]

CLINICAL ISSUES. Oncologic and pathologic conditions in the presence of BMPs casts a sinister shadow over an exciting clinical therapeutic. This issue merits clinical concern in light of the fact that administered doses of BMP are manyfold greater than levels encountered developmentally and endogenously. It is noteworthy, however, that BMPs are cell-differentiating factors rather than factors promoting or sustaining cell transformation. Moreover, to date, there have not been any reports of either oncologic or pathologic responses from BMPs.

Another clinical issue is whether BMPs will promote

preferential responses in bone derived from different embryologic pathways. Preclinical studies have been accomplished in endochondral and intramembranous bone with persuasive results.

Currently, one clinical study describing rhBMP-2 has been published.[9] In the study, the maxillary sinuses in 12 patients were treated with a collagen sponge and rhBMP-2 to promote bone formation suitable for dental implants.[9] Observations after 16 weeks appeared to indicate a satisfactory prosthetic result; however, a realistic long-term assessment must be made.

OUTCOMES

The field of bone repair and bone regeneration is rapidly changing. Many options are available at this writing that were not available a few years ago. A case in point would be mandible reconstruction for congenital deformities. Although a rib graft may be used for a specific deformity, such as mandibular ramus reconstruction, now with the option for distraction osteogenesis, specific treatment may be tailored to individual requirements. Outcome studies are important and help focus treatment in a cost-effective and efficacious manner. Discussion of specific treatment outcomes regarding complications, aesthetic results, function, quality of life, economics, and patient satisfaction for each individual site in the craniofacial skeleton is beyond the scope of this chapter, and we defer to the authors of the individual chapters.

Many materials and techniques for bone regeneration are presented throughout this chapter. Some of them have been well received by reconstructive surgeons and others are still undergoing further clinical studies. Each method requires close evaluation and follow-up in the postoperative period.

POSTOPERATIVE CARE FOR CRANIOFACIAL DEFECTS

Management should continue with close follow-up to evaluate the craniofacial reconstruction with clinical examination and films by the multidisciplinary team. Clinical examination will allow aesthetic and skeletal stability evaluation. Plain radiographs and three-dimensional CT scans also assist with evaluation of reconstructed segments, which may lead to further intervention. Postoperative failure can occur by several means. Loss of skeletal stability promotes motion at the osseous wound and thus potentiates poor vascularization. Other means of vascular impairment can lead to a soft tissue interface preventing osseous healing. Inflammation at the interface can be due to bacterial seeding or alloplastic implant mobility, which can promote resorption, soft tissue breakdown, and possibly implant extrusion.[35] Further surgical intervention may require débridement, reestablishment of rigid fixation, implant removal, and further staged operations.

SUMMARY

Many new materials and techniques are under investigation, and these alternatives may offer advantages, especially in cases of limited donor autogenous bone. Bone substitutes have constituted one arena of reconstructive advancement, and the osteoinductive bone morphogenetic proteins will play an important role as clinical trials continue. Distraction osteogenesis and guided bone regeneration research have also provided a second advancement for reconstructive surgery. It is possible that a combination of these advancements will allow for optimal bone regeneration in human craniofacial reconstruction.

ACKNOWLEDGMENTS

The authors would like to express their gratitude for the technical and scholarly contributions of their colleagues. Special thanks are extended by the authors to associates at Oregon Health Sciences University. Financial support for JOH and for some of the work described was from the National Institutes of Health (NIAMSD:R01-HD31451 and NIDR:R01-DE11416).

REFERENCES

1. Alberius P, Dahlin C, Linde A: Role of osteopromotion in experimental bone grafting to the skull: a study in adult rats using a membrane technique, *J Oral Maxillofac Surg* 50:829-834, 1992.
2. Altobelli DE, Kikinis R, Mulliken JB, et al: Computer-assisted three dimensional planning in craniofacial surgery, *Plast Reconstr Surg* 92:576-585, 1993.
3. Aronson J: Experimental and clinical experience with distraction osteogenesis, *Cleft Palate Craniofac J* 31:473-480, 1994.
4. Aronson J: The biology of mechanical distraction osteogenesis. In Bianchi Maiocchi A, Aronson J, editors: *Operative principles of Ilizarov-fracture treatment, nonunion, osteomyelitis, lengthening, deformity correction,* Baltimore, 1991, Williams & Wilkins.
5. Becker W, Becker B, Caffesse RA: A comparison of demineralized freeze-dried bone and autologous bone to induce bone formation in human extraction sockets, *J Periodontol* 1994;65:1128-1133, 1994.
6. Bellows CG, Heersche JN, Aubin JE: Determination of the capacity for proliferation and differentiation of osteoprogenitor cells in the presence and absence of dexamethasone, *Dev Biol* 1990:132-138, 1990.
7. Bianchi Maiocchi A, Aronson J: Indications. In Bianchi Maiocchi A, Aronson J, editors: *Operative principles of Ilizarov-fracture treatment, nonunion, osteomyelitis, lengthening, deformity correction,* Baltimore, 1991, Williams & Wilkins.
8. Bosch C, Birte M, Vargervik K: Guided bone regeneration in calvarial bone defects using polytetrafluoroethylene membranes, *Cleft Palate Craniofac J* 32:311-317, 1995.

9. Boyne PJ, Marx RE, Nevins M, et al: A feasibility study evaluation rhBMP-2/absorbable collagen sponge for maxillary sinus augmentation, *Int J Periodont Restor Dent* 17:11-25, 1997.

10. Brighton CT, Lorich DG, Kupcha R, et al: The pericyte as a possible osteoblast progenitor cell, *Clin Orthop* 275:287-299, 1992.

11. Brownell AG: Osteogenesis inhibitory protein: a preview, *Connect Tissue Res* 24:13-16, 1990.

12. Buser D, Bragger U, Lang NP, et al: Regeneration and enlargement of jaw bone using guided tissue regeneration. *Clinical Oral Implant Research* 1:22-32, 1990.

13. Caffesse R, Quinones CR: Guided tissue regeneration: biologic rationale, surgical technique, and clinical results, *Compendium* 13:166-178, 1992.

14. Callahan DP, Rohrer MD: Use of bovine-derived hydroxyapatite in the treatment of edentulous ridge defects: a human clinical and histologic case report, *Am Acad Periodontol* 64:575-581, 1993.

15. Campbell JT, Kaplan F: The role of morphogens in endochondral ossification, *Calcif Tissue Int* 50:283-289, 1992.

16. Celeste AJ, Song JJ, Cox K, et al: Bone morphogenetic protein-9, a new member of the TGF-β superfamily, *J Bone Miner Res* 9:S137, 1994.

17. Celeste AJ, Taylor R, Yamaji N, et al: Molecular cloning of BMP-8: Present in bovine bone which is highly related to BMP-5/6/7 subfamily of osteoinductive molecules, *Keystone Symposium* 100, 1992.

18. Chin M, Toth BA: Distraction osteogenesis in maxillofacial surgery using internal devices: review of five cases, *J Oral Maxillofac Surg* 54:45-53, 1996.

19. Constantino P, Friedman C, Jones K, et al: Experimental hydroxyapatite cement cranioplasty, *Plast Reconstr Surg* 90: 174-185, 1992.

20. Constantino PD, Friedman CD, Lane A: Synthetic biomaterials in facial plastic and reconstructive surgery, *Facial Plastic Surgery* 9:1-15, 1993.

21. Constantz BR, Ison IC, Fulmer MT, et al: Skeletal repair by in situ formation of the mineral phase of bone, *Science* 267:1796-1799, 1995.

22. Cornell CN: Current assessment of fracture healing. In Brighton CT, Freidlander GE, Lane JM, editors: *Bone formation and repair*, Rosemont, Ill, 1994, American Academy of Orthopaedic Surgeons.

23. Cornell CN, Lane JM, Chapman M, et al: Multicenter trial of Collagraft as a bone substitute, *J Orthop Trauma* 5:1-8, 1991.

24. Coulier F, Pontarotti P, Roubin R, et al: Of worms and men: an evolutionary perspective on the fibroblast growth factor (FGF) and FGF receptor families, *J Mol Evol* 44:43-56, 1997.

25. Dahlin C, Linde A, Gottlow J, et al: Healing of bone defects by guided tissue regeneration, *Plast Reconstr Surg* 81:672-676, 1988.

26. Dal Monte A, Donzelli O: Tibial lengthening according to Ilizarov in congenital hypoplasia of the leg, *J Pediatr Orthop* 7:135-138, 1987.

27. David DJ, Hemmy DC, Cooter RD: Craniofacial deformities. In *Atlas of three dimensional reconstructions from computed tomography,* New York, 1990, Springer Verlag.

28. Eppley BL, Sadove M: Aesthetic facial applications of HTR polymer grafts: experimental and clinical results, *Int J Aesthet Reconstr Surg* 2:111-118, 1994.

29. Eppley BL, Sadove AM, German RZ: Evaluation of HTR polymer as a craniomaxillofacial graft material, *Plast Reconstr Surg* 86:1085-1092, 1990.

30. Fetner AE, Hartigan MS, Low SB: Periodontal repair using PerioGlas in nonhuman primates: clinical and histological observations, *Compend Contin Educ Dent* 15:935-938, 1994.

31. Folkman J, Klagsburn M: Angiogenic factors, *Science* 235: 442-447, 1987.

32. Folkman J, Klagsburn M, Sasse J, et al: A heparin-binding angiogenic protein—basic fibroblast growth factor—is stored within basement membrane, *Am J Pathol* 130:393-400, 1988.

33. Francis PH, Richardson MK, Brickell PM, et al: Bone morphogenetic proteins and a signalling pathway that controls patterning in the developing chick limb, *Development* 120: 209-218, 1994.

34. Friedlaender G: Bone banking and clinical applications, *Transplant Proc* 17:99-104, 1985.

35. Friedman CD, Costantino PD: General concepts in craniofacial skeletal augmentation and replacement, *Otolaryngol Clin North Am* 27:847-857, 1994.

36. Gottlow J, Laurell L, Rylander H, et al: Treatment of infrabony defects in monkey with bioresorbable and non-resorbable guided tissue regeneration devices, *J Dent Res* 72:206, 1993 (abstract).

37. Gottlow J, Lundgren D, Nyman S, et al: New attachment formation in the monkey using GUIDOR®, a bioabsorbable GTR-device, *J Dent Res* 71:297, 1992 (abstract).

38. Gottlow J, Nyman S, Karring T: New attachment formation as the result of controlled tissue regeneration, *J Clin Periodontol* 11:494-503, 1984.

39. Habal MB: Bone grafting in craniofacial surgery, *Clin Plast Surg* 1994;21:349-363, 1994 (review).

40. Hall BK, Miyake T: The membranous skeleton: the role of cell condensations in vertebrate skeletogenesis, *Anat Embryol* 186:107-124, 1992.

41. Hanson LJ, Donovan MG, Hellstein JW, et al: Experimental evaluation of expanded polytetrafluoroethylene for reconstruction of orbital floor defects, *J Oral Maxillofac Surg* 52:1050-1055, 1994.

42. Hardesty RA, Marsh JL: Craniofacial onlay bone grafting: a prospective evaluation of graft morphology, orientation, and embryonic origin, *Plast Reconstr Surg* 85:5-14, 1990.

43. Hogan LB: Bone morphogenetic proteins in development, *Curr Opin Genet Dev* 1996;6:432-438, 1996.

44. Hollinger JO, Brekke J, Gruskin E, et al: The role of bone substitutes, *Clin Orthop* 324:55-65, 1996.

45. Hollinger JO, Buck DC, Bruder S: Biology of bone healing: its impact on clinical therapy. In Lynch S, editor: *Tissue engineering in dentistry,* San Diego, 1999, Quintessence.

46. Huerzeler MB, Quinones CR, Schuepback P, et al: Treatment of furcated molars in monkeys with a synthetic bioabsorble barrier, *J Dent Res* 73:380, 1994 (abstract).

47. Huggins CB: Experimental osteogenesis—influence of urinary tract mucosa on the experimental formation of bone, *Proc Soc Exp Biol Med* 27:349-353, 1930.

48. Ilizarov GA: The tension-stress effect on the genesis and growth of tissues. Part I, *Clin Orthop* 238:249-281, 1989.

49. Ilizarov GA: The tension-stress effect on the genesis and growth of tissues. Part II, *Clin Orthop* 239:263-285, 1989.

50. Ilizarov GA: The principles of the Ilizarov method, *Bull Hosp Jt Dis* 48:1-11, 1988.

51. Karp NS, Thorne CHM, McCarthy JG: Bone lengthening in the craniofacial skeleton, *Ann Plast Surg* 24:2, 1990.

52. Kingsley D: What do BMPs do in mammals? Clues from the mouse short-ear mutation, *Trends Genet* 10:16-21, 1994.

53. Kingsley DM: The TGF-beta superfamily: new members, new receptors, and new genetic tests of function in different organisms, *Genes Dev* 8:133-146, 1994.

54. Klinge B, Alberius P, Isaksson S, et al: Osseous response to implanted natural bone mineral and synthetic hydroxylapatite ceramic in the repair of experimental skull bone defects, *J Oral Maxillofac Surg* 50:241-249, 1992.

55. Kocialkowski A, Wallace WA, Prince HG: Clinical experience with a new artificial bone graft: preliminary results of a prospective study, *Injury* 21:142-144, 1990.

56. Kusiak JF, Zins JE, Whitaker LA: The early revascularization of membranous bone, *Plast Reconstr Surg* 76:510-514, 1985.

57. Kveton JF, Friedman CD, Constantino PD: Indications for hydroxyapatite cement reconstruction in lateral skull base surgery, *Am J Otolaryngol* 16:465-469, 1995.

58. Laufer E, Nelson CE, Johnson RL, et al: Sonic hedgehog and Fgf-4 act through a signaling cascade and feedback loop to integrate growth and patterning of the developing limb bud, *Cell* 79:993-1003, 1994.

59. Laurell L, Falk H, Fornell J, et al: Clinical use of a bioresorbable matrix barrier in guided tissue regeneration therapy, *J Periodontol* 65:967-975, 1994.

60. Levander G: A study of bone regeneration, *Surg Gynecol Obstet* 67:705-714, 1938.

61. Levin SS, Prewett AB, Cook SD: The use of a new form of allograft bone in implantation or osseointegrated dental implants—a preliminary report, *J Oral Implantol* 18:366-371, 1992.

62. Marx RE, Kline SN: Principles and methods of osseous reconstruction, *International Advances in Surgical Oncology* 6:167-228, 1983.

63. Mayer M, Ellenbogen R, Hollinger J, et al: Rigid skeletal fixation of the immature craniofacial skeleton in the non-human primate, *International Conference of Craniofacial Surgery* 1995 (abstract).

64. McCarthy JG: Discussion: distraction osteogenesis in maxillofacial surgery using internal devices: review of five cases, *J Oral Maxillofac Surg* 54:54, 1996.

65. McCarthy JG: Commentary on distraction osteogenesis: experimental and clinical experience with distraction osteogenesis, *Cleft Palate Craniofac J* 31:481-482, 1994.

66. McCarthy JG, Schreiber J, Karp N, et al: Lenthening the human mandible by gradual distraction, *Plast Reconstr Surg* 89:1-8, 1992.

67. Meek'ren JJV: Observations, *Medico-Chirurgicaae* 6, 1668.

68. Melcher AH, Dreyer CJ: Protection of the blood clot in healing circumscribed bone defects, *J Bone Joint Surg* 44:424-430, 1962.

69. Michieli S, Miotti B: Lengthening of mandibular body by gradual surgical orthodontic distraction, *J Oral Surg* 35:187, 1977.

70. Neigel JM, Ruzicka PO: Use of demineralized bone implants in orbital and craniofacial reconstruction and a review of the literature, *Ophthal Plast Reconstr Surg* 12:108-120, 1996.

71. Neuhof H: Fascia transplantation into visceral defects, *Surg Gynecol Obstetr* 24:383-427, 1917.

72. Newman SA: Lineage and patterning in the developing vertebrate limb, *Trends Genet* 4:329-332, 1988.

73. Nishitoh H, Ichijo H, Kimura M, et al: Identification of type I and type II serine/threonine kinase receptors for growth/differentiation factor-5, *J Biol Chem* 271:21345-21352, 1996.

74. Nyman S, Gottlow J, Lindhe J, et al: New attachment formation by guided tissue regeneration, *J Periodonl Res* 22:252-254, 1987.

75. Onishi H, Kushitani S, Yasukawa E, et al: Particulate bioglass compared with hydroxyapatite as a bone graft substitute, *Clin Orthop* 334:316-325, 1997.

76. O'Reilly MS, Holmgren L, Sing Y, et al: Angiostatin: a novel angiogenesis inhibitor that mediates the suppression of metastasis by a Lewis lung sarcoma, *Cell* 79:315-328, 1994.

77. Owen M: Lineage of osteogenic cells and their relationship to the stromal system. In Peck WA, editor: *Bone and mineral research,* Amsterdam, 1985, Elsevier Science Publishers.

78. Owsley TG, Taylor CO: The use of Gore-Tex for nasal augmentation: a retrospective analysis of 106 patients, *J Plast Reconstr Surg* 94:241-248, 1994.

79. Özkaynak E, Schnegelsberg PN, Jin DF, et al: Osteogenic protein-2. A new member of the transforming growth factor-beta superfamily expressed in early embryogenesis, *J Biol Chem* 267:25220-25227, 1992.

80. Paley D: Current techniques of limb lengthening, *Journal of Pediatric Orthopedics* 8:73-92, 1988.

81. Paralkar VM, Weeks BS, Yu MY, et al: Recombinant human bone morphogenetic protein 2B stimulates PC12 cell differentiation: potentiation and binding to type IV collagen, *J Cell Biol* 119:1721-1728, 1992.

82. Peltier LF: The use of plaster of Paris to fill defects in bone, *Clin Orthop* 21:1-31, 1961.

83. Quinones CR, Caffesse RG: Current status of guided periodontal tissue regeneration, *Periodontology 2000* 9:55-68, 1995.

84. Quinones CR, Huerzeler MB, Schuepback P, et al: Treatment of infrabony defects in monkeys with a synthetic bioabsorbable barrier, *J Dent Res* 73:380, 1994 (abstract).

85. Reddi AH: Bone and cartilage morphogenesis: cell biology to clinical applications, *Curr Opin Genet Dev* 4:737-744, 1994.

86. Reddi AH, Kuettner KE: Vascular invasion of cartilage: correlation of morphology with lysozyme, glycosaminoglycans, and protease-inhibitory activity during endochondral bone formation, *Dev Biol* 82:217-223, 1981.

87. Riddle RD, Johnson R, Laufer E, et al: Sonic hedgehog mediates the polarizing activity of the ZPA, *Cell* 75:1401-1416, 1993.

88. Ripamonti U, Ma SS, Reddi AH: Induction of bone in composites of osteogenin and porous hydroxyapatite in baboons, *Plast Reconstr Surg* 89:731-739, 1992.

89. Rose EH, Norris MS, Rosen JM: Application of high-tech three-dimensional imaging and computer-generated models in complex facial reconstructions with vascularized bone grafts, *Plast Reconstr Surg* 91:252-264, 1993.

90. Rosen V, Nove J, Song JJ, et al: Responsiveness of clonal limb bud cell lines to bone morphogenetic protein-2 reveals a sequential relationship between cartilage and bone cell phenotypes, *J Bone Miner Res* 9:1759-1768, 1994.

91. Scantlebury TV: 1982-1992: a decade of technology development for guided tissue regeneration, *J Periodontol* 64:1129-1137, 1993.

92. Schmitt JM, Buck DC, Joh SP, et al: Comparison of porous bone mineral and biologically active glass in critical-sized defects, *J Periodontol* 68:1043-1053, 1977.

93. Schmitz JP, Hollinger JO: The critical size defect as an experimental model for craniomandibulofacial nonunions, *Clin Orthop* 205:299, 1986.

94. Smiler DG, Johnson PW, Lozada JL, et al: Sinus lift grafts and endosseous implants, *Dent Clin North Am* 36:151-186, 1992.

95. Smith JD, Abramson M: Membranous vs endochondral bone autografts, *Arch Otolaryngol* 99:203-205, 1974.

96. Snyder CC, Levine GA, Swanson HM, et al: Mandibular lengthening by gradual distraction: preliminary report, *Plast Reconstr Surg* 51:506, 1973.

97. Song JJ, Celeste A, Kong FM, et al: Bone morphogenetic protein-9 binds to liver cells and stimulates proliferation, *Endocrinology* 136:4293-4297, 1995.

98. Storm EE, Huynh TV, Copeland NG, et al: Limb alterations in brachypodism mice due to mutations in a new member of the TGF-beta superfamily, *Nature* 368:639-643, 1994.

99. Taylor S, Folkman J: Protamine is an inhibitor of angiogenesis, *Nature* 297:307-312, 1982.

100. Thaller SR, Hoyt J, Borjeson K, et al: Reconstruction of calvarial defects with anorganic bovine bone mineral (Bio-Oss®) in a rabbit model, *J Craniofac Surg* 4:79-84, 1993.

101. Tickle C: On making a skeleton, *Nature* 368:587-588, 1994.

102. Tomford W: Current concepts review. Transmission of disease through transplantation of musculoskeletal allografts, *J Bone Joint Surg* 77-A:1742-1754, 1995.

103. Tomizawa K, Matsui H, Kondo E, et al: Developmental alteration and neuron-specific expression of bone morphogenetic protein-6 (BMP-6) mRNA in rodent brain, *Mol Brain Res* 28:122-128, 1995.

104. Urist MR: Bone: formation by autoinduction, *Science* 150:893-899, 1965.

105. Urist MR, Strates BS: Bone morphogenetic protein, *J Dent Res* 50:1392-1406, 1971.

106. Vukicevic S, Kopp J, Luton FP, et al: Induction of nephrogenic mesenchyme by osteogenic protein 1 (bone morphogenetic protein 7), *Proc Natl Acad Sci USA* 93:9021-9026, 1996.

107. Wang EA, Isreal DL, Luxenberg DP: Bone morphogenetic protein-2 causes commitment and differentiation in C3H10T1/2 and 3T3 cells, *Growth Factors* 9:57-71, 1993.

108. Wang EA, Rosen V, Cordes P, et al: Purification and characterization of other distinct bone-inducing factors, *Proc Natl Acad Sci USA* 85:9484-9488, 1988.

109. White E, Shors EC: Biomaterial aspects of Interpore 200 porous hydroxyapatite, *Dent Clin North Am* 30:49-66, 1986.

110. Woodburne RT, Crelin ES, Kaplan FS: *Musculoskeletal system,* Summit, NJ, 1994, Ciba-Geigy Corp.

111. Wozney J: Bone morphogenetic proteins and their expression. In Noda M, editor: *Cellular and molecular biology of bone,* San Diego, 1993, Academic Press.

112. Wozney JM, Rosen V, Celeste AJ, et al: Novel regulators of bone formation: molecular clones and activities, *Science* 242:1528, 1988.

113. Yaremchuk MJ: Experimental studies addressing rigid fixation in craniofacial surgery, *Clin Plast Surg* 21:517-524, 1994 (review).

114. Yaremchuk MJ, Fiala TGS, Barker F, et al: The effect of rigid fixation on craniofacial growth in rhesus monkeys, *Plast Reconstr Surg* 93:1-10, 1994.

115. Yaremchuk MJ, Gruss JS, Manson PN, editors: *Rigid fixation of the craniomaxillofacial skeleton,* Boston, 1992, Butterworth-Heinemann.

116. Zardiackas LD, Teasdall RD, Black J, et al: Torsional properties of healed canine diaphyseal defects grafted with fibrillar collagen and hydroxyapatite/tricalcium phosphate composite, *J Appl Biomat* 5:277-283, 1994.

117. Zdeblick TA, Cooke ME, Kunz DN, et al: Anterior cervical discectomy and fusion using a porous hydroxyapatite bone graft substitute, *Spine* 19:2348-2357, 1994.

118. Zerwekh JE, Kourosh S, Scheinberg R, et al: Fibrillar collagen-biphasic calcium phosphate composite as a bone graft substitute for spinal fusion, *J Orthop* 10:562-572, 1992.

119. Zins JE, Whitaker L: Membranous versus endochondral bone: implications for craniofacial reconstruction, *J Plast Reconstr Surg* 72:778-784, 1983.

CHAPTER

Distraction Osteogenesis: Remodeling the Hypoplastic Mandible

Fernando Molina

INTRODUCTION

Mandibular hypoplasia is a current problem in craniofacial and maxillofacial surgery, and its correction is crucial for the final aesthetic results.[2,5,6,8,13-15] Mandibular hypoplasia, unilateral or bilateral, may result from disturbed embryogenesis or may be acquired as a sequela of condylar fractures suffered at an early age with secondary ankylosis of the temporomandibular joint.

Bone lengthening, or distraction osteogenesis using osteotomies and circumferential gradual distraction, was described by Ilizarov in 1954 to align fracture segments of long bones and later to elongate these bones avoiding the use of bone grafts.[3,4] Although initially the technique was developed to lengthen the long bones, not until 1973 did Snyder,[17] using an extraoral device, reported mandibular lengthening in a canine model, and a similar report on two dogs using an intraoral device followed from Italy.[10] More recently, Karp and McCarthy[7] reported membranous bone lengthening with external devices and found that cortical bone formed in the expanded area of the mandible. Histologic examination of the zone revealed a highly organized biologic process. In 1992, McCarthy et al[9] presented their preliminary clinical results, in which they successfully elongated the mandible in four young patients using a bicortical osteotomy and a rigid external fixator.

INDICATIONS

In Mexico since 1990, I have been performing mandibular distraction using external corticotomy and flexible unidirec-
tional and bidirectional external devices to achieve simultaneous skeletal and soft tissue correction with minimal surgery.[11,12] My philosophy is to elongate and remodel the hypoplastic mandible. During the last 6 years, 234 mandibular corticotomies and distractions have been performed: 192 patients with hemifacial microsomia (HM) and 42 patients with micrognathia (Treacher Collins syndrome, Pierre Robin syndrome, and Nager's syndrome).

In the HM group, the age varied from 2 to 17 years old, 110 patients were female and 82 male, and the mandibular hypoplasia has been classified according to the Pruzanski's[16] and Murray and Mulliken's[14] system: grade I, in which the hypoplasia affects only the gonial angle; grade II-A, in which the angle and the ascending ramus are affected; and grade II-B, in which the hypoplasia more severely affects the angle and ascending ramus, which has a flat and rudimentary condyle (Figure 46-1). In patients with grade III, who show a complete absence of the ramus and condyle, mandibular distraction is not indicated.

OPERATIONS

Preoperatively lateral and anteroposterior (AP) cephalometric studies are done. Panorex views are used to compare both sides of the mandible and to locate the tooth buds and dental nerve to avoid their injury during surgery. In the first cases the superimposing method of Björk[1] was used to obtain a mandibular growth prediction, to assess the ideal dimension of the mandible, and to reproduce the rotational movements (anterior and posterior) that it performed during growth.

Under general anesthesia a 3-cm incision is made on the lateral vestibule oral mucosa. A subperiosteal dissection is performed, exposing the gonial angle and the neighboring area of the ascending ramus. The site of the planned external corticotomy and of the pin insertion is marked with gentian violet, avoiding the nerve and the tooth buds.

The corticotomy is done with a side cutting burr. Beginning at the retromolar angle, its medial and lateral buttress are cut, followed by the lateral aspect of the mandibular angle, including all of the cortex to the cancellous layer. Inferiorly, the corticotomy is extended widely around the angle, where the bone is very thick. Only 6 to 8 mm of the internal cortical layer remains intact, protecting the nerve and artery. In fact, different zones of bone resistance are encountered: minor resistance at the angle and major resistance at the alveolar ridge, which will be elongated differently under a perpendicular distraction vector (Figure 46-2). The orientation of the corticotomy and the position of the pins will determine the distraction vector. The distraction vector is different in each patient according to the grade of mandibular hypoplasia (Figure 46-3).

PROCEDURE IN HEMIFACIAL MICROSOMIA

In patients with grade I HM, the corticotomy extends obliquely from the posterior edge of the hypoplastic gonial angle to the retromolar angle in the alveolar ridge. The pins must be placed perpendicular to the corticotomy, obtaining an oblique vector distraction that produces a larger bone elongation in the angle and a minor bone elongation in the alveolar ridge.

In patients with grade II-A HM, the distraction process must remodel and elongate the angle and the initial portion of the ascending ramus. For this reason the corticotomy is placed obliquely at the junction of the angle and ramus and the pins must be inserted in an intermediate position between a vertical and oblique vector distraction. In patients with grade II-B HM, the corticotomy is placed horizontally at the base of the ascending ramus and the pins must follow a vertical vector distraction to obtain more elongation in the hypoplastic ascending ramus.

Two stainless steel screws, 2.0 to 3.5 mm in diameter (age depending), are introduced percutaneously through the whole thickness of the mandible 3 to 5 mm in front of and behind the corticotomy. The diamond tip design of the pins makes it unnecessary to drill a hole before its introduction in the bone. Care must be taken to position the pins parallel to each other and facilitate their fixation to the distraction device.

The mucosa is closed with a fine absorbable suture, and the distraction device is applied. This is made of two hollow plates with a central perforation to allow the entrance of the mandibular pins. The two plates are joined by another stainless steel screw running free in one of them and transversing the whole length of the plate at the other, so when it is turned, the distance between the plates is increased or decreased (Figure 46-4). The steel resistance of the distractor device is softer than the pins; this produces a flexible device that can bend under the

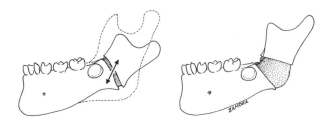

Figure 46-2. Diagram of the elongated and remodeled mandible. The corticotomy extended widely around the angle and has produced different zones of bone resistance. Two pins were introduced through the full thickness of the mandible. Bone elongation was more pronounced at the angle and less at the retromolar triangle.

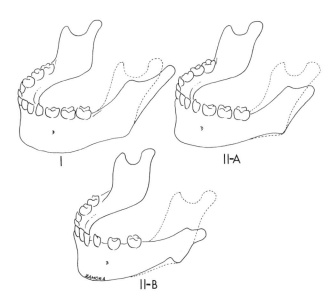

Figure 46-1. Grades of bone hypoplasia in hemifacial microsomia according to Pruzansky and Murray and Mulliken classification, in which mandibular distraction is indicated.

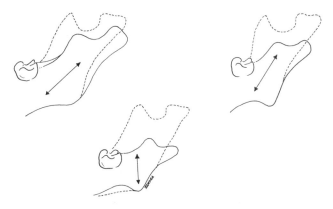

Figure 46-3. The distraction vector is different in each grade of bony hypoplasia. The mark in the mandibular angle shows the different vectors. Notice the vertical position in grade II-B.

masticatory muscle action and externally reflects the shape of the elongated area.

I start the elongation at the fifth postoperative day (latency period) at a rate of about 1 mm per day (rhythm). This is done by the patient's parents with minimal discomfort. The elongation is usually completed in 3 to 4 weeks (distraction period), and the device is left in place for 6 to 8 weeks more (consolidation period) until radiologic evidence of new cortical bone formation is found. At that time the screws are removed under sedation.

PROCEDURE IN MICROGNATHIA

The patients with micrognathia present a different bone hypoplasia problem from patients with HM. In these patients the deformity is bilateral and both the mandibular body and the ascending ramus are affected. For this reason, micrognathic patients require a bilateral and bidirectional distraction. This concept is also true for patients with Treacher Collins, Pierre Robin, Nager's, and bilateral microsomia syndromes.

In this group, two corticotomies are done, one vertical in the mandibular body and the other horizontal in the ascending ramus. Three pins are used: a central one is introduced at the mandibular angle between the two corticotomies, a second into the mandibular body, and a third into the central aspect of

the ascending ramus. One bidirectional device is used on each side, each one with two distraction plates to allow independent and more precise elongation of each segment, using the central pin as the fixed pivot for both of them (Figure 46-5).

Measurements of the distance between the pins and soft tissue structures (external canthus–buccal commissure and the inferior orbital rim–buccal commissure) are recorded weekly. Dental casts and x-rays are taken at the end of the distraction period and 6 to 8 weeks later to assess osteogenesis at the site of the corticotomy and occlusal changes. The results of mandibular distraction are evaluated at the end of the distraction period, at the time of removal of the device (end of the consolidation period), and subsequently every 6 months.

OUTCOMES

In patients with grade I HM, the elongation varied from 12 to 18 mm (mean 16 mm). Dental occlusion remained stable without posterior open bite. No active functional orthodontic appliances were used. The aesthetic results were excellent, the facial symmetry was restored with descent of the buccal commissure to the level of the contralateral one, and the menton became horizontal and located at the midline. The long-term follow-up shows stable results clinically and occlusally.

In grade II-A HM, mandibular elongation ranged from 14 to 22 mm (mean 19 mm). The dental occlusion was disrupted, and a contralateral crossbite and a posterior open bite of 1 to

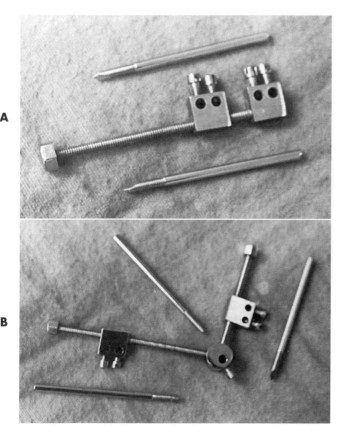

Figure 46-4. A, The unidirectional external device. **B,** The bidirectional external device.

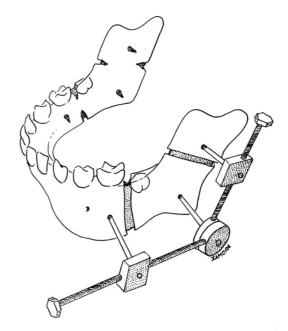

Figure 46-5. Diagram showing two corticotomies for bidirectional elongation. A central screw introduced at the angle serves as a pivot for independent vertical and horizontal distraction.

3 mm were produced in half of the patients. Posterior bite blocks and dynamic orthodontic appliances were used to maintain the elongation and to stabilize the occlusion. The aesthetic results were excellent with restoration of facial symmetry and horizontalization of the chin and the buccal commissure (Figure 46-6).

The group of patients with grade II-B HM characteristically had a stable but incorrect dental occlusion with marked deviation of the mandibular midline teeth to the affected side. During the distraction, bite blocks were required to maintain the posterior open bite; the blocks were gradually reduced to allow vertical maxillary growth. Dynamic orthodontic appliances were also used in all of the patients at an early stage. After the distraction the initial occlusion was reproduced in the opposite direction on the contralateral side as a result of overcorrection. The aesthetic improvement and the restoration of symmetry have also been impressive in these patients.

In the patients with micrognathia, 6 to 9 mm of vertical elongation of the ramus and a 10-to 16-mm increase in length of the mandibular body were obtained. Dental occlusion was acceptable in most of the cases. Eleven of the posttrauma cases were asymmetric, requiring more elongation on one side, which was easily achieved because the distraction was manipulated in two different directions on both sides, all independent from each other. The aesthetic results were excellent with improved gonial angle, good projection of the chin, and remarkable expansion of the soft tissues of the lower face and upper neck (Figure 46-7).

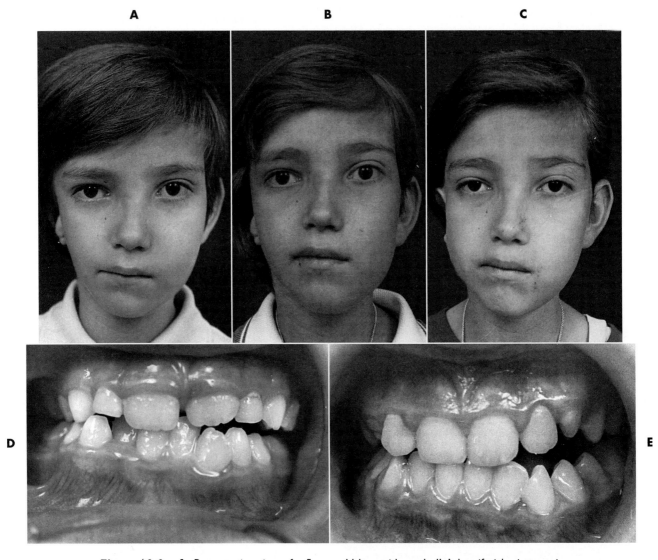

Figure 46-6. **A,** Preoperative view of a 5-year-old boy with grade II-A hemifacial microsomia showing facial asymmetry with deviation of the buccal commissure and the chin. **B,** Six months after the removal of the pins showing descent of the buccal commissure and medialization of the chin. **C,** Four years later with stable facial symmetry. **D,** Preoperative dental occlusion of the patient. **E,** Postoperative view showing overcorrection with displacement of the incisors midline to the right. *Continued*

Mandibular distraction has been extremely benign for the patients. Morbidity is limited to the presence of skin scars slightly enlarged by the distraction, which have evolved satisfactorily with time and no revisions have been necessary.

On the temporomandibular joint, no symptom of functional disruption has been detected; however, from x-ray studies I have observed in the unidirectional cases, the condylar head uprighted and increased in size and volume, and because of the bone remodeling in the gonial angle, the condyle laterally displaced moves to a medial and correct position that resembles the contralateral side. This change in condylar morphology occurred during the consolidation period. The contralateral unexpanded condyle maintained its size and shape and did not show evidence of deformational changes.

SUMMARY

Distraction osteogenesis is a technique that is becoming more common for the reconstruction of deficient mandibles and has simplified the treatment for congenital mandibular hypoplasia. Technically, it is a minor surgical procedure preserving the integrity of the nerve and vascular supply. Careful planning of the corticotomy and the position of the pins produces a vector distraction that follows closely the direction of normal mandibular growth.

An enormously important benefit of bone distraction is the simultaneous expansion of the soft tissues of the face (skin, muscles, fascia, vessels, and nerves). In fact, we were surprised

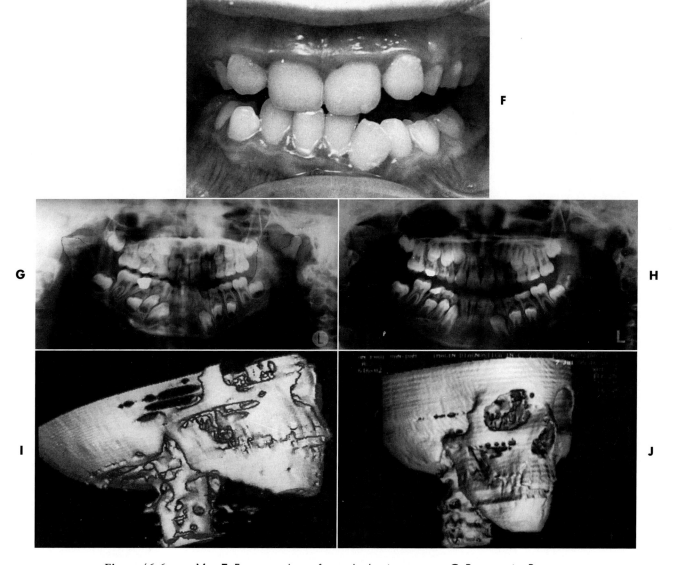

Figure 46-6, cont'd. **F,** Four years later after orthodontic treatment. **G,** Preoperative Panorex view of the patient. **H,** One year later showing the final elongation and remodeling of the angle and ascending ramus. **I,** Preoperative tridimensional reconstruction of the mandible. **J,** Postoperative tridimensional reconstruction of the mandible showing the remodeling of the angle and the new proportions of the ascending ramus. Notice the increased vertical dimension of the maxilla and the horizontalization of the menton.

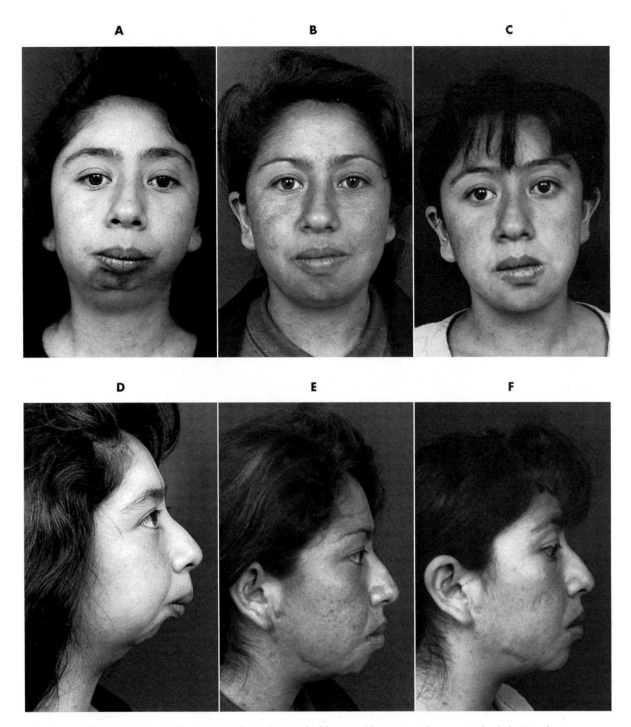

Figure 46-7. **A,** Preoperative frontal view of a 22-year-old patient with congenital ankylosis and resulting asymmetric micrognathia. **B,** One year later, notice the simultaneous soft tissue expansion and its distribution in the inferior third of the face and upper neck. **C,** Three years later, the result is stable. **D,** Preoperative lateral view of the patient. **E,** One year later, showing the skin scars that represent the major complication. **F,** Three years later, the soft tissue expansion is maintained because the distraction has produced a solid neomandible. *Continued*

to see the rapid descent of the buccal commissure to a normal position, the horizontalization of the chin, the increase in the distance between the buccal commissure and the external canthus–inferior orbital rim, and the remarkable improvement in facial symmetry in all the unilateral cases.

All the patients with micrognathia presented the typical "bird face" deformity with deficient soft tissue at the lower third of the face and at the neck, absence of the neck angle, and shortened suprahyoid muscles. The overall aesthetic results obtained with bilateral and bidirectional distraction have been

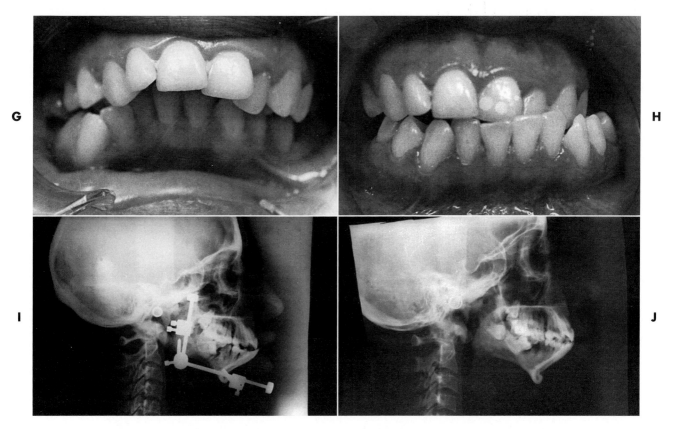

Figure 46-7, cont'd. G, Preoperative occlusion. **H,** The occlusion 3 years later. Orthodontic treatment is required that must include transverse expansion and teeth alignment. **I,** Lateral cephalogram during the consolidation period. Notice the separation between the molars and that the vector of distraction at the mandibular body is parallel to the occlusal plane, avoiding production of an anterior open bite. **J,** Lateral cephalogram 3 years later, showing a solid and mature neomandible.

spectacular, beyond the patients' and our expectations. The neck took a normal shape with a well-defined angle; the muscles and soft tissues of the floor of the mouth, as well as the masseter insertion and the muscle volume, expanded; and the chin took a more prominent position. All of these changes in position and shape would not be possible with conventional orthognathic surgery using the sagittal split osteotomy procedure.

The operation can be performed on an outpatient basis and requires only weekly follow-up visits. Further refinements in surgical technique and other external or intraoral devices will be necessary. A well-coordinated orthodontic-surgeon team is necessary to obtain optimal results.

REFERENCES

1. Björk A, Skieller V: Normal and abnormal growth of the mandible: a synthesis of longitudinal cephalometric implant studies over a period of 25 years, *Eur J Orthod* 5:1, 1983.

2. Converse JM, Horowitz SL, Coccaro PJ, et al: The corrective treatment of the skeletal asymmetry in hemifacial microsomia, *Plast Reconstr Surg* 52:221, 1973.

3. Ilizarov GA, Soybelman LM, Chirkova AM: Some roentgenographic and morphologic data on bone tissue regeneration in distraction epiphysiolysis in experiment, *Orto Traumato Protol* 31:26, 1970.

4. Ilizarov GA, Devyatov AA, Kamerin VK: Plastic reconstruction of longitudinal bone defects by means of compression and subsequent distraction, *Acta Chir Plast* 22:32, 1980.

5. Iñigo F, Rojo P, Ysunza A: Aesthetic treatment of Romberg's disease: experience with 35 cases, *Br J Plast Surg* 46:194, 1993.

6. Kaban LB, Moses MH, Mulliken JB: Surgical correction of hemifacial microsomia in the growing child, *Plast Reconstr Surg* 82:9-19, 1988.

7. Karp NS, Thorne CH, McCarthy JG, et al: Bone lengthening in the craniofacial skeleton, *Ann Plast Surg* 24:231, 1990.

8. Lauritzen C, Munro IR, Ross RB: Classification and treatment of hemifacial microsomia, *Scand J Plast Reconstr Surg* 19:33, 1985.

9. McCarthy JG, Schreider J, Karp N, et al: Lengthening the human mandible by gradual distraction, *Plast Reconstr Surg* 89:1, 1992.

10. Michieli S, Miotti B: Lengthening of mandibular body by gradual surgical orthodontic distraction, *J Oral Surg* 35:187, 1977.

11. Molina F, Ortiz Monasterio F: Mandibular elongation and remodeling by distraction: a farewell to major osteotomies, *Plast Reconstr Surg* 96:4, 825-842, 1995.

12. Molina F, Ortiz Monasterio F: Extended indications for mandibular distraction: unilateral, bilateral and bidirectional. In Ortiz Monasterio F, editor: *Craniofacial surgery,* ed 5, Bologna, Italy, 1993, Monduzzi Editore.

13. Munro IR: One stage reconstruction of the temporomandibular joint in hemifacial microsomia, *Plast Reconstr Surg* 66:669, 1980.

14. Murray JE, Mulliken JB, Kaban LB, et al: Twenty-year experience in maxillocraniofacial surgery: an evaluation of early surgery on growth, function and body image, *Ann Surg* 190:320, 1979.

15. Ortiz Monasterio F: Early mandibular and maxillary osteotomies for the correction of hemifacial microsomia, *Clin Plast Surg* 9:509-517, 1982.

16. Pruzansky S: Not all dwarfed mandibles are alike, *Birth Defects* 1:120, 1969.

17. Snyder CC, Levine GA, Swanson HM, et al: Mandibular lengthening by gradual distraction: preliminary report, *Plast Reconstr Surg* 51:506, 1973.

PART II

CRANIOFACIAL SURGERY

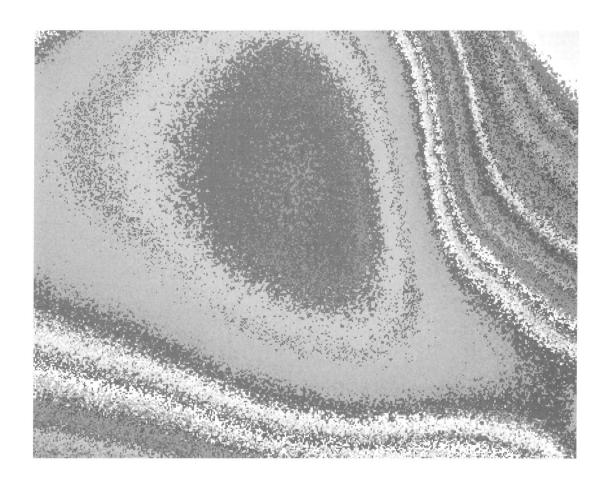

CHAPTER 47

Nonsyndromic Craniosynostosis

J. Kerwin Williams
Steven R. Cohen
Fernando D. Burstein
Roger J. Hudgins
William R. Boydston

INDICATIONS

Craniosynostosis refers to the premature fusion of one of the six major sutures of the craniofacial vault. Functionally, craniosynostosis may be defined as the premature conversion of a *dynamic* region of growth and resorption between two adjacent bones of the cranial vault into a *static* region of bony union. The final result is the formation of a single bony plate from two smaller segments. The term *craniostenosis* is used interchangeably but actually describes the consequences of craniosynostosis. The first description of the morphologic changes created by premature fusion was recorded by Hippocrates.[60] Galen[91] also described a patient with craniosynostosis and coined the term *oxycephaly*. Sommering[86] first recognized that skull growth occurred at the sutures and fusion of these "growth areas" would create a deformity. Subsequently, Virchow[92] initiated the use of the word *craniosynostosis* to describe the premature suture fusion and further established what is known as Virchow's law for compensatory cranial vault growth after suture fusion.

CLASSIFICATION

Premature suture fusion may be characterized as described by Cohen.[14] Nonsyndromic, or isolated, craniosynostosis predominates and is defined as suture fusion that creates functional impairments related to local effects of the fusion, that is, intracranial hypertension or ophthalmoplegia. Occurrences are usually sporadic, but rare familial tendencies have been reported.[32] Furthermore, craniosynostosis in two members of the immediate family will increase the chance the next child will develop a premature suture fusion.[70] Craniosynostosis associated with craniofacial syndromes (e.g., Apert's syndrome, Crouzon's disease, Pfeiffer's syndrome) may be autosomal dominant or autosomal recessive and have second-ary anomalies not directly associated with the suture fusion.[15] These may include the cardiovascular, genitourinary, or vertebral organs. Craniosynostosis may also be classified as simple (one suture) or complex (two or more sutures) and primary or secondary as a reflection of the underlying cause.

The most commonly affected nonsyndromic suture fusion usually involves the sagittal suture.[63] It is characterized by an increased anteroposterior position and decreased biparietal width (scaphocephaly). Presentation may be variable, but generally anterior sagittal fusion will present with significant frontal bossing; posterior sagittal fusion is characterized by an occipital bulge.

Coronal sutures may have unilateral (anterior plagiocephaly) or bilateral (brachiocephaly) involvement.[70] The primary dysmorphology involves the forehead and the supraorbital region, which includes the zygomatic process of the frontal bone (lateral orbital rims) and the temporal area. In unilateral coronal synostosis, the forehead is flattened and there is retrusion of the ipsilateral superior orbital rim. If both coronal sutures are involved, the lateral dimensions of the skull are widened and the superior orbital rim is displaced bilaterally. There may also be an associated increase in the height of the forehead (turricephaly).

Trigonocephaly from metopic suture fusion is probably the most obvious deformity of the craniosynostoses. The occurrence is uncommon (7.9% to 10.0%),[28,84] and the presentation may range from a simple midline ridge to full expression, including a prominent keel-shaped forehead, bitemporal narrowing, and hypotelorism. Associated intracranial midline anomalies may also be seen in these patients.

Lambdoid sutures are paired and may be involved unilaterally or bilaterally. The subsequent deformity is often referred to as an occipital or posterior plagiocephaly and posterior brachiocephaly, respectively. The deformity usually occurs on the right side and may have compensatory bossing of the contralateral anterior skull. Bilateral involvement is characterized by a widened biparietal width and occipital flattening.

Vertex elongation is present in both unilateral and bilateral suture fusions. Lambdoid suture fusion must be differentiated from deformational plagiocephaly, which also presents with a flattened occiput. True lambdoid synostosis is extremely rare, with reports being 1% to 2% of all craniosynostoses.[90]

Plagiocephaly without Synostosis

Craniosynostosis should be differentiated from plagiocephaly resulting from external forces on an otherwise normal cranial vault complex. Often called *deformational plagiocephaly,* or *plagiocephaly without synostosis* (PWS), shaping of the skull may come from intrauterine constraint and/or postnatal positioning.[43] The incidence has been sited as being as low as one in 300 births[11] to as high as 48% of otherwise healthy newborns.[6] Postnatal forces may come from supine positioning favoring one side or mild flattening of the occiput during birth, which is accentuated in the supine position from head turning by force of gravity.[79] Muscular torticollis, a fixed head position from vertebral malformations,[49,101] and extraocular motor dysfunction[35] have also been related to plagiocephaly.

Deformational plagiocephaly is uniquely different from craniosynostosis-induced plagiocephaly and may be determined by the physical examination. Frontal examination of the patient with deformational plagiocephaly reveals retrusion of the ipsilateral frontal bone and superior orbit with a narrow palpebral fissure, lower eyebrows, angulation of the nasal root, and a slightly inferior position of the ipsilateral ear. There is bossing of the contralateral frontal area. The vertex view demonstrates a "pushed" posterior position of the ipsilateral chin and ear associated with a parallelogram shape of the skull.

Unilateral coronal craniosynostosis is characterized by a widened palpebral fissure and a superiorly placed eyebrow and supraorbital rim. The ipsilateral ear may be higher, and the nasal root is deviated to the flattened side. The vertex view demonstrates a trapezoid shape to the skull and an anterior displacement of the chin and ear.

NORMAL DEVELOPMENT AND ANATOMY

Sites of suture formation in the neurocranium are thought to be determined by dural reflections.[85] Cranial bone expands from intramembranous ossification centers within a fibrous membrane called the *ectomeninx.* The leading edge of these bone plates, referred to as osteogenic fronts, contains a wedge-shaped proliferation of osteoprogenitor cells.[22] A syndesmosis (no interposing cartilage) is formed through apposition of these bony plates. In contrast, a synchondrosis, which contains a cartilage interposition, is seen in cranial base sutures.[21]

A suture contains the leading edge of the bony plates and the intervening radiolucent fibrous tissue. Five distinct layers of the cranial suture were identified by Pritchard[74] and include two cambial and two capsular layers of the periosteum with a middle vascular layer. The interposed fibrous tissue between the bony fronts has been shown to contain collagen types I, III, and V,[13] fibronectin, osteoprogenitor cells, and osteonectin.[33]

The bony edges may approximate in an end-to-end relationship, as seen in the midline sagittal and metopic sutures, or overlap, as seen in the coronal, lambdoid, sphenozygomatic, and squamosal sutures. Initially all the bone edges are smooth,[42] but as the time of suture patency increases, the number of interdigitations also increases.[46] Studies have not demonstrated an association between the number of interdigitations and the onset of suture fusion. Facial sutures formed in the absence of dura have different developmental and growth patterns from those seen in sutures of the cranial vault.[68,74]

Cranial vault sutures usually close in early adult life, with the exception of the metopic suture, which begins to close at age 2.[13] Initial bone bridging is usually seen on the endocranial surface, although it can also begin on the ectocranium.[58] There is a single focus of suture fusion that may occur anywhere along the course of the suture and is especially true for the sagittal suture.[1] In contrast, metopic suture fusion progresses from inferior to superior.[50] During suture fusion, there is a zone of osseous obliteration characterized by nonlamellar bone across the preexisting suture. As one progresses away from the site of fusion, an area of both connective tissue and osseous union exists, followed by areas of thinned connective tissue (impending suture fusion) and, eventually, an area of uninvolved sutures with normal-appearing connective tissue.[45]

PATHOGENESIS

The specific cause of premature suture fusion is unclear and may be multifactorial. Nonsyndromic suture fusion may be related to extrinsic causes, such as metabolic disorders (e.g., vitamin D deficiency, hyperthyroidism) or brain malformations (e.g., microcephaly, encephalocele, corrected hydrocephalus). Chromosomal abnormalities and exposure to teratogens (e.g., aminopterin, diphenylhydantoin, retinoic acid, valproic acid) are usually associated with syndromic fusion (Box 47-1).[16]

Three general theories of the pathogenesis of craniosynostosis have been described. Virchow[92] suggested that the primary abnormality was localized to the affected suture and translated to the cranial base. Moss[61] theorized that the cranial base was the source of the pathogenesis. Tension translated from the cranial base to the cranial vault sutures (presumably by the dura) cause a premature fusion of the suture. Finally, Park and Powers[66] suggested that the defect was secondary to an abnormality in the local mesenchymal blastema. It is important to understand that the latter theory of mesenchymal cell dysfunction does not stand in conflict with the initial two theories. The pathology, as proposed by Moss and Virchow, reflects the initial *site* of abnormal growth, not the primary *cause* of the abnormality.

The biochemical activities at the cellular and molecular levels are not well understood, but some possible mechanisms have been suggested. The predominant cell type in fused sutures has been found to be osteoprogenitor cells.[27] The dura in proximity to the suture is necessary to maintain pa-

Box 47-1.
Known Causes of Craniosynostosis

Monogenic conditions
Chromosomal syndromes
Metabolic disorders
   Hyperthyroidism
   Rickets
Mucopolysaccharidoses
   Hurler's syndrome
   Morquio's syndrome
   β-Glucuronidase deficiency
Mucolipidoses
   Mucolipidosis III
Hematologic disorders
   Thalassemias
   Sickle cell anemia
   Congenital hemolytic icterus
   Polycythemia vera
Teratogens
   Aminopterin
   Diphenylhydantoin
   Retinoic acid
   Valproic acid
Malformations
   Microcephaly
   Encephalocele
   Shunted hydrocephalus
   Holoprosencephaly

From Cohen MM: *Craniosynostosis: diagnosis, evaluation and management,*
New York, 1986, Raven Press.

tency.[36,64] Growth factors have been suggested as a regulator of osteogenesis and may be temporally and spatially specific to this task.[53,80] Recently, cells at sites of active suture fusion have demonstrated "programmed" cell death, or apoptosis.[29,87] Controlled cell death may be an avenue of normal suture fusion that is misregulated at a gene level in craniosynostosis. Finally, Cohen[13] has suggested that a migration of osteoprecursor cells may occur at suture sites, causing a fusion to occur prematurely.

MORPHOGENESIS

In 1851, Virchow[92] described the principle that growth is restricted in the plane parallel to the prematurely fused suture. This explanation was challenged by Moss[61] based on observations that abnormal skull shapes occur in the absence of suture fusion and that cranial vault suture fusion was often associated with a cranial base deformity. He concluded that the initiating event for premature suture fusion was an abnormality in the cranial base. He also expanded the concept that the approximating soft tissue plays an active role in the shape and size of the associated bone. In light of these principles, Delashaw et al[23] outlined four components of compensatory cranial

vault growth that more fully explain morphologic findings seen clinically.

With the assumption that sutural edges may have asymmetric growth activities, they proposed the following:

1. Cranial vault bones that are prematurely fused act as a single bone plate with decreased growth potential.
2. Abnormal asymmetric bone deposition occurs at perimeter sutures with increased bone deposition directed away from the bone plate.
3. Perimeter sutures adjacent to the prematurely fused suture compensate in growth more than perimeter sutures distant to the sutural stenosis.
4. A nonperimeter suture that is contiguous to the prematurely fused suture undergoes enhanced symmetric bone deposition along both edges.

These four principles of cranial vault restriction and compensation have been supported by clinical findings in nonsyndromic craniosynostosis.

POTENTIAL FUNCTIONAL COMPLICATIONS

Functional disability is an ill-fitting term in plastic surgery, especially in the area of craniofacial abnormalities. It not only includes anatomically related disabilities but should also incorporate psychologic and developmental issues. In isolated craniosynostosis, concerns related to exorbitism; speech; and associated neurologic anomalies, such as hydrocephalus and Chiari's malformations, may be minimal.

Intracranial Hypertension

The primary concern with premature suture fusion relates to brain growth. The brain volume of the infant increases twofold by age 1 and threefold by age 3. This rapid brain growth is paralleled by an equally rapid accommodating increase in the size of the cranial vault (Table 47-1). The major functional problem associated with restrictive craniostenosis is the development of increased intracranial pressure (ICP). Elevated ICP may manifest in two forms. The first is the well-recognized global increase in ICP subsequent to a restrictive cranium. Late radiographic signs may include "fingerprinting" or "copper beating" of the endocranial surface or loss of the cisternae on two-dimensional CT scans. If severe and untreated, intracranial hypertension can translate to the optic nerve with development of papilledema; nerve ischemia; and, eventually, optic atrophy.

Elevated ICP may also occur transiently and be limited to a region of the brain near the fused suture. Focal regions of pressure and ischemia associated with areas of suture fusion have been identified using technetium 99 cerebral flow studies.[82] Focal hypertension probably has less dramatic consequences than are seen with overt elevations in ICP, but the effects may correlate more with long-term brain function, such as mental development, learning disabilities, and intelligence quotients.

Aside from the potential for optic atrophy, some forms of craniosynostosis may lead to other ocular disturbances. A

Table 47-1.
Cranial and Brain Growth during the First 20 Years of Life

AGE	VOLUME OF BRAIN (cm³)	CRANIAL CAPACITY (cm³)
Newborn	330	350
3 mo	550	600
6 mo	575	775
9 mo	675	925
1 yr	750	1000
2 yr	900	1100
3 yr	960	1225
4 yr	1000	1300
6 yr	1060	1350
9 yr	1100	1400
12 yr	1150	1450
20 yr	1200	1500

From Blinkov SM, Glezer II: *The human brain in figures and tables: a quantitative handbook,* New York, 1968, Plenum Press and Basic Books.

significant decrease in the volume of the orbit may cause exorbitism and subsequent corneal abrasions from exposure. Likewise, suture fusion associated with orbital hypertelorism may cause restricted binocular vision. The most common intrinsic ophthalmoplegia associated with coronal synostosis is either a divergent or convergent nonparalytic strabismus or exotropia. This is related to the misshapen orbital roof and subsequent malalignment of the extraocular muscles.

CONSENT

The importance of informed consent for any procedure has been well established (Figure 47-1). It does not relieve any physician of responsibility, but it does provide a format for discussing aspects of the procedure, including potential complications and the magnitude of the surgery. Specific complications related to corrective surgery are discussed in this chapter. The parents or legal guardians should be aware of the potential for blood transfusions and provide donor-directed blood, if possible. Complications associated with the intracranial components of the procedure should also be discussed in conjunction with the neurosurgeon. A lumbar drain may be necessary if there is potential for dural compromise (for instance, during a reoperation) or evidence of elevated ICP and should be included in the preoperative review. Finally, the expected scar, postoperative course (including recovery period in the intensive care unit), and potential donor sites should be discussed.

OPERATIONS

The first recorded surgical approach for craniosynostosis was performed by Lannelongue[48] in 1890 and Lane[47] in 1892, who completed strip craniectomies of fused sutures. The classic neurosurgical techniques developed over the ensuing decades were geared toward resecting the synostotic suture. It was thought that a new suture line would be created that would permit normalization of the cranial vault as further growth occurred. With the realization that this goal was rarely achieved, attempts were made to further fragment the cranial vault surgically, replacing the bone as autogenous grafts that would improve preoperative cranial shape. Uncontrolled postoperative skull molding during the healing process often resulted in skull distortions. Skull reossification by the technique of calvarectomy and morcellation was found to be unpredictable and associated with substantial residual cranial vault deformity.[71] In 1967, Tessier[88] described a new approach to the management of Crouzon's disease and Apert's syndrome. His landmark presentation and publications were the beginning of modern craniofacial surgery. Tessier combines an intracranial-extracranial approach with the use of a coronal incision, extensive periorbital subperiosteal dissection, autogenous bone grafting, and ingenious osteotomies. The concept of calvarial suture resection combined with skull reshaping in infancy was later pioneered by Hoffman,[37] Whitaker,[98] and Marchac.[51] Hoffman[37] reported lateral canthal advancement of the supraorbital margin as a new corrective technique in the treatment of coronal synostosis in 1976. This heralded reports by Whitaker[98] in 1977 and the classic article by Marchac and Renier,[51] which presented the floating forehead technique combined with frontoorbital advancement.

It has become accepted clinical practice with patients with nonsyndromic and single-suture craniosynostosis for clinicians to perform the primary operative procedure—frontoorbital advancement with cranial vault remodeling—at an early age to improve craniofacial form and function and lead to satisfactory long-term growth and development of the calvaria. Our current approach to single-suture and nonsyndromic craniosynostosis varies with the underlying sutural fusion. In general, once a diagnosis has been established by physical examination and appropriate radiologic studies, a surgical treatment plan is recommended. It is critical that children undergo multidisciplinary evaluation by a craniofacial team. The team geneticist rules out associated abnormalities that can occur to a greater or lesser proportion in a number of craniosynostosis patients. In children with bicoronal synostosis, it is especially important to rule out syndromic involvement because this will not always be

Do not sign this form until you have read it and fully understand its contents.

Patient's Name_____ Date_____

The following has been explained to me in general terms, and I understand that:

1. The diagnosis requiring this procedure is:

   _____

2. The nature of the procedure is:

   _____

3. The purpose of this procedure is:

   _____

4. Material risks of the procedure: As a result of this procedure being performed, there may be material risks of infection, allergic reaction, disfiguring scar, severe loss of blood, loss or loss of function of any limb or organ, paralysis, paraplegia or quadraplegia, brain damage, cardiac arrest, or death.

5. In addition to these material risks, there may be other possible risks involved in this procedure, including, but not limited to:

   _____
   _____

6. The likelihood of success of the above procedure is:
   ( ) Good   ( ) Fair   ( ) Poor

7. Practical alternatives to this procedure include:

   _____
   _____

8. If I choose not to have the above procedure, my prognosis (future medical condition) is:

   _____
   _____

9. I understand that the physician, medical personnel, and other assistants will rely on statements about the patient, the patient's medical history, and other information in determining whether to perform the procedure or the course of treatment for the patient's condition and in recommending the procedure that has been explained.

10. I understand that the practice of medicine is not an exact science and that no guarantees or assurances have been made to me concerning the results of this procedure and that sometimes a patient's expectations may be greater than the reality of the treatment.

11. I understand that during the course of the procedure described above it may be necessary or appropriate to perform additional procedures that are unforeseen or not known to be needed at the time this consent is given. I consent to and authorize the persons described herein to make the decision concerning such procedures. I also consent to and authorize the performance of such additional procedures as they may deem necessary or appropriate.

12. I consent to diagnostic studies, tests, local and/or general anesthesia, x-ray examinations, and any other treatment or courses of treatment relating to the diagnosis or procedures described herein as may be deemed advisable.

13. I consent that any tissues, specimens, organs, or limbs removed from the patient's body in the course of any procedure may be tested or retained for scientific or teaching purposes and then disposed of within the discretion of the physician, facility, or other health care provider.

14. I consent to the taking of photographs before and after this operation or treatment, as well as in the course of this operation or treatment. I understand and give my permission for the photographs to be used for the purpose of medical or instructional purposes, including lectures and/or publications.

15. By signing this form, I acknowledge that I have read or had this form read and/or explained to me, that I fully understand its contents, that I have been given ample opportunity to ask questions, and that any questions have been answered satisfactorily. All blanks or statements requiring completion were filled in and all statements I do not approve of were stricken before I signed this form. I also have received additional information, including, but not limited to, the materials listed below, related to the procedures described herein.

16. Additional materials used, if any, during the informed consent process for this procedure include:

17. I voluntarily allow _____ along with any physician designated or selected by him or her and all medical personnel under him or her and all medical personnel under the direct supervision and control of such physician and all other personnel who may otherwise be involved in performing such procedures to perform the procedures described or otherwise referred to herein.

Signature of person giving consent:_____

Relationship to patient if not the patient:_____

Patient unable to sign because of:_____

Date:_____ Time:_____ Witness:_____

Figure 47-1.   Informed consent.

apparent on preliminary examination yet has important prognostic implications for the family and patient. An ophthalmologist routinely sees each patient preoperatively to determine whether associated ocular adnexal problems exist and to rule out papilledema. The neurosurgeon ensures that associated brain parenchymal abnormalities are not present and evaluates the patient for the possibility of subclinical or overt intracranial hypertension.

The decision to operate on cases of single-suture synostosis should not be based solely on aesthetic considerations, but concerns regarding local or regional increases in ICP on brain function should also be raised with parents. By the same token, families with children in whom more minor degrees of skull deformity exist, such as mild metopic synostosis, should not be frightened into surgery because of the prospect of brain damage secondary to undetected elevations of ICP. These children can be followed in a craniofacial team setting to optimize the chances for normal development and outcome. The diagnosis of elevated ICP in children with single-suture craniosynostosis must be made from a constellation of clinical findings supported by the measurement of ICP in selected cases. Children with a history of developmental delay, headaches, and other neurologic symptoms of elevated ICP should be referred to a pediatric ophthalmologist for funduscopic evaluation. The presence of papilledema and other findings consistent with elevated ICP should be noted. It is important, however, to remember that increased ICP may be present in the absence of papilledema, which is often a later finding. Two- and three-dimensional computed tomography (CT) scans should be routinely obtained. We rarely order plain films of the skull, but occasionally these are brought by patients from outside settings and should be reviewed for evidence of craniosynostosis and digital printing or copper-beaten appearances of the calvaria. In children less than 1 year of age with isolated synostosis of the sagittal, metopic, or lambdoid suture whose parents already wish to proceed to normalize skull shape, ICP monitoring is unlikely to contribute to clinical management. For children in these categories whose parents do not desire surgical intervention, the measurement of ICP, if indicated, may provide a means of excluding potentially damaging consequences of the synostosis. In children with unicoronal synostosis of any age, surgical intervention is generally recommended because of facial growth problems accompanying this type of sutural fusion. Children presenting with craniosynostosis later than 1 year of age, particularly those with developmental delay or other signs of ICP, may be referred for ICP monitoring. It is important that all factors be taken into account before proceeding with surgical interventions. The family should be appraised as best as possible and given realistic expectations regarding improvement in developmental delays.

Eppley and Sadove[28] paved the way for the use of biodegradable plates and screws in infant craniofacial surgery. Our own center's experience with these have been extremely positive. They do require more patience than conventional metallic plates and screws and, once positioned, if changes are necessary, the biodegradables must usually be discarded and replaced with new hardware. They are also more expensive than metallic plates and screws; however, the decreased reoperation rate for removal will more than likely make up for the added initial expense. Metallic plates and screws are still useful, however, in infant craniofacial surgery, provided that the parents are appraised of their need. Consideration can also be given to removing them at a later date on a routine basis, although we do not advocate this in most patients. Provided that the plate lengths are kept small and the configuration simple, migration may be less likely. Also, it is preferable to avoid using metallic plates in the midline and especially the nasofrontal region because this is where most clinical cases associated with migration have been found.

PATIENT PREPARATION

In children undergoing simple sagittal or lambdoid synostectomies, two intravenous lines are used, but a Foley catheter and intraarterial line are not routinely inserted. Our preference is to perform synostectomies from 2 to 4 months of age, if at all possible. When performing simple synostectomies for cases of sagittal and true lambdoid synostosis, earlier surgery results in the best chance for normalization of calvarial shape. Simple sagittal and lambdoid synostectomies are performed with the patient in prone position on a horseshoe headrest. Attention is taken to ensure that no pressure on the eyes occurs because this is a known cause of blindness. For the smaller infants, typically chest rolls are not used because they may impede ventilation. In patients undergoing either a Pi procedure[41] or major cranial vault reconstruction for sagittal synostosis, the modified prone position with the neck hyperextended is used. In these cases, a cervical spine x-ray is obtained before putting the child in this position. In addition, because of the potential for increased bleeding secondary to jugular venous hypertension, an intraarterial line is inserted, as is a Foley catheter in those children undergoing major cranial vault reconstruction. For patients with metopic, unicoronal, and bicoronal synostosis, the patient is operated on in the supine position. In addition to two intravenous lines, an intraarterial line is routinely used, as is a Foley catheter. In the standard team approach, the neurosurgeon begins the operation. The child undergoes a 10-minute head scrub and a povidone-iodine (Betadine) preparation. We do not routinely shave the hair. The incision is marked with a pen and generally performed in a wavy S-shaped fashion behind the hairline. A Shaw scalpel is used with the skin incision made at 110 degrees and the deeper dissection performed at 260 degrees. Michel clips are used to attach sponges to the wound edges for hemostasis. Continuing with the Shaw scalpel, the dissection is performed in the subgaleal plane. This is carried out down to the level of the supraorbital rims, and then the periosteum is incised along the insertions of the temporal muscles and then horizontally at the level of the anterior fontanelle. This permits subperiosteal elevation of a generous tongue of periosteum and galea. Subperiosteal dissection is then performed to expose the supraorbital rim and lateral orbital rim down to the body of the zygoma, and intraorbitally to the level of the inferior orbital foramen. In patients undergoing correction of metopic, unicoronal, and bicoronal synostosis, a bifrontal craniotomy is always carried out. The anterior cranial fossa is then exposed to perform the frontoorbital osteotomies. All children undergoing correction of craniosynostosis at our institution are typed and crossed for either donor-directed or banked blood. Before beginning the surgical procedure, the blood is transported to the refrigerator in the operating room, where it is immediately available at the commencement of the case.

SAGITTAL SYNOSTOSIS

Depending on the degree of deformity and the age of the patient, a variety of operations have been used for correction of sagittal synostosis. In young infants with mild scaphocephaly, a simple sagittal synostectomy is carried out. With the skull exposed, an incision is made with the Shaw scalpel 2.5 cm off the midline and carried from the coronal suture posteriorly through the lambdoid suture. This pericranial incision then continues well past the lambdoid sutures into the occiput. The extent of the posterior bone removal will depend on the severity of the posterior deformity. A burr hole is made in the pericranial incision at the level of the vertex. With the Midas Rex drill (Midas Rex, Fort Worth, Tex.), it is unnecessary to strip the pericranium. A second pericranial incision is made in front of the lambdoid suture on either side 2.5 cm off the midline. The bone is removed from side to side, just in front of the lambdoid suture using either a fine Rongeur or the M-8 attachment of the Midas Rex. The pericranium is then incised along the posterior border of the anterior fontanelle. A curette opens the interval between the bone and dura. The B-5 attachment, which is the pediatric craniotome of the Midas Rex, is used to make a linear osteotomy. The parasagittal osteotomy is made from the coronal suture to the lambdoid suture on both sides. Typically the bone is stuck to the dura, especially over the sagittal sinus. A sharp periosteal elevator is used to dissect the remaining midline suture away from the sinus. Bleeding from the pacchionian granulations and draining veins are common, and the dissection must be performed quickly but carefully. Once the bone is removed, the dura is immediately covered with a wet sponge to stop significant bleeding. The bipolar cautery is then used to coagulate significant bleeders remaining on the dura. Now the bone has been removed from the coronal suture to just in front of the lambdoid. Dissecting underneath the lambdoid sutures and across the midline with periosteal elevator, the Midas Rex drill is then used to remove any significant occipital deformity. The bipolar is turned to 45, and the dura directly over the sagittal sinus is coagulated swiftly in order not to thrombose the sinus but rather to retard the dural osteoclast in the midline. The wound is then copiously irrigated with bacitracin, and the skin is closed with 4-0 Vicryl and staples. We have gotten away from using head wraps and prefer to place mupirocin (Bactroban) over the incision. The child is then carefully rolled back into supine position and taken to the recovery room.

This synostectomy procedure allows for significant improvement in head shape. It works especially well on large

occipital knobs and in correcting the biparietal narrowing. The downside to the technique is that it fails to address significant forehead bossing. For children who present with moderate frontal prominence without saddling deformities or significant occipital abnormalities, a Pi procedure[41] is used. This procedure is carried out in the modified prone position with the neck hyperextended. A cervical spine x-ray is obtained before putting the child in this position. Bilateral parasagittal strips of bone are removed between the coronal and lambdoid sutures. An osteotomy is then performed the length of the coronal suture on each side. This completes the formation of the Pi. A 3-0 silk is threaded through a twist drill hole between the midline construct and the forehead. When this is tied down, it foreshortens the forehead. Before tightening the suture, vertical osteotomies in the parietal bone are carried into the temporal fossa. Thus when the forehead is pulled back, the dura bulges laterally, correcting the biparietal narrowing. The procedure takes longer than a sagittal synostectomy and has a larger blood loss. Children who undergo strip craniectomy typically go home the following morning, and only 5% or less require a blood transfusion. Children undergoing the Pi procedure generally stay longer simply because they are sicker in the first day or so. Typically a higher percentage require blood transfusions, as well.

A major cranial vault reconstruction in an infant is reserved for children with severe skull deformities. In children under 7 months of age with severe sagittal synostosis, conventional strip craniectomy and even the Pi procedure fail to correct late deformities characteristic of severe scaphocephaly. The components of the deformity that require correction include extreme elongation, frontal and occipital bossing, temporal pinching, and angulatory apical skull deformations. Several investigators[8,39] have reported unsatisfactory results in children of any age when the scaphocephalic deformity is severe, particularly when associated with large occipital shelves and marked frontal bossing. To improve surgical results, we prefer total cranial vault reconstruction (Figure 47-2) in these children.[8,39] After

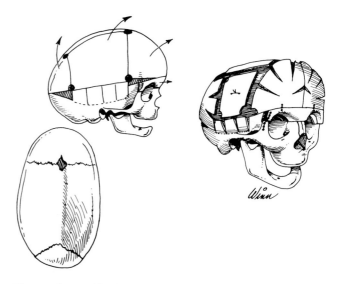

Figure 47-2. Total cranial vault reconstruction in children younger than 2 years old.

general anesthesia is induced, the endotracheal tube is secured to the mandible with a circummandibular wire. Two large intravenous catheters are placed, as is a Foley, to monitor urine output. An arterial line is used. The patient is placed in prone position with the head position maintained using an Olympic Vac positioning system (Sizell, Olympic Medical, Seattle) chin support. The neurosurgical and craniofacial portions of the procedure are carried out in sequential fashion. First, a frontal craniotomy is performed with a supraorbital osteotomy below the frontal boss. The posterior osteotomy is placed in front of the coronal suture, and the frontal bone is carefully removed. The two lateral temporoparietal bone segments are removed, staying just lateral to the sagittal suture. The occiput is removed, keeping the posterior osteotomy below the occipital shelf. A burr hole is placed adjacent to the midline of the occiput to facilitate stripping of the dura mater. Barrel-Stave osteotomies are performed in a vertical fashion along the remaining temporal bone and occipital bone and infractured to permit lateral expansion of the cranium. Plication sutures are placed diagonally in two rows in the bulging frontal dura mater. The frontal bone is split into halves and expands in the transverse plane with radial osteotomies and interposition bone grafts. A wedge of bone is removed from the frontal bone at its junction with a supraorbital osteotomy to allow posterior rotation of the frontal bone. Biodegradable plates, titanium or Vitallium microplates, or wire osteosynthesis are used to link the two halves of the frontal bone in the supraorbital osteotomy site. The occiput is split in half, allowing for lateral expansion in the same fashion as the frontal bone.

While the craniofacial surgeon reconstructs the frontal and occipital bones on a side table, the neurosurgeon inserts an ICP monitor through the right side of the large sagittal bone strip, which has been left between the osteotomized frontoparietal and occipital bone segments. This central strip serves as an anchor for the anteroposterior correction. Two small drill holes are placed in the central portion of the occipital and frontal bone plates. The central bone segment covering the sagittal sinus is then dissected free of the dura and sinus. A section of the central strip is removed according to the amount of anteroposterior correction deemed necessary, which averages 2.5 cm. A corresponding strip of the lateral temporoparietal bone segment is also removed. Small drill holes are placed through the central sagittal bone strip. The frontal bone segment is replaced using biodegradable plates, metallic plates, or wires along the supraorbital rim. Posteriorly, the occipital bone is replaced in a similar manner. Then 28-gauge wire is passed through the osteotomized occipital and frontal bone segments and attached to the central sagittal bone strip. While carefully monitoring the ICP, the right and left wires are slowly twisted on the frontal segment until bone contact occurs between the frontal bone and the central sagittal strip. As anteroposterior correction proceeds, bulging of the dura mater laterally is noted. The occipital correction is carried out by slowly twisting the wires, advancing the occipital bone segment toward the central sagittal strip until bone contact is achieved. ICP is maintained at 15 mm Hg with normocapnia. The anteroposterior correction is carried out slowly, often over

30 to 45 minutes in some cases. This permits equilibration of the ICP. Two small holes are drilled into the lateral temporoparietal bone segments, and these are then sutured directly to the dura mater with a horizontal mattress suture.

After all the osteotomized segments have been replaced, attention is then turned to the anterior temporal fossa region. Preoperatively this area is often pinched. To correct these depressions, excess bone that has been trimmed from the calvaria is cut and contoured to fit the temporal fossa. These may be attached with biodegradable screws or microscrews to the lateral orbital rim. The temporalis muscle is then advanced and resuspended to the lateral orbital rim. The large pericranial flaps, which had been elevated at the time of craniotomy, are replaced, covering the frontal bone and lateral orbital regions. In cases of total cranial vault reconstruction, we routinely insert a closed-system drain through a separate stab incision in the posterior occipital flap. The galea is closed using absorbable sutures in the skin with staples. Postoperatively, the patient is extubated in the recovery room and sequential neurologic examinations are performed. Patients undergoing total cranial vault reconstruction are placed in the intensive care unit for 24 to 48 hours. Careful monitoring of serum sodium is carried out over the first 72 hours. Transfusion of donor-directed blood, usually from parents, is begun intraoperatively and continues postoperatively for the first 24 hours as required. The drain is removed when its output has been reduced to less than 10 mm per day. The skin staples are removed from 7 to 10 days postoperatively.

Patients presenting after 2 years of age with significant scaphocephaly and sagittal synostosis undergo either three-quarters calvarial vault reconstruction or total calvarial vault reconstruction (Figure 47-3), depending on the degree of deformity. The main difference in technique in these patients

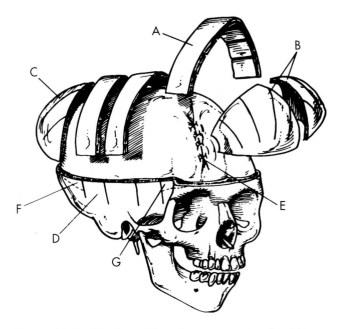

Figure 47-3. Total cranial vault reconstruction in children older than 2 years. (From Burstein FD, Hudgins RH, Cohen SR, et al: *J Craniofac Surg* 5:228-235, 1994.)

is that calvarial defects are not left. When performing total cranial vault reconstruction, the calvaria between the frontal and occipital bones is usually removed in three transverse bands of approximately equal width. The lateral osteotomies for these bands are made just above the squamosal suture. The osteotomy across the midline is accomplished via three slightly off-center central drill holes to protect the sagittal sinus. In contrast to the early cases in which the bone over the majority of the sagittal sinus is left intact, in the later cases the bone is removed in its entirety. Each one of the three central bony segments is taken to the side table, where multiple partial-thickness osteotomies are made with a cutting burr on the inner surface of the bone. Next, gentle greenstick fractures are made along each of the partial-thickness osteotomies with a bone-contouring forceps. To expand the transverse dimensions of the skull, frequently these plates are split down the center, and an interposition bone graft is inserted. Biodegradable plates and/or microplates are used for stabilization of the interpositional bone. An average of 1.5 cm of bone is removed from the anterior and posterior skeletal bands to allow appropriate anteroposterior correction. The occipital and frontal bones, which have been typically split down the midline and enlarged transversely with placement of an interpositional bone graft, are reattached to the supraorbital and posterior occipital ledges with biodegradable plates or microplates. The central bone segment is then secured with biodegradable plates or microplates to the lateral temporal bone to allow it to act as a central post. Next, the anterior and posterior bands are replaced. The frontal bone is connected to the anterior strut either with 28-gauge wire or biodegradable plates or microplates, while careful attention is paid to ICP. The occipital bone is treated in a similar fashion. Lateral dural bolting into the Barrel-Stave osteotomies that have been placed along the lateral temporal and parietal bones permit increased transverse dimensions (Figure 47-4).

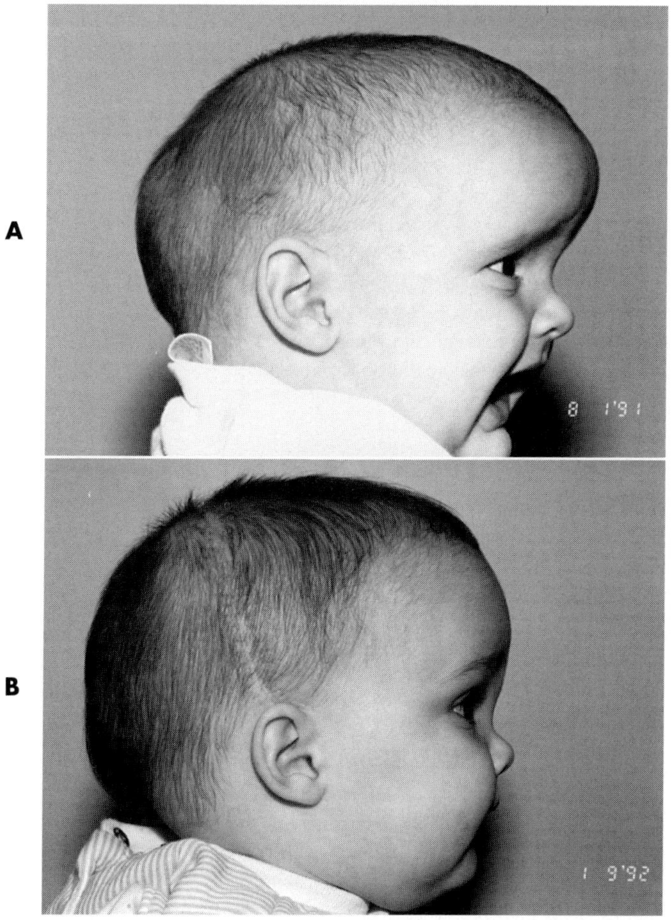

METOPIC SYNOSTOSIS (Figures 47-5 and 47-6)

Although some variation of technique is used depending on the degree of deformity, in general the surgical approach is fairly routine for correction of metopic synostosis.[20] After frontal craniotomy, bilateral supraorbital rim osteotomies are performed without a temporal tenon or Z-plasty unless wires are being used for stabilization. The supraorbital bar is split vertically with a reciprocating saw, and the deformed metopic suture is completed resected. A bone graft is routinely used in the midline to increase the transverse dimensions of the supraorbital bar. If hypotelorism is present, the nose is split in the midline and bone grafted as first described by Marchac and Renier[51] and later by Sadove et al.[81] In patients with severe hypotelorism, correction may be incomplete with the above technique. In such cases, we have used a modified medial orbital osteotomy (Figure 47-7) to increase the degree of interorbital separation. In these cases, the osteotomies are performed in situ. A Smith separator is placed in the osteotomy gap along the zygomatic temporal junction and gently spread to separate and advance the superior and lateral orbital rim to correct the triangular-shaped deformity of the skull. Partial-

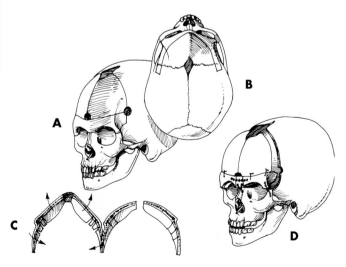

Figure 47-4. A, Eight-month-old with sagittal synostosis and severe scaphocephaly. **B,** Postoperative result after total cranial vault reconstruction.

Figure 47-5. Technique used for correction of metopic synostosis. **A** and **B,** Deformity and osteotomies. **C,** Osteotomies. **D,** Reconstruction.

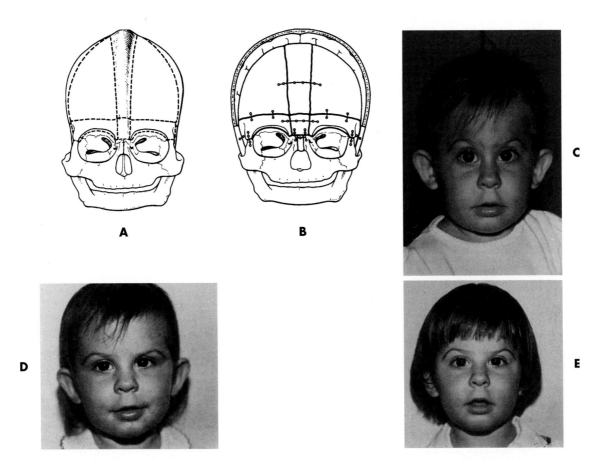

Figure 47-6. **A,** Lines of osteotomy for resection of synostosed metopic suture. Note that the osteotomy extends down to the nasofrontal region and is then continued along the midline of the nose. Segments are then differentially advanced laterally and transversely expanded. **B,** Artist's version of the craniofacial reconstruction for metopic synostosis. Note the two-hole microplate on the lateral orbital rim to temporal bone region. This is fixed anteriorly only and left floating posteriorly. Also note the bone graft wedged in the midline after the nasal osteotomy and transverse expansion, plus anterior advancement of the lateral supraorbital bar. Posteriorly, the forehead is left floating. **C,** Preoperative frontal and lateral photograph of an 8-month-old girl with metopic synostosis. **D,** Postoperative frontal photograph 6 months after frontoorbital remodeling. **E,** At 16 months after frontoorbital remodeling, grade I surgical result with minimal aesthetic irregularities.

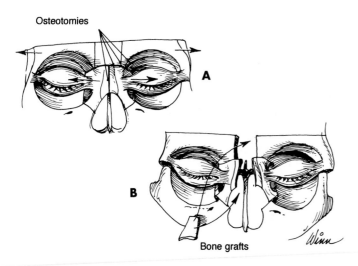

Figure 47-7. Modified medial orbital osteotomy used for patients with severe hypotelorism and metopic synostosis. **A,** Osteotomies. **B,** Bone grafts. Supraorbital rims are advanced in situ.

thickness osteotomies are performed along the undersurface of the lateral orbital rim to allow appropriate bending, which softens the lateral supraorbital rim, giving a more natural curvature. Then a spreader is inserted in the midline, and the entire construct, which includes the medial canthal tendons, is separated. An interposition bone graft is inserted along this osteotomy gap and plated into position. The recontoured supraorbital bar is stabilized with biodegradable plates or titanium microplates at the frontonasal region and lateral orbital rims. Typically, the supraorbital bar is advanced at the lateral orbital rims and maintained either flush or slightly advanced at the frontonasal region. The transition area of the advanced lateral orbital rim is smoothed with a burr. The squamosal portions of the temporal bone are recontoured and plated anteriorly to the posterior lateral aspect of the advanced lateral orbital rim. The frontal bone is then reconstructed with appropriately contoured bone graft or grafts, which are fixed with biodegradable plates or microplates to the advanced supraorbital bar. When additional projection is necessary, the frontal bone may be onlaid over the advanced supraorbital rim and held in place with positional microscrews or biodegradable screws—the advancement-onlay technique. Typically stabilization with plates and screws is sufficient such that in children under 2 the frontal bone graft is left floating posteriorly. In older patients (>18 to 24 months), craniectomy defects are filled with bone grafts. The temporalis muscles are advanced and resuspended to the lateral orbital rim with Vicryl sutures.

UNICORONAL SYNOSTOSIS
(Figures 47-8 to 47-10)

The surgical approach to unicoronal synostosis again depends on the degree of deformity. Again, after a bifrontal craniotomy, an osteotomy of both supraorbital rims is carried out. The entire complex is then removed. In children with malar recession, the osteotomy along the lateral orbital rim may be carried into the zygoma and even include the inferior orbital rim. In cases in which the nasal deviation is severe, the osteotomy may be performed low across the nasal dorsum. We have not used nasal maxillary osteotomies to correct deviation in this region in this age-group after this deviation improves over time. It is not easy to predict which patients will go on to develop facial scoliosis secondary to synostosis along the cranial base. Current surgical techniques do little to prevent this outcome. When compensatory changes of the contralateral forehead are severe, the contralateral "unaffected orbit" will be lowered, in addition to the peaked harlequin orbit of the affected side. In such cases, it is important to reposition the entire supraorbital bar in a manner that normalizes the horizontal position of the orbital roofs. In milder cases, the transverse deficiency of the affected orbit can be corrected by carving out the area along the nasal junction. However, in more severe cases, a vertical osteotomy is usually performed through the affected supraorbital rim and an interpositional bone graft placed. The supraorbital bar in unicoronal synostosis must be inspected carefully because the curvature is frequently abnormal when viewed from the undersurface. Rather than the normal convexity of the curve at the midportion of the orbital roof, a concavity in this area is present. Partial-thickness wedge osteotomies will allow proper recontouring with the bone-contouring forceps. When an interposition bone graft is used, it is rigidly fixed with biodegradable plates or microplates into position. Once the supraorbital bar is recontoured, it is stabilized along the inferior portion of the lateral orbital rims. The temporal region is taken off as a separate strut rather than as a tenon so that it may be segmentally reconfigured. This allows for maximum flexibility in correcting the temporal region, which is often the site of residual deformity. Once the supraorbital rim has been adequately stabilized and the temporal region corrected and stabilized to the advanced supraorbital rim, the frontal bone is recontoured. Often by rotating the frontal bone 180 degrees, a more acceptable contour will be achieved. However, the region that had developed compensatory bossing will require multiple wedge osteotomies to allow proper recontouring. Generally, the frontal bone can be recontoured by the combination of

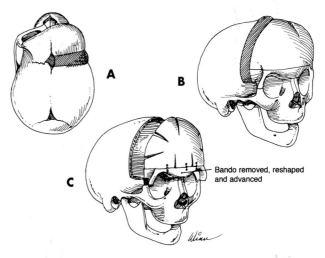

Figure 47-8. Artist's depiction of operative correction of unicoronal synostosis. **A,** The deformity. **B,** Osteotomy. **C,** Reconstruction.

Bando removed, reshaped and advanced

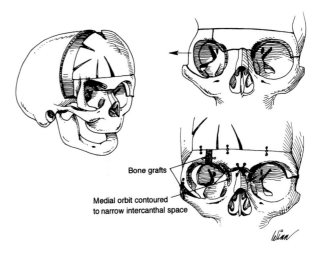

Bone grafts

Medial orbit contoured to narrow intercanthal space

Figure 47-9. Artist's rendition of recontouring the supraorbital bar to achieve symmetry in shape.

wedge osteotomies and bone remodeling with the bone-bending forceps. Occasionally, however, it will need to be osteotomized into segments, which are then rigidly fixated to each other with biodegradable plates or microplates. The forehead is then reattached to the supraorbital rim, either flush or, if additional projection is necessary, as an advancement-onlay technique.[19] Occasionally, additional bone grafts will be necessary to augment the affected supraorbital rim. Once the frontal bone has been restabilized, the peaked lateral aspect of the orbital roof is corrected with a contoured bone graft, as well. In cases of large advancements, the bone graft is actually wedged into the osteotomy gap created at the lateral superior aspect of the rim. The supraorbital rim is also stabilized at the nasal bridge either with a biodegradable plate or occasionally with Vicryl sutures affixed directly to the periosteum. This is done to prevent superior rotation of the rim. Occasionally a bone graft will need to be inserted along the nasal bridge to ease the transition at the nasofrontal junction. A lateral canthopexy may be necessary, depending on the final position of the lateral canthus with respect to the contralateral side. The temporalis muscle is then resuspended. Once in a while, additional contoured bone grafts are inserted under the temporalis muscle to add further augmentation to the temporal region. Generally the forehead is left floating; however, in older children or in cases in which significant advancement has been performed, bone struts may be used for posterior stabilization, as well.

BICORONAL SYNOSTOSIS
(Figures 47-11 to 47-13)

Again, a frontal craniotomy that includes the fused coronal sutures is performed. The supraorbital bar is removed with a reciprocating saw. Some degree of turribrachycephaly may be present, even in nonsyndromic patients.[17] In such cases, a craniotomy is carried posteriorly along the inferior portion of the parietal bone on both sides. Just proximal to the

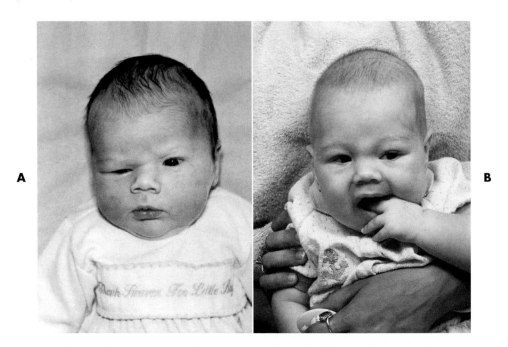

Figure 47-10. **A,** Preoperative photographs of a 6-month-old boy with unicoronal synostosis. **B,** Postoperative photograph following technique illustrated in Figure 47-11.

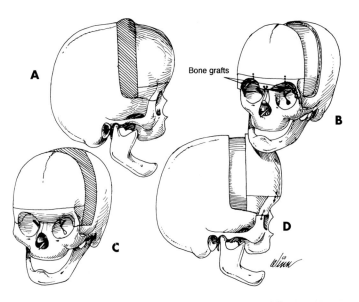

Figure 47-11. **A** to **D,** Technique used to correct bicoronal synostosis without turricephaly.

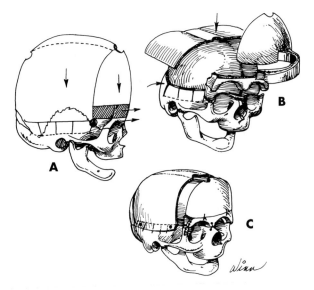

Figure 47-12. **A** to **C,** Technique used when turricephaly is present. (From Cohen SR, de Chalain TM, Burstein FD, et al: *Ann Plast Surg* 35:627-630, 1995.)

lambdoids, the craniotomy proceeds superiorly toward the sagittal sinus. The bone across the midline is carefully removed with a ronguer. With the maneuver repeated on the opposite site, a visor of bone still attached at the midline over the sinus may be gently compressed, overlapping the superior portion of the parietal bones over the inferior cranium. This lowers the vault, pushing the brain and dural coverings forward to fill out the forehead and supraorbital rims.[17]

Stabilization of the supraorbital rims and forehead is carried out with biodegradable plates and screws placed at the lateral orbital rims and nasofrontal junction. The frontal bone is reattached to the advanced supraorbital rim with biodegradable plates and screws. Often a cranial bone graft is placed along the nose to case the stepoff at the nasofrontal junction.

LAMBDOID SYNOSTOSIS AND POSITION-RELATED HEAD DEFORMITIES

The diagnosis and treatment of posterior plagiocephaly and true lambdoid synostosis is one of the most controversial aspects of craniofacial surgery.[3,12,38,67,89] The features of true lambdoidal synostosis versus those of positional or deformational plagiocephaly are inadequately described in the literature. This has resulted in many infants across the United States undergoing major intracranial surgery to treat nonsynostotic plagiocephaly.

Patients with true lambdoid synostosis have a thick ridge over the fused suture with compensatory contralateral parietal and frontal bossing, as well as an ipsilateral occipitomastoid bulge (Figure 47-14). The skull base has an ipsilateral inferior tilt, with a corresponding inferior and posterior displacement of the ipsilateral ear. The skull, when viewed from above, takes on a trapezoidal appearance. These characteristics are opposite to findings in patients with positional molding and open lambdoid sutures.[38] In positional molding, the head takes on a parallelogram shape with flattening of the occiput and contralateral frontal bossing.

Treatment of true lambdoid synostosis is surgical. In younger infants, a broad strip of craniectomy is performed. In older children (<2 years) or those with severe deformities, skull vault remodeling is carried out. The treatment of mild

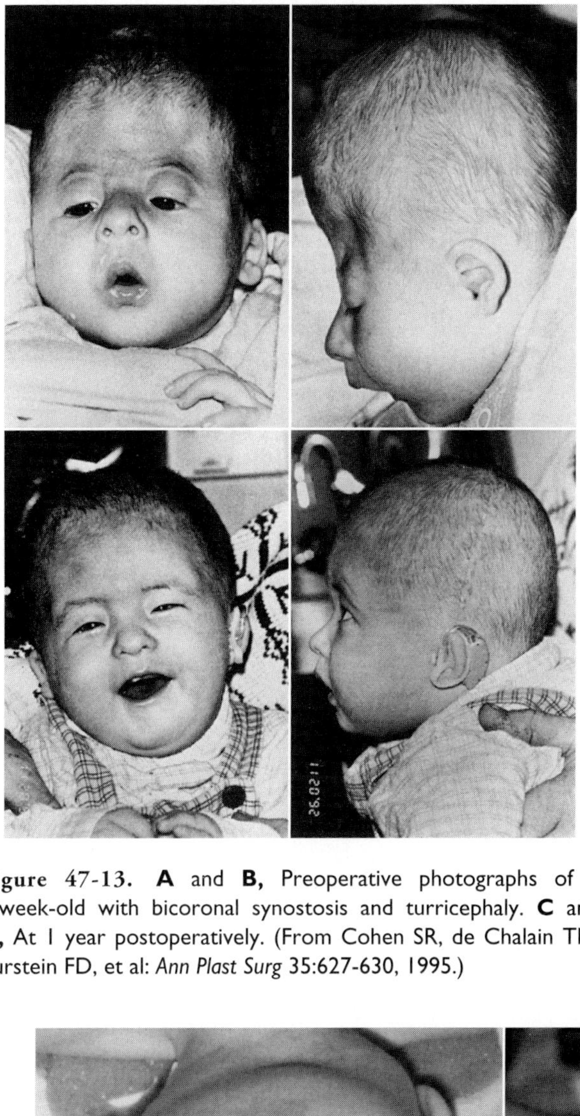

Figure 47-13. A and **B,** Preoperative photographs of a 6-week-old with bicoronal synostosis and turricephaly. **C** and **D,** At 1 year postoperatively. (From Cohen SR, de Chalain TM, Burstein FD, et al: *Ann Plast Surg* 35:627-630, 1995.)

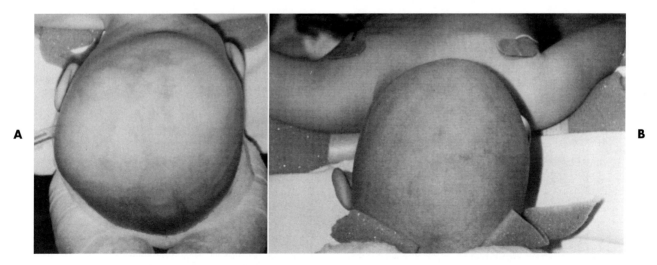

Figure 47-14. Vertex views. **A,** Infant with positional molding. Observe right occipitoparietal flattening, left occipital bossing, anterior displacement of right ear, and lack of right occipitomastoid bulge. **B,** Infant with left lambdoid synostosis. Observe right parietal bossing, left occipitomastoid bossing, and posterior displacement of left ear.

positional molding is repositioning. Moderately severe deformities are treated as early as possible with helmet therapy[12] or dynamic orthotic cranioplasty.[78]

POSTOPERATIVE MANAGEMENT

The vast majority of children undergoing correction of nonsyndromic single-suture craniosynostosis are admitted first to the recovery room and then transferred to either the surgical floor or intensive care unit. At our institution, only those patients undergoing major cranial vault reconstruction and/or those patients with associated congenital disorders (e.g., cardiac disease) are admitted to the intensive care unit. Approximately 70% of the children are transferred directly to the surgical floor. When a head dressing is used, it is typically removed on the third postoperative day. Patients are given intravenous antibiotics until the time of discharge and begun on a clear liquid, progressing to an age-appropriate regular diet once awake and alert. A complete blood count (CBC) and electrolytes are routinely drawn in the recovery room and on the first postoperative morning. In children undergoing major cranial vault reconstruction, serum electrolytes are followed for the first 72 hours. The majority of children leave the hospital by the fourth postoperative day. The family is instructed to care for the suture or staple lines. Typically, the staples are removed 7 to 10 days after operation. Children return 4 to 6 weeks later, after which time routine follow-up is established at the craniofacial center. Children are typically followed every 4 to 6 months until their third birthday, when annual follow-up begins. Children are monitored for normal neurologic development, and symptoms and signs of elevated ICP are closely monitored.

SECONDARY PROCEDURES

In the Outcomes section of this chapter, the frequency and types of secondary procedures are listed. In patients undergoing correction of metopic synostosis, secondary procedures may be necessary to treat residual or recurrent temporal depressions. In such cases, any metallic hardware is removed, and hydroxyapatite or paste (bone source) is used for reconstruction. We have been pleased with the outcomes after simple recontouring using hydroxyapatite and recently reported our results in a small group of patients.[7] Occasionally, as noted in the next section on outcomes, total reoperation is necessary. When total reoperation is carried out, generally the cases are longer and associated with higher blood loss. The same basic principles, however, are adhered to, as described above. Rarely, a patient will present with residual calvarial defects. Typically these children are given until around age 2 to develop new bone. If residual defects are present by this time, bone grafting is carried out. Although some authors have noted improvement in hypotelorism associated with metopic synostosis over time, others have found residual hypotelorism.[20] In cases in which redundant epicanthal folds are associated with intercanthal narrowing, a simple cranial bone graft to the nose

may take up the extra tissue, and medial osteotomies are not usually necessary.

In patients with sagittal synostosis treated by strip craniectomy, a small proportion may ultimately require total or subtotal cranial vault remodeling. Patients who have undergone total calvarial reconstruction may require secondary cranial reconstruction for (1) hardware removal; (2) hardware removal and recontouring; and (3) rarely, redoing total cranial vault reconstruction. We have recently had good experience with bone source, a hydroxyapatite paste with which it is easy to work.

Patients with unicoronal synostosis may require secondary surgery for minor temporal depressions and supraorbital rim asymmetry. A small percentage, who may have more extensive involvement of cranial base sutures, will go on to develop a clinical picture that has been referred to as *facial scoliosis*.[55] Significant nasal deviation and zygomatic-maxillary deformities are often associated with occlusal cants and even mandibular asymmetry. Correction requires a complex craniofacial approach combined with orthognathic procedures to realign the jaws.

Patients undergoing correction of bilateral coronal synostosis usually do well. It is likely, however, that a percentage of children with "nonsyndromic" craniosynostosis have an undiagnosed craniofacial syndrome leading to a higher frequency of recurrent deformity, which may require partial or total reoperation.[93]

Secondary procedures to expand the cranial vault may be necessary in a few patients with nonsyndromic craniosynostosis who develop increased ICP after frontoorbital advancement. We follow all children annually in the Center for Craniofacial Disorders to monitor skull growth and neuropsychiatric development.

OUTCOMES

Outcome analysis functions to determine the efficacy and reasonability of a service or product. This model is complicated in health care by the balance of cost containment to patient satisfaction and quality. Even so, application of outcome analysis provides the medical community a method of comparing and adjusting practice modalities to meet specific demands. It can also provide a means of establishing and communicating standard of care levels to those involved in the health care industry.

COMPLICATIONS

Cranial vault remodeling is usually completed within the first 12 to 15 months of age. The magnitude of the surgery is dictated by the sutures involved. The age of the patient and the intracranial component of the procedure carry inherent risks. Anesthetic risks are not significantly increased in the patient population compared with adults. But the introduction of venous and arterial lines, as well as central venous monitoring ports, may be difficult in some cases. Because of the diminished size of the airway and the small oxygen reserve in these patients, potential airway problems should always be considered. Finally, the increased surface area of the pediatric patient can cause a quick decrease in the core body temperature if active steps to maintain body temperature are not taken.

Specific complications associated with craniosynostosis may be classified as either perioperative or postoperative. In a review of 204 patients treated for nonsyndromic craniosynostosis at Scottish Rite Children's Medical Center, the overall perioperative complication rate was 9.8% (20/204) (Box 47-2). Major

complications were seen in total cranial vault remodeling for sagittal synostosis in which four experienced hypovolemic shock. One patient had a transection of the sagittal sinus, and one death was recorded. This was the only death in our series. Seven patients were found to have syndrome of inappropriate antidiuretic hormone (SIADH) in the immediate postoperative period (four in the total cranial vault remodeling group). Other perioperative or immediate postoperative complications included severe chemosis (one case), wound infection (one case), and urethritis (one case). Perioperative complications, including air embolism after a venous tear, infarction, and damage to the unprotected brain, have also been reported.[34]

Blood loss may be acute, but transfusions are usually necessary because of insidious losses throughout the case. Blood transfusions are required in almost all total cranial vault remodeling procedures. Transfusion requirements have been reported from 15% to 90% of the patient's estimated red blood cell volume.[26,57] Variability is seen based on the type of synostosis (Table 47-2). Acute complications of blood transfusion are well known and include hypocalcemia, hyperkalemia, coagulopathies, and transfusion incompatibility. Delayed complications of blood transfusions usually involve the potential for transmission of viral infections.

REOPERATION RATES

The rate of reoperation is an important outcome variable in the surgical treatment of craniosynostosis. Although quantitative changes in craniofacial remodeling are critical to understanding operative results, the decision to reoperate on a particular child is determined primarily from subjective measures of outcome, most commonly aesthetic appearance. Longitudinal studies of reoperation rates from a variety of centers are beginning to appear in the literature.[55,56,95,97]

A prospective statistical study of reoperation rates was reviewed in the treatment of 167 consecutive children with nonsyndromic and syndromic craniosynostosis over a 6-year

---

Box 47-2.
Complications Requiring Reoperation

SAGITTAL
Early strip craniectomy (<7 mos): none
Late strip craniectomy (>7 mos): none
Early vault remodeling (<7 mos): none
Late vault remodeling (>7 mos): significant relapse

METOPIC
Suboptimal cranial contouring

BICORONAL
Suboptimal cranial contouring ×2
Significant relapse ×2

UNICORONAL
Residual plagiocephaly
Suboptimal cranial contouring

MULTIPLE
Significant relapse

SYNDROMIC
Marked brachioturricephaly
Significant relapse

Table 47-2.
Mean (SD) Percentage of Patient's Estimated Red Cell Volume Lost and Type of Skull Deformities

TYPE OF SYNOSTOSIS	DURING OPERATION	AFTER OPERATION	TOTAL
Oxycephaly	49.1 (22.9)	−3.7 (16.8)*	45.4 (36.9)
Plagiocephaly	59 (37.4)	27.7 (41.7)	86.7 (56.2)
Trigonocephaly	92.4 (49.7)	11.7 (16.6)	104.1 (49.2)
Brachycephaly	105.3 (48.45)	25.5 (56.5)	130.9 (69.1)
Scaphocephaly	92.1 (65.2)	35.9 (38.4)	121.7 (78.2)
Complex	198.5 (165)	44.5 (97.6)	243.1 (259.4)

From Meyer P: *Br J Anaesth* 71:854-857, 1993.
*Negative value indicates postoperative overtransfusion.

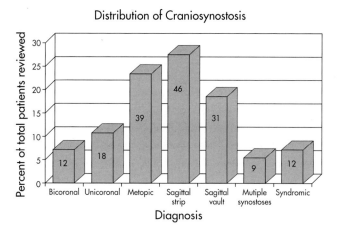

Figure 47-15. Craniosynostoses at Scottish Rite Children's Medical Center, Atlanta. (From Williams JK, Cohen SR, Burstein FD, et al: *Plast Reconstr Surg* 100:305-310, 1997.)

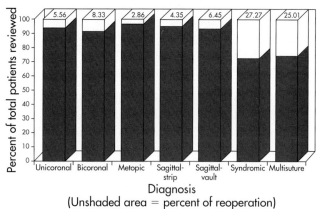

Figure 47-16. Reoperation rates. (From Williams JK, Cohen SR, Burstein FD, et al: *Plast Reconstr Surg* 100:305-310, 1997.)

period at Scottish Rite Children's Medical Center[99] (Figure 47-15). Mean length of follow-up was 2.8 years. Frontoorbital remodeling with a floating forehead was completed at 4 to 6 months of age for nonsyndromic synostosis other than sagittal synostosis. This approach is similar to treatment of isolated synostosis in several centers.[71,95,97] Bilateral frontoorbital remodeling has been shown to be comparable with or better than unilateral remodeling and was done in all cases.[52,97] Strip craniectomies were limited to sagittal synostosis with mild-to-moderate deformities. Total cranial vault remodeling was completed for severe deformities if the patient was greater than 7 weeks old. Patients with syndromic craniosynostosis underwent frontoorbital advancement and cranial reshaping in 4 to 6 months unless increased cranial pressures required decompression.

Reoperation equal to or exceeding the magnitude of the original procedure occurred in 7% of cases (Figure 47-16). Total reoperation rates for syndromic and nonsyndromic synostoses were 27.3% and 5.9%, respectively. Five of the 12 reoperative cases (41.6%) were completed for significant relapse, as demonstrated clinically and radiographically. Neither early nor late sagittal strip craniectomies required reoperations; only one patient in the late cranial vault remodeling group for sagittal synostosis (>7 months) demonstrated relapse and required reoperation. Relapse was seen in two patients with bicoronal synostosis, requiring reoperation, and two more patients in this group underwent a second procedure for suboptimal cranial contouring. The rates of total reoperation significantly differed by gender (Fisher exact test $p = .029$). Of the female patients, 13.8% required reoperation compared with 3.8% of males.

The highest reoperative rate in nonsyndromic children was found in bicoronal synostosis. Of children with single-suture synostosis, reoperative rates were highest in those with sagittal suture fusion requiring total vault remodeling (6.45%). Reoperative rates in metopic synostosis were 2.86% with an average follow-up of 42 months. No statistical significance

was found in reoperative rates for the various single-suture synostoses.

Multiple regression analysis revealed female patients and children with syndromic synostoses were more likely to require reoperation (Table 47-3). The reason for the increased odds ratio associated with female patients is unknown. Age did not appear to have an effect on reoperation rates. A 1-year increase in age at operation was not statistically significant after controlling for diagnostic group. The effect on reoperation rate of a 100-mm increase in estimated blood loss was not significant after controlling for diagnostic group. Similarly, length of hospital stay, length of surgery, intensive care unit admission, and the amount of transfusion were not statistically significant after controlling for diagnostic category.

Whitaker's classification[97] of clinical results after a craniofacial procedure includes Category III (C-III), requiring major bone grafting or other osteotomies, and Category IV (C-IV), requiring duplication of the previous craniofacial procedure. Total reoperations in our review were classified into the latter group. The increase in reoperation rates of syndromic were consistent with previous reviews. Whitaker[96,97] showed a C-IV reoperation rate of 3% for asymmetric lesions (isolated synostosis) and 64% for the symmetric lesions (95% in Apert's syndrome). Excluding strip craniectomies, McCarthy had a 6.7% reoperation rate for isolated synostosis[55] and 28.3% for syndromic deformities.[56] Surgical approaches similar to ours were used in each of the aforementioned studies.

In most studies, no differences were seen in reoperative rates for treatment of single-suture synostosis as related to age (Table 47-4);[24,73] recommendations for primary intervention ranged from 2 to 18 months. Wall et al[95] showed an increased reoperation rate of 20% in nonsyndromic synostosis when primary treatment was in patients less than 6 months of age compared with 5.6% in patients greater than 6 months old. In syndromic disorders, patients less than 6 months old had a 30.2% reoperation rate compared with 9.1% when older than

Table 47-3.
Multivariable Analysis of Total Reoperation Rates

CONTROL VARIABLE	SYNDROMIC VERSUS NONSYNDROMIC	SAGITTAL VAULT VERSUS OTHER	ONLY CONTROL VARIABLE (p value)
None	6.0	1.1	–
Female gender	5.9	1.3	3.9 (0.04)
Age at surgery (1 yr)	9.7	0.7	0.6 (0.19)
Blood loss (each 100 units)	6.4	0.4	1.1 (0.31)
Length of stay (days)	1.3	0.5	1.2 (0.07)
Length of surgery (each 100 minutes)	5.2	0.5	1.3 (0.53)
Months of follow-up	5.7	1.1	1.1 (0.74)
Any ICU stay	9.1	1.7	0.6 (0.59)
Any transfusion	6.3	0.5	2.3 (0.46)
Any complications	4.2	0.9	5.7
Early complications	4.4	0.8	2.4
Late complications	5.0	1.4	6.2

From Williams JK, Cohen SR, Burstein FD, et al: *Plast Reconstr Surg* 100:305-310, 1997.

Table 47-4.
Age-Related Reoperation

	TOTAL REOPERATIONS	
	YES	NO
Number of patients	11	144
Mean age of initial operation	0.57 yr	1.0 yr
Standard deviation	0.52 yr	1.27 yr
Standard error	0.16 yr	0.11 yr

From Williams JK, Cohen SR, Burstein FD, et al: *Plast Reconstr Surg* 100:305-310, 1997.

6 months (40.9-month follow-up). Other reviews have shown no relationship of age to reoperative rates.[99]

FUNCTIONAL OUTCOME

Increased Intracranial Pressures

The first major study attempting to measure ICP in children with craniosynostosis was by Renier et al.[77] Defining normal ICP as below 10 mm Hg and elevated as above 15 mm Hg, ICP were recorded preoperatively by an epidural sensor for 12 to 24 hours. Of 92 patients, 14% with nonsyndromic suture fusion had evidence of elevated ICP. After surgery, the ICP decreased to within normal limits in all but 7% of patients (Table 47-5). The review eventually consisted of 358 patients.[76] Using Renier's criteria for normal and abnormal levels of ICP, Thompson[44] also found 12.9% of patients with single-suture fusion, and 57% of patients with nonsyndromic multiple suture fusion, to have elevated ICP (Table 47-6). The latter study used subdural monitoring devices, which are thought to be more accurate.

The association between increased ICP and craniosynostosis is well established, but a direct corollary between the two is not clear in every patient.[44,100] Recent advances in imaging techniques have provided a method of intracranial volume analysis that demonstrates a more complicated relationship between craniosynostosis and ICP. Several studies have demonstrated that suture fusion does not always cause a decrease in the volume of the cranial vault in nonsyndromic suture fusion.[31,54,72] Furthermore, studies using intracranial-invasive monitoring did not find a consistent correlation between intracranial hypertension and decreased cranial volume. In one study, 13 of 66 patients were found to have elevated ICP, of whom 12 had decreased intracranial volume. In contrast, only 5 of 13 patients with the most severe reduction in volume demonstrated intracranial hypertension (above 15 mm Hg).[30]

Late postoperative increases in ICP were seen in 2% of patients at our institution. One patient developed elevated ICP

Table 47-5.
Baseline Intracranial Pressure in Patients Subdivided according to Skull Shape and Syndrome, Used in This Study

TYPE	BASELINE ICP		
	≤10 mm Hg	10-15 mm Hg	≥15 mm Hg
31 Trigono	21 (28%)	8 (26%)	2 (6%)
118 Scapho	76 (64%)	33 (28%)	9 (8%)
65 Plagio	40 (62%)	17 (26%)	8 (12%)
34 Brachy	17 (50%)	8 (24%)	9 (26%)
66 Oxy	23 (35%)	7 (11%)	36 (54%)
9 Crouzon	3	0	6
16 Apert	3	6	7

From Renier D: Intracranial pressure craniosynostosis: pre and postoperative recording/correlation with functional results. In Persing J, editor: *Scientific foundation on surgical treatment of craniosynostosis,* Baltimore, 1989, Williams & Wilkins.

Table 47-6.
Elevated Intracranial Pressures in Craniosynostosis*

STUDY	SINGLE SUTURE FUSION % (n)	MULTIPLE SUTURE FUSION % (n)	CROUZON'S DISEASE % (n)	APERT'S SYNDROME % (n)
Thompson (1995)[89a]	12.9 (8/62)	57.0 (12/21)	65.0 (13/20)	38.5 (5/13)
Gault (1992)[30]	3.9 (2/51)	71.4 (8/11)	67.0 (2/3)	100.0 (1/1)
Renier (1989)[76]	8.9 (19/124)	45.0 (45/100)	66.7 (6/9)	43.8 (7/16)
Renier (1982)[77]	13.5 (5/37)	43.3 (13/30)	100 (2/2)	50.0 (3/6)

From Williams JK, Longaker MT, Wisoff J, et al: *J Craniofac Surg* 8:373-378, 1997.
*All studies used 15 mm Hg as upper limit of normal pressure.

requiring decompression after a cranial vault remodeling. Recurrent intracranial hypertension after previous corrective surgery has been reported and requires a secondary cranial vault remodeling.[18,77]

Mental Development

Studies on the effects of isolated craniosynostosis on mental development are difficult to interpret because of differences in the definitions of mental delay, variability of inclusion criteria, and differences in testing methods. Two questions exist: (1) does nonsyndromic synostosis cause a decrease in mental development? and if so, (2) does surgical intervention prevent the delay in mental development? Earlier studies have reported a prevalence of mental delay ranging from 0% to 20% in metopic synostosis,[2,4,25] 10% to 66% in sagittal synostosis,[4,9,25,83] and 0% to 27% in coronal synostosis.[4,40,59,62]

Recent studies elucidating the relationship of craniosynostosis and mental development have been conflicting. Recognizing the problems with the definitions of normal and abnormal ICP, Renier et al[76] obtained ICP (using an epidural sensor) in 358 patients with various types of craniosynostosis. Some 229 patients with nonsyndromic suture fusion underwent intelligence testing. Excluding trigonocephaly, more than 90% of the patients with single-suture fusion tested within the normal range. The proportion was lower in trigonocephaly (83%) because of the presence of syndromic anomalies. Patients with multiple-suture fusion had a lower number of patients in the normal range (brachycephaly 78%, oxycephaly 69%). Also interesting was the overall decrease in the number of normal patients over 1 year old in the normal range compared with patients less than 1 year old. When stratified for ICP, patients with scaphocephaly did *not* show a decrease in the proportion of normal intelligence associated with elevated ICPs. In unicoronal plagiocephaly the percentage of patients testing within the normal range decreased from 97% to 86%, and the decrease was even more dramatic in patients with multiple-suture fusion.

A longitudinal study by Kapp-Simon et al[44] following mental development in patients with nonsyndromic suture fusion failed to confirm these findings. A review of 45 patients demonstrated no differences in terms of mental development between patients with synostosis and a normal control group. No decrease in mental development when analyzed for suture type, single-suture versus multiple sutures, timing of repair, or severity of deformity (4-point severity scores from patient and radiographic review) were found. Furthermore, no differences were noted between patients in the operative group and the nonoperative group. Mental developmental scores were actually higher in patients with multiple-suture synostosis compared with single-suture fusion. The major criticism of this study was the low number of patients who were assessed.[75]

Improvement in behavior has been reported with resolution of papilledema as an indicator of decreased ICP.[10] Using "monitor-proven" decreases in ICP after surgery, Renier et al did not conclusively demonstrate an improvement in intelligence compared with nonoperated controls.[76] It was concluded that the effective decrease in ICP after the operative intervention could possibly arrest the deterioration in intelligence. Therefore surgical intervention should be within the first year of life (during the maximal growth conflict stage). In contrast, Kapp-Simon found no improvement in mental development of patients with surgical intervention compared with the nonoperative group.[44]

Aesthetics

Recognizing the potential functional complications associated with nonsyndromic synostosis, operative intervention is usually undertaken because of aesthetic concerns. The acquired deformity of the various synostoses has been discussed previously. The importance of appearance in social interactions and the social advantages associated with attractiveness have been established. Few studies have attempted to clarify the impact of congenital malformation on psychosocial well-being. Pertshuk and Whitaker[69] evaluated the psychosocial impact of congenital craniofacial malformations in two groups of children between ages 6 and 13, categorized by having early surgery (before age 4) or later surgery (after age 4). The earlier group demonstrated "no differences" to matched healthy subjects regarding psychosocial adjustment. In contrast, the later group expressed poorer self-concept, greater anxiety, more problematic behaviors, and more introversion. The psychosocial adjustments in this group appeared "limited." A final group of adolescent adult patients with uncorrected craniofacial malformations underwent similar analysis and was found to have obvious disturbances in social adjustment and self-concept. The analysis was not stratified for specific disorders, but general conclusions regarding the importance of improving appearance for psychosocial adjustment were demonstrated.

Table 47-7. Results after Initial FOA-CVR		
GRADE	NO. PATIENTS	%
I	10	45
II	3	14
III	9	41
TOTAL	22	100

FOA, Frontal orbital advancement; *CVR*, calvarial vault remodeling.
From Wagner J, Cohen S, Maher H, et al: *J Craniofac Surg* 6:32-37, 1995.

Table 47-8. Results after FOA-CVR versus Age at Operation				
AGE AT INITIAL FOA-CVR	NO. PATIENTS			
	GRADE I	GRADE II	GRADE III	TOTAL
≤5 mo	5	0	8	13
≥6 mo	5	3	1	9

FOA, Frontal orbital advancement; *CVR*, calvarial vault remodeling.
From Wagner J, Cohen S, Maher H, et al: *J Craniofac Surg* 6:32-37, 1995.

Standardized clinical assessments of aesthetic outcome in cranial vault remodeling are limited. Wagner et al[93] reviewed 22 patients with bicoronal synostosis who underwent cranial vault remodeling. Using the grading system proposed by Whitaker et al, 45% (10) were judged to have satisfactory results, 14% were classified as grade II requiring minor revisions, and 41% required major reoperation rates (Tables 47-7 and 47-8). In a similar study,[55] 17 patients with trigonocephaly requiring cranial vault remodeling underwent review using a similar grading scale. Some 53% of the patients were found to have none or mild deformities (grade I), 35% had moderate deformities (grade II), and 12% had severe deformities requiring major reoperation (grade III).

Risk Stratification for Reoperation—Quantitative CT Scan Analysis

Current diagnosis and surgical correction of craniofacial anomalies benefited from accurate quantitative CT analysis as described by Waitzman and Posnick.[94] Clinically useful growth information may be obtained, and the treating clinician may calculate preferred osteotomy movements to be achieved at operation. The intraoperative execution of the calculated changes at operation can be verified by analysis of postoperative CT scans.

Child's Name: _____ Account Number: _____

Note: This pathway is a tool to be used in progressing the patient through a hospitalization. This document is maintained as a part of the chart during hospitalization only. It is not to be considered as a prescription for services, but rather as a guide. **THE PATHWAY IS *NOT* TO BE A PART OF THE PERMANENT RECORD.**

Instructions: Record the appropriate variance type (coded as: A = Practitioner, B = Patient, C = System, D = Other) in the blanks provided. *Check marks are not acceptable.* For each variance, document the cause of the variance in the table at the bottom of each page with the date, day, variance type (again), and your signature. NOTE: Blanks are provided for documentation of variances *only*. If there are no variances, check the box for no variances. In addition, when the review for the day is complete, check the box for review completed and sign as reviewer.

Hospital Day	Dx/Tx Measures	Medications	Nursing Services	Anesthesia/Resp. Care	Nutrition/Diet
Preop	___ CBC ___ Type and cross-match one unit of PRBC ___ UA	___ Anesthesia preop	Nursing Assessment: ___ Allergies ___ Immunization history ___ Medical/surgical history ___ General health weight ___ Support system Preop Teaching: ___ NPO times ___ Arrival time, day of surgery ___ Day surgery procedures ___ Preop checklist ___ Reinforce preop teaching, prn	Anesthesia Assessment: ___ History ___ Physical exam ___ Respiratory/cardiac assessment	___ NPO as instructed
	☐ No variances ☐ Review completed Reviewed By:	☐ No variances ☐ Review completed Reviewed By:	☐ No variances ☐ Review completed Reviewed By:	☐ No variances ☐ Review completed Reviewed By:	☐ No variances ☐ Review completed Reviewed By:

Variation Types: A = Practitioner   B = Patient   C = System   D = Other

DATE	DAY	VARIANCE TYPE	VARIANCE/CAUSE	SIGNATURE

Figure 47-17. Sagittal synostosis critical pathway. Strip craniectomy patients only.

We recently performed a quantitative CT scan analysis in patients with metopic synostosis to determine if preoperative findings are predictive of the need for reoperation.[65] In 35 children with metopic synostosis, measurements of the cranial length, cranial width, anterior intercoronal distance, anterior interorbital distance (intercanthal distance), lateral orbital distance, and interzygomatic buttress distance were taken from the preoperative CT scans and normalized relative to each child's age.[94] Abnormal measurements were defined as those that fell outside of the age-appropriate mean by greater than or equal to 5% of the mean. To separate overall facial hypoplasia from regional hypoplasia, a ratio of intercanthal distance to interzygomatic buttress distance was determined. These prognostic factors were analyzed using chi-squared or Fisher's exact test with respect to length of hospital stay, transfusion requirement, postoperative complications, and reoperation rate. Some 29% of the children underwent reoperation (5% total reoperation and 24% recontouring) for correction of residual contour deformities. All of the reoperations occurred in children with abnormally small intercanthal distance ($p = 0.16$). The ratio of intercanthal distance to midfacial width was significantly related to reoperation rate with those children who had a ratio of less than or equal to 0.80, having a reoperation rate of 43.8% ($p = 0.05$). This relationship suggests that the preoperative CT scan measurements can be used as a means of risk stratification in outcome analyses of the surgical treatment of craniosynostosis. In children treated for metopic synostosis, a foreshortened intercanthal distance compared with interzygomatic buttress distance was significantly related to reoperation rate, particularly in those children who were under 12 months of age when treated.

Economic Issues

Critical pathways are case management mechanisms. From 1994 to 1995, Scottish Rite Children's Medical Center adopted a variety of critical pathways. Patients undergoing sagittal synostectomies were included in one such critical path. In an environment in which multiple clinical disciplines provide patient care services, case management through the use of critical paths is one of the more efficient ways to ensure continuity of care. Critical pathways are class project-management and industrial-engineering tools that are simple, visual, and two-dimensional. They plot time along one axis and staff actions-tasks, interventions, and orders along another to form a "schedule of events within time periods."[5] The pathway development model Scottish Rite adopted is an integrated model developed by interdisciplinary teams and supported by the quality improvement structure.

The critical path is a clinical tool for achieving better quality and cost outcomes by outlining and sequencing the usual and/or desired care for particular groups of patients. At its core, the critical path is a communication tool, facilitating coordination among a wide variety of clinicians and departments. As Bruce Campbell, Director of Medical Liaison at Scripps Memorial Hospital in San Diego, observed, "Care is so complex now, and variable from patient to patient, that if the

essential components of care are not 'blueprinted,' they are either forgotten or not done on time."[102] As a result, patient outcomes are jeopardized.[102] Critical paths create a matrix that profiles interventions on one axis and time on another. Second-generation critical paths, which are called care maps, incorporate usual patient problems, desired clinical outcomes, and intermediate goals into the matrix. Critical paths are generally used in high-volume, high-cost, high-risk, or high-interest patient populations. They involve physicians in all stages of critical path development. The variances for critical pathways are used to stimulate discussion among practitioners and to identify opportunities to improve organizational systems and care practices.

Economic issues are discussed in terms of hospitalization costs rather than surgical fees. Every effort has been made with the individual surgeon's fees to remain competitive. At our center, discussions are underway to develop package pricing for craniosynostosis services. The cost of hospitalization for nonsyndromic craniosynostosis patients was assessed through a biopsy of the hospital bills of 197 patients operated on from 1988 to 1996 at our institution. The costs range from $5130.30 to $120,121. The mean costs range from $52,381 in 1990 to $14,225 in 1996. In 1990 and 1994, costs exceeded $100,000 in two patients who had suffered complications. The patients' diagnoses included sagittal, bicoronal, unicoronal, and metopic synostoses. After surgery the presence or absence of an early complication was noted. When an early complication occurred, the mean hospital charge was $75,995 compared with $22,293 ($p = .03$).

In 1995 a critical pathway was introduced for patients undergoing sagittal synostectomies. Figure 47-17 shows an example of the sagittal synostectomy critical pathway. Variances in variation types are recorded. Variation types may be related to the practitioner, patient, system, or other. Although the number of observations is small, the mean cost of hospitalization dropped substantially, but numbers are still too small for meaningful statistical analysis.

REFERENCES

1. Albright AL, Byrd RP: Suture pathology in craniosynostosis, *J Neurosurg* 54:384, 1981.
2. Anderson FM, Greiger L: Craniosynostosis: a survey of 204 cases, *J Neurosurg* 22:229, 1965.
3. Argenta LC, David L, Wilson J, et al: An increase in infant cranial deformity with supine sleeping position, *J Craniofac Surg* 7:5, 1996.
4. Bertelson TI: The premature synostosis of the cranial sutures, *Acta Ophthalmol Suppl* 51(suppl 1), 1958.
5. Bower KA: Developing and using critical paths. In Lord J, editor: *The physician leader's guide,* Rockville, Md, 1996, The Quality Letter.
6. Bruneteau RJ, Mulliken JB: Frontal plagiocephaly: synostotic, compensatory, or deformational, *Plast Reconstr Surg* 89:21, 1992.

7. Burstein F, Cohen S, Hudgins R, et al: The use of granular hydroxyapatite in secondary orbitocranial reconstruction. In Marchac D, editor: *Craniofacial surgery,* vol 6, Proceedings of the Sixth Congress of the International Society of Craniofacial Surgery, Bologna, Italy, 1996, Monduzzi Editore.

8. Burstein F, Hudgins R, Cohen SR, et al: Surgical correction of severe scaphocephalic deformities, *J Craniofac Surg* 5:228-235, 1994.

9. Butti G, Locatelli D, Caccialanza E, et al: Surgical treatment of craniosystoses, *J Neurosurg Sci* 32:41, 1988.

10. Campbell JW, Albright AL, Losken HW, et al: Intracranial hypertension after cranial vault decompression for craniosynostosis, *Pediatr Neurosurg* 22:270, 1995.

11. Clarren SK: Plagiocephaly and torticollis: etiology, natural history, and helmet treatment, *J Pediatr* 98:92, 1981.

12. Clarren SK, Smith DW, Hansen JW: Helmet treatment for plagiocephaly and congenital muscular torticollis, *J Pediatr* 94:43, 1979.

13. Cohen MM Jr: Sutural biology and the correlates of craniosynostosis, *Am J Med Genet* 47:581, 1993.

14. Cohen MM Jr: *Craniosynostosis: diagnosis, evaluation, and management,* New York, 1986, Raven Press.

15. Cohen MM Jr: Craniostenoses and syndromes with craniosynostosis: incidence, genetics, penetrance, variability and new syndrome updating, *Birth Defects* 15:13, 1979.

16. Cohen MM Jr: The etiology of cranial synostosis, *Childs Brain* 1:22, 1975.

17. Cohen S, de Chalain T, Burstein F, et al: Turribrachycephaly: a technical note, *Ann Plast Surg* 35:6, 1995.

18. Cohen SR, Dauser RC, Newman MN, et al: Surgical techniques of cranial vault expansion for increase in intracranial pressure in older children, *J Craniofac Surg* 4:167, 1993.

19. Cohen SR, Kawamoto HK Jr, Burstein F, et al: Advancement onlay: an improved technique of fronto-orbital remodeling in craniosynostosis, *Childs Nerv Syst* 7:264, 1991.

20. Cohen SR, Maher H, Wagner JD, et al: Metopic synostosis: evaluation of aesthetic results, *Plast Reconstr Surg* 94:759-767, 1994.

21. Cormack DH: *Ham's histology,* Philadelphia, 1987, JB Lippincott.

22. Decker JD, Hall SH: Light and electron microscopy of the newborn sagittal suture, *Anat Rec* 212:81, 1985.

23. Delashaw JB, Persing JA, Broaddus WC, et al: Cranial vault growth in craniosynostosis, *J Neurosurg* 70:159, 1989.

24. DiRocco C, Marchese E, Velardi F: Craniosynostosis: surgical treatment during the first year of life, *J Neurosurg Sci* 36:129, 1992.

25. Dominiquez R, Oh KS, Bender T, et al: Uncomplicated trigonocephaly, *Radiology* 140:681, 1981.

26. Eaton AC, Marsh JL, Pilgram TK: Transfusion requirements for craniosynostosis surgery in infants, *Plast Reconstr Surg* 95:277-283, 1995.

27. Engstrom C, Wergeda JE, Engstrom H, et al: Characterization of cells isolated from synostotic suture and skull bone from neonatal humans (Abstract 24), *J Dent Res* 67:115, 1988.

28. Eppley B, Sadove AM: Surgical correction of metopic synostosis, *Clin Plast Surg* 21:555, 1994.

29. Furtwangler JA, Hall SH, Koskinen-Moffett LK: Sutural morphogenesis in the mouse calvaria: the role of apoptosis, *Acta Anat* 124:74, 1985.

30. Gault DT, Renier D, Marchac D, et al: Intracranial pressure and intracranial volume in children with craniosynostosis, *Plast Reconstr Surg* 90:377-381, 1992.

31. Gault DT, Renier D, Marchac D, et al: Intracranial volume in children with craniosynostosis, *J Craniofac Surg* 1:1-3, 1990.

32. Gorlin RJ, Pindborg JJ, Cohen MM: *Syndromes of the head and neck,* ed 2, New York, 1976, McGraw-Hill.

33. Hall SH, Decker JD: Light and electron microscopic immunocytochemistry of osteonectin and a bone-specific proteoglycan, *J Bone Miner Res* 1:136, 1986.

34. Harrop CW, Avery BS, Marks SM, et al: Craniosynostosis in babies: complications and management of 40 cases, *Br J Oral Maxillofac Surg* 34;158-161, 1996.

35. Helveston EM: Symposium: head posture and strabismus, *Am Orthoptic J* 33:1, 1983.

36. Hobar PC, Schreiber JS, McCarthy JG, et al: The role of the dura in cranial bone regeneration in the immature animal, *Plast Reconstr Surg* 92:405, 1993.

37. Hoffman HJ, Mohr G: Lateral canthal advancement of the supraorbital margin. A new corrective technique in the treatment of coronal synostosis, *J Neurosurg* 45:376, 1976.

38. Huang MHS, Gruss J, Clarren S, et al: The differential diagnosis of posterior plagiocephaly: true lambdoid synostosis versus positional molding, *Plast Reconstr Surg* 98:766-774, 1996.

39. Hudgins R, Burstein F, Boydston W: Total calvarial reconstruction for sagittal synostosis in older infants and children, *J Neurosurg* 78:119, 1993.

40. Hunter AGW, Rudd NL: Craniosynostosis: II. Coronal synostosis: its familial characteristics associated with clinical findings in 109 patients lacking bilateral polysyndactyly or syndactyly, *Teratology* 15:310, 1977.

41. Jane JA, Edgarton MT, Futrell JW, et al: Immediate correction of sagittal synostosis, *J Neurosurg* 49:705-710, 1978.

42. Johanson V, Hall SH: Morphogenesis of the mouse coronal suture, *Acta Anat* 114:58, 1982.

43. Kane AA, Mitchel LE, Craven KP, et al: Observations on a recent issue in plagiocephaly without synostosis, *Pediatrics* 97:877, 1996.

44. Kapp-Simon KA, Figueroa A, Jocher CA, et al: Longitudinal assessment of mental development in infants with nonsyndromic craniosynostosis with and without cranial release and reconstruction, *Plast Reconstr Surg* 92:831, 1993.

45. Kokich VG, Moffett BC, Cohen MM Jr: The cloverleaf skull anomaly: an anatomic and histologic study of two specimens, *Cleft Palate J* 19:89, 1982.

46. Koskinen L, Isotupa K: A note on craniofacial sutural growth, *Am J Phys Anthropol* 45:511, 1976.

47. Lane LC: Pioneer craniectomy for relief of mental imbecility due to premature sutural closure and microcephalus, *JAMA* 18:49, 1892.

48. Lannelongue M: De la craniectomie dans la microcephalie, *Compte-Rendu Academic des Sciences* 110:1382, 1890.

49. Lawrence WT, Azizkhan RG: Congenital muscular torticollis: a spectrum of pathology, *Ann Plast Surg* 23:523, 1989.

50. Manzanares MC, Goret-Nicaise M, Dhem A: Metopic sutural closure in the human skull, *J Anat* 161:203, 1988.

51. Marchac D, Renier D: "Le front flotant." Traitement precoce des facio-craniostenoses, *Ann Chir Plast* 24:121-126, 1979.

52. Marchac D, Renier D, Broumand S: Timing of treatment for craniosynostosis and faciocraniosynostosis: a 20-year experience, *Br J Plast Surg* 47:211, 1994.

53. Markens IS: Embryonic development of the coronal suture in man and rat, *Acta Anat* 93:257, 1975.

54. Marsh JL: Discussion: metopic and sagittal synostosis: intracranial volume measurements prior to and after cranio-orbital reshaping in childhood, *Plast Reconstr Surg* 96:312-315, 1995.

55. McCarthy JG, Glasberg SB, Cutting CB, et al: Twenty-year experience with early surgery for craniosynostosis: I. Isolated craniofacial synostosis—results and unsolved problems, *Plast Reconstr Surg* 96:272, 1995.

56. McCarthy JG, Glasberg SB, Cutting CB, et al: Twenty-year experience with early surgery for craniosynostosis: II. The craniofacial synostosis syndromes and pansynostosis—results and unsolved problems, *Plast Reconstr Surg* 96:284, 1995.

57. Meyer P, Renier D, Arnaud E, et al: Blood loss during repair of craniosynostosis, *Br J Anaesth* 1993;71:854, 1993.

58. Miroue M, Rosenberg L: *The human facial sutures: a morpholic and histologic study of age changes from 20 to 95 years,* master's thesis, Seattle, 1975, University of Washington.

59. Mohr G, Hoffman HJ, Munroe IR, et al: Surgical management of unilateral and bilateral coronal synostosis: 21 years of experience, *Neurosurgery* 2:83, 1978.

60. Montaut J, Stricker M: *Dysmorphies craniofaciales: les synostoses prematuries (craniostenoses et faciostenoses),* Paris, 1977, Masson.

61. Moss ML: The pathogenesis of premature cranial synostosis in man, *Acta Anat* 37:351, 1959.

62. Noezel MJ, Marsh JL, Palkes H, et al: Hydrocephalus and mental retardation in craniosynostosis, *J Pediatr* 107:885, 1985.

63. Ocampo RV, Persing JA: Sagittal synostosis, *Clin Plast Surg* 1994;21:563, 1994.

64. 64. Opperman LA, Sweeney TM, Redmond J, et al: Tissue interactions with underlying dura mater inhibit osseous obliteration of developing cranial sutures, *Dev Dyn* 198:312, 1993.

65. Paige K, Cohen S, Simms C, et al: Risk stratification for reoperation in metopic synostosis: a quantitative CT analysis. In Whitaker L (ed): *Proceedings of the 7th International Congress of the International Society of Craniofacial Surgery,* Bologna, Italy, 1997, Monduzzi.

66. Park EA, Powers GF: Acrocephaly and scaphocephaly with symmetrically distributed malformations of the extremities, *Am J Dis Child* 20:235, 1920.

67. Persing JA, Delashaw JB, Jane JA, et al: Lambdoid synostosis: surgical considerations, *Plast Reconstr Surg* 81:852, 1988.

68. Persson M, Roy W: Suture development and bony fusion in the fetal rabbit palate, *Arch Oral Biol* 24:283, 1979.

69. Pertshuk MJ, Whitaker LA: Psychosocial considerations in craniofacial deformity, *Clin Plast Surg* 14:163, 1987.

70. Posnick JC: Unilateral coronal synostosis (anterior plagiocephaly): current clinical perspectives, *Ann Plast Surg* 36:430, 1996.

71. Posnick JC: The craniofacial dystosis syndromes: current reconstructive strategies, *Clin Plast Surg* 21:585-598, 1994.

72. Posnick JC, Armstrong D, Bite U: Metopic and sagittal synostosis: intracranial volume measurements prior to and after cranio-orbital reshaping in childhood, *Plast Reconstr Surg* 96:299-309, 1995.

73. Prevot M, Renier D, Marchac D: Lack of ossification after cranioplasty for craniosynostosis: a review of relevant factors in 592 consecutive patients, *J Craniofac Surg* 4:247, 1993.

74. Pritchard JJ, Scott JH, Girgis FG: The structure and development of cranial and facial sutures, *J Anat* 90:73-86, 1956.

75. Renier D: Longitudinal assessment of mental development in infants with nonsyndromic craniosynostosis with and without cranial release and reconstruction: discussion, *Plast Reconstr Surg* 92:840, 1993.

76. Renier D: Intracranial pressure in craniosynostosis: pre-and postoperative recordings—correlation with functional results. In Persing J, Edgerton MT, Jane JA, editors: *Scientific foundations and surgical treatment of craniosynostosis,* Baltimore, 1989, Williams & Wilkens.

77. Renier D, Sainte-Rose C, Marchac D, et al: Intracranial pressure in craniostenosis, *J Neurosurg* 57:370-377, 1982.

78. Ripley CE, Pomatto J, Beals SP, et al: Treatment of positional plagiocephaly with dynamic orthotic cranioplasty, *J Craniofac Surg* 5:150, 1994.

79. Robson P: Persisting head turning in the early months: some effects in the early years, *Dev Med Child Neurol* 10:82, 1968.

80. Roth DA, Longaker MT, McCarthy JG, et al: Studies in cranial suture biology: Part I. Increase immunoreactivity for TGF-b isoforms (B1, B2, and B3) during rat cranial suture fusion, *J Bone Miner Res* 71:622, 1997.

81. Sadove AM, Kalsbeck JE, Eppley B, et al: Modifications in the surgical correction of trigonocephaly, *Plast Reconstr Surg* 85:853, 1990.

82. Sen A, Dougal P, Padhy AK, et al: Technetium-99m-HMPAO SPECT cerebral blood flow study in children with craniosynostosis, *J Nucl Med* 36:394, 1995.

83. Shillito J Jr, Matson DD: Craniosynostosis: a review of 519 surgical patients, *Pediatrics* 41:829, 1968.

84. Shuper A, Merlob P, Grunebaum M, et al: The incidence of isolated craniosynostosis in the newborn infant, *Am J Dis Child* 139:85, 1985.

85. Smith DW, Tondury G: Origin of the calvaria and its sutures, *Am J Dis Child* 132:662, 1978.

86. Sommering ST: *Vom Baue des Menschlichen Korpers. Erster Heil: Knochenlehre.* Frankfort am Main, Germany, 1839, Voss Leipzig.

87. Ten Cate AR, Freeman E, Dickinson JB: Sutural development: structure and its response to rapid separation, *Am J Orthodont* 71:622, 1977.

88. Tessier P: Osteotomies totales de le face. Syndrome de Crouzon, Syndrome d'apert: oxcephalies, scaphocephalies, turricephalies, *Ann Chir Plast* 12:273, 1967.

89. Turk AE, McCarthy JG, Thorne CHM, et al: The "back to sleep" campaign and deformational plagiocephaly: is there cause for concern? *J Craniofac Surg* 7:12, 1996.

89a. Thompson DN, Harkness W, Jones B, et al: Subdural intracranial pressure monitoring in craniosynostosis: its role in surgical management, *Childs Nerv Syst* 11:269-275, 1995.

90. Vander Kolk C, Carson B: Lambdoid synostosis, *Clin Plast Surg* 21:575, 1994.

91. Virchow R: Uber den Cretinismus, nametlich in Franken und uber pathologische Schadelforamen, *Verhandlungen Physikalische-Medizinische Gesellschaft in Wurzburg* 2:230, 1881.

92. Virchow R: Uber den Cretinismus, nametlich in Franken und uber pathologische Schadelforamen, *Verhandlungen Physikalische-Medizinische Gesellschaft in Wurzburg* 2:230, 1851.

93. Wagner J, Cohen S, Maher H, et al: Critical analysis of results of craniofacial surgery for nonsyndromic bicoronal synostosis, *J Craniofac Surg* 6:32-37, 1995.

94. Waitzman A, Posnick JC, Armstrong DC, et al: Craniofacial skeletal measurements based on computed tomography: part II. Normal valves and growth trends, *Cleft Palate Craniofac J* 92:118-127, 1992.

95. Wall SA, Goldin JH, Hockley AD, et al: Fronto-orbital reoperation in craniosynostosis, *Br J Plast Surg* 80:195, 1994.

96. Whitaker LA, Bartlett SP: The craniofacial dystoses: guidelines for management of the symmetric and asymmetric deformities, *Clin Plast Surg* 14:73, 1987.

97. Whitaker LA, Bartlett SA, Schut L, et al: Craniosynostosis: an analysis of the timing, treatment, and complications in 164 consecutive patients, *Plast Reconstr Surg* 80:195, 1987.

98. Whitaker LA, Schut L, Kerr LP: Early surgery for isolated craniofacial dystosis, *Plast Reconstr Surg* 60:575, 1977.

99. Williams J, Cohen S, Burstein F, et al: A longitudinal, statistical study of reoperation rates in craniosynostosis, *Plast Reconstr Surg* 100:305-310, 1997.

100. Williams JK, Longaker MT, Wisoff J, et al: The presence of elevated intracranial pressures in a patient with craniodysostosis and patent sutures, *J Craniofac Surg* 8:373-378, 1997.

101. Wolfort FG, Kanter MA, Miller LB: Torticollis, *Plast Reconstr Surg* 84:682, 1988.

102. Zander K: *Physicians, caremaps and collaboration: the new definition,* South Natick, Mass, 1992, Center for Case Management.

CHAPTER 48

Syndromic Craniosynostosis: Craniofacial Dysostosis

Craig A. Vander Kolk
Bryant A. Toth

INTRODUCTION

Craniofacial dysostosis is a term used in this chapter to describe a group of patients with complex craniofacial abnormalities. These abnormalities go beyond those seen in the manifestations of multiple cranial suture synostosis,[32,41] extending from the cranial base to the facial growth centers.[18,22] In addition, this group frequently has anomalies distant to the craniofacial region. With this constellation of findings, these patients are usually categorized as having syndromic craniosynostosis. Therefore this chapter provides an overview of the indications, operations, and outcomes of patients with Apert, Crouzon, Pfeiffer, and Saethre-Chotzen syndromes.[3,9]

Because the cranium, cranial base, and facial regions are all involved in these syndromes, there is an exponential increase in the complexity of the problems facing the craniofacial surgeon. Usually the involvement is so extensive and severe that these patients present with problems related to the local anatomic abnormality. This is seen in the calvaria, orbital, and midface region, which affects each of those structures' development and function. Problems can be seen with development of the brain and potentially intelligence,[29] visual disturbances or extraocular muscle movement problems, and airway disturbance along with occlusal and mastication irregularities.[4]

These functional problems are further exacerbated by changes that occur with growth abnormalities. Although not progressive in the sense that they worsen as time goes on, they do, however, have an effect as each of the various developing structures comes into focus during development. Therefore problems with airway and midfacial growth are seen in infancy, childhood, and adolescence. Irregularities in occlusion and mastication occur in the primary, mixed, and permanent dentition phases. Most of the orbital problems occur early on because the majority of orbital growth occurs over the first 5 to 8 years. Patients can have problems with sinus development as these structures begin to develop in late childhood and adolescence. Treatment options therefore need to consider all of these aspects in a growing, developing child.

In single-suture synostosis, it appears that once the abnormality is corrected, the growth of the craniofacial region is unlocked and progresses in a relatively normal fashion. In contrast, in craniofacial dysostosis the subsequent growth does not follow a normal pattern. This frequently results in the need for multiple operations. Many of the craniofacial procedures listed in the Chapter 47 can be, and are frequently, necessary for reconstruction in these cranial dysostosis patients. However, a coordinated individual plan that carefully evaluates the indications, treatment options, and ultimate outcomes is very important.

Recent landmark breakthroughs in molecular genetics have begun to provide us with understanding of the etiology of craniofacial dysostosis. It is now known that most of these patients fall into several syndromes that all have now been categorized as to specific genetic mutations. They all appear to be related to growth factor receptor genes, which have a multitude of effects on growth and development. This appears to be mostly related to fetal development, which then has a long-term effect on growth and development of the structures mentioned above.

To date, however, this research has not brought us from the mutation, which is the overall underlying cause, to the actual pathogenesis that is occurring with the mutation. This appears to be the major limiting factor in further understanding these deformities. It is hoped that new techniques in molecular biology will bring us from the genetic abnormality into a paradigm and model for the pathogenesis, which then can lead to further refinements in treatment.[31] Ideally, if individual mutations can be further categorized, perhaps the phenotypic outcome of this type of mutation can then be further categorized, allowing us to understand the individual presentation and long-term growth and development of the patients. Ultimately this not only will help determine the phenotypic presentation and the subsequent indications for surgery but it also will allow us to refine surgical techniques and improve the final outcomes.

INDICATIONS

Generally the indications for procedures need to be individually considered within a craniofacial team environment. Early evaluation of the patient by a craniofacial team allows understanding of the underlying etiology provided by genetic evaluation and mutation confirmation. Early team evaluation includes neurosurgery for understanding the neurologic and neurosurgical aspects of the patient. Primarily, this is focused on the first year of life and, to a lesser extent, the first 5 years, after which there are less complex neurosurgical issues as the child grows. Ophthalmology is an important part of the evaluating team, particularly with gross deformities of the fronto-orbital region, in which exposure of the eyes can lead to injuries to the cornea and the underlying eye itself. In addition, frequently these patients have abnormalities of extraocular muscle movements. Crouzon syndrome, in particular, has retinal detachment, blindness, and other potential ophthalmologic problems that need frequent evaluation and follow-up.

Otolaryngology and pulmonary specialists can be important adjunctive services when significant midfacial hypoplasia occurs and the airway needs to be further investigated. Because patients can have sleep apnea related to obstructive and central components, this team evaluation concept can be helpful in understanding options for treatment. The availability of hand surgery consultations is important for reconstructive options in regard to the congenital hand deformities. Often these abnormalities provide the initial information to make the clinical diagnosis, which is subsequently confirmed with genetic markers. With further growth and development, dental concerns and orthodontic treatment are extremely important in preserving the health of the teeth and maximizing occlusive relationships, with the final goal of treatment to provide good occlusion and skeletal position at an older age. Within the multidisciplinary craniofacial team, the plastic surgeon, having the most experience with all of the areas that are functionally and structurally compromised, directs the team and the evaluations and treatment concepts.

Craniofacial dysostosis patients present with five major craniofacial issues that need to be considered. The first is fronto-orbital retrusion, a manifestation secondary to the frequent presentation of coronal synostosis, which affects the fronto-orbital region. A second area is the posterior constraint that can occur with growth disturbances in the parietal and occipital bones through the lambdoidal and squamosal sutures. Many of the more severe syndromic patients develop a presentation known as towering of the skull, or turricephaly. Turricephaly is the third indication or consideration for treatment in these patients because this problem is related not

only to the anterior and posterior growth disturbance but also to the disturbance of the cranial base and perhaps the brain development itself.[30] The fourth major area of concern is midfacial hypoplasia. Again, this is related not only to the calvarial growth disturbances and craniofacial disturbances but also to midfacial growth disturbances. The fifth group is miscellaneous abnormalities. These include hypertelorism, which can be associated with Apert and, to a lesser extent, Crouzon syndromes. The patient can have brain abnormalities, including hydrocephalus and a Chiari malformation. Other miscellaneous abnormalities include cleft palate, abnormalities of extraocular muscle movements, and ocular abnormalities. All of these miscellaneous problems illustrate the need for patients to be followed in the multidisciplinary craniofacial clinic.

To understand craniofacial dysostosis within the limitations of this chapter, we attempt to identify worst-case scenarios for the indications, operations, and outcomes for treatment. This begins with the functional problems that can be seen. Initial concerns are issues of the airway and the brain. Airway issues can frequently present at an early age in the more severe cases. Midfacial hypoplasia is seen in these patients at birth. Because the airway can also affect feeding, the two evaluations often work in conjunction. Currently, midface advancement in infants is not recommended, although it is hopeful that in the future this will be possible with distraction osteogenesis. Therefore, for patients who fail sleep studies and are unable to feed when placed in the supine position, a tracheostomy may be needed. Usually this will also necessitate a feeding gastrostomy or jejunostomy to assist in nutrition of the patient with the tracheostomy. Occasionally the airway issues present later in development and initial treatment attempts can include adjunctive measures, such as bilevel positive airway pressure (BiPAP) and tonsillectomy and adenoidectomy, although this is rarely sufficient to prevent the need for the tracheostomy in severe cases.

Hydrocephalus occasionally occurs with severe craniofacial dysostosis.[20] In these patients, the decision to proceed with a ventricular peritoneal shunt is complex. Although it is important to decrease the chances of having problems with increased intracranial pressure related to the hydrocephalus, the effects of the shunt on further reconstruction and more complex issues of infection and need for multiple procedures further complicate the later cranial reconstructions. Once the decision is made for ventricular peritoneal shunting, the appropriate pressure needs to be carefully controlled so that the shunt is of the highest pressure type possible. This prevents the formation of dead space after craniofacial advancement and reconstruction.[33] New advances in adjustable-pressure shunts may be appropriate for the future to control pressure and possible dead space in the perioperative period.

Once the patient has been evaluated and treated for ancillary problems that can occur in the first few months, the major issue for reconstruction becomes the fronto-orbital deformity. Typically this is a manifestation of the coronal suture synostosis, occasionally complicated by metopic synostosis or even hypertelorism. In Apert syndrome, a widely patent anterior fontenel usually extends down the metopic suture. This extension can then affect the interorbital region, resulting in hypertelorism. Treatment of fronto-orbital retrusion traditionally involves a bifrontal craniotomy and fronto-orbital advancement. This corrects the deformity and probably has some effect on limiting the restrictive growth that is thought to occur without treatment. The amount of growth potential that is unlocked with the fronto-orbital advancement is under great debate. Proponents for early surgery believe the greatest growth potential is achieved when surgery is performed at 3 to 6 months. However, a fronto-orbital advancement at 3 to 6 months of age is more difficult than one at 6 to 12 months of age because of the thin, fibrous bone. Therefore some surgeons think that the best, most stable result occurs when surgery is performed at 9 to 12 months of age. Rigid fixation is helpful in obtaining a stable advanced construct and does not appear to significantly affect growth. We prefer surgery at 7 to 9 months as the ideal time for obtaining the best possible stability in advancement and obtaining the most growth potential.[23]

After fronto-orbital advancement, usually there is a significant improvement in craniofacial form. The patient needs to be carefully observed for early signs of growth limitation of the posterior cranium or even recurrent anterior deformity.[8] When the former occurs, consideration for early release of the posterior cranium is indicated.[1] This will help limit the potential for turricephaly. When posterior reconstruction is necessary, it is usually performed between 12 and 24 months of age.

In the more severe syndromic children, turricephaly often continues to be a problem. In these patients, it is probably related to not only a growth restriction of the calvarial sutures but also an extensive involvement in the cranial base. These patients often are ones with significant midfacial hypoplasia and have had a tracheostomy. When these patients present to the craniofacial team, particularly after a posterior expansion, conservative treatment should first be considered. We prefer a molding helmet to limit the amount of cephalad growth and promote anterior, posterior, and lateral circumferential growth. When this conservative therapy fails, a secondary procedure of total calvarial reconstruction may need to be considered.[5]

Midfacial growth abnormalities tend to be one of the more complex problems related to craniofacial dysostosis. The calvarial treatments that have been mentioned so far follow a fairly standard protocol and usually result in reasonable form. Calvarial reconstruction may require several treatments, but ultimately growth abnormalities stabilize and the shape and growth are more or less complete at a young age. This is not the case, however, with midfacial abnormalities. These midfacial abnormalities, because of the nature of the overall growth of the midface in relationship to the lower face and calvaria, are complex and of long duration. Indications for procedures depend on the age of the patient and the functional limitations that are occurring. Throughout all of the evaluations, the aesthetic considerations need to be kept in mind.

Midfacial treatment typically is considered from age 4 to adulthood, depending on the individual presentation.[16] Early correction is indicated for those patients with tracheostomy and occasionally can be considered for occlusal and aesthetic considerations. However, most of the time growth abnormalities can continue and require secondary revisions at a later date, culminating in definitive treatment at age 14 to 18 for the female or male patient, respectively.

Midfacial treatment is easier as the patient gets older. Bones are stronger and there is less of a problem with developing tooth follicles. Bones are different in their overall composition, being more fibrous and flexible at earlier ages as opposed to later on, when the bone is more compact and rigid. This allows osteotomies to be more accurately performed and advanced into position and stabilized.

Since the beginning of treatment of these complex deformities by Paul Tessier in the 1960s,[34-38] surgery has been performed at an earlier and earlier age. More recently, advances in distraction osteogenesis have allowed us to reexamine the limitations and the timing issues that have influenced options in the past. With this in mind, the Operations section concentrates on the treatment indications that we have discussed with a focus on outcomes that are currently available with the new advances in distraction for treatment of younger patients. Several cases are shown to demonstrate these procedures, along with the current thoughts on treatment protocols.

OPERATIONS

Craniofacial surgery began in the mid-1960s with the pioneering work of Paul Tessier. At that time, the results of reconstruction of complex craniofacial anomalies had been limited by the orbital region. Once he demonstrated that the orbits could be safely incorporated into the surgical procedure, he found and demonstrated to the world that there were better overall results. This has held up through time and was one of the early examples of the benefits of outcome analysis. The majority of the work that Tessier did was in adults with well-established facial deformities. These adults underwent one-stage repairs because growth and development did not need to be taken into account. One-stage treatment of craniofacial dysostosis in infants has been a more difficult path to travel because of their size, anatomy, and growth.

Controversy exists as to the type of procedure that is performed at an early age. This issue is centered around the safety of the monoblock, or frontofacial advancement, advanced by Ortiz-Monasterio.[21] The major concern is the potential for infection of the anterior cranial base, which is in direct contact with the nasal airway and sinuses. This is further complicated by the dead space that is created with advancement. Although there is a significant risk of this morbidity, which can even result in mortality, there are significant advantages to this technique. This is most commonly seen in patients with significant residual frontal orbital retrusion. In a similar fashion, a facial bipartition, originated by Vander Meulen, may be necessary for patients with extensive vertical and horizontal discrepancies. The choice of operations requires a careful evaluation of the patient's presenting abnormalities on a global and segmental basis. Each of these more extensive procedures may be safer and better to perform than performing two or more segmental procedures. Several surgeons have demonstrated that this procedure can be safely performed and provides dramatic results.[28] The reader is advised to refer to several articles by Posnick for details of these procedures.[25-27,39] Other centers have chosen to perform the procedures in a staged fashion. The protocols for this chapter follow the latter approach for all but the most severe functionally compromised patients.

ORBITAL ADVANCEMENT

The orbital advancement has been modified over the years based on improvement in techniques and advancements in technology.[10] In craniofacial dysostosis, the deformity is usually relatively symmetric and bilateral. This necessitates a bilateral orbital advancement with the attendant orbital, frontal, and temporal remodeling. Although Marchac[13,15] demonstrated improvement with the floating forehead concept, this has not become a universal technique. The idea behind the floating forehead was that it would unlock the potential for growth and any posterior fixation could perhaps limit growth and development. However, this did not appear to occur, and therefore most surgeons have gone to overcorrection and fixation to hold the reconstruction in position.

The other advances and changes in technique have been based on technology. In the past, Tessier needed stable bone to hold the segments in position, which were then held in place with wire and augmented with autologous bone grafts. Today rigid fixation, originally provided with titanium microplates and screws and now with resorbable plates and screws, can provide rigid three-dimensional construct stabilization. No longer do temporal tenons or a frontal bandeau need to be incorporated into the osteotomy segment; this allows segments to be individually osteotomized, subsequently contoured, and held rigidly in place.

Our preferred technique involves a combined neurosurgery/plastic (craniofacial) surgery approach (Figure 48-1, *A* to *E*). The craniofacial procedure begins with a zig-zag bicoronal incision followed by a subperiosteal dissection down to the brow region. A frontal craniotomy is performed, followed by a lateral temporal and anterior parietal extension. The craniotomy is performed to allow for advancement of these areas and more extensive remodeling of the forehead, temporal, and anterior parietal regions. The anterior cranial base is exposed and the brain gently retracted. Occasionally this requires the use of mannitol; however, most of the time the exposure can be assisted with lowering carbon dioxide. Spinal drainage is no longer used because pharmacologic manipulation usually allows adequate exposure.

Subperiosteal dissection is further extended by the craniofacial surgeon down over the supraorbital ridge and brow, down into the nasofrontal region, and along the lateral orbital rim down to the zygomatic arch. The temporalis muscle is included with the subperiosteal dissection, which limits the need for repositioning the temporalis at the completion of the procedure. Because the advancement of the orbital segments in the temporal area pushes the soft tissues forward, the muscle routinely redrapes into the appropriate position and has less potential for atrophy with a separate dissection. The osteotomy can extend into the temporal region because rigid fixation can bridge a defect in this region and provide stable fixation, which is augmented with a bone graft at the completion of the advancement.

The orbital osteotomy is accomplished by first cutting the anterior cranial base. This is accomplished by protecting the orbital contents and retracting the periorbita. The osteotomy can be performed 1 cm behind the orbital rim with a Lindeman burr. This side-cutting burr allows easy osteotomy of the anterior cranial base under direct vision. This is extended medially and laterally. Next, the osteotomy along the nasofrontal region is accomplished as low as possible without extending into the nose. Usually this is at the nasofrontal suture. This can be accomplished with a Lindeman burr, although an oscillating saw creates a smaller osteotomy gap. The lateral osteotomy begins as a Z osteotomy. This allows the maximum amount of advancement and recruitment of bone. The Z allows the osteotomy to be performed low down in the lateral orbital rim and allows some stable fixation below to the osteotomized segment above. The connection between this Z osteotomy on the lateral orbital rim into the temporal area is accomplished with either the Lindeman burr or a reciprocating saw at approximately 7 to 10 mm behind the rim. The segment is then fractured and brought out of the field.

The brain and periorbita are checked for any irregularities or any cerebrospinal fluid (CSF) leakage. The orbital segment is then contoured. This requires minimal contouring, usually in the craniofacial dysostosis patients, except for perhaps some bending and rounding. In severe cases of asymmetry or other abnormalities, resorbable plates can be placed on the bone surface to get an improved three-dimensional shape.

The osteotomized segment is then advanced to a normal position. Often this requires 20 mm of advancement. Originally, fixation was established with microplates and screws. This has been eliminated by the use of resorbable plates and screws. Occasionally, to get a large advancement, microplates and screws are used first to stabilize the advanced segment, then resorbable plates are placed around the construct to stabilize it and the microtitanium plates and screws are removed. Because systems such as the Synthes resorbable system allow contouring of the plate in situ, the plates can be placed onto the orbital segment on the back operating table and then brought up to the field, where they can be contoured and held in place with screws that are placed after drilling and tapping.

Because the procedure is performed at a young age, a portion of the temporoparietal bone can be used as a bone graft behind the advanced orbital segment and connected to the resorbable plate in the temporal advancement area. Following

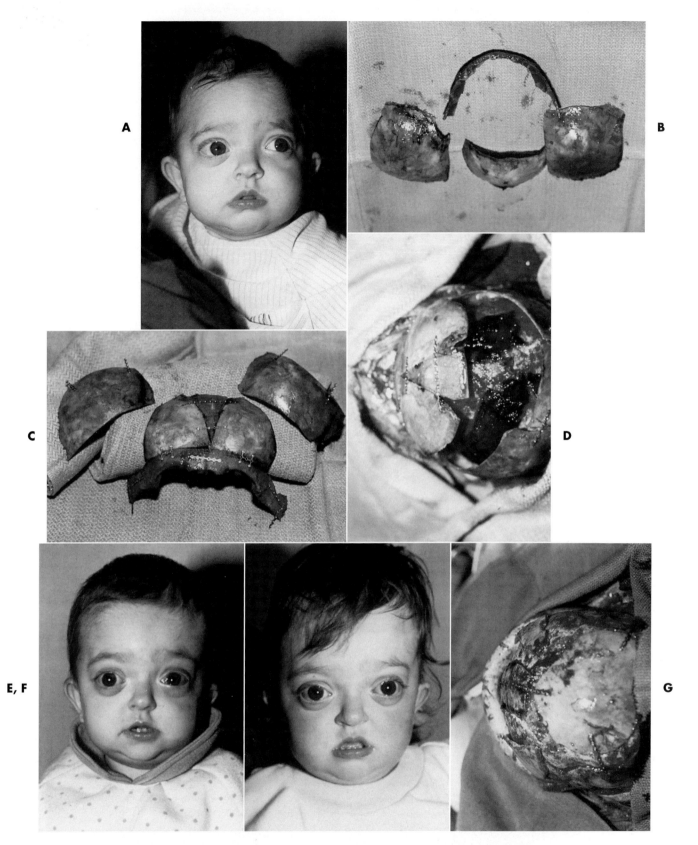

Figure 48-1. Crouzon syndrome patient who demonstrated orbital retrusion and brachycephaly, cranial growth limitation and early turricephaly, and midfacial hypoplasia. She has undergone staged recontructive management over the past 9 years, including orbital advancement, posterior expansion, and midface distraction. **A,** Appearance at 7 months before orbital advancement. **B,** Osteotomy segments removed. **C,** Reshaped segments with placement of rigid fixation. **D,** Orbital advancement and frontal reshaping fixed in position. **E,** Postoperative appearance at 10 months of age. **F,** At 15 months the patient exhibited significant towering. **G,** Intraoperative photograph of posterior reconstruction with occipital recontouring and parietal and occipital advancement.

Continued

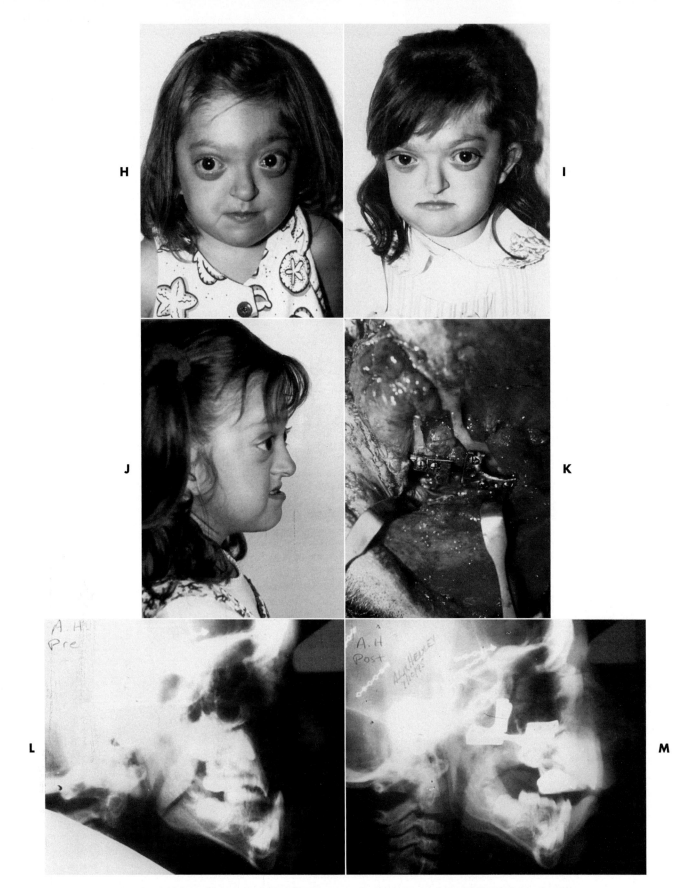

Figure 48-1, cont'd. H, Postoperative appearance at 3½ years of age. **I,** Before midface advancement the patient had a series of abnormal sleep studies and failed conservative treatment with BiPAP and therefore underwent distraction-assisted Le Fort III advancement at 4⅓ years of age. **J,** Lateral view of patient before midface advancement. **K,** Intraoperative photograph of distractor in place on the left lateral orbital/zygomatic osteotomy site. Some 9 mm of advancement was completed in the operating room and 10.5 mm postoperatively. **L,** Preoperative lateral cephalometric radiograph demonstrating significant midface retrusion and Class III occlusion. **M,** Lateral cephalometric radiograph 1 month postoperatively demonstrating the device in place and the advancement achieved.

Continued

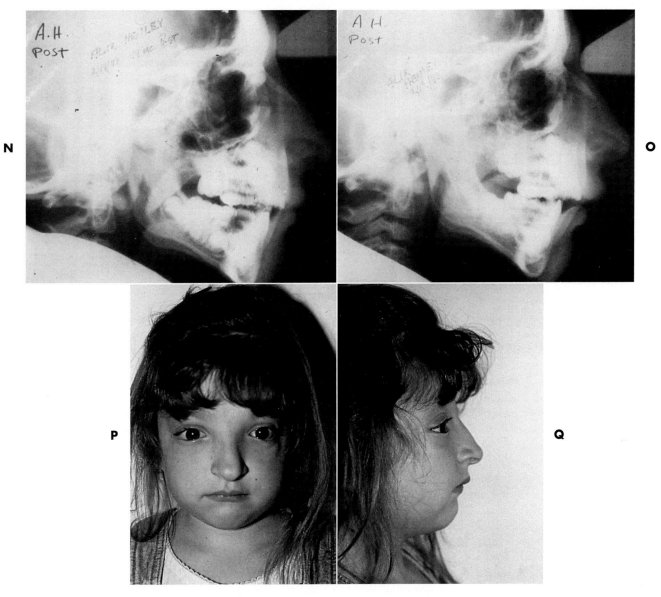

Figure 48-1, cont'd. N, Eight months postoperative cephalometric radiograph. **O,** Three-year follow-up cephalometric radiograph with stable advancement. **P,** Three-year follow-up appearance with excellent improvement in appearance. **Q,** The patient in lateral view. She does not need any additional pulmonary support.

this, the frontal bone is contoured and attached to the orbital segment with wires or resorbable plates. The temporal segments are then attached to the forehead and orbital segments. If an extensive advancement has been performed, then the temporal segments are fixed to the native temporal bone to counteract the forces for closure that may be excessive.

Closure proceeds in a routine fashion after establishing that there is no bleeding or CSF leakage. Standard postoperative care includes monitoring the patient in the intermediate care unit, and discharge usually is accomplished after 4 to 5 days. Erythropoietin injections decrease the need for transfusion. This is further supplemented by the use of the cell saver during the procedure, although frequently not enough blood is lost to require this unless there is excessive bleeding from the sagittal sinus. Throughout the procedure, the patient is monitored

for air embolism with central venous catheter in place for treatment.

POSTERIOR RECONSTRUCTIONS

Posterior reconstructions follow a similar pattern to the anterior cranial expansions (see Figure 48-1, *F* to *H*). Occasionally it is advantageous to use an occipital bar for advancement similar to the orbital bar.[40] Asymmetries are corrected by rotating the various segments. Rigid fixation or resorbable fixation is particularly helpful in this region because an extensive amount of recontouring is necessary and the patient will lie on his or her back postoperatively. The general goal of the procedure is to advance the posterior segment as much as possible along with some expansion in width to decrease the towering. Occasionally the vertex cranial portion needs to be lowered to allow for expansion posteriorly. This can be accomplished with wires twisted down to the native bone and the reconstructed segments. This is similar to the total calvarial reconstruction recommended for sagittal synostosis.[6,11]

LE FORT III ADVANCEMENT

Le Fort III advancement has been a major advance in craniofacial reconstruction. When the reconstruction has been staged in the protocol we used, the Le Fort III can be performed as a subcranial osteotomy with distraction. Distraction osteogenesis has been a major revolution in craniofacial reconstruction, pioneered by McCarthy with the treatment of unilateral and bilateral mandibular deformities. The goals of distraction at an early age are to improve shape, begin to control dental eruption and occlusion, reposition soft tissues, and open the airway. Bone reconstruction is accomplished in a natural way, with new bone being formed rather than the requirement for bone grafts between the osteotomized segments. This appears to provide a more stable reconstruction with lower potential for relapse. In addition, there has been recent evidence that soft tissues respond favorably to this procedure in improving overall symmetry and shape.

Distraction osteogenesis of the midface region has been more difficult to accomplish than that of the mandible. There has been reluctance to place external devices on the cheek because of the scarring, which is more noticeable than along the mandible. On the other hand, the advantages that have been identified with a mandibular distraction osteogenesis would be even greater for the midface. In particular, osteotomy segments are difficult to graft and stabilize, and relapse is more of a problem. In addition, extensive advancements at the time of surgery are difficult to accomplish in the young child's bone.

Not infrequently, Le Fort III osteotomies can result in fracture of the orbital or the palatal segments, resulting in disturbance in the final advancement and shape. Distraction osteogenesis increases the amount of advancement that can be performed and allows it to be accomplished slowly with movement and stretching of soft tissues. As always, growth and development need to be considered, and the long-term outcome of these procedures being performed at an earlier age will need to be monitored.

We have chosen distraction osteogenesis of the midface to provide better overall results with advancement (see Figure 48-1, *I* to *Q*). The advancement is more controlled with better potential for stabilization, there is less relapse, and the surgery can be performed at an earlier age in a more reproducible fashion. The ability to do a midface distraction has occurred because of an advancement in technology. There are numerous devices currently available; however, the ones developed by Bryant Toth and Martin Chin are key to this procedure (Figure 48-2).

The old bicoronal incision is utilized for exposure along with gingival-buccal incisions for exposure of the anterior maxilla and pterygoid junction. Dissection is carried down over the frontal bone, supraorbital ridge, and lateral orbital ridge. Dissection proceeds below the deep temporal fascia to preserve the frontal branch of the facial nerve. The dissection is carried down to the zygomatic arch, malar eminence, and lateral orbital rim. Dissection medially occurs over the nasofrontal region, behind the nasolacrimal system and medial canthal tendon. Complete dissection along the floor of the orbit is accomplished from medial and lateral approaches. Dissection also connects between the lateral malar dissection and the gingival-buccal dissection up along the maxilla.

The osteotomy sites are determined preoperatively from three-dimensional computed tomography (3D CT) scans, cephalometric analysis, and patient examination (Figure 48-3, *A* to *D*). The osteotomy of the nasofrontal region needs to be in the area where the deformity is most noticeable. Frequently

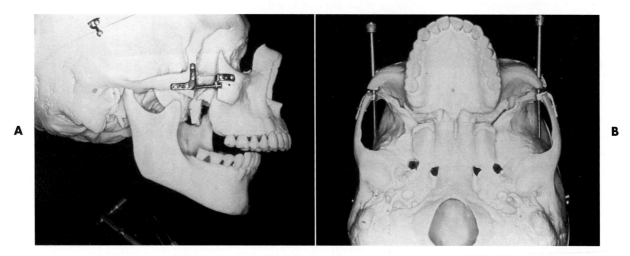

Figure 48-2. Distraction devices utilized in midfacial advancement. **A,** This photograph demonstrates the device in place, the location, and the vector of advancement. **B,** Basilar view demonstrates the location of the advancing screw mechanism behind the zygomatic arch and the activating percutaneous pin.

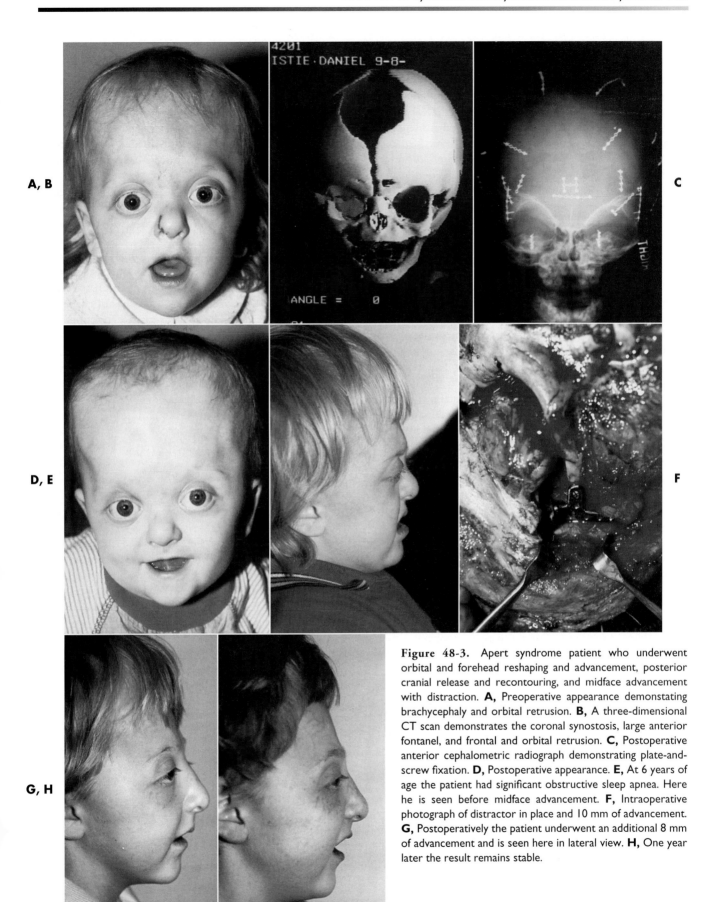

Figure 48-3. Apert syndrome patient who underwent orbital and forehead reshaping and advancement, posterior cranial release and recontouring, and midface advancement with distraction. **A,** Preoperative appearance demonstating brachycephaly and orbital retrusion. **B,** A three-dimensional CT scan demonstrates the coronal synostosis, large anterior fontanel, and frontal and orbital retrusion. **C,** Postoperative anterior cephalometric radiograph demonstrating plate-and-screw fixation. **D,** Postoperative appearance. **E,** At 6 years of age the patient had significant obstructive sleep apnea. Here he is seen before midface advancement. **F,** Intraoperative photograph of distractor in place and 10 mm of advancement. **G,** Postoperatively the patient underwent an additional 8 mm of advancement and is seen here in lateral view. **H,** One year later the result remains stable.

there is a step-off from the previous orbital advancement. Care should be taken to analyze the level of the cranial base to prevent the osteotomy in this region from causing injury to the brain or CSF leakage. A lateral osteotomy is likewise performed along the lateral orbital rim where the deformity begins. Laterally and inferiorly, the osteotomy is performed along the zygomatic arch in a position to allow for placement of the distracting device. Osteotomy along the floor of the orbit extends from the lateral osteotomy through the inferior fissure, medially up to the area behind the nasolacrimal system and the posterior lacrimal crest. Inferiorly the osteotomy is performed at the pterygoid region.

The reciprocating saw is used for the lateral zygomatic osteotomy and for the lateral orbital osteotomy. An oscillating saw can be used for the transverse cut across the lateral rim and the nasofrontal region. A small osteotome can be used then to complete the osteotomy along the floor of the orbit. A curved osteotome is used to perform the osteotomy from the nasofrontal region down along the perpendicular plate of the ethmoid and the vomer osteotomy. The pterygoid osteotomy is accomplished with a curved osteotome and palpating the medial aspect of the palate to make sure a sufficient osteotomy is accomplished without overextension medially. Rowe disimpaction forceps are placed and care taken to carefully complete the osteotomy. If the osteotomy sites have undue resistance, all of the osteotomies are rechecked because excessive pressure can result in fracture or separation of the palate or orbital floor.

The distraction device is then fashioned into the osteotomy connecting the maxilla and the lateral zygoma. The bone is contoured to fit the device and the predetermined direction of distraction in the axial, coronal, and sagittal planes. This is rechecked with the preoperative cephalometrics and 3D CT scan. The device is placed first by making a small stab incision in the skin at the malar–lower lid skin junction for the activator pin. The device is then placed into the osteotomy gap and held in place with titanium screws. The distractor is created as a rigid device that holds segments in position and is activated by a screw and a pin that penetrates the skin.

Once the device is positioned, it can be activated. When a large distraction is required, a portion is accomplished on the operating table. This is performed until there is an extensive amount of pressure and the force required is excessive. Usually this is in the neighborhood of 13 to 15 mm. While the distraction device provides stable fixation and bone fills in behind it, often this early part of the fixation can be filled in with bone grafts to decrease the need for complete new bone formation. Iliac crest is frequently used for the nasofrontal bone defect that occurs with the distraction. The bone is thin here, and the amount of new bone formation with distraction is thought to be limited. 3D CT scans have demonstrated bone formation at the region of the zygomatic arch after distraction despite the fact that a lot of the distraction is performed in the acute phase according to this protocol. The rest of the planned distraction is accomplished in the early postoperative period in the intensive care unit with the patient sedated during the distraction process (Figure 48-3, E to H).

At the completion of the procedure the surgical field is copiously irrigated with saline and checked for CSF leakage or bleeding. Frequently the patient needs a transfusion because reoperation in the cranial region results in a moderate amount of blood loss. The osteotomies are performed under hypotensive anesthesia, if at all possible, to decrease the blood loss. The scalp incision is closed over a drain in a standard fashion. The patient is transferred to the intensive care unit for monitoring and for sedation for the early postoperative rapid distraction phase.

Although this procedure is not a classic form of distraction osteogenesis because it does not gradually separate the osteotomy segments, it does overcome many of the disadvantages of standard osteotomy techniques. In addition, in our experience, new bone forms in the osteotomy and distraction gap and provides stable fixation. It is important to remember that the thin, compact bone in the midfacial region does not contain a medullary space and may not create new bone as seen in the mandible with classic distraction. It is hoped that, with the development of new internal devices, more extensive procedures can be performed in a classic fashion. This would perhaps even include frontal facial advancements in selected patients. This may also decrease the potential for infection and the attendent morbidity.

OUTCOMES

The first issues to be considered in outcomes are the side effects or complications that can be encountered in craniofacial reconstructions in dysostosis patients. Several articles have reported the overall incidence of complications in a wide range of craniofacial reconstructions. In general, these have reported a low level of morbidity and mortality (6.5%). In a detailed analysis of complication and outcomes, Whitaker[43] reported that when dysostosis patients were compared with asymmetric synostosis patients, the former group had a threefold increase in complications (10.8% vs. 32.9%). In the next article to appear in that issue of *Plastic and Reconstructive Surgery*, David[6a] had similar findings and reported that factors that resulted in an increase in infectious complications included secondary procedures, adults as opposed to children, and patients with craniofacial dysostosis.

Outcomes of distraction osteogenesis of the midface are summarized in an article by Toth and Chin.[2] They reported nine patients undergoing this technique at ages 4 to 13. The procedure was well tolerated and provided excellent aesthetic improvement and stable, long-term results. In addition, the procedure was instrumental in allowing a previously placed tracheostomy to be removed and in several patients has prevented tracheostomy. Morbidity is low and thought to be lower than reported morbidity for standard Le Fort III osteotomies.

The major issue in regards to craniofacial reconstruction and craniofacial dysostosis patients is what type of outcome can be obtained from both an aesthetic and a functional consideration.[24] As mentioned in the beginning of this chapter, these are very complex problems for which we do not have all of the answers for controlling growth and development. We can attempt to unlock growth, and this appears to be advantageous; however, it does not completely ameliorate the problem, and recurrent treatment is necessary to obtain the best possible final result. This is further complicated by the fact that there is a broad spectrum of presentations of these patients within each syndrome and between diagnostic syndromes.[45] All of this needs further investigation. The best way to approach this would be with a multiinstitutional study to obtain outcomes. This would be similar to the single-suture craniosynostosis project being performed by the American Society of Maxillofacial Surgeons, supported in part by the Plastic Surgery Educational Foundation and AO North America.

In the literature, Ortiz-Monasterio,[21] Posnick,[25-27] and Wolfe[46] have published the results of frontal facial advancement. They documented many advantages, and their outcomes had low morbidity and mortality. In a counterpoint to these articles are the results of other authors and surgeons (Muehlbauer,[19] Marchac,[14] Fearon and Whitaker[7]), who believe that the morbidity and mortality is higher, decreasing the indications for these types of procedures to only those patients who have severe proptosis, midfacial hypoplasia, and neurologic brain issues.

Outcome studies that have discussed the results in an analytic and organized fashion have been done by Whitaker[42-44] and McCarthy.[12,17] They point out the increased need for multiple operations in craniofacial dysostosis patients compared with synostosis patients. Whereas Whitaker suggests that this is an indication for delaying surgery if possible, McCarthy believes that early surgery is the key to obtaining the best results.

SUMMARY

Craniofacial dysostosis patients are usually syndromic multiple suture synostosis patients. As such, they present with extensive functional, anatomic, and growth abnormalities that require a comprehensive, coordinated approach to treatment. A mainstay in the treatment of these patients is to approach them in a way in which their individual problems can be addressed with reconstructive procedures that correct the problem as early as possible to obtain the best possible result.

REFERENCES

1. Campbell JW, Albright AL, Losken HW, et al: Intracranial hypertension after cranial vault decompression for craniosynostosis, *Pediatr Neurosurg* 22:2, 1995.

2. Chin M, Toth BA: Le Fort III advancement with gradual distraction using internal devices, *Plast Reconstr Surg* 100:819, 1997.

3. Cohen MM Jr: Sutural biology and the correlates of craniosynostosis, *Am J Med Genet* 47:581, 1997.

4. Cohen MM Jr: Cranistenoses and syndromes with craniosynostosis: incidence, genetics, penetrance, variability and new syndrome updating, *Birth Defects* 15:13, 1979.

5. Cohen S, de Chalain T, Burstein, F, et al: Turribrachycephaly: a technical note, *Ann Plast Surg* 35:6, 1995.

6. Cohen SR, Dauser RC, Newman MN, et al: Surgical techniques of cranial vault expansion for increase in intracranial pressure in older children, *J Craniofac Surg* 4:167, 1993.

6a. David DJ, Cooter RD: Craniofacial infection in 10 years of transcranial surgery, *Plast Reconstr Surg* 80:2-3, 1987.

7. Fearon J, Whitaker L: Complications with facial advancement: a comparison between the Le Fort III and monoblock advancements, *Plast Reconstr Surg* 91:990, 1993.

8. Gault DT, Renier D, Marchac D, et al: Intracranial pressure and intracranial volume in children with craniosynostosis, *Plast Reconstr Surg* 90:377-381, 1992.

9. Gorlin RJ, Pindborg JJ, Cohen MM: *Syndromes of the head and neck*, ed 2, New York, 1976, McGraw-Hill.

10. Hoffman HJ, Mohr G: Lateral canthal advancement of the supraorbital margin. A new corrective technique in the treatment of coronal synostosis, *J Neurosurg* 45:376, 1976.

11. Hudgins R. Burstein F, Boydston W: Total calvarial reconstruction for sagittal synostosis in older infants and children, *J Neurosurg* 78:119, 1993.

12. Marchac D: Twenty-year experience with early surgery for craniosynostosis: results and unsolved problems (discussion), *Plast Reconstr Surg* 96:296, 1995.

13. Marchac D, Renier D: "Le front flotant." Traitement precoce des faciocraniostenoses, *Ann Chir Plast* 24:121-126, 1979.

14. Marchac D, Renier D, Broumand S: Timing of treatment for craniosynostosis and faciocraniosynostosis: a 20-year experience, *Br J Plast Surg* 47:211, 1994.

15. Marchac D, Renier D, Jones BM: Experience with the "floating forehead," *Br J Plast Surg* 41:1, 1988.

16. McCarthy JG, La Trenta GS, Breibart AS, et al: The Le Fort III advancement osteotomy in the child under 7 years of age, *Plast Reconstr Surg* 86:633, 1990.

17. McCarthy JG, Glassberg SB, Cutting CB, et al: Twenty-year experience with early surgery for craniosynostosis: II. The craniofacial synostosis syndromes and pansynostosis—results and unsolved problems, *Plast Reconstr Surg* 96:284, 1995.

18. Moss ML: The pathogenesis of premature cranial synostosis in man, *Acta Anat* 37:351, 1959.

19. Muehlbauer W, Anderl H, Marchac D: Complete frontofacial advancement in infants with craniofacial dysostosis. In *Transactions of the Eighth International Congress of Plastic and Reconstructive Surgery*, Montreal, 1983.

20. Noezel MJ, Marsh JL, Palkes H, et al: Hydrocephalus and mental retardation in craniosynostosis, *J Pediatr* 107:885, 1985.

21. Ortiz-Monasterio F, Fuente de Campo A, Carrillo A: Advancement of the orbits and midface in one piece combined with frontal repositioning for the correction of Crouzon's deformities, *Plast Reconstr Surg* 61:507, 1978.

22. Park EA, Powers GF: Acrocephaly and scaphocephaly with symmetrically distributed malformations of the extremities, *Am J Discomfort Child* 20:235, 1920.

23. Persing J, Babler W, Winn HR, et al: Age as a critical factor in the success of surgical correction of craniosynostosis, *J Neurosurg* 54:601, 1981.

24. Pertshuk MJ, Whitaker LA: Psychosocial considerations in craniofacial deformity, *Clin Plast Surg* 14:163, 1987.

25. Posnick JC: The craniofacial dystosis syndromes: current reconstructive strategies, *Clin Plast Surg* 21:585-598, 1994.

26. Posnick JC, Al-Quattan MM, Armstrong D: Monobloc and facial bipartition osteotomies: quantitative assessment of presenting deformity and surgical resuts based on computed tomography scans, *J Oral Maxillofac Surg* 53:358, 1995.

27. Posnick JC, Lin KY, Jhawar BJ, et al: Crouzon syndrome: quantitative assessment of presenting deformity and surgical results bases on CT scans, *Plast Reconstr Surg* 92:1027, 1993.

28. Raulo Y, Tessier P: Fronto-facial advancement for Crouzon and Apert syndromes, *Scand J Plast Reconstr Surg* 15:245, 1981.

29. Renier D: Longitudinal assessment of mental development in infants with nonsyndromic craniosynostosis with and without cranial release and reconstruction (discussion), *Plast Reconstr Surg* 92:840, 1993.

30. Renier D, Sainte-Rose C, Marchac D, et al: Intracranial pressure in craniostenosis, *J Neurosurg* 57:370-377, 1982.

31. Roth D, Longaker MT, McCarthy JG, et al: Studies in cranial suture biology: Part I. Increase immunoreactivity for TGF-β isoforms (β1, β2, and β3) during rat cranial suture fusion, *J Bone Miner Res* 71:622, 1997.

32. Sommering ST: *Vom Baue des Menschlichen Korpers. Erster Heil: Knochenlehre,* Frankfort am Main, Germany, 1839, Voss Leipzig.

33. Spinelli HM, Irizarry D, McCarthy JG, et al: An analysis of extradural dead space after fronto-orbital surgery, *Plast Reconstr Surg* 93:1372, 1994.

34. Tessier P: Relationship of craniosynostosis to craniofacial dysostosis and to faciosynostosis: a study with therapeutic implications, *Clin Plast Surg* 9:531, 1982.

35. Tessier P: The definitive plastic surgical treatment of the severe facial deformities of craniofacial dysostosis. Crouzon and Apert diseases, *Plast Reconstr Surg* 48:419, 1971.

36. Tessier P: Total osteostomy of the middle third of the face for faciostenosis or for sequelae of the Le Fort III fractures, *Plast Reconstr Surg* 48:533, 1971.

37. Tessier P: Traitement des Dysmorphies Faciales Propres aux Dysostoses Craniofaciales (DGF), Maladies de Crouzon et d'Apert, *Neurochirurgie* 17:295, 1971.

38. Tessier P: Osteotomies Totales de le Face. Syndrome de Crouzon, Syndrome d'Apert: Oxcephalies, Scaphocephalies, Turricephalies, *Ann Chir Plast* 12:273, 1967.

39. Vander Kolk C: Commentary on monoblock and facial bipartition osteotomies, *J Craniofac Surg* 7:251, 1996.

40. Vander Kolk CA, Carson BS, Robertson BC, et al: The occipital bar and internal osteotomies in the treatment of lambdoidal synostosis, *J Craniofac Surg* 4:112, 1993.

41. Virchow R: Uber den Cretinismus, Nametlich in Franken and Uber Pathologische Schadelforamen, *Verhandlungen Physikalische-Medizinische Gesellschaft in Wurzburg* 2:230, 1852.

42. Whitaker LA, Bartlett SP: The craniofacial dystoses: guidelines for management of the symmetric and asymmetric deformities, *Clin Plast Surg* 14:73, 1987.

43. Whitaker LA, Bartlett SP, Schut L, et al: Craniosynostosis: an analysis of the timing, treatment and complications in 164 consecutive patients, *Plast Reconstr Surg* 80:195, 1987.

44. Whitaker LA, Schut L, Kerr LP: Early surgery for isolated craniofacial dysostosis, *Plast Reconstr Surg* 60:575, 1977.

45. Williams J, Cohen S, Burstein F, et al: A longitudinal, statistical study of reoperation rates in craniosynostosis, *Plast Reconstr Surg* 100:305-310, 1997.

46. Wolfe SA, Morrison G, Page LK, et al: The monoblock frontofacial advancement: do the pluses outweight the minuses? *Plast Reconstr Surg* 91:977, 1993.

CHAPTER 49

Orbital Hypertelorism

Kenneth E. Salyer

Eric H. Hubli

INTRODUCTION

Orbital hypertelorism is a condition in which the interorbital distance, as measured from dacryon to dacryon, is greater than the expected age-appropriate normative values (adult normative values range from 25 to 30 mm). The normative values used to make the diagnosis of orbital hypertelorism have been brought forward by Tessier,[20,21] who stratified the interorbital dimensions as a means of rating the severity of each presenting deformity. Tessier's classification describes a grade I deformity as a medial osseous interorbital distance (MOIOD) of 30 to 34 mm; grade II as a MOIOD of 35 to 39 mm; and a grade III as any MOIOD greater than 40 mm. The base values for this system are derived from adult measurements taken in 1933 by Gunther.[6] As such, they must be modified in an age-appropriate, growth-relative manner if they are to be effectively applied to a pediatric population.

The severity and degree of orbital displacement varies from case to case and may be symmetric or asymmetric in any or all of the three-dimensional axes of the cranium. The deformity is termed *true hypertelorism* when the increased MOIOD is associated with an increased lateral IOD (7.0 cm in the newborn and 11.3 cm in adults[7]), or when the angle between the lateral orbital walls, when assessed by computerized axial tomography, is greater than 90 degrees.

It is important to differentiate this condition from pseudohypertelorism, a state in which the measured interpupillary and osseous interorbital distances are normal, but the measured soft tissue interorbital distance is increased. Pseudohypertelorism may have a congenital cause, as in blepharoptosis, or it may arise secondarily resulting from lateralization of the medial canthal structures. These changes can occur posttraumatically or through the distractive forces generated by the presence of a tumor. Regardless of the causative agent, the management of nonosseous pseudohypertelorism is dramatically different from that of true hypertelorism in that surgical repair is usually limited to the medial orbital wall and the medial canthal tendon.

ETIOLOGY

The etiologic basis for true orbital hypertelorism is unknown. However, it is safe to assume that an error in the genetic coding sequence contributes to the deformity. This is borne out by the fact that orbital hypertelorism is a characteristic finding in Apert's and Crouzon's diseases. The cause of these craniosynostosis syndromes is known and has been traced back to the FGFR-2 locus on the chromosome number 10.

Other entities that present with orbital hypertelorism as associated clinical findings are Saethre-Chotzen syndrome, Grieg's syndrome, frontonasal dysplasia,[1] and central or paramedian clefting syndromes.

ANATOMY/PATHOPHYSIOLOGY

Orbital hypertelorism is not a diagnosis in and of itself; it is a descriptive term that can be associated with many different syndromal and nonsyndromal deformities. As such, a "classic" anatomic presentation is not possible. Other than the presence of wide-set orbits and the associated nasal disharmony, the defining characteristics vary in each case. Careful clinical examination combined with detailed photographic and radiographic evaluation is essential if one is to arrive at an accurate diagnosis and create a comprehensive surgical plan.

One constant in all cases of orbital hypertelorism is the associated nasal deformity. Excessive growth and development of the ethmoid air cells contributes to the nasal deformity by widening the upper one third of the nose. This leads to lateral displacement of the nasal bones, the columella, and the lower lateral cartilages, thus creating a nose that is both short and wide. The nasolabial angle tends to be obtuse, and internal examination reveals a septum that is thick because of cartilage duplication. These two factors, combined with moderate to severe turbinate hypertrophy, can lead to partial or complete nasal airway obstruction. The extent and complexity of the nasal deformity varies greatly from case to case, but its constant presence must be taken into account. As such, any well-planned orbital hypertelorism correction will include or set up definitive nasal repair.

Orbital hypertelorism reflects a significant deformity of the facial skeleton. Although lateral displacement of the bony orbits is always present, the patient may also present with an asymmetric cranium and/or maxillary hypoplasia. Soft tissue anomalies are also prevalent, including a skin redundancy around the nasal radix and dorsum, the presence of prominent epicanthal folds, and an underdevelopment or absence of one or both of the nasolacrimal systems. The opening of the palpebral fissures may be increased or decreased as a result of an associated exophthalmus or enophthalmus, respectively. A complete preoperative ophthalmologic examination with accurate documentation of visual acuity, eye muscle balance, and globe positioning is essential.

TIMING/PATIENT COUNSELING

As with any surgical intervention, the optimal time for planning and execution of an orbital hypertelorism repair must be individualized. Obvious considerations include the general health of the patient and the effect that any other comorbid deformity may have on the ability to achieve a safe and effective outcome. Generally, we do not perform an orbital hypertelorism correction on any patient under 2 years of age. Before this age the diminutive size of the facial skeleton, along with the associated osseous immaturity, makes intracranial reconstruction technically difficult because of the thinness of the orbits and the fragile nature of the bone. Coupled with this is the finding that the immature skeleton may not be able to maintain the repair.[10]

As with every rule, there are exceptions. Early surgical intervention may be warranted in situations in which the severity of the deformity progresses so rapidly that the projected deformity will be extremely difficult, if not impossible, to correct. Indications for early surgical intervention (between 1 and 2 years of age) include rapid expansion of the interorbital distance with associated widening of the bizygomatic distance and/or an interorbital distance greater than 40 mm.

Preoperative counseling is an essential part of every operative intervention. In the setting of orbital hypertelorism, there are many unique points to cover. Generally, we start by educating the patient on the extent and nature of the deformity. We outline any comorbid diagnoses and indicate how each will affect the operative procedure and the outcome of the planned intervention. Next, we emphasize the team approach to comprehensive craniofacial care, introducing the relevant team members and outlining how each will be involved with the patient. We indicate that blood loss is expected and that a transfusion may be needed. Preoperative donor-directed blood is used when applicable. The patient is walked through the intensive care unit if he or she is of sufficient age to grasp the significance of the surroundings. After this, we discuss the problems that may arise during surgery, indicating the close proximity of the brain, the optic nerve, and the globes to the operative instruments. The

possibility of injury to these structures is discussed. After all questions have been answered, the consultation is concluded.

OPERATIONS

PREOPERATIVE PLANNING

Orbital hypertelorism represents a complex three-dimensional deformity. Discrepancies in orbital positioning can occur in any of the craniofacial axes. The wide range of possible deformities makes planning of the surgical procedure very difficult. As such, three-dimensional computerized axial tomography, anthropometric measurements, and detailed photographic and artistic representations are extremely helpful. Dental models are required if a facial bipartition is planned.[9]

The degree of hypertelorism and the severity of the comorbid deformities dictate the type of surgical intervention to be used. In some cases, optimal results can be achieved with a single procedure. However, in cases of severe deformity, a staged approach is necessary. In this setting, the first operation corrects the orbital hypertelorism, and subsequent operations are aimed at correcting the associated deformities. Generally, excellent aesthetic results can be obtained using a three-wall or four-wall orbital osteotomy. These initial maneuvers involve medial and lateral canthal repositioning and correction of any existing enophthalmus or exophthalmus. At times, this initial correction will also encompass a frontocranial vault remodeling with an associated primary nasal reconstruction. The extent of the nasal reconstruction is wholly dependent on the severity of the initial deformity (Figure 49-1).

SURGICAL TECHNIQUE

There are many approaches to the surgical correction of orbital hypertelorism. Regardless of technique, our initial considerations are always focused on the anesthetic preparation. We use controlled hypotension (mean arterial pressure 50 to 55 mm Hg) with hemodilution as a means of minimizing blood loss. In this way, we maintain a fairly bloodless operative field and decrease the necessity for the transfusion of bank blood. Our antibiotic of choice is cefotaxime (Claforan) 1 g given 5 minutes before the initial incision.

The procedure begins with the identification and isolation of the medial canthal tendons bilaterally. We approach the tendon through a Fuente Del Campo type of incision,[4] which not only gives us excellent access but also allows for correction of any epicanthal folds that may be present. The medial canthal tendons are then identified and tagged with a suture so that they can be easily retrieved at the time of medial canthal reconstruction. Attention is then turned to the scalp, where a serpentine bicoronal incision is made through the skin and the galea. Dissection is carried forward in a subgaleal plane up to the supraorbital bar. At this point, the periosteum is incised around the lateral orbital rims.[13] If it is anticipated that a flap will be needed to close over a potential space or defect in the

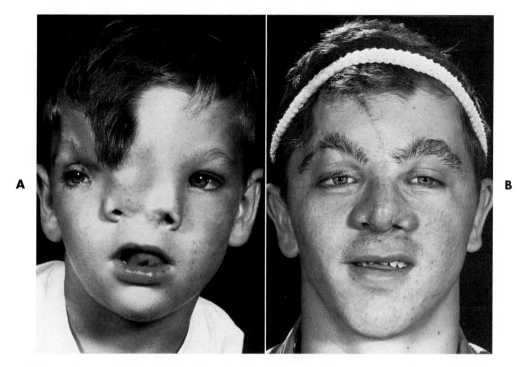

Figure 49-1. **A,** Preoperative frontal view of 5-year-old patient with 65-mm intraorbital distance requiring hypertelorism correction and nasal reconstruction. **B,** Postoperative frontal view after intracranial hypertelorism correction and nasal reconstruction multistage procedure at 19 years of age.

anterior cranial fossa, a pericranial flap may be raised based on either the anterior or lateral perforators. In this setting, one must tailor the pericranial flap to accommodate the anticipated transposition. In our standard approach, we incise the pericranial flap across the supraorbital rim. This allows for the supraorbital and supratrochlear nerves to be turned down with the globe, thus preserving sensation to the forehead. Once this is done, dissection proceeds caudally, freeing the soft tissue completely from the dorsal nasal structures, the zygomatic arch, and the malar eminence. Complete dissection of the orbital contents is accomplished in a circumferential fashion. The inferior orbital fissure is identified, and the infraorbital nerve is visualized from above. At this point, the neurosurgical and craniofacial teams must be in close coordination if an intracranial hypertelorism correction is desired. The craniofacial surgeon identifies the osseous anomalies and then diagrams the patterns for bony resection. Generally, this will include the creation of a frontal bone plate, a supraorbital bandeau, and the parameters of the orbital osteotomies. The team will confer on the location of the burr holes, after which the neurosurgical team proceeds with removal of the frontal bone plate. Next, under neurosurgical guidance the supraorbital bandeau is cut. Care must be taken to leave an adequate amount of bone on the cranial aspect of the orbital rim to ensure the integrity of the orbit during the transposition phase. At this point, the surgeon has the option of proceeding to a three-wall or four-wall intracranial orbital hypertelorism correction. If the patient is young and the maxillary dentition is at risk, we will proceed to a three-wall, inverted U-shaped osteotomy.[10] This approach will always preserve the integrity of the inferior

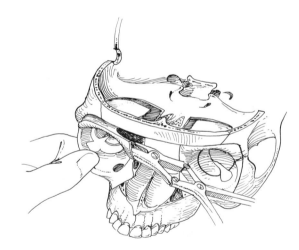

Figure 49-2. Rotation of the bony orbital windows with total removal of the ethmoid sinus using rongeur and pituitary types of forceps to remove all of the mucosa of the ethmoid. (From Salyer KE: Orbital hypertelorism. In Goodrich JT, Hall CD, editors: *Craniofacial anomalies: growth and development from a surgical perspective,* New York, 1995, Thieme Medical Publishers.)

orbital nerve. If, however, the procedure is performed on a more mature patient, our procedure of choice is the classic four-wall correction as described by Tessier[20,21] and later modified by Converse.[19] In mild cases of hypertelorism, those requiring less than 10 mm of medial orbital translocation, we perform bilateral medial orbital wall osteotomies with complete ethmoidectomy followed by bilateral medial canthopexy (Figure 49-2).

In cases of facial dysraphia in which the maxilla is narrow, vaulted, and V-shaped, the facial bipartition procedure may be successfully used.[23] In this manner, we can correct both the orbital and maxillary discrepancies with a single procedure. In brief, the procedure combines superior, medial, and lateral orbital wall osteotomies with a palatal split and a pterygomaxillary dysjunction to create two hemifacial osseous segments. These segments are then rotated toward the midline to decrease interorbital distance while gaining maxillary and palatal expansion. The move is then secured with rigid fixation.[22]

FOUR-WALL OSTEOTOMY

After exposure to the anterior cranial fossa, the olfactory nerves are identified and preserved via careful dissection of the nasal mucosa to which the olfactory fibers are attached. The frontal lobes of the brain are retracted, and an intracranial osteotomy is performed through the orbital roof 1 to 2 cm from the supraorbital rim. This osteotomy is carried forward just medial to the medial orbital wall. A transverse osteotomy is then made just posterior to the inner table of the cranium. In this way, the cribriform plate is isolated from the reconstruction and kept intact. Next, the orbital roof undergoes osteotomy, after which the reciprocating saw is placed into the inferior orbital fissure just posterior to the inferior orbital rim. The lateral orbital wall osteotomy is then cut. This may be cut as one unit or split laterally depending on the thickness of the orbit and the degree of deformity. Next, attention is turned medially, where a paramedian osteotomy is made along the medial border of the orbit. This osteotomy rises from the maxilla posterior to the nasal lacrimal duct up to the nasofrontal junction. Through the lateral incision, the inferior orbital rim is approached and then cut along the horizontal plane. The osteotomies are then connected so that a circumferential osteotomy has been created. The orbit should be completely mobile. The medial wall osteotomy is generally the most difficult osteotomy to perform because of the presence of the nasal lacrimal system in the medial orbital wall. In many instances this structure is damaged during orbital hypertelorism correction. To prevent any complications associated with this structure, we have developed a technique in which we remove the bone overlying the nasal lacrimal duct. This increases the mobility of the duct and allows for the translocation of the entire nasal lacrimal system without any kinking or osseous obstruction. This technique has reduced our nasal lacrimal duct obstruction rate from 33% to 10%.[12]

Having completed the osteotomies, the redundant medial nasal bone is defined and then resected. In some instances, a complete ethmoidectomy and sacrifice of the lateral cribriform plate may be required if one is to obtain the appropriate interorbital distance. When all the intervening structures have been appropriately reduced, the orbits are translocated towards the midline and held in place with rigid fixation. Care must be taken to identify any enophthalmus

or exophthalmus that may be created by this move. Exophthalmus can be corrected by expanding the medial orbital content via medial wall resection and ethmoidectomy. Enophthalmus can be corrected by decreasing orbital volume via the placement of split cranial bone grafts into the bony orbit. In this way, the orbital volume will be decreased and the enophthalmus corrected. It is important to note that the initial deformity will usually create orbits of different geometric shapes and dimensions. As such, it may be very difficult to achieve the desired symmetry on initial translocation. In many cases, segmental orbital osteotomies are required to achieve the balance and harmony desired. Single orbital movement should never be attempted because it is impossible to achieve a symmetric result.

Once the orbits are in their appropriate aesthetic and anthropometric position, the medial canthal tendons are brought into the operative field. A transnasal medial canthopexy is then performed using an awl to pass the medial canthal wire from one orbit to the other. The wire must be positioned so that it transverses the nasal region in a deep posterior-superior arc. The awl must be insinuated with great care because its passage is just below the anterior cranial base. The medial canthal wire should be slightly overtightened to compensate for the wire's natural tendency to stretch.

At this juncture, one should consider the possibilities of nasal reconstruction. If needed, a cantilevered split cranial bone graft can be placed to reconstruct the nasal dorsum. This should be tunneled subcutaneously to the tip of the nose to achieve an aesthetic result. Release of the midline skin using a V-Y advance may be necessary if one is to achieve adequate projection. Soft tissue and tip reconstruction can be performed at this time; however, secondary procedures may be necessary (Figure 49-3).

Completion of the hypertelorism correction requires bilateral lateral canthopexies. These are usually secured to the lateral orbital rim through two lateral drill holes. The frontal bandeau is then positioned appropriately, after which the forehead is reshaped and inset. Any osseous defects are filled with split cranial bone grafts. The pericranium, if it has not been used to line the anterior cranial vault, is then draped over the reconstruction, after which the scalp is closed in layers (Figure 49-4).

THREE-WALL OSTEOTOMY

The three-wall osteotomy is used in any patient who presents during the primary or mixed dentition stages. We also use this procedure in patients whose orbital rims show significant architectural discrepancies. In these cases, each orbit is so uniquely shaped that a symmetric four-wall movement will not create a symmetric orbit reconstruction. As such, the limited osteotomy allows for greater degrees of positioning freedom. The technique for this procedure mirrors that described for the four-wall osteotomy save for the cutting of the inferior orbital wall. The inferior orbital nerve is left intact. Reconstruction

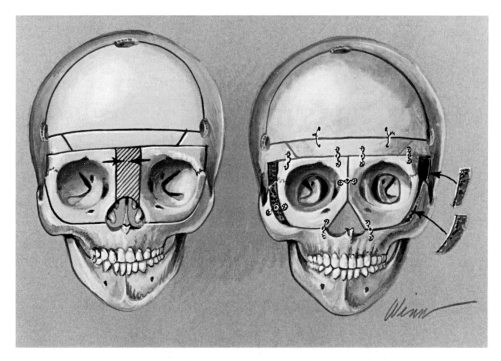

Figure 49-3. Hypertelorism with increased interorbital distance. Correction of hypertelorism performed through intracranial approach and four-wall osteotomy. On the left side the bandeau is outlined while planning the translocation of the bony orbital window. On the right side, correction of the hypertelorism is accomplished and miniplate fixation stabilizes the bone grafts in the split lateral orbital wall. This approach prevents subsequent displacement of the bony fragments and creates a good contour. (From Salyer KE: Orbital hypertelorism. In Goodrich JT, Hall CD, editors: *Craniofacial anomalies: growth and development from a surgical perspective,* New York, 1995, Thieme Medical Publishers.)

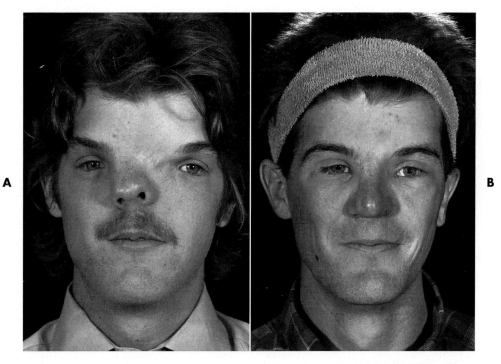

Figure 49-4. A, Preoperative frontal view of 21-year-old patient with hypertelorism and asymmetric orbital displacements. Intraorbital distance is 50 mm with short nose deformity. **B,** Postoperative frontal view of the same patient 4 years after intracranial correction of hypertelorism with nasal elongation produces good facial balance.

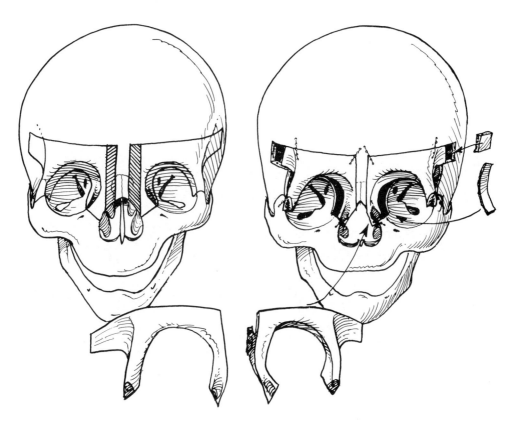

Figure 49-5. Schematic indicating the osteotomes and movements used in the inverted U three-wall osteotomy. (From Salyer KE: *Techniques in aesthetic craniofacial surgery,* New York, 1989, Gower Medical Publishing.)

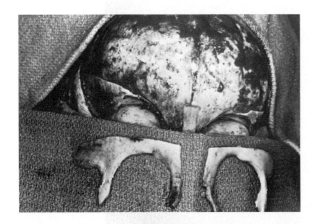

Figure 49-6. U osteotomy performed intracranially and simultaneously with remodeling of the forehead. (From Salyer KE: Orbital hypertelorism. In Goodrich JT, Hall CD, editors: *Craniofacial anomalies: growth and development from a surgical perspective,* New York, 1995, Thieme Medical Publishers.)

is as described for the four-wall osteotomy (Figures 49-5 to 49-7).

MEDIAL ORBITAL WALL OSTEOTOMY WITH ETHMOIDECTOMY

In cases of mild orbital hypertelorism or pseudohypertelorism, a limited surgical approach is used. In this setting, lateral orbital wall positioning is adequate or only slightly wide. As such, the focus of the surgical procedure is the medial orbital wall and its associated structures. On opening, a standard bicoronal approach is used. Complete periorbital dissection is accomplished, after which a triangular medial orbital wall osteotomy is performed. Next, using a pituitary rongeur, the ethmoid sinuses are completely removed. In this manner, significant medial orbital volume expansion is created. Medial translocation of the orbital contents is accomplished via a medial canthopexy that is performed under direct vision. A standard closure completes the procedure.

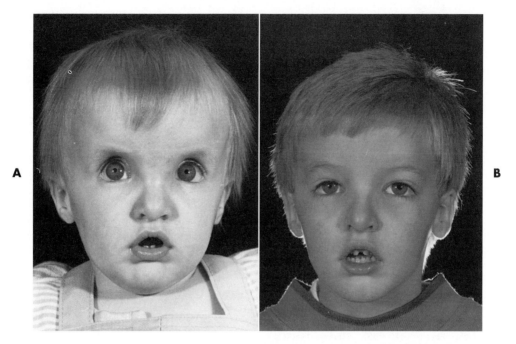

Figure 49-7. **A,** Preoperative frontal view of an 8-month-old patient with dysmorphic syndrome, which includes hypertelorism and retrusion of the supraorbital area and deformity of the forehead. **B,** Postoperative frontal view 2 years after cranial vault remodeling, remodeling of the forehead, and inverted U osteotomy for correction of the hypertelorism. This technique preserves the tooth buds and prevents damage of the intraorbital region on young children.

LAMELLAR SPLIT ORBITAL OSTEOTOMY

Remodeling of the forehead, supraorbital bandeau, and orbital rims can be accomplished using the lamellar split technique.[14,16] In this operation, the outer osseous table is separated from the inner table while in situ. The split is created by a reciprocating saw that is passed through the cancellous portion of the facial skeleton that is to be manipulated. Once the segments are free, they can be effectively translocated and fixed into a new position while the preoperative bony landmarks are maintained. In this fashion an anatomic reference "template" is created. This template serves two purposes. First, it serves as an accurate point of reference; and second, it serves as a base for osseous fixation. Used alone, this approach does not correct true orbital hypertelorism, but it can serve as a useful adjunctive procedure in pseudohypertelorism and can be used to safely refine the orbital slope performing a classic four-wall or three-wall osteotomy or a facial bipartition when treating true hypertelorism (Figures 49-8 to 49-10).

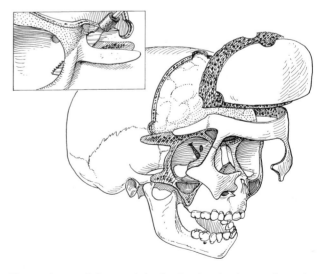

Figure 49-8. Splitting of the forehead and orbits in the malar region down to the intraorbital nerve. In this particular case, the orbits are primarily advanced but may also be moved in any direction. (From Salyer KE: Orbital hypertelorism. In Goodrich JT, Hall CD, editors: *Craniofacial anomalies: growth and development from a surgical perspective,* New York, 1995, Thieme Medical Publishers.)

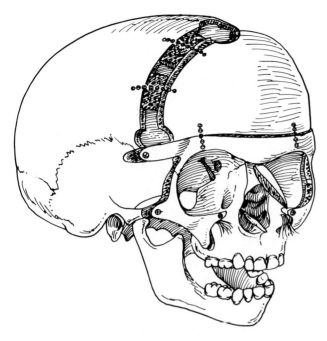

Figure 49-9. Completion of the lamellar split procedure for orbital repositioning, including reconstruction of the forehead and malar region. (From Salyer KE: Orbital hypertelorism. In Goodrich JT, Hall CD, editors: *Craniofacial anomalies: growth and development from a surgical perspective,* New York, 1995, Thieme Medical Publishers.)

POSTOPERATIVE MANAGEMENT

All orbital hypertelorism patients spend at least 1 night in the intensive care unit to ensure patient safety. On arrival, a limited test of visual acuity is performed to confirm normal function. If vision is absent, aggressive evaluation and treatment are required. The patients are maintained on antibiotics for 7 days postoperatively and are discharged to home when their orbital swelling has decreased enough to allow for near-normal vision. Follow-up is within 1 week.

OUTCOMES

Orbital hypertelorism is a rare and extremely difficult craniofacial anomaly whose correction requires a coordinated craniofacial team approach. We believe that this type of surgery should only be attempted in centers accustomed to the nuances of treating these complex patients. Over the past 5 years, we have performed 20 orbital hypertelorism corrections. The overall results have been excellent, with complete retention of the corrected interorbital distances. We have had a few patients who underwent procedures before 1991 return

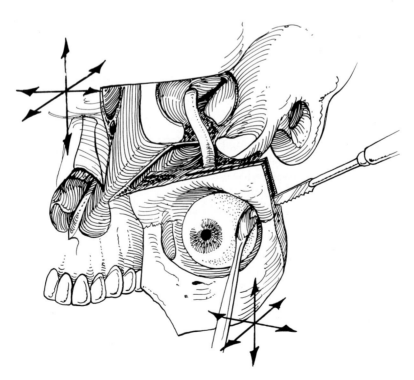

Figure 49-10. Lamellar split technique can be used to refine the final results of the classic four-wall orbital hypertelorism correction. The lamellar split can be performed either before or after the four-wall osteotomy. (From Salyer KE: *Techniques in aesthetic craniofacial surgery,* New York, 1989, Gower Medical Publishing.)

with a slight increase in interorbital diameter. This has generally been associated with patient growth and development and the associated enlargement of the ethmoid air cells. In these cases, we have used the medial orbital wall/ethmoidectomy approach as a means of correcting any significant interorbital width discrepancies. This approach, when used as a secondary treatment, has proven very effective, and to date, we have not had any subsequent recurrences of increased interorbital dimensions.

Achieving "normal" attractive facies may be impossible in severe cases of orbital hypertelorism. In spite of this, our patients uniformly express satisfaction with their postoperative results. Although symmetries created by osseous transposition are uniformly excellent, the technical challenges associated with nasal soft tissue deficiencies have yet to be overcome. As such, secondary procedures are necessary if optimal aesthetic results are to be achieved. Our patients understand our staged approach to orbital hypertelorism correction and have readily accepted secondary procedures to refine nasal shape and contour. We believe that this approach has yielded consistently positive results.

REFERENCES

1. Cohen M: Craniosynostoses: phenotypic/molecular correlations, *Am J Med Genet* 56:334-339, 1995.

2. Cohen M, Sedano H, Gorlin R, et al: Frontonasal dysplasia (median cleft face syndrome): comments on etiology and pathogenesis, *Birth Defects: Original Article Series* 8:117-119, 1971.

3. Converse JM, Ransohoff J, Mathews ES, et al: Ocular hypertelorism and pseudohypertelorism, *J Plast Reconstr Surg* 7:39, 1970.

4. Fuente Del Campo A: Surgical treatment of the epicanthal fold, *J Plast Reconstr Surg* 73:566-570, 1984.

5. Gorlin R, Cohen MM Jr, Levine S: *Syndromes of the head and neck,* ed 3, New York, 1990, Oxford University Press.

6. Gunther H: Konstitutioelle anomalien der augenabstandes und der interorbitalbriete, *Virchows Arch* 290(pt A):373, 1933.

7. Laestadois N, Aase J, Smith D: Normal inner canthal and outer orbital dimension, *J Pediatr* 74:465-468, 1969.

8. McCarthy J, LaTrenta G, Breitbart A, et al: Hypertelorism correction in the young child, *J Plast Reconstr Surg* 86:214-228, 1990.

9. Monasterio F, Medina O, Musolas A: Geometrical planning for the correction of orbital hypertelorism, *J Plast Reconstr Surg* 7:39, 1970.

10. Mulliken J, Kaban L, Evans C, et al: Facial skeletal changes following hypertelorbitism correction, *J Plast Reconstr Surg* 77:7-16, 1986.

11. Mustarde J: Epicanthus, telecanthus, and blepharophimosis. In Tessier P, Callahan A, Mustarde J, et al, editors: *Symposium on plastic surgery in the orbital region,* St Louis, 1976, Mosby.

12. Salyer K: Orbital hypertelorism. In Goodrich J, Hall C, editors: *Craniofacial anomalies: growth and development from a surgical perspective,* New York, 1995, Thieme Medical Publishers.

13. Salyer K: *Techniques in aesthetic craniofacial surgery,* Philadelphia, 1989, JB Lippincott.

14. Salyer K, Gudmundsen A: Facial balance and harmony through the use of split bone techniques. In Ousterhout DK, editor: *Aesthetic contouring of the craniofacial skeleton,* Boston, 1991, Little, Brown.

15. Salyer K, Hall J: Bandeau—the focal point of frontocranial remodeling, *J Craniofac Surg* 1:18-31, 1990.

16. Salyer K, Hall C, Joganic E: Lamellar split osteotomy: a new craniofacial technique, *J Plast Reconstr Surg* 86:845-853, 1990.

17. Sedano H, Cohen M, Jurisek J, et al: Frontonasal dysplasia, *J Pediatr* 76:906-913, 1970.

18. Sedano H, Gorlin RJ: Frontonasal malformation as a field defect in syndromal associations, *Oral Surg* 65:704-710, 1988.

19. Tessier P: Orbital hypertelorism. In Tessier P, Callahan A, Mustarde J, et al, editors: *Symposium on plastic surgery in orbital regions,* St Louis, 1976, Mosby.

20. Tessier P: Orbital hypertelorism: I. Successive surgical attempts, material and methods, causes and mechanism, *Scand J Plast Reconstr Surg* 53:1, 1974.

21. Tessier P, Guiot G, Rougerie J: Osteotomies cranio-naso-orbital-faciales, *Hypertelorisme Ann Chir Plast* 12:103-118, 1967.

22. Tessier P, Tulasne J: Stability in correction of hypertelorbitism and Treacher Collins syndromes, *Clin Plast Surg* 16:195-204, 1989.

23. Van der Meulen JCH, Vaandrager J: Surgery related to the correction of hypertelorism, *J Plast Reconstr Surg* 71:6-17, 1983.

24. Whitaker L, Katowitz J: Facial anomalies involving the nasolacrimal apparatus. In Tessier P, Callahan A, Mustarde J, et al, editors: *Symposium on plastic surgery in orbital regions,* St Louis, 1976, Mosby.

CHAPTER

Craniofacial Tumors and Fibrous Dysplasia

Yu-Ray Chen
Chia Chi Kao

INTRODUCTION

Craniofacial tumors originate from a variety of cell types present in the specialized structures in and around the skull base area. They may originate intracranially, involving the craniofacial bones secondarily, or they may begin as soft tissue lesions that spread and invade intracranially. In rare instances these tumors originate from within the craniofacial bone itself (Table 50-1). Benign tumors typically expand along the path of least resistence, usually spreading through foramina, to gain direct access to other areas. They can be locally destructive and can erode through soft tissue and bone to invade or encroach on other anatomic structures.[13] Malignant tumors are not only locally destructive but also they frequently extend along or within nerves or vessels to contiguous anatomic sites or may metastasize via the lymphatic or vascular system to distant sites. For most malignant and benign tumors of the craniofacial region, complete excision is the therapeutic modality of choice. Adjuvant radiation and chemotherapy is often indicated in the management of malignant tumors. Tumors involving the orbit, midface, nasopharynx, and skull base were once considered inaccessible, hazardous, and prohibitive. However, wide exposure of these difficult areas is now safely accessed through a combined transcranial and facial approach. Surgical strategies to particular types of tumors have been refined by using standard osteotomies to provide wide exposure and by reconstructing the defect with a combination of bony and soft tissue replacement that optimizes appearance and function while minimizing complications. Thus the surgery is becoming safer, the operations shorter, and the results better both oncologically and reconstructively. The boundaries of operability continue to slowly expand. This is certainly true in the management of craniofacial fibrous dysplasia. Management of intracranial tumors and malignant soft tissue tumors has been well described in the standard neurosurgery and head and neck literature. The purpose of this chapter is to highlight the principles of craniofacial tumor surgery in the context of fibrous dysplasia. The emphasis is placed on the operative indications, a systematic approach to operative decision

making, tumor exposure, concepts of immediate reconstruction, and surgical outcomes. General management principles that are described here can be applied to other locally aggressive benign tumors of the craniofacial region.

INDICATIONS

Fibrous dysplasia (FD) is a benign disease of the bone representing approximately 2.5% of all bone tumors. It is characterized by the replacement of normal bone matrix with a fibroblastic proliferation that contains irregular trabeculae of partially calcified osteoid. The exact etiology of FD and its histologic origins remain unclear; however, it appears to be a congenital anomaly that produces dysplastic growth of bone along with incomplete maturation of mesenchymal tissue.[17] FD may be classified as monostotic, involving one site in the body, or polyostotic, involving two or more noncontiguous sites. Monostotic forms are about four times more common than the polyostotic variety and tend to involve most frequently the ribs, femur, tibias, and bones of the craniofacial region.[6] A small subset of patients with FD include those with Albright's syndrome, a condition characterized by cutaneous pigmentation, endocrine disorders, precocious puberty, and premature skeletal maturation along with the associated FD.

In contrast to FD at other sites, most cases of craniofacial FDs represent the polyostotic form, with skull involvement occurring in 27% of monostotic and up to 50% of polyostotic patients.[11] The frontal and sphenoidal bones are most frequently involved, followed by maxillary, temporal, parietal, and occipital bones.

CLINICAL FEATURES

Craniofacial FD is typically first noted at 10 years of age, with progression of the disease throughout adolescence. It was once

Table 50-1.
Tumors of the Craniofacial Region

	INTRACRANIAL	SKIN/SOFT TISSUE	BONY ELEMENTS
Benign	Meningioma Chordoma	Neurofibroma Juvenile hemangioma Salivary pleomorphic adenomas	Osteoma Fibrous dysplasia
Malignant	Neuroblastoma Neurofibrosarcoma	Squamous cell carcinoma Basal cell carcinoma Melanoma Chondrosarcoma Liposarcoma	Osteogenic sarcoma

thought to become inactive after childhood, but there are numerous reports of continuing activity of disease into adult life. Leeds and Seaman[15] found radiologic evidence of continuous progression in 13 of 15 patients followed for periods up to 39 years. The rate of growth is generally slow; however, it may show aggressive behavior, exhibiting exuberant growth and bony erosion despite being histologically benign. Depending on the anatomic location and extent and duration of the bony involvement, the clinical behavior of craniofacial FD can vary from a painless local swelling producing only a slight facial asymmetry to a grotesque deformity associated with proptosis and ocular complications. Progressive disease in the frontal bone often causes proptosis. When the sphenoid or ethmoid is involved, the globe can be displaced downward and either outward or inward depending on the vector of the force. Dysplastic sphenoid bone can also encroach on the optic nerve and chiasm, leading to optic atrophy and loss of vision. A complete ophthalmologic examination, including visual acuity, visual fields, color perception, and cortical visual evoked potentials (VEPs), is mandatory when the orbit is involved. Involvement of the base of the skull may lead to extraocular muscle palsies and trigeminal neuralgia. If maxillary dysplasia involves the bony nasolacrimal duct, persistent epiphora can occur. Other neurologic complications, such as hearing loss resulting from acoustic nerve compression and seizure disorders, have been reported, as well.

DIAGNOSIS

Except for Albright's syndrome, the diagnosis of FD is seldom made on clinical, radiographic, or histologic criteria alone but on consideration of all three factors. Radiologic appearance is nonspecific for the diagnosis of FD. Plain radiography typically reveals radiolucent lytic lesions with an homogenous ground-glass appearance and ill-defined borders. Occasionally, the radiograph may demonstrate a predominantly sclerotic appearance or a mixture of both sclerotic and lytic characteristics. The radiologic appearance may be confused with other conditions, such as ossifying fibroma, Paget's disease, hyperparathyroidism, and meningioma. Ossifying fibroma is a distinctly different clinical entity from FD. It is monostotic and rarely multiple, and, in contrast to FD, it is more common in the third or fourth decade of life. It is a well-circumscribed radiolucent lesion (eggshell rim) that can be easily shelled out. FD, on the other hand, is relatively difficult to remove at surgery.[24] The earliest manifestation of Paget's disease of the bone is detected in the skull and the ends of the long bones. The osteolytic lesions of Paget's disease, termed *osteoporosis circumscripta,* are well circumscribed and radiolucent in appearance. The condition is usually associated with hyperphosphatemia and bowing of the femurs.[32]

FD confined to the sphenoid is difficult to distinguish from meningioma of the en plaque type. Meningiomas are soft tissue tumors that may involve the bone secondarily and represent up to 1.4% of intracranial tumors.[21] Meningioma should be suspected if a bony lesion on computed tomography (CT) scan is seen in conjunction with soft tissue abnormalities. However, the absence of soft tissue involvement does not necessarily exclude meningioma.[10] In the intraosseous type of disease, the tumor arises and spreads through the bone in a plaquelike manner. These tumors provoke a vigorous bony response, leading to thickening and distortion and a radiologic picture indistinguishable from FD. Some have suggested helpful radiographic features, such as soft tissue plaque, inwards (intracranial) bulging, cerebral edema, surface irregularity, and subdural ossification.[14] None of these signs is reliable. However, unlike FD, meningioma is rare in children, accounting for only 0.4% to 4.6% of all intracranial neoplasms in this patient population.[12]

To assess tumor extent and optic canal involvement, and to plan treatment, CT scan is the study of choice (Figure 50-1, *A-B*). Few studies report the use of magnetic resonance imaging (MRI) for diagnosis of craniofacial FD.[1,33] Lesions were characterized by a decreased signal on both T1-weighted and T2-weighted images with sharply demarcated borders. MRI may thus be helpful in preoperative assessment and surgical planning of FD, but its accuracy and cost-effectiveness await further investigation.

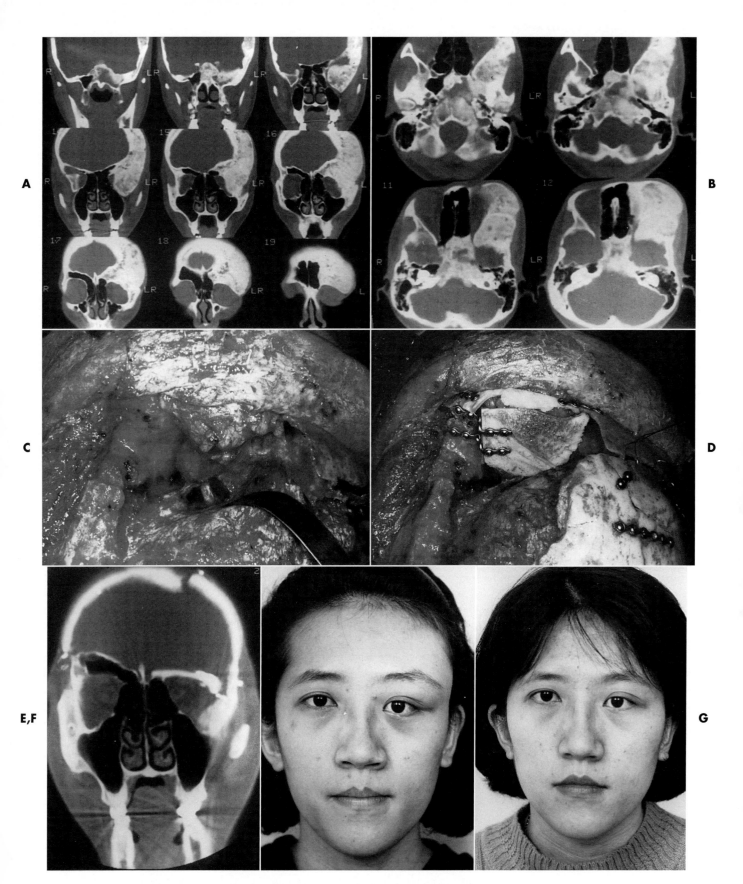

Figure 50-1. A 22-year-old woman with left frontoorbital fibrous dysplasia, who underwent radical resection, prophylactic decompression of the left optic nerve, and primary bone graft. **A,** Preoperative coronal CT scans. The optic nerve is not clearly visualized on the left. **B,** Preoperative axial CT scans. The left optic nerve is tightly compressed despite normal visual acity. **C,** Intraoperative transcranial view of left optic nerve decompressed through the orbital roof. The left frontal lobe is being retracted. **D,** The resected left orbital roof and frontoorbital rim were reconstructed with calvarial bone graft fixed with miniplates and screws. **E,** Postoperative CT scan. **F** and **G,** Preoperative and postoperative facial views. (From Chen Y-R, Breidahl AF, Chang C-N: *Plast Reconstr Surg* 99:22-30, 1997.)

RISK OF MALIGNACY

Malignancy in FD, though rare, can occur in either monostotic or polyostotic FD and the risk is greatest in males with polyostotic disease. Clinical signs and symptoms of developing malignancy are pain, rapid swelling, and elevation of the alkaline phosphotase level. The mean interval between the diagnosis of FD and malignant degeneration is 13.5 years, with the frequency ranging from 0.5% in monostotic disease to 4% in Albright's syndrome.[29] A review of 1122 cases of FD at the Mayo Clinic, Rochester, Minnesota, in 1993 found 28 cases of malignant degeneration. Sarcoma occurred in 19 cases of monostotic FD and 9 cases of polyostotic disease (only one being in a patient with Albright's syndrome).[26] The most common histotype was osteosarcoma, followed by fibrosarcoma, chondrosarcoma, and malignant fibrohistiocytoma. Most of these sarcomas occurred in the craniofacial bones, followed by the proximal femur. Significantly, half of all patients developing malignancy had received earlier treatment with radiotherapy. Radiation should never be used to treat FD.

TREATMENT STRATEGY

The treatment options for craniofacial FD include observation, conservative shaving/contouring, and radical resection and immediate reconstruction. The choice of these options is influenced by (1) anatomic location and rate of growth of lesions, (2) extent of cosmetic and functional disturbance, (3) the patient's preference and the ability to withstand surgery, and (4) the surgeon's own experience, as well as the availability of a multidisciplinary team encompassing neurosurgery, ophthalmology, otolaryngology, and orthodontics.

In 1990, the experience at the Chang Gung Craniofacial Center (CGCC), Taipei, Taiwan, was used to devise a classification of the craniofacial bones into four major zones (Figure 50-2).[4] Recommendations for various treatment modalities of craniofacial FD were then based on its anatomic location, its propensity for cosmetic disturbance or functional impairment, and the ease of resection and reconstruction.

Zone 1 is the facial area above the maxillary alveolar bone, including the frontal bone and zygomatic maxillary complex and the bones of the orbital wall. It is the most aesthetically obvious region, and FD in this area may lead to visual problems from displacement of the globe or optic nerve compression. This is the region in which modern craniofacial surgical techniques make the greatest contribution in safely performing radical resection and reconstruction, with excellent functional and cosmetic outcome.

Zone 2 is the hair-bearing cranium. FD in this region causing a small contour deformity is usually well camouflaged, and it is unlikely to impinge on any vital structures. The treatment may range from observation, or conservative shaving, to radical excision and reconstruction, based on the experience of the surgeon, tumor characteristics, and the individual patient.

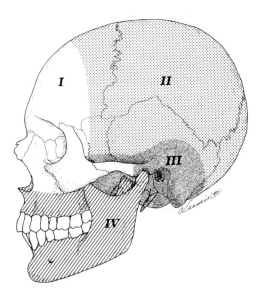

Figure 50-2. Craniomaxillofacial bones are devided into four zones. (From Chen Y-R, Noordhoff MS: *Plast Reconstr Surg* 86:835-842, 1990.)

Zone 3 is the central cranial base, petrous, mastoid, and pterygoid region, where cranial nerves and vital vessels are located. Because surgical resection in this region is hazardous, most lesions here are best observed if they are asymptomatic. If optic nerve compression occurs, the optic canal should be decompressed, in association with an aggressive resection.

Zone 4 includes the teeth-bearing areas of the maxillary alveolar bone and mandible. Resection of these bones will require the use of prosthesis and dentures. For this reason, conservative shaving is favored over resection. However, occasionally orthognathic surgery is required for realignment of the occlusal plane distorted by FD or correcting gross protrusion of the mandible.

These treatment principles serve only as a general guidelines; each case should be individualized. For Zone 1 lesions in younger patients or in patients with a history of continual tumor growth, complete excision and reconstruction is the treatment of choice. In patients 35 years and older with no recent history of growth, radical contouring may be more appropriate, and if the tumor recurs, excision may be offered at that time.[20] Another important factor to consider is the effect of surgical repositioning on the compressed eye. In frontoorbital dysplasia, the eye is displaced downward and forward. These patients usually have binocular vision, and sudden eye repositioning will cause diplopia, which may be irreversible in older people. For athletes, this may not be acceptable. Although the sudden elevation of the eye will also produce diplopia in children and adolescents, it will usually disappear after several months.[19,20] The highest priority must be given to Zone 1 FD involving the optic canal. Once visual impairment is noted, it is generally progressive.[7,16] Sassin and Rosenberg[28] reported on 10 patients with radiographic evidence of narrowing of the optic canal, with progressive visual loss in eight. The absolute indications for therapeutic optic nerve decompression are ongoing gradual visual loss or the patient presenting within 1 week of acute visual loss. The goal is to stop any further progression of visual loss; the recovery of visual acuity is less likely but still worthy of attempt.[2]

A new treatment strategy slowly gaining acceptance is the prophylactic decompression of the optic nerve for children and adults with progressive FD who are currently asymptomatic but have radiographic evidence of optic canal reduction.[2,22,27] The experience at CGCC suggests that if the optic canal is radiologically involved, the incidence of blindness in that eye is 33% and the presence of detectable visual disturbance is as high as 67%.[2] There are also reports of a sudden loss of vision resulting from hemorrhage or mucocele associated with FD in the optic canal. Prophylactic optic nerve decompression should be performed only at specialized craniofacial centers using a team of plastic surgeons, neurosurgeons, ophthalmologists, psychiatrists, otolaryngologists, and social workers. This multi-disciplinary approach helps minimize perioperative complications so that the benefit of prophylactic optic nerve decompression outweighs the risk.

INFORMED CONSENT

The primary risk of observation is progression of disease with subsequent increased deformity and possible impairment of vital function. Tumors treated by shaving and contouring have a high incidence of recurrence and allow for the small possibility of malignant degeneration. Radical resection involves the risk of anesthesia, blood loss (these tumors tend to be vascular), extradural abscess, bone graft resorption, and infection. In frontoorbital dysplasia, therapeutic decompression of the impinged optic nerve may result in no improvement or worsening of already impaired visual acuity. Prophylactic decompression of the optic nerve carries the inherent risk of injuring the nerve. Patients with frontoorbital dysplasia tend to have binocular vision even though the eye is displaced downward and forward, and sudden eye repositioning can cause diplopia, which may be irreversible in adults. In children and adolescents, this diplopia often resolves after several months.

OPERATIONS

Modern surgical techniques have greatly expanded the boundaries of operability of craniofacial tumors. In 1972, Derome[5] applied the concept of radical excision and immediate reconstruction to include the treatment of four cases of craniofacial FD. Tessier described refinement of the technique of excision and immediate reconstruction for the frontoorbital region in 1977. In 1981, Munro and Chen[19,25] further supported the concept of radical excision with immediate reconstruction by reporting on five patients with extensive frontoorbital FD successfully treated using this technique. In 1985, Moore and Munro[18] described 16 children with orbital FD who were safely resected and reconstructed using rib or cranial graft. During the same time period, the CGCC reported similar success in eight patients with frontoorbito-sphenoidal FD using split rib grafts for reconstruction.[3] Recently, the CGCC further reported on the prophylactic treament of patients with orbital FD.[2]

SURGICAL EXPOSURE

The coronal flap is the mainstay of craniofacial exposure. The entire skull, all of the frontal bone (including the superior orbital rim and orbital roof extending down into the medial and lateral orbital walls), the nasal skeleton, the zygoma, and the upper maxilla can all be widely exposed through this single incision. The involved bone can be easily recognized because it is more vascular in appearance. For maxillary and mandibular involvement, an intraoral, upper and lower buccal sulcus approach gives good exposure.[13] For patients with frontal bone, orbital roof, or sphenoid involvement, a combined intracranial approach with the help of a neurosurgeon provides the best exposure.

RESECTION AND RECONSTRUCTION

For Zone 1 involvement, en bloc or block excision of all diseased bone with microsaw or osteotomes should be attempted whenever possible. In anatomically critical areas containing vital stuctures in close proximity (e.g., sphenoid, ethmoid, and palatine bone inferior to the superior orbital fissure and optic canal; central base of the skull, including cribriform plate and sella turcica; the maxillary alveolar ridge containing permanent teeth), a rongeur should be used to avoid thermal and vibratory injury. The entire excised area can be reconstructed with cranial bone graft (see Figure 50-1), split thickness rib graft (Figure 50-3), or iliac bone graft. The split cranial grafts are obtained from frontal, temporal, and parietal regions that have diploë separating inner and outer cortex. The inner cortex is used as a graft, and the outer cortex is returned to its original site. All bones are rigidly fixed into position with miniplates or microplates and screws, which ensures revascularization within 2 weeks with minimal resorption or loss of contour. The "chain link fence" technique of split rib graft is useful for reconstructing a large area of the defect in the frontal bone and the lateral orbital wall when cranial bone graft is not available.[19] A full-thickness rib is excellent for reconstruction of the smooth, rounded contour of the superior orbital rim.

Alternatively, Edgerton and Persing[6] advocate removal, remodeling, and reimplantation of dysplastic bone. Their series using this technique demonstrated excellent bony healing, good postoperative contours, and no clinical evidence of recurrence of bone enlargement.

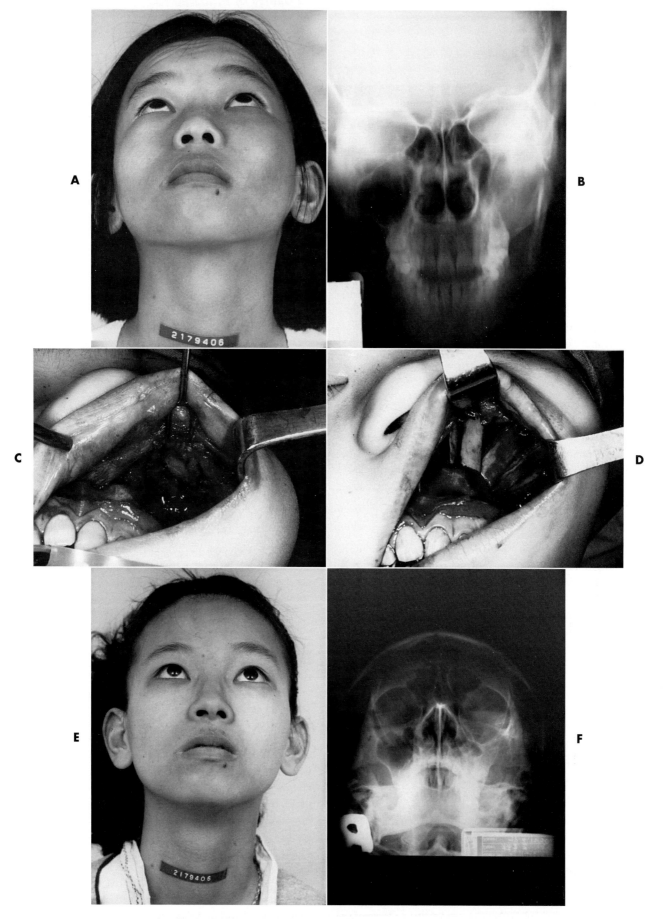

Figure 50-3. Fifteen-year-old girl with Zone I fibrous dysplasia at left zygomaticomaxillary area. **A,** Preoperative face-up view. **B,** Preoperative x-ray film. **C,** Intraoperative transoral view of the resected zygomaticomaxillary area. **D,** The resected part was reconstructed with split rib bone graft. **E,** Five years after radical resection, face-up view. **F,** Postoperative x-ray film. (From Chen Y-R, Noordhoff MS: *Plast Reconstr Surg* 86:835-842, 1990.)

A large frontoorbital tumor can make the orbit smaller and can push the orbital floor downward compared with its normal contralateral side. In the reconstruction of this situation, it is necessary to ensure that the new orbital roof is at the height of the opposite orbit, and the orbital floor is raised by a bone graft to bring the eye upward. The orbital volume is enlarged only sufficiently to correct the proptosis. The orbital contents have usually been compressed for many years and are thus smaller than in the opposite orbit. Although the new orbital roof may be reconstructed at the correct height, the eye often will not move upward unless pushed from below by a graft[19,20] (Figure 50-4).

In maxillary and mandibular (Zone 4) FD, conservative shaving or recontouring with osteotomes, rongeur, or burr is advocated. A 5-mm rim of bone surrounding the tip of the root and the side of the tooth must be preserved to ensure its viability. The surgeon should anticipate that the axis of the dental roots may be tilted outward. A preoperative Panorex film is paramount. On occasion, when severe protrusion of the jaw or the occlusal plane is tilted because of FD, orthognathic maxillary or mandibular osteotomies are required. We have used Le Fort I wedge resection, segmental osteotomies, sagittal split of the mandibular rami, genioplasty, or resection of the lower mandibular border to correct these problems (Figure 50-5).

ORBIT INVOLVEMENT AND OPTIC NERVE DECOMPRESSION

In FD involving the optic canal, the objective is decompression and also to remove as much diseased bone as possible because any residual disease can potentially recur and threaten the optic nerve again. The tightest point in the optic canal is the exit of the nerve from the canal or the *optic ring*.[8,9] The optic ring bone is also the thickest. If the decompression is to be complete, the optic ring should be included. Therefore it is important to have a combined intraorbital and intracranial approach to the optic canal. The intraorbital approach can be accomplished either by subperiosteal frontal bone dissection extending into the roof of the medial walls of the orbit or by a frontoorbitotomy through the roof of the orbit, lateral to the optic nerve. This dual approach also decreases the likelihood of damage to the nerve because it enables the surgeon to identify the nerve within normal tissue rather than finding the nerve within the tightly narrowed canal. Extreme caution must be exercised when unroofing the optic canal. Munro[20] has reported sudden and permanent loss of vision 24 hours after the operation when the initial postoperative visual acuity was normal. He attributed this occurrence to late edema and subsequent vessel compression as a result of vibration from the diamond burr used for unroofing. He recommended using pituitary rongeurs for the final unroofing of the optic canal to avoid this defect. The blood supply of the optic nerve is derived from branches of the ophthalmic artery, which lie within the pia mater and pass into the nerve via fibrous septae. Within the optic canal, the optic nerve is enclosed within the

optic sheath, which consists of the fused layers of pia, arachnoid, dura mater, and periosteum. The ophthalmic artery lies closely bound to the nerve within this sheath, inferolateral to the nerve. Thus if the dissection progresses from intracranially external to the dura and from intraorbitally at the subperiorbital level, the blood supply will be protected. If any region of the optic canal is to be left undisturbed, it should be the inferolateral quadrant, where the ophthalmic artery lies.

OUTCOMES

At CGCC, 71 patients (male 29, female 42) were treated for craniofacial FD between 1978 and 1995. Their age at presentation was 4 to 55 years (mean 19 years) and the age at onset of first symptoms was 1 to 24 years (mean 9 years). Two patients had Albright's syndrome, and one had associative pituitary adenoma. The choice of operation was determined based on the anatomic location of the dysplastic bones, aggressiveness of disease, and patient characteristics as described above. Nineteen (26%) had conservative recontouring resection, 28 (40%) had partial resection and bone graft, and 24 (34%) received radical resection and bone graft.

It is clear from our experience that conservative shaving will lead to a high incidence of recurrence. More than 50% of patients with FD of the alveolar bone (Zone 4) developed recurrence or residual deformity requiring repeated shaving or formal orthognathic surgery. Similarly, Ramsey et al[23] reported 47 cases of craniofacial FD. They used a conservative therapeutic approach with debulking of the bony overgrowth for relief of symptoms. They reported on 12 of 12 patients with complete resection of mandibular disease with no recurrence, whereas 4 of 10 with limited resection had symptomatic recurrence. No patients with disease in the maxillary and ethmoid region with radical resection had a recurrence, and 60% of patients with disease at the sphenoid had no recurrence or progression after radical resection. It appears that total excision of the involved bone is the most successful form of treatment.

Thirteen patients at CGCC with craniofacial FD underwent 16 procedures for optic nerve decompression for both therapeutic (10) and prophylactic (6) indications.[2] All patients who underwent therapeutic decompression experienced a break in the progression of visual loss. Two patients sustained clinically useful improvement in vision in response to therapeutic decompressions. All those who underwent a prophylactic decompression experienced no change in their visual acuity postoperatively except for one patient. This patient developed a temporary deterioration in visual acuity after a prophylactic decompression, which fully recovered within 6 months. In patients with complete blindness of over 1 month's duration, decompression of the optic nerve has universally failed to improve vision. No patient experienced a permanent deterioration of vision as a result of either

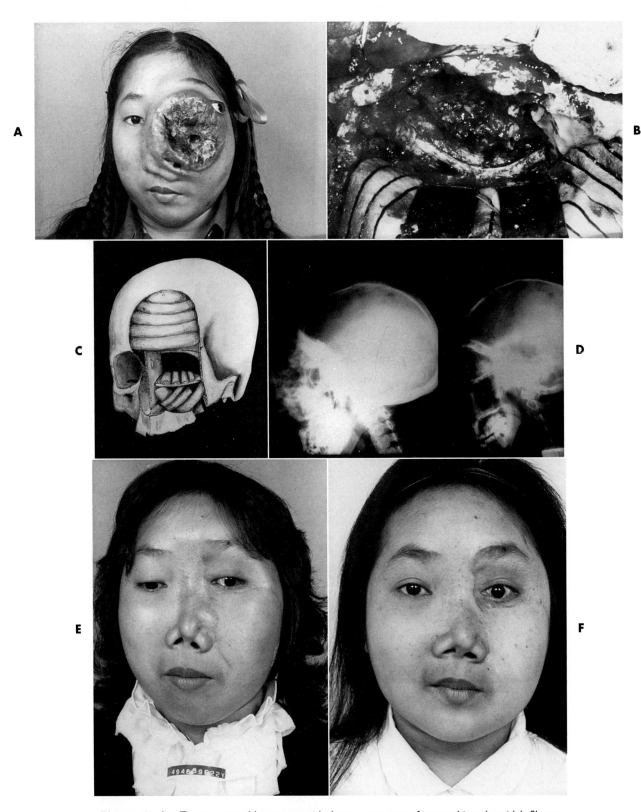

Figure 50-4. Twenty-year-old woman with huge, grotesque frontoorbitoethmoidal fibrous dysplasia of 16-year duration. **A,** Preoperative facial view, the skin over the central part of the tumor mass was ulcerated after herb drug application. **B,** Intraoperative transcranial view of bilateral optic nerve and optic chiasm after decompression. **C,** Diagramatic illustration of the resected frontoorbitoethmoidal area, which was reconstructed with rib and iliac bone grafts. **D,** Preoperative and postoperative lateral skull x-ray film. **E,** Four years after initial bony reconstruction and 2 years after revision of scar and nose. The long mid-face was subsequently shortened with two-jaw surgery. **F,** Seven years after initial bony reconstruction and 1 year after Le Fort I maxillary wedge resection with bilateral sagittal split of mandibular rami and genioplasty. (From Chen Y-R, Fairholm D: *Ann Plast Surg* 15:190-203, 1985.)

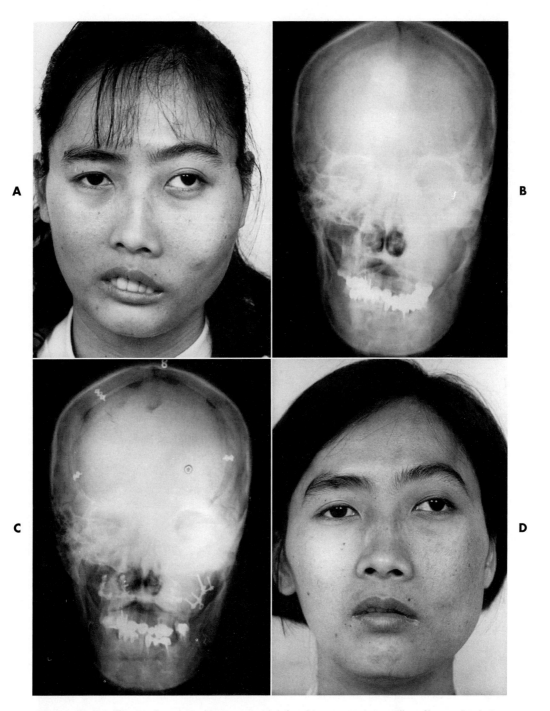

Figure 50-5. Twenty-five-year-old woman with left orbitozygomaticomaxillary fibrous dysplasia. **A,** Preoperative facial view, left eye visual acuity decreased with dystopia. **B,** Preoperative posteroanterior cephalometry. Frontocraniotomy, optic nerve decompression, and left orbital zygomatic contouring in June 1992; Le Fort I wedge resection and anterior segmental osteotomy of the maxilla and bilateral sagittal split of mandibular rami to relevel the occlusal plane in May 1993. **C,** Postoperative posteroanterior cephalometry. **D,** Two years after second operation, facial view.

therapeutic or prophylactic decompression. Others have reported successful prophylactic optic nerve decompression, as well.[22,27]

In general, complications of surgery include cerebrospinal fluid (CSF) leak, intracranial infection, bone graft resorption, contour irregularities, nasolacrimal obstruction, and oculomotor dysfunction. CSF leak can occur especially with resection of dysplastic bone that abuts against the dura. A team approach for this type of lesion with a neurosurgeon is recommended. Careful repair of dural tears by direct suture or pericranial patch covered with highly vascularized tissues helps prevent this problem. Intracranial infections, prevalent in the early days of craniofacial surgery, are minimized by use of the robust, highly vascular galea frontalis flap or free tissue transfer to obliterate intracranial dead space.[13] Attention to the craniofacial principles of rigid fixation and adequate coverage with well-vascularized tissues are key to avoid bone graft loss caused by infection. Osteotomies performed in the region of the nasolacrimal duct should be done with care.

Oculomotor dysfunction may occur after radical orbital resection, elevation of the periorbita, and bone graft reconstruction. In Munro's series,[18] 5 of 16 children after surgery for orbital FD experienced diplopia postoperatively. Several mechanisms have been cited to play a role in its development. Transient superior oblique palsy may result from extensive stripping of the periorbita, causing damage to the superior oblique muscle or detachment of the trochlea from the medial orbital wall. The inferior oblique insertion may be damaged during excision of FD of the maxilla. Vertical and horizontal recti function may be compromised by edema or small hematoma. Finally, placement of the bone grafts to reconstruct the orbital roof and floor or correct displacement of the globe may change the mechanical actions of the cyclovertical muscles. Whatever causes the diplopia, most patients eventually improve spontaneously, so any strabismus surgery should be deferred at least 6 months and until the deviation is stable.[18]

CURRENT AREAS OF RESEARCH

The evolution in the management of craniofacial FD exemplifies the advancements made in craniofacial tumor surgery within the past 20 years in terms of improving the safety of the procedures, expanding the limits of operability, and refinements in reconstruction with an emphasis on cosmesis and function. There remain many unanswered questions in the etiology of this bony disorder. Recently, a postzygotic mutation in the guanine nucleotide-binding regulatory protein of adenyl cyclase has been identified in patients with Albright's syndrome.[30,31] However, it is still unclear whether this mutation is specific for Albright's syndrome or if it can be found in nonsyndromic FD. The postzygotic mutation produces a mosaic distribution throughout the body, giving some insight into the mechanism of polyostotic FD. The role of endocrine manipulation to retard the growth of the lesion needs to be explored and may be an extremely useful modality in aggressive cases of polyostotic fibrous dysplasia. Future research efforts in this area should focus on the genetic and molecular aspects of this disease.

REFERENCES

1. Casselman JW, De Jonge I, Neyt L, et. al: MRI in craniofacial fibrous dysplasia, *Neuroradiology* 35:234-237, 1993.

2. Chen YR, Breidahl A, Chang CN: Optic nerve decompression in fibrous dysplasia: indications, efficacy, and safety, *Plast Reconstr Surg* 99:22-30, 1997.

3. Chen YR, Fairholm D: Fronto-orbito-sphenoidal fibrous dysplasia, *Ann Plast Surg* 15:190-203, 1985.

4. Chen YR, Noordhoff MS: Treatment of craniomaxillofacial fibrous dysplasia: how early and how extensive? *Plast Reconstr Surg* 86:835-842, 1990.

5. Derome PJ: Sphenoid-ethmoidal tumors. Possibilities for exeresis and surgical repair, *Neurochirurgie* 18:1-164, 1972.

6. Edgerton MT, Persing JA, Jane JA: The surgical treatment of fibrous dysplasia, *Ann Surg* 202:459-479, 1985.

7. Finney HL, Roberts TS: Fibrous dysplasia of the skull with progressive cranial nerve involement, *Surg Neurol* 6:341-343, 1976.

8. Habal MB: Discussion: optic nerve decompression in fibrous dysplasia: indications, efficacy, and safety, *Plast Reconstr Surg* 99:31-33, 1997.

9. Habal MB: Optic nerve decompression: commentary, *J Craniofac Surg* 6:14, 1995.

10. Hansen-Knarhoi M, Pool MD: Preoperative difficulties in differentiating intraosseous meningiomas and fibrous dysplasia around the orbital apex, *J Craniomaxillofac Surg* 22:226-230, 1994.

11. Harris WH, Dudly HR, Barry RJ: The natural history of fibrous dysplasia, *J Bone Joint Surg* 44A:207-212, 1962.

12. Herz DA, Shapiro K, Shulman K: Intracranial menigiomas of infancy, childhood and adolescence: review of the literature and addition of 9 case reports, *Childs Brain* 7:43-56, 1980.

13. Jackson IT: Craniofacial tumors, *Clin Plast Surg* 21:633-648, 1994.

14. Kim KS, Rogers LF, Goldblatt D: CT features of hyperostosing meningioma en plaque, *Am J Neuroradiol* 8:853-859, 1987.

15. Leeds N, Seaman WB: Fibrous dysplasia of the skull and its differential diagnosis, *Radiology* 78:570-577, 1962.

16. Liakos GM, Walker CB, Carruth JAS: Ocular complications in fibrous dysplasia, *Br J Opthalmol* 63:611-616, 1979.

17. Lichtenstein L, Jaffe HL: Fibrous dysplasia of bone: etc, *Arch Pathol* 33:777-816, 1942.

18. Moore AT, Buncic JR, Munro IR: Fribrous dysplasia of the orbit in childhood. Clinical features and management, *Ophthalmology* 92:12-20, 1985.

19. Munro IR, Chen YR: Radical treatment for fronto-orbital fibrous dysplasia: the chain link fence, *Plast Reconstr Surg* 67:719-729, 1981.

20. Munro IR: Discussion: treatment of craniomaxillofacial fibrous dyasplasia: how early and how extensive? *Plast Reconstr Surg* 86:843-844, 1990.

21. Nakasu S, Hirano A, Shimura T, et al: Incidental meningiomas in autopsy study, *Surg Neurol* 27:319-322, 1987.

22. Papay F, Morales L, Flaharty P, et al: Optic nerve decompression in cranial base fibrous dysplasia, *J Craniofac Surg* 6:1-10, 1995.

23. Ramsey HE, Strong EW, Frazell EL: Fibrous dysplasia of the craniofacial bones, *Am J Surg* 116:542-547, 1968.

24. Rompaey DV, Schmelzer B, Verstraete W, et al: Fibrous dysplasia in the frontoethmoidal complex: diagnosis and surgical aspects, *Acta Otorhinolaryngol Belg* 48:37-40, 1994.

25. Rougier J, Tessier P, Hervouet, et al: Orbit-palpebral plastic surgery, *Bulletins et Memoires de la Societe Francaise d Ophtalmologie* 1-25, 1977.

26. Ruggieri R, Sim FH, Bond JR: Malignacies in fibrous dysplasia, *Cancer* 73:1411-1424, 1994.

27. Saito K, Suzuki Y, Nehashi K, et al: Unilateral extradural approach for bilateral optic canal release in a patient with fibrous dysplasia, *Surg Neurol* 34:124-128, 1990.

28. Sassin JF, Rosenberg RN: Neurological complications of fibrous dysplasia of the skull, *Arch Neurol* 18:363-369, 1968.

29. Schwartz DT, Alpert M: The maligant transformation of fibrous dysplasia, *Am J Med Sci* 247:1-20, 1964.

30. Schwindinger WF, Francomano CA, Levine MA: Identification of a mutation in the gene encoding the alpha subunit of the stimulatory G protein of adenylyl cyclase in McCune-Albright syndrome, *Proc Natl Acad Sci USA* 89:5152-5156, 1992.

31. Weinstein LS, Shenker A, Gejman PV, et al: Activating mutations of the stimulatory G protein in the McCune-Albright syndrome, *N Engl J Med* 325:1688-1695, 1991.

32. Wyngaarden JB, Smith LH: *Cecil textbook of internal medicine*, ed 18, Philadelphia, 1988, WB Saunders.

33. Yano M, Tajima S, Tanaka Y, et al: Magnetic resonance imaging findings of craniofacial fibrous dysplasia, *Ann Plast Surg* 30:371-374, 1993.

CHAPTER

Craniofacial Clefts and Other Related Deformities

51

Louis C. Argenta
Lisa R. David

INDICATIONS

GENERAL PRINCIPLES

The surgical correction of craniofacial clefts is an extremely difficult series of procedures that frequently encompasses many specialists. Because of the rarity of these conditions, most plastic surgeons will confront very few of these conditions in their careers. The treatment of craniofacial clefts should be restricted to those craniofacial teams that have experience in their treatment. Initiating reconstruction in these patients requires a commitment to be willing to treat and follow these patients until late adolescence because problems will invariably occur until complete development of the facial structures. Optimizing functional and aesthetic results in these patients determines whether they will be productive citizens. The temptation to perform only the initial soft tissue or only the hard tissue reconstruction and refer these patients "later" is detrimental to the overall welfare of the patient. This results in ethical problems and multiple medical problems. Compromise or loss of tissue, damage to vital structures, and neurologic impairment during an ill-advised first procedure frequently compound the patient's problems and increase the number of procedures required for successful reconstruction.

A myriad of structures are frequently involved in these clefts, and multiple specialists must be included in their treatment. The development of computed tomography (CT) and magnetic resonance imaging (MRI) scans and the increase in the radiologist's understanding of these problems allow better definition of the problem preoperatively. This greatly diminishes the length of the surgical procedure and, more importantly, makes the procedure safer for the patient. Aesthetic reconstruction is of no value if severe neurologic complications occur. Therefore neurologists, neurosurgeons, and ophthalmologists should evaluate these patients carefully preoperatively and participate actively in their surgery and later in the course of their growth. Maximal recovery of these patients will require audiologic, otolaryngologic, orthodontic, and psychologic specialists in the course of their development. Adhering to basic principles allows many of these patients, the

vast majority of whom have normal neurologic capability, the ability to lead normal and productive lives.

Craniofacial clefts comprise some of the most difficult and debilitating problems that exist in plastic surgery. Patients afflicted with such disorders face a lifetime of surgical reconstruction, socioeconomic depravation, and psychologic difficulty. Although the severity and extent of craniofacial clefts and malformations varies extraordinarily, a predictable variety of patterns occurs. Understanding of these patterns is helpful in moving toward an understanding of the etiology and the potential treatment for these deformities. A craniofacial cleft is both a soft tissue and a bony disruption in the normal growth pattern of the face often with significant functional impairment.

Because of the difficulty in conceptualizing and classifying a wide variety of craniofacial clefts, the precise incidence of these clefts and their related craniofacial malformations is poorly documented in the literature. The lack of a concise system to document and classify these deformities, a relatively low incidence, and a great degree of variability in occurrence in various regions of the world have made these conditions a curiosity. Most of the literature is filled with solitary case reports, and only few individuals with very large, specialized practices have personal experiences with a significant number of each cleft.[41,42] The incidence of each of these major facial deformities is probably significantly higher than reported because a large number do not survive birth or die in the neonatal period.[29,43] Social and economic factors in various parts of the world also result in many of these children being abandoned to die in the early neonatal period. With the development of surgical techniques to reconstruct an affected individual and gradual changes in social and medical acceptance, many more of these children are surviving. In addition, better prenatal care, postoperative care, and management of respiratory and neurologic difficulties have rendered many of these children viable who previously would have expired.[10] Simultaneously, as ultrasound and other intrauterine procedures become more reliable, it is possible that some parents will elect termination of pregnancies when major craniofacial anomalies are present.

MORPHOGENESIS OF CRANIOFACIAL CLEFTS

Given the complexity of embryonic development of the cranial and facial structures, it is difficult to understand why abnormalities are not more frequent. Development of the face occurs between 3 and 8 weeks of fetal development in an extremely complex series orchestrated events[31] (Figure 51-1). The third and fourth weeks of gestation are characterized by the nasal frontal prominence of the forebrain, with early development of the nasal and olfactory placodes. These placodes subsequently become the medial and lateral processes. Between the fifth and sixth weeks of gestation, the nasal processes enlarge, migrate, and coalesce in the midline to unite with the developing maxillary facial process to form the upper lip. The nasal tip, columella, philtrum, and premaxilla derive from the medial nasal process, whereas the nasal ala derive from the lateral nasal process.

Concurrently, the mandibular arch bifurcates in the fourth week to form the mandibular processes. These processes move toward the midline to form the lower mouth. Union of the maxillary processes with the nasal processes completes the

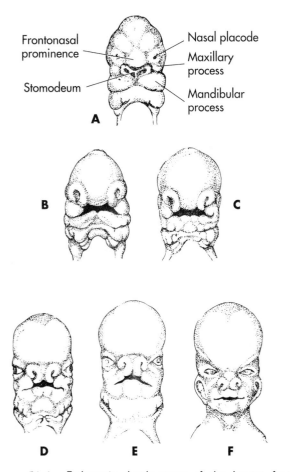

Figure 51-1. Embryonic development of the human face. **A,** 4-week embryo. **B,** 5-week embryo. **C,** 6-week embryo. **D,** 6½-week embryo. **E,** 7-week embryo. **F,** 8-week embryo. (From Kawamoto H, Jr: Rare craniofacial clefts. In McCarthy J, editor: *Plastic surgery: cleft lip and palate and craniofacial anomalies,* vol 4, Philadelphia, 1990, WB Saunders.)

growth of the midface and by 6 weeks of gestation the base and structure of the face is established. By the eighth week of gestation, the face is fully developed.

Facial clefts occur when any of a wide diversity of factors interfere with development, migration, adhesion, or coalescence of these processes. The classic fusion theory developed by Dursey and Aschia[9] postulated that clefts were caused by failure of fusion of facial processes as they developed and migrated. The mesodermal penetration theory was advanced by Pohlman and Veau.[33] This concept postulates that clefts are formed by failure of the mesenchyme to migrate into areas of fusion after epidermal contact has occurred. Although both of these concepts have value in explaining the basic etiology of craniofacial clefts, the recent discovery of genetic factors, apoptosis, and microbiologic influences need to be further developed.[16]

In our experience, the vast majority of such clefts occur in third world countries and are largely centered in Hispanic and Asiatic groups. Although many teratogens have been incriminated in experimental procedures to create clefts and craniofacial deformity, very few agents have been directly incriminated in human teratogenesis. Tranquilizers, steroids, alkalizing agents, and anticonvulsants have all been directly related to the formation of clefts in humans.[30,34,37,44] The well-known teratogenic effects of isotretinoin (Accutane),[6,19] the anticonvulsant phenytoin (Dilantin),[30,37] and thalidomide[22,35] all have been associated with clefting. An extremely diverse group of other agents, including infection, radiation, and steroids, although having clefting potential in animal models, have not been directly related to human teratology in this area.[12,13,20,32] The fact that the preponderance of these unusual clefts occur in third world countries points to other investigations that need to be focused in malnutrition and misnutrition. Concentration of these clefts in Hispanic and Asiatic groups points to the need for further investigation into genetic abnormalities and genetic predispositions.

OPERATIONS

INDIVIDUAL CLEFTS

The wide array of craniofacial clefts makes classification difficult. Previously, multiple terms denoting dysmorphia have been applied to these conditions. Van der Meulen[42] has attempted to classify these clefts on an embryologic basis (Figure 51-2). Tessier's classification[41] is based on anatomic findings related to his very wide surgical and clinical experience (Figures 51-3 to 51-5). At times, however, both of these classifications become cumbersome and difficult to conceptualize for the clinical surgeon. For this reason, we would propose dividing the craniofacial clefts into four general groups, each of which include specific subgroups as described by Tessier and Van der Meulen.[41,42] Based on physical findings and general surgical principles, craniofacial clefts can be divided into four categories: (1) the oral-nasal clefts, (2) the oral ocular clefts,

(3) the lateral facial clefts, and (4) the orbital cranial clefts. The oral-nasal group includes those with disruptive elements of the nose and lip and include Tessier clefts numbers 0, 1, 2, and 3. The oral ocular clefts encompass those that disrupt the lip and orbit and include Tessier clefts numbers 4, 5, and 6. Lateral clefts include those that are lateral to the mouth and orbit and includes Tessier clefts numbers 7, 8, and 9. The cranial clefts include those that affect the cranium, Tessier clefts numbers 10, 11, 12, 13, and 14. The general principles for reconstruction of each group of clefts is conceptually related.

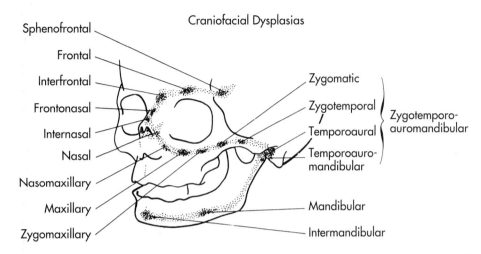

Figure 51-2.   Van der Meulen et al classification. (From Van Der Meulen J, Mazzola, Stricer M, et al: Classification of craniofacial malformations. In Stricker M, Van Der Meulen J, Raphael B, editors: *Craniofacial malformations,* Edinburgh, 1990, Churchill Livingstone.)

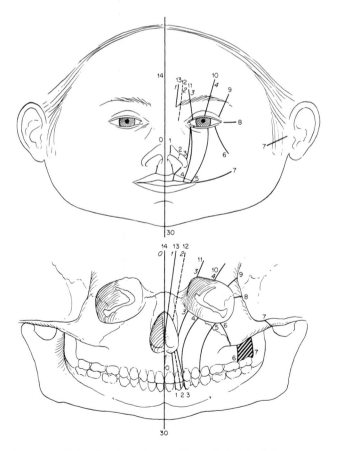

Figure 51-3. Tessier classification of facial clefts. (From Kawamoto H Jr: Rare craniofacial clefts. In McCarthy J, editor: *Plastic surgery: cleft lip and palate and craniofacial anomalies,* vol 4, Philadelphia, 1990, WB Saunders.)

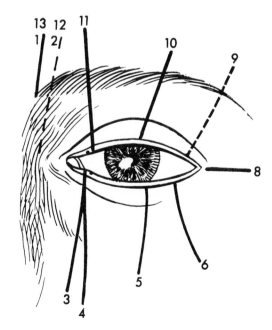

Figure 51-4.   Location of clefts in relation to the eyelids and eyebrow. (From Kawamoto H Jr: Rare craniofacial clefts. In McCarthy J, editor: *Plastic surgery: cleft lip and palate and craniofacial anomalies,* vol 4, Philadelphia, 1990, WB Saunders.)

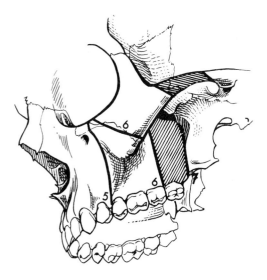

Figure 51-5. Lateral view of the facial clefts on the zygomatico-maxillary skeletal complex. (From Kawamoto H Jr: Rare craniofacial clefts. In McCarthy J, editor: *Plastic surgery: cleft lip and palate and craniofacial anomalies,* vol 4, Philadelphia, 1990, WB Saunders.)

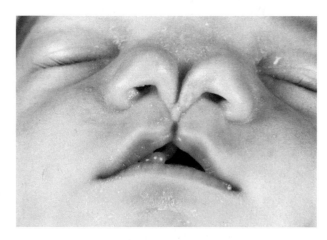

Figure 51-6. No. 0 cleft. Patient with a bifid nose and median cleft of the upper lip. Orbital hypertelorism is also noted.

Oral-Nasal Clefts

This group is characterized by clefts that occur between the midline and the Cupid's bow and disrupt the integrity of both the lip and the nose. They can occur alone or in combination with extensions into the cranium and are discussed later. All of these clefts demonstrate abnormalities in both the lip and the nose.

CLEFT NO. 0. The No. 0 midline cleft of Tessier occurs directly in the midline of the lip and nose.[41] This cleft includes most of the midline deformities as described in earlier classifications, including internasal dysplasia.[42] This cleft can occur as a failure of closure of the anterior neuropore, resulting in widening and displacement of structures of the midface, or as a true agenesis, resulting from an absence or decreased formation of the midface, a "false cleft."[5] When a true cleft exists secondary to failure of closure of the neuropore, a distinct clinical entity is formed. There is a deficiency in the central upper lip, the degree of severity of which can range from minimal notching of the vermilion border to a complete cleft (Figure 51-6). The cleft may continue through the mid-premaxilla and may involve the secondary palate. The nose is usually bifid with irregularity and thickening in the columella. Scarring retracts the nose in a cephalad direction, and the cartilages are displaced laterally. The osseous component of this deformity is manifest as a diastasis between the central incisors, a sclerotic irregularity or a true cleft of the central gingiva, and a flattening and widening of the nasal bridge. The septum may be irregular, duplicated, or occasionally absent. Depending on the severity of the cleft, it may extend into the forehead and upper middle face as a No. 14 cleft.

If true dysgenesis of the midline structures occurs, a false median cleft may arise in which tissue is deficient or absent in the midline. Partial or total absence of the philtrum, columella,

and premaxilla may occur, resulting in a midline defect with maldevelopment of the nose. The nose is present in varying degrees and may exist as a central proboscis or as total nasal aplasia. The lifespan of these children is usually compromised because of frequently associated brain dysgenesis. In such cases, death usually occurs before an attempt at reconstruction. Infants with minimal forms of false zero clefts can approach mental normality with a normal life expectancy.[8]

The median cleft can extend cephalad as a No. 14 cleft or caudad as a central cleft of the mandible. Tessier[41] classified this entity as a No. 30 cleft, whereas Van der Meulen[42] classifies it as an inframandibular dysplasia. Such anomalies are extremely rare and may vary from a small coloboma of the lower lip to a complete cleft of the lower lip, mandible, and tongue with scar extending toward the hyoid and thyroid cartilages.

CLEFT NO. 1. The Nos. 1, 2, and 3 clefts all have in common a cleft through the lateral margin of the Cupid's bow. The No. 1 cleft has been previously classified as a nasoschizis, a subtype of nasal dysplasia,[42] and was described as a separate clinical entity by Tessier in 1973.[41] This cleft may continue into the cranium as a No. 13 cranial cleft.

The cleft originates at the lateral Cupid's bow and progresses into the nose through the parasagittal dorsum on one side (Figure 51-7). The No. 1 cleft can occur as a result of dysgenesis or as a true cleft. If dysgenesis occurs, complete absence of half of the nose may be present (Figure 51-8). In such cases, the nasal airway, ethmid, and frontal sinuses may be hypoplastic and replaced by sclerotic bone. In milder cases, the nasal bone is hypoplastic while the nasal spine and septum are normal.

Unilateral nasal aplasia with proboscis is thought to be a rare form of No. 1 cleft and occurs when the involved soft tissue attempts to form a false nasal structure. The proboscis

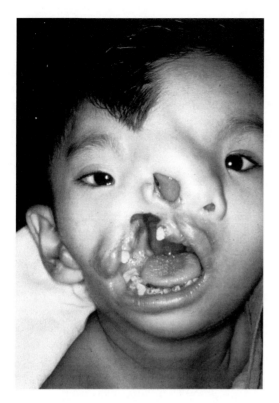

Figure 51-7. Nos. 1 and 3 clefts. The cleft in the dome of the nostril is a classic feature for the No. 1 cleft. The cleft is continued into the cranium as a No. 13 cleft.

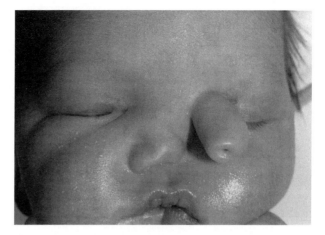

Figure 51-9. Proboscis lateralis, a rare form of cleft No. 1. The mucosal lined tube ends blindly.

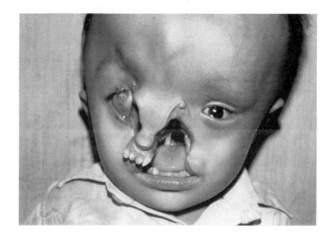

Figure 51-10. No. 2 cleft on left and No. 3 cleft on the right. Orbital hypertelorism is seen.

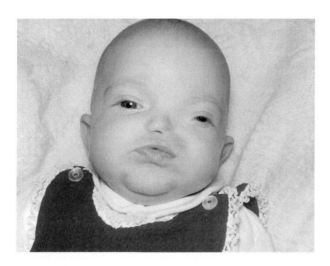

Figure 51-8. Nasal dysgenesis with complete absence of one of the nares.

contains the sweat glands, sebaceous tissue, striated muscle fibers, nerve endings, and cartilage that normally would be in the nose. The proboscis is a mucosal lined tube and almost always ends blindly with sclerotic bone (Figure 51-9). The nasal bone and cartilages of the involved side are not present as distinct entities.

CLEFT NO. 2. These clefts are extremely rare and were initially only theorized by Tessier.[41] A very few rare cases show

unique soft and hard tissue characteristics that distinguish them from a No. 1 or No. 3 cleft. The cleft originates at the lateral margin of the Cupid's bow and extends into the middle third of the nostril as a deficiency and flattening of the soft tissue of the nose rather than as a true cleft (Figure 51-10). The absence of a true cleft helps distinguish it from a No. 1 cleft. There is no palpebral fissure involvement in this cleft; however, orbital hypertelorism may be present when it extends in a cephalad direction as a No. 12 cleft.

Bony abnormalities include sclerosis and hypoplasia of the bones on the involved sides that extends toward the medial canthus but does not enter the orbit. In Van der Meulen's classification, this is classified as a nasomaxillary dysplasia.[42]

CLEFT NO. 3. This is a relatively common form of craniofacial cleft that has been previously described as a nasal ocular cleft, oblique facial cleft, or nasomaxillary dysplasia.[28,42] The cleft can be unilateral or bilateral and varies considerably depending on the degree involvement of the tissue medial to the orbit (Figure 51-11). This cleft can continue above the orbit as a No. 10 or No. 11 cleft. The lip portion of the cleft

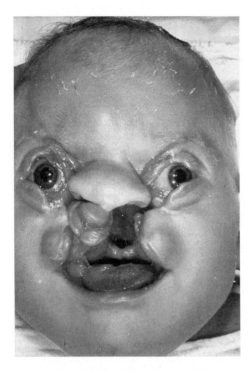

Figure 51-11. Bilateral No. 3 cleft. The nasal alae are displaced, and a coloboma is present in the lower eyelids.

has a common origin, as do clefts Nos. 1 and 2, from the lateral margin of the Cupid's bow. This cleft then extends across the base of the nasal ala and extends into the region of the normal union between the medial nasal process and the maxillary process. It extends through the nasolacrimal duct and into the lacrimal groove. There is a deficiency of tissue between the alar base and the medial canthus, resulting in a contracture of this area. In severe cases, the nose, mouth, and maxillary sinus are contiguous. Colobomas of the lower eyelid medial to the punctum, as well as displacement and hypoplasticity of the medial canthal ligament, may also occur. Involvement of the globe itself is unusual. Functional impairment of the lips may be significant secondary to downward displacement of the medial structures.

The bony compartment of this cleft passes through the alveolus between the lateral incisor and the canine tooth. The lateral border of the pyriform aperture is involved, and there is division between the nasal cavity and maxillary sinus. The frontal process of the maxilla may be disrupted or absent.

OPERATIONS FOR THE ORAL-NASAL CLEFTS. The surgical management of the oral-nasal clefts may become extremely difficult and may be complicated by changes that occur with growth and development of this area. The treatment of No. 0 clefts is usually staged. The central lip cleft can be closed usually in a straight-line vertical manner, carefully approximating muscle, mucosa, and skin. Occasionally because of loss of vertical height, rotation from the lateral segments of the lip may be necessary. The initial nasal deformity is repaired at the time of lip repair by approximating the nasal ala in the midline and excising redundant soft tissue. This leaves a vertical midline scar that heals with good cosmetic

results. These noses grow irregularly and require further surgery later in life. Surgery of the nasal septum is best delayed until adolescence to minimize growth disturbances.

When the No. 0 cleft is the result of aplasia and significant tissue is truly absent, reconstruction becomes more difficult. The lip is closed primarily in the midline, taking care to carefully approximate muscle. Abbe flaps are reserved for secondary revisions and are usually not necessary.[1] Nasal reconstruction is usually staged. If sufficient soft tissue is available, it can be encouraged to grow by successive cantilever bone grafts placed at intervals of every 2 to 3 years. Severe soft tissue deficiencies are treated with subtotal or total nose reconstructions from the forehead when the child enters school.[33] The forehead flap reconstruction is serially expanded using repeat cantilever bone graft. Should the nose fail to develop appropriately, a second total nose reconstruction can be accomplished by expanding the forehead and taking tissue from the contralateral side.

Reconstruction of clefts Nos. 1 and 2 are basically hemirhinoplasties. Attempts at producing patent airways almost always result in constriction and failure. Progressive enlargement of the involved side by soft tissue serial cantilevered bone graft is helpful until adolescence. When a proboscis exists, this soft tissue can be used in the hemirhinoplasty, but such tissue does not usually grow commissural with the opposite side. In adolescence, hemirhinoplasty, or total reconstruction with a forehead flap, is usually required and often will produce excellent cosmetic results. Attempts at producing a patent lacrimal system in these patients is usually futile.

Repair of the No. 3 cleft requires mobilization of the lateral facial tissue using wide undermining of the involved side. Occasionally, total cheek flaps may be necessary. Closure should be with multiple Z-plasties as described by Van der Meulen aimed at reconstructing an adequate lower lid and lengthening the deficient distance between the canthus and the lip.[42] Every attempt should be made to mobilize sufficient soft tissue to achieve satisfactory lower lid reconstruction so that the eye is protected. Attempts at reconstructing a true lacrimal system in these clefts usually fail, and recurrent infections are common. There is usually enough tissue to reconstruct the nose and return the base of the nose to a normal position using a Reiger flap placed on the opposite side. This moves tissue from the central forehead to the nose for reconstruction without compromising the possibility of later forehead flaps. Approximation of the skin and facial musculature over the cleft usually results in narrowing of the bony defect over time. Bone grafting of the defect with cranial grafts is usually delayed until early adolescence.

Multiple secondary surgeries are the rule with this type of cleft. Secondary distortion of the lip and nose with growth, infection, and scarring are common. Secondary surgeries of the lid are frequent.

Oral Ocular Clefts

This group incorporates clefts that connect the oral and orbital cavities without disrupting the integrity of the nose. These clefts occur lateral to the Cupid's bow, and the central facial

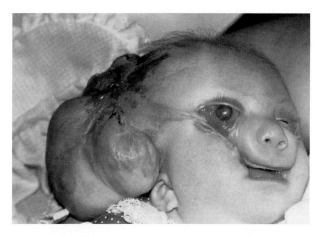

Figure 51-13. No. 5 cleft in combination with a No. 9 cleft. The No. 5 cleft extends from the medial to the lateral eyelid. The No. 9 cleft is seen at the superolateral angle of the orbit.

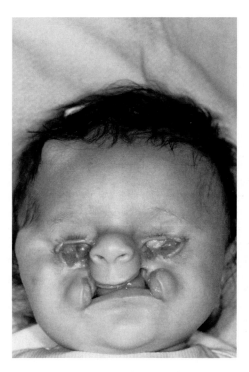

Figure 51-12. Bilateral No. 4 cleft. Cephalad rotation of the central portion of the face.

structure is largely intact. These clefts extend through the soft tissue of the cheek and maxillary process and are sometimes termed *oblique facial clefts* or *meloschises*. This group incorporates Tessier clefts Nos. 4, 5, and 6.[41]

CLEFT NO. 4. The No. 4 cleft is one of the most disruptive and complicated of the facial clefts. It exists in multiple degrees of severity. This group includes medial maxillary dysplasia of Van der Meulen and the general classification of oblique facial cleft.[42]

The No. 4 cleft begins lateral to the Cupid's bow between the commissure of the mouth and the philtral crest. The cleft passes onto the cheek, lateral to the nasal ala, and curves into the lower eyelid, terminating medial to the punctum. The lower canaliculus is usually disrupted, although most of the lacrimal apparatus is intact. The medial canthal ligament is intact, but most of the inferior supporting structures to the eye are disrupted.[38] Varying degrees of eye deformity ranging from a normal eye to total anophthalmia can be observed.

The No. 4 cleft results in significant osseous and soft tissue disruption. It usually begins between the lateral incisor and canine teeth and extends onto the anterior surface of the maxilla lateral to an intact pyriform aperture. It always extends medial to the infraorbital nerve and never through the infraorbital foramen. The medial and inferior portions of the orbital wall are disrupted, and considerable bone may be absent. When bilateral forms of cleft No. 4 occur, the entire central portion of the face rotates in a cephalad direction (Figure 51-12). These clefts may be unilateral, bilateral, or combined with other oral ocular clefts. Kawamoto[18] notes that six of nine patients with bilateral No. 4 clefts that he reviewed had other craniofacial clefts on opposite side of the face.

CLEFT NO. 5. This group incorporates the lateral maxillary dysplasia described by Van der Meulen[42] in 1983 and the Boo-Chai[4] No. 2 oral ocular cleft. This group constitutes the rarest of the oral ocular clefts, with less than 15 reported in the literature.[3,4] They usually occur with other rare clefts in the opposite side.[18]

The lip is cleft medial to but very near to the commissure and then extends laterally on to the cheek into the lateral third of the lower eyelid (Figure 51-13). The intervening soft tissue is hypoplastic. Various degrees of ocular involvement, including anophthalmia, microphthalmia, or a normal eye, may occur.

The skeletal deformities of the No. 5 cleft reveal an origin lateral to the canine that extends lateral to the infraorbital foramen. The cleft then enters the orbit in its lateral half. Significant amounts of bone in the infraorbital rim can be missing or highly sclerotic, resulting in prolapse of the orbital contents.

CLEFT NO. 6. This cleft includes the maxillozygomatic dysplasia of Van der Meulen and the incomplete forms of Treacher Collins syndrome.[7,11,42] It represents a transition form between the oral ocular clefts and the lateral facial clefts. This cleft is distinguished by a more subtle soft tissue deformity than usually occurs in true Treacher Collins syndrome. This cleft extends from the tissue immediately lateral to the oral commissure and across the lateral portion of the maxilla and zygoma to terminate in a coloboma or soft tissue deformity of the lower lid in the lateral third (Figure 51-14). Irregularities in the deficiency of soft tissue are frequently present. The ear is normal in this cleft.

The skeletal deformity is more obvious in the No. 6 cleft than the soft tissue abnormality. True clefts of the alveolus are unusual, but the molar area on the involved side is usually hypoplastic and deficiency extends into the zygomatic maxillary suture. The malar portion of the zygoma is hypoplastic but present, and a zygomatic arch is intact. Extending into the orbit, a cleft is frequently present in the lateral third, but these can be extremely minor.

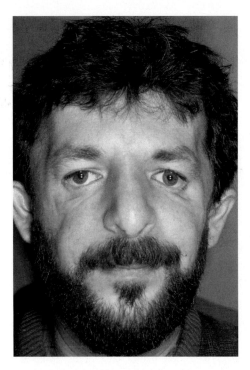

Figure 51-14. No. 6 cleft on the right. This is an incomplete form of the Treacher Collins malformation.

OPERATIONS FOR THE ORAL OCULAR CLEFTS. Surgical correction of the nasal ocular clefts is extremely difficult and is frequently a multiple-stage procedure. Careful consultation with ophthalmologists is necessary because abnormalities of the eye itself are frequently present. Primary emphasis is placed on preservation of the globe and normal vision. Lubrication of the eye early in life is necessary to prevent the eye from desiccating. Partial tarsorrhaphies that do not totally occlude vision are frequently necessary. The high possibility of developing visual impairment makes reconstruction of these clefts urgent rather than elective cases. At the time of surgical correction, extensive mobilization of the soft tissues of the face are usually necessary. Tissue expansion of the lateral segments can facilitate movement of the lateral facial tissue across defects. Extensive undermining as far as the auricle is frequently necessary. Rotations of the skin and soft tissue from the lateral and inferolateral face may be needed.[24] Multiple Z-plasties at the cleft site are usually performed so as to increase the distance between the orbit and the mouth and to avoid later contractures.[38] Soft tissues, including muscles, subcutaneous tissue, and skin, are closed at the primary operation. There may be a significant amount of tissue between the Cupid's bow and the actual clefts that needs to be discarded so that the final suture line will come to rest along the philtral column and nasolabial groove. This tissue can be discarded at the initial operation if there is sufficient lateral tissue to close the cleft. More frequently, this segment of tissue is discarded at the time of revisional surgery after the lateral facial tissues have had the opportunity to "expand." The use of a constriction device may be helpful to bring a free-floating central portion of the face into alignment. This is superior to performing a formal

osteotomy, attempting to move the central segment into position. We prefer to delay formal bone grafting until the child is 8 to 10 years of age because most of these faces grow normally. The use of costal, auricular, or cadaver cartilage in the orbital floor at the initial surgery is extremely useful to prevent herniation of the orbital contents. Further reconstruction of the lower lid using conchal or composite conchal grafts is helpful in maintaining lower lid continuity, particularly when a prosthesis is required.[26] Because most of the lacrimal apparatus is intact, attempts at reconstruction of the inferior canaliculus can be attempted but are usually not necessary if the superior canaliculus is intact.

Multiple secondary procedures and revisions are the rule in these types of clefts rather than the exception. With growth, there is frequent secondary deformity of the soft tissues, particularly because it involves the lower lid. Augmentation of the central face using cranial bone grafts is usually delayed and may require multiple procedures. When ocular prostheses are required, reconstruction of a lower lid with sufficient integrity to maintain the prosthesis must be accomplished. Reconstruction of cranial deformity No. 6 (minimal Treacher Collins syndrome) is addressed in reconstruction of the lateral facial clefts.

Lateral Facial Clefts

Tessier clefts Nos. 7, 8, and 9 constitute the lateral facial clefts and include the previously described entities of Treacher Collins syndrome, Goldenhar's syndrome, hemifacial microsomia, and necrotic facial dysplasia. Clefts Nos. 6, 7, and 8 usually occur in combination to produce Treacher Collins syndrome.[7,11,27] Cleft No. 7 is an extremely common abnormality. Cleft No. 8 is rare, and cleft No. 9 is extremely rare. Cleft No. 6 is a transitional cleft that bridges the oral ocular clefts and the lateral facial cleft, and cleft No. 9 is a transitional cleft that bridges the lateral facial clefts and the cranial clefts.

CLEFT NO. 7. The No. 7 cleft is the most common of all the craniofacial clefts. It has been described extensively under the terms *hemifacial microsomia, otomandibular dysostosis,*[11] *first and second brachial arch syndrome,*[23] and *zygotemporal dysplasia.*[42] Tessier[41] has postulated that the cleft is centered over the zygomatic temporal suture. Descriptions of this syndrome were first seen in early writings from Mesopotamia.[2] Males are affected more frequently then females,[15] and the cleft is bilateral in approximately 10% of cases. The No. 7 cleft occurs in approximately in 1 to 6 of 8000 births in a sporadic fashion.[15] Poswillo[34] postulated that this cleft was the result of injury or disruption of the stapedial artery early in embryogenesis.

The No. 7 cleft is the most widely variant of the craniofacial clefts and can exist as a form fruste with very minimal soft tissue or bone deformity (Figure 51-15). In such forms, there is only a widening of the commissure. The cleft originates in the lip at the oral commissure and extends laterally toward the ear, usually ceasing at the anterior border of the masseter muscle. Soft tissue depressions may exist laterally. In its fullest form, this cleft is manifest by various degrees of maldevelopment of

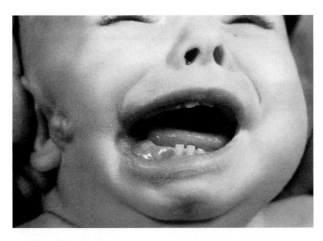

Figure 51-15. No. 7 cleft with ear deformity compatible with hemifacial microsomia.

the external ear. The middle ear, zygoma, and maxilla are all affected. The mandible is usually most affected with deficiencies in the condyle, ascending ramus, and temporomandibular joint. Occlusion is usually manifest as an open bite or crossbite with overeruption of the maxilla on the involved site. Soft tissue deficiencies are frequent in the parotid area, tongue, and palate. These deficiencies can be compounded by paresis of cranial nerves 5 and 7. In very severe forms, severe hypoplasia of the maxilla may result in a vertical orbital dystopia.

CLEFT NO. 8. Unlike cleft No. 7, cleft No. 8 is unusual and almost always exists in combination with another form of rare cleft. This cleft was described as zygofrontal dysplasia by Van der Meulen[42] and is isolated largely to the orbital area. Soft tissue components of this cleft may be very subtle and may be visible only as a lateral canthal irregularity often accompanied by a dermoid. The osseous form of this cleft also varies considerably in intensity and lies in the frontozygomatic suture. This cleft is usually associated with Goldenhar's syndrome.[14]

CLEFT NO. 9. This cleft represents a transition from the lateral facial clefts into the orbital cranial clefts. This is an extremely rare cleft, and only a few have been described in the literature.[36] This cleft involves the superolateral orbit dividing the eyelid in the lateral third and frequently the brow (see Figure 51-13). Osseous defects occur in the superior orbital rim and temporal bone. It can extend laterally into the temporal area and may be accompanied by encephaloceles.

TRUE TREACHER COLLINS SYNDROME (COMBINED CLEFTS NOS. 6, 7, AND 8). Treacher Collins syndrome is a bilateral combination of clefts Nos. 6, 7, and 8 (Figure 51-16). The condition is almost universally bilateral, although very rare occasions of unilateral manifestations may exist. All three clefts as previously described surround the zygoma on the maxillary, temporal, and frontal sides, resulting in severe dysplasia or absence of the zygoma. This anomaly has been described since antiquity, but its description was formalized by Treacher

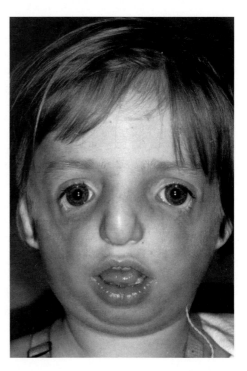

Figure 51-16. Child with the complete form of the Treacher Collins malformation.

Collins in the 1900s.[7] The soft tissue deformities of Treacher Collins syndrome include a coloboma and retraction of the lower lid, usually accompanied by a hypoplasia of lashes on the lower lid, as well. The upper lid frequently is redundant in its lateral half and gives the false impression of ptosis. The lateral canthus is displaced inferiorly. Soft tissue deficiencies associated with cleft No. 7 are manifested as absence of the zygomatic arch, hypoplasia of the temporalis muscle, ear malformations, and abnormalities of the hairline. Absence of the lateral inferior orbital rim is the manifestation of cleft No. 8.

OPERATIONS FOR THE LATERAL FACIAL CLEFTS. Surgical correction of the lateral facial clefts includes a very wide variety of procedures to correct two of the most complicated syndromes in craniofacial surgery. The lateral oral cleft of the No. 7 cleft is best repaired early in life by reapproximation of the skin, mucosa, and most critically the orbicularis oris muscle and surrounding muscles to create a normal commissure.[23] The lateral extent of the lip can be determined by finding the end of the white line of the lip or in unilateral cases by measuring from the philtral column to the commissure. The lateral cleft of the soft tissue is then closed in a running Z-plasty to minimize scar formation. The vast array of concomitant problems, including microtia, mandibular hypoplasia, and bony asymmetry, require a myriad of procedures that are described elsewhere in this text.

Correction of the lateral orbital clefts Nos. 8 and 9 usually involves reconstruction of the lateral canthus and proper positioning of the canthus at the lateral orbital rim. If the lateral rim is absent, cranial bone grafts are required for reconstruction to maintain proper positioning of the canthus.

The surgical correction of Treacher Collins syndrome encompasses the entire scope of craniofacial surgery. Ocular colobomas require grafts, transposition flaps from the upper lid, or rotation flaps from lateral facial area to reconstruct the coloboma.[17,26] Positioning of the lateral canthus requires adequate reconstruction of the lateral and inferior orbital rim so that position is maintained. This is usually accomplished with cranial bone graft. Timing for bony reconstruction of the zygoma, lateral inferior orbital rim, and deficient maxilla is debated. Most surgeons approach these conditions at 6 to 8 years of age with a full knowledge that multiple serial bone grafts will usually be required into adolescence. The severe mandibulomaxillary malpositioning that has occurred has previously required extensive combined maxillary and mandibular osteotomies. The use of multidimensional distraction osteosynthesis of the ascending ramus and maxilla may make correction of this deformity much easier in the future. It is critical to remember when operating on patients with Treacher Collins syndrome that the infraorbital nerve usually enters directly from the orbit and that no infraorbital foramen is present.[40]

Cranial Clefts

This group encompasses clefts extending superiorly from the lateral orbit to the midline and proceeds through the frontal bone and often into the base of the cranial vault. These clefts may be associated with specific clefts of the lower face or may occur in isolation. In general, when cranial clefts occur in combination with clefts Nos. 0 to 6, the deformity is much more severe, probably secondary to the distracting effect of the growing brain on the face. Van der Meulen[42] categorized the vast majority of these clefts as part of the frontal dysplasia group. This group encompasses Tessier clefts Nos. 10 to 14.[41] Manifestations of these clefts vary depending on the severity of the cleft. The larger the defect, the greater the cerebral herniation that occurs, and the more pronounced the malpositioning of the orbits which results in hypertelorism. These clefts present many of the more formidable corrections required in craniofacial surgery. Because of abnormal brain involvement, severe neurologic compromise may exist. Significant neurologic impairment may be present, and correction of these defects should be handled in conjunction with appropriate neurosurgeons.

CLEFT NO. 10. This cleft corresponds to the cranial branch of the No. 4 cleft. It is positioned in the center of the upper lid, brow, and orbit. Soft tissue manifestations are usually a coloboma in the mid-upper lid and an irregular retracted central brow (Figure 51-17). The osseous component of this cleft divides the central superior orbital rim, the underlying cranial base, and the frontal bone. Disruption of the skull, particularly when a large encephalocele occurs, results in an inferolateral rotation of the orbit, often with significant hypertelorism.

CLEFT NO. 11. The No. 11 cleft is almost invariably found in combination with a No. 3 cleft, and there is question as to whether or not it ever occurs in isolation. Soft tissue manifestations are a cleft in the medial eyebrow and lid with some soft tissue irregularity over the forehead. The osseous deformity extends through the cranial base and into the ethmoid sinuses. Orbital hypertelorism frequently occurs in combination with an encephalocele.

CLEFT NO. 12. The No. 12 cleft is an extension of the No. 2 cleft of the lower face. Soft tissue deformities include an encephalocele and a disruption of the eyebrow at its medial margin (Figure 51-18). The bony cleft is usually more severe

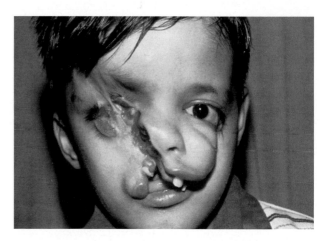

Figure 51-17. No. 3 cleft combined with a No. 10 cleft extending up onto the right cranium.

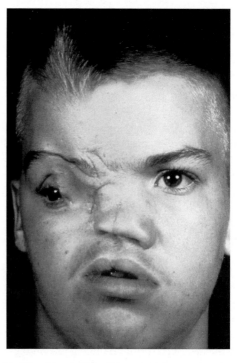

Figure 51-18. No. 2 cleft with a cranial extension as a No. 12 cleft.

and is almost invariably accompanied by orbital hypertelorism. The bony abnormality of this cleft involves the frontal bone extending inferiorly to the frontal process of the maxilla and deep into the ethmoid labyrinth. The cribriform plate is relatively normal in these cases because the cleft is lateral to the olfactory groove.

CLEFT NO. 13. This cleft is the cranial extension of the No. 1 cleft that occurs in the lower face. In the cranium, it extends through the olfactory groove, resulting in a widening of the cribriform plate. Large defects in the frontal bone and cribriform plate may result in massive encephaloceles, particularly when these clefts occur bilaterally. Soft tissue manifestations of the No. 3 cleft demonstrate an irregularity of the medial eyebrow, usually with some displacement into the orbit (Figure 51-19). Coloboma of the lids may occur but is rare.

CLEFT NO. 14. This group includes the midline facial clefts in the cranial region accompanying central nervous system abnormalities. They are included in Van der Meuler's classification as the interophthalmic dysplasia group.[42] This cleft is the cranial extension of the zero cleft in lower in the face and may occur with or without it. Like the zero cleft in the midline, the No. 14 cleft can be produced by a dysgenesis or agenesis of the midline cranial structures or by a true cleft, resulting in herniation of the intracranial contents. When a true cleft exists, herniation of the intracranial contents results in a morphokinetic arrest of the normal migration of the orbit.

The orbits remain in their embryonic position, resulting in hypertelorism and cranium bifida. The cribriform plate is displaced inferiorly, allowing herniation of the intracranial contents into the lower portion of the face. The olfactory grooves are widely separated. Depending on the degree of brain herniation, the nose and ethmoid sinuses can be widely separated, producing gross distortion of the midline structures (Figure 51-20). The osseous deformity reveals a cranium bifida with a frontal nasal encephalocele and wide displacement of the orbits.

When dysgenesis or agenesis occurs in the midline, severe malformations of the midline are accompanied by gross abnormalities of nose and orbital development. In the most severe case, cyclopia, or cebocephaly, may result. Holoprosencephaly manifest as hypotelorism, microcephaly, and severe central nervous system anomalies may occur (Figure 51-21). Life expectancies in these children are extremely limited.

Operations for the Cranial Clefts

Surgical treatment of the cranial clefts is directed at preserving brain integrity and function, reestablishing the cranial vault, and repositioning of displaced facial and orbital structures.[25] The degree of deformity is directly related to the size of the cleft and the amount of central nervous tissue that herniates through the defect. Correction of cranial cleft should be accomplished early in life before rupture or contamination of the meninges occur. CT and MRI scans in these cases are invaluable. Careful neurosurgical and ophthalmologic consultation is required. The dissection of the central nervous system

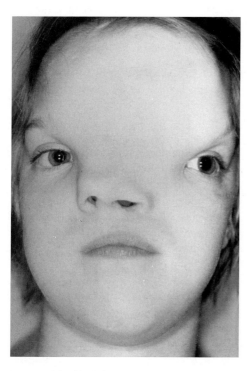

Figure 51-19. No. 13 cleft on the right is demonstrated. A No. 2 cleft with extension onto the cranium as a No. 12 cleft is also seen on the left.

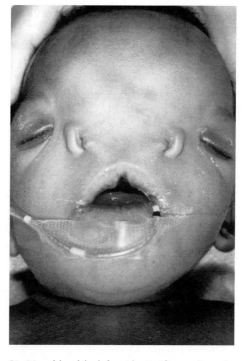

Figure 51-20. No. 14 cleft with significant distortion of the midline structures.

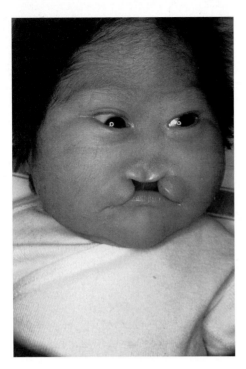

Figure 51-21. A child with holoprosencephaly with hypotelorism.

structures from these clefts may be extremely difficult and may require wide exposure. Combined intracranial-extracranial procedures are almost always needed.

Once the dura and brain have been mobilized from the cleft, the cranial defect is closed either by direct bone graft, when intraorbital distance is normal, or by repositioning the orbit to a more midline position, thus closing the cranial defect. Tessier's pioneering work on combined intracranial-extracranial correction of hypertelorism has made reconstruction of these deformities feasible.[39] All of the dura within the cranial cleft defect should be covered with bone. This is achieved by mobilization of the lateral and posterior cranial skull. If osseous defects are to be left in the skull, as they can be for the first year of life, they should be left posteriorly in an area not involved with abnormal dura. Osseous defects left over previous sites of cranial clefts will recur. In cases in which cranial clefts exist in combination with a lower facial cleft, correction of hypertelorism and axillary abnormalities with a midline facial bipartition may be necessary. This procedure allows simultaneous correction of the encephalocele, hypertelorism, and lower facial osseous deformity. Correction of such deformities requires extensive experience, and such surgery should be undertaken only by trained craniofacial surgeons.

Surgical correction of the holoprosencephalic group of patients necessitates ethical and technical considerations. Most of these children live for only a few weeks, although some patients have been reported to live into adulthood. Because there is minimal brain development, hypertelorism and its associated deformity should be deferred indefinitely.

OUTCOMES

Outcomes and treatment of patients with rare craniofacial clefts vary greatly. Results are directly related to the severity of the cleft; the experience of individuals treating these patients; the number of secondary reconstructive procedures; and the availability of all of the supporting specialties that are critical in craniofacial clinics, such as audiology, speech therapy, psychology, ophthalmology, otorhinolaryngology, anesthesiology, and radiology. Better preoperative delineation of abnormality and better anesthetic control of blood pressure and airway has greatly decreased the length of time most surgical reconstructions previously required. Advances in neurologic and ophthalmologic techniques have been critical in maintaining normal mental and visual capacities in these children. Increased psychologic and sociologic support has provided an important impetus toward encouraging these patients and families to pursue more secondary reconstructive surgery procedures knowing that normalcy can be an achievable goal.

In general, children with these rare craniofacial clefts do quite well if repaired appropriately. Some of the malformations are associated with CNS developmental problems, and these children especially need to be started in therapy early. It must not be forgotten that these children require a multiple-discipline approach so as to best promote their growth, both physically and psychologically.[21] This craniofacial team approach includes the involvement early on of a speech therapist; dentist; oral surgeon; ear, nose, and throat specialist; social worker; and craniofacial surgeon. This team approach will best prevent deficiencies from happening in the treatment plan of each of the individual children with these craniofacial clefts.

SECONDARY PROCEDURES

Unfortunately, most of these complex clefts are repaired in a single operation. The initial soft tissue repairs are key to the child's early development. Bony repairs need to be performed later on once development and growth will not be adversely affected. Recontouring of scars and adjustments for lack of growth must be expected. On counseling the patient's family, this should be a component of their informed consent. They should be aware that this is a process that will take several years and most of the child's adolescence will be involved in continual procedures to optimize functional and aesthetic results. Bearing this in mind, it is important to remember that the child, once old enough, should be involved in the decision-making process as to what he or she may want done and what he or she may be willing to accept as the functional and aesthetic result. This will ultimately lead to a better-adjusted child and family.

Multiple recent treatment options, including tissue expansion, distraction osteogenesis, plating systems, and synthetic bone substitute, have dramatically improved the potential for treating these individuals. Distraction osteogenesis in particular has the potential of allowing many deformities that previously could be approached only after full facial development had occurred to be attacked very early in life with exciting results. The lack of symmetry of these deformities and the creativity of physicians treating these deformities are a tribute to the triumph of modern medicine.

REFERENCES

1. Abbe R: A new plastic operation for the relief of deformity due to double harelip, *Med Rec Ann* 53:477, 1898.

2. Ballantyne JW: The teratological records of Chaldea, *Teratologia* 127:1, 1894.

3. Boo-Chai K: The transverse facial cleft: its repair, *Br J Plast Surg* 22:119-124, 1969.

4. Boo-Chai K: The oblique facial cleft: a report of 2 cases and a review of 41 cases, *Br J Plast Surg* 23:352, 1970.

5. Braithwaite F, Watson J: Three unusual clefts of the lip, *Br J Plast Surg* 2:38, 1949.

6. Braun JT, Franciosi RA, Drake AR, et al: Isotretinoin dysmorphic syndrome (Petter), *Lancet* 1:506, 1984.

7. Collins ET: Case with symmetrical congenital notches in the outer part of each lower lid and defective development of the malar bones, *Transactions of the Ophthalmological Society of the UK* 20:190, 1900.

8. Converse JM, McCarthy JG, Wood-Smith D: Orbital hypotelorism: pathogenesis, associated faciocerebral anomalies and surgical correction, *Plast Reconstr Surg* 56:389, 1975.

9. Dursy E: Zur Entwicklungsgeschichte des Kopfes des Menschen und der hoherern Wirbeltheire, *Tubingen* 99, 1869.

10. Fogh-Anderson P: Rare clefts of the face, *Acta Chir Scand* 129:275, 1965.

11. Francheschetti A, Zwahlen P: Un Syndrome nouveau: Ladysostose mandibulo-faciale, *Bull Schweiz Akad Med* 1:60, 1944.

12. Frazer FC, Fainstat TD: Production of congenital defects in offspring of pregnant mice treated with cortisone, *Pediatrics* 8:527, 1951.

13. Frazer FC, Chew D, Verusio AC: Oligohydramnios and cortisone-induced cleft palate in the mouse, *Nature* 214:417, 1967.

14. Goldenhar M: Associations malformations de l'oeil et de l'oreille, en particulier le syndrome dermoide epibulbaire-appendices auriculaires-fistula auris congenita et ses relations avec la dysostose mandibulo-facile, *J Gen Hum* 1432, 1952.

15. Grabb WC: The first and second branchial arch syndrome, *Plast Reconstr Surg* 36:485, 1965.

16. Hoepke H, Maurer H: *Z Anat Entwicklungsgesch* 108:768, 1939.

17. Jackson IT: Reconstruction of the lower eyelid defect in Treacher Collins Syndrome, *Plast Reconst Surg* 67:365, 1981.

18. Kawamoto HK Jr: The kaleidoscopic world of rare craniofacial clefts: order out of chaos (Tessier classification), *Clin Plast Surg* 3:529, 1976.

19. Lammer EJ, Chen DT, Hoar RM, et al: Retinoic acid embryopathy, *N Engl J Med* 313:837, 1985.

20. Langman J, Van Faassen F. Congenital defects in rat embryos after partial thyroidectomy of the mother animal: a preliminary report on eye defects, *Am J Ophthalmol* 40:65, 1955.

21. Lefebvre A, Barclay S: Psychosocial impact of craniofacial team, *Can J Psychiatry* 27:576, 1982.

22. Livingstone G: Congenital ear abnormalities due to thalidomide, *Proc R Soc Med* 58:493, 1965.

23. Longacre JJ, DeStefano A, Holmstrand K: The early versus the late reconstruction of congenital hypoplasia of the facial skeleton and skull, *Plast Reconstr Surg* 27:489, 1961.

24. Mansfield OT, Herbert DC: Unilateral transverse facial cleft—a method of surgical closure, *Br J Plast Surg* 25:29, 1972.

25. Marchac D: Radical forehead remodeling for craniostenosis, *Plast Reconstr Surg* 61:823, 1978.

26. Marks MW, Argenta LC, Freidman RJ, et al: Conchal cartilage and composite grafts for correction of lower lid retraction, *Plast Reconstr Surg* 83:629, 1989.

27. Marsh JL, Celin SE, Vannier MW, et al: The skeletal anatomy of mandibulofacial dysostosis (Treacher Collins Syndrome), *Plast Reconstr Surg* 78:460, 1986.

28. Morian R: Ueber die schrage Gesichtsspalte, *Arch Klin Chir* 35:245, 1887.

29. Nishimura HJ: Incidence of malformations in abortion. In *Congenital malformations* (Proceedings of the 3rd International Conference, Netherlands, 1969), Amsterdam, 1969, Excerpta Medica.

30. Pashayan H, Pruzansky D, Pruzansky S: Anticonvulsanta teratogenic, *Lancet* 2:702, 1971.

31. Patten BM: *Human embryology,* ed 3, New York, 1986, McGraw-Hill.

32. Pederson LM, Thigstrop I, Pederson J: Congenital malformation in newborn children of diabetic women, *Lancet* 1:790, 1964.

33. Pohlmann EH: Die embryonale Metamorphose der Physiognomie und der Mundhohle des Katzenkopes, *Morphol Jahrbuch (Leipzig)* 41:617, 1910.

34. Poswillo D: The etiology and surgery of cleft palate with micrognathia, *Ann R Coll Surg* 41:61, 1968.

35. Poswillo D: Otomandibular deformity. Pathogenesis as a guide to reconstruction, *J Maxillofac Surg* 2:64, 1974.

36. Sanvenero-Rosselli G: Developmental pathology of the face and the dysrhaphia syndromes —an essay of interpretation based on experimentally produced congenital defects, *Plast Reconstr Surg* 11:36, 1953.

37. Spidel BD, Meadow SR: Maternal epilepsy and abnormalities of the fetus and newborn, *Lancet* 2:839, 1972.

38. Tessier P: Colobonas: vertical and oblique complete facial clefts, *Panminerva Med* 11:95, 1969.

39. Tessier P: Orbital hypertelorism. Successive surgical attempts, materials and methods, causes and mechanisms, *Scand J Plast Reconstr Surg* 6:135, 1972.

40. Tessier P: Personal communication, 1975.

41. Tessier P: Anatomical classification of facial, craniofacial and latero-facial clefts, *J Maxillofac Surg* 4:69, 1976.

42. Van der Meulen J, Mazzola B, Stricker M, et al: Classification of craniofacial malformations, *Craniomalformations* 149, 1990.

43. Warburton D, Frazier FC: Genetic aspects of abortion, *Clin Obstet Gynecol* 2:22, 1956.

44. Wilson JG: Abnormalities of intrauterine development in non-human primates, *Acta Endocrinol (Kbh)* 166(suppl):261, 1972.

CHAPTER

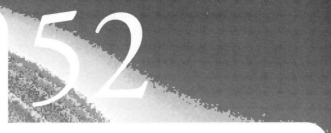

Unilateral Cleft Lip Repair

Don LaRossa

INTRODUCTION

A cleft lip is more accurately described as a cleft lip and nose deformity or perhaps even better as a cleft lip, nose, and alveolar deformity because all of these anatomic structures of the primary palate are affected to some degree in all but the most minor clefts. Even in these form fruste clefts, one can appreciate subtle differences in the shape and position of the nostril on the cleft side. As the deformity worsens, the effect on the lip, nose, and alveolar structures becomes more apparent. The alar base is displaced laterally as the two halves of the lip become more widely separated. Likewise, the two halves of the bony platform on which the alar base rests widen as the alveolar cleft deepens. With eventual complete separation of the lip structures, the floor of the nose dissolves, the alar cartilages become increasingly distorted, the caudal septum shifts toward the normal side while the nasal bones and maxilla on the cleft side shift laterally, and the alveolar cleft extends back to the incisive foramen. Teeth within the cleft site are displaced, rotated, or duplicated or are occasionally missing. In complete clefts of the lip and palate the defect extends to involve the structures of the secondary palate, the remaining hard and soft palate posterior to the incisive foramen. This chapter concerns itself with the deformity of the primary palate only.

INDICATIONS

INCIDENCE AND EPIDEMIOLOGY

It is evident from studies of homogeneous and heterogeneous populations that ethnic variations exist in the incidence of clefting. Fogh-Anderson[16] reported the occurrence as 1:750 live births in an essentially homogeneous population in Scandinavia, and Ivy[23] reported an incidence of 1:760 in a heterogeneous population in Pennsylvania. Burdi[7] and Habib[19] further defined this information and described an incidence of 2.1:1000 live births in Asians, 1:1000 in Caucasians, and 0.41:1000 in African-Americans in more

recent data. Clefts of the lip only occur in 21% of affected populations, whereas 46% involve clefts of the lip and palate and 33% are isolated clefts of the palate only.[17] Increasing parental age is apparently a risk factor, particularly the father's age and when both parents are over 30 years of age.[19] Clefts of the lip are more commonly left-sided and show a male predominance.[20]

ETIOLOGY

Although hereditary factors and specific drugs, such as phenytoin (Dilantin) and isotretinoin (Accutane), substance abuse of alcohol, and now smoking, have been directly implicated as causative agents, most of the evidence points to a multifactorial cause for clefting. Clearly hereditary factors play a role, with approximately 33% to 36% of cases having a positive family history for clefting.[16]

OPERATIONS

EVOLUTION OF SURGICAL PRINCIPLES OF CLEFT LIP REPAIR

The evolution of surgical repair of cleft lip can be viewed as occurring in five stages: simple closure of the lip defect, refinement of skin repair, functional muscle repair, restoration of the bony platform, and management of the cleft nasal deformity.

Because of the relative simplicity of repairing a cleft of the lip compared with a cleft of the palate, recorded instances of surgical correction appear quite early in medical history. The first documented cheiloplasty occurred in approximately 390 ad in China, and the earliest report in Western medical literature was by Yuperman, a Flemish surgeon (1295-1350).[11,65] Perhaps the best known of the early repairs was by the noted Renaissance surgeon Ambrose Paré.[44] Surgeons of that era used needles (hare lip needles) around which were twisted figure-of-eight sutures of horsehair, flax, or waxed linen thread because sutures could not be sterilized and were used only by medical "quacks." The medial margins of the cleft were simply freshened and reapproximated. Rose[51] in 1891 and later Thompson[61] (1912) used a modified straight line repair. They were able to achieve lengthening of the shortened vertical height of the cleft side by using curved, convex lines bordering the cleft. This method is still useful for minor or form fruste unilateral clefts but not for more serious ones (Figure 52-1, A). Malgaigne,[32] a noted French surgeon of his era, is credited with introducing the concept of flaps in 1843, although his flap was more of a back-cut into the lateral and medial lip, which lengthened the pared edges. One year later, Mirault[38] first used a flap of vermilion from the lateral lip

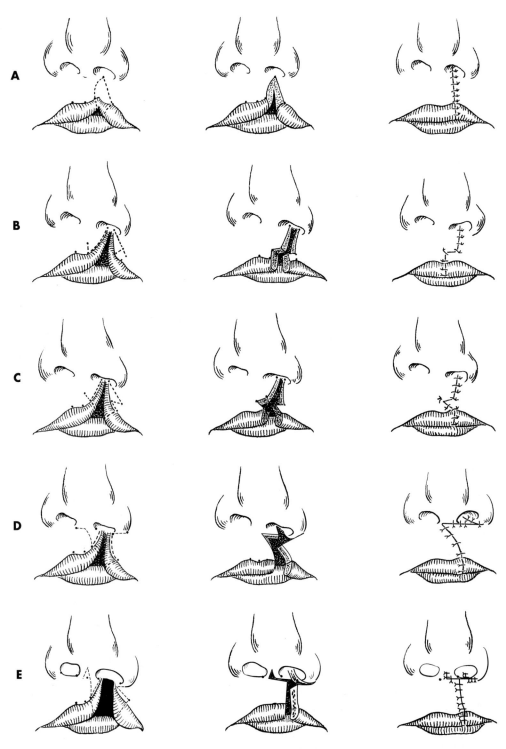

Figure 52-1.   **A,** Rose-Thompson repair. **B,** Quadrangular flap repair (Hagedorn, LeMesurier). **C,** Triangular flap repair (Tennison, Randall). **D,** Rotation-advancement repair (Millard). **E,** Mohler modification of rotation-advancement repair.

element in the repair. Blair[3] and Brown and McDowell[6] further modified the straight line repair with a triangular flap of vermilion and lower lip skin in the 1930s and 1940s in the United States. This era in the evolution of cleft lip repair emphasized the *first principle of management of the defect: lengthening of the shortened vertical height of the cleft side to match the normal side.* However, the straight line repairs with their multiple modifications neglected a critical anatomic feature of the unrepaired cleft lip: that it retained the Cupid's bow within the medial lip element. Cardoso[10] was one of the first to emphasize the importance of retaining this structure, although this was not possible until the development of the triangular flap repairs as described below.

The seminal step of transferring tissue from the lateral lip to lengthen the medial lip occurred when Hagedorn[21] used a quadrangularly shaped flap in 1884. LeMesurier[30] refined and popularized this approach beginning in 1949. In these repairs, a quadrangular flap of lower lip skin and adjacent vermilion from the lateral lip was inserted into the medial lip to lengthen it and to recreate a Cupid's bow (see Figure 52-1, *B*). Almost simultaneously, Tennison[60] described the use of a triangular flap of lower lip skin adjacent to the vermilion inserted into a back-cut in the medial lip to accomplish the same effect at the Meeting of the American Association of Plastic Surgeons at the Broadmoor in Colorado Springs, Colorado, in 1950; he reported it in the literature in 1952. He used a wire bent into thirds to outline a triangular flap of precise dimensions to accomplish the desired lengthening. Randall[48] described the geometric measurements used to attain the same result (see Figure 52-1, *C*). Their combined efforts produced an understandable and reproducible method that dominated cleft lip repair around the world for several decades. Wynn,[65] Marcks,[33] Cronin and Brauer,[5] and others added their modifications to the technique. This era in cleft lip repair focused *two additional principles* of all cleft lip repairs: *bringing a flap of tissue from the lateral lip where it is abundant into the medial lip where it is missing,* and *retaining the normal anatomic Cupid's bow.*

In further refining the skin repair of the clefted lip, Millard[37] introduced the *fourth principle of cleft lip repair, the rotation-advancement concept,* in 1955. The benefits were twofold: the incision lines follow the natural anatomic position of the philtral ridge and avoided placement of scars across the philtrum in the lower part of the lip (see Figure 52-1, *D*). However, the technique is more challenging to learn, perform, and reproduce. Nonetheless, it has displaced the triangular flap repair, becoming the more commonly used method because of its obvious aesthetic advantages. Millard and many other authors have modified the basic principles of the repair to permit adjustments to the multitude of anatomic variations inherent in lip clefts. A particularly useful one was described by Mohler[39] in 1984 (see Figure 52-1, *E*). By bringing the medial incision into the base of the columella, one can achieve a more rectangularly shaped philtrum, a more common variant than the shield-shaped one created by Millard's rotation advancement design.

Skoog[59] and Trauner[62] later introduced the use of two triangular flaps, one bordering the vermilion as in the triangular flap repair and the other beneath the nostril sill as in the rotation advancement technique.

Lip function became the focus in the quest for the "normal lip," ushering in the era of *muscle reconstruction* and the *fifth principle of cleft lip repair.*

In carefully documented fetal dissections, Fara[15] described the displacement of the normal course of the orbicularis muscle fibers and its vascular supply. He pointed out that muscle bundles parallel the margin of the cleft to insert medially at the base of the columella and laterally at the alar base and periosteum of the piriform aperture. He suggested that the abnormal pull was responsible for the orbicularis muscle bulge typical of the unrepaired cleft, the distortion of the ala nasi, and the deflection of the nasal septum. In contrast, Dado and Kernahan[12] described a more chaotic pattern of the muscle fibers in the cleft margin rather than the more orderly pattern of muscle bundles found by Fara. These differences are perhaps reconciled by a further elucidation of the complex anatomy of the orbicularis oris muscles by Nicolau, Latham, DeMey, and others. Nicolau[41] pointed out that the orbicularis is not simply a circular sphincter but has a well-defined deep and superficial portion. Intertwined are fibers from the paraoral and paranasal muscles, which work in concert with the orbicularis to produce the myriad of lip motions that are distinctly human. Nicolau suggested that the deep portion of the orbicularis does not reach the margin of the cleft vermilion but simply stops before reaching it. DeMey et al[13] further described the muscular anatomy in complete and incomplete lip clefts. They pointed out that the deep muscular component is interrupted at the level of the submucosa in both complete and incomplete clefts. In complete clefts the superficial muscular component parallels the margin of the cleft, although it is more sparse on the medial side; whereas in incomplete clefts, it alone crosses the cleft. Latham[29] and Nicolau described the intricate and complex muscle arrangements that help form the philtral ridges. Long and short fibers of the superficial component of the orbicularis crisscross in the midline to insert medial and lateral to the ridges and seem to create a mobile architectural infrastructure to support and move this region of the lip. Additional details of the microanatomic and macroanatomic interplay of the muscle and skin of the cleft region is provided by Mulliken.[40] Normally, the anterior projection of pars marginalis of the superficial portion of the orbicularis gives rise to the vermilion-cutaneous junction. However, in the cleft specimen, there is hypoplasia and disorientation of this portion of the muscle associated with a disappearance of the vermilion-cutaneous ridge (white roll of Gilles). As one proceeds orally from the vermilion-cutaneous junction, a gradual thickening of the epithelium is noted until an abrupt change to nonkeritinized epithelium is noted at the so-called "red line" of Noordoff.[42] On the medial side the width of the vermilion is narrower, whereas on the lateral side it is wider than normal, creating a disparity in the distance of the red line from the vermilion-cutaneous junction between the medial and lateral lip margins.

Fara[15] recommended turning down muscle stumps from the margin of the cleft in lip repair to counteract the displacement of the muscle bundles. Randall described reorientation of the bundles, dissecting them out from within the substance of the lip and crisscrossing them across the repair. In an attempt to more precisely reconstruct the normal configuration of the muscles, Randall and LaRossa[49] have interdigitated slips of muscle, whereas Park[45] has dissected out the superficial and deep portions of the muscle in his reconstructions. Others[36,45,49] have described the importance of reconstruction of the nasolabial bundles and the alar base. Although these steps are important in the evolution of creating a normally functioning lip, this ultimate goal has not yet been achieved.

The *sixth principle* in the evolution of the surgical management of the cleft lip deformity is *restoration of the bony platform.* Clefting of the alveolus and disruption of the dentoalveolar and adjacent maxilla varies with the degree of clefting. In more minor clefts the bone may be indented, whereas in more severe ones the bone gap extends to the incisive foramen. Clefts posterior to the incisive foramen are considered clefts of the secondary palate, as is seen in complete clefts of the lip and palate. The lateral incisor teeth at the margins of the cleft are affected to a variable extent and may be missing, diminutive, duplicated, or rotated except in minor clefts, in which the underlying bone is either unaffected or only minimally affected. The lateral incisor may erupt mesial, distal, or palatal to the cleft. Complete habilitation of the patient with a cleft that involves the alveolus may require repositioning of the displaced alveolar segments and bone grafting of the alveolar cleft. Although debate persists over timing of these procedures, most experts in the field agree that restoration of a normal dentoalveolar architecture is an important goal.

Presurgical orthopedic repositioning of the malpositioned alveolar segments with passive or active appliances can facilitate lip repair by bringing the cleft margins closer together. Burston,[8] McNiel,[36] and Hubner, Goinski, and Hotz[22] promoted the use of passive appliances that gradually nudged the segments into alignment. Latham,[28] Georgiade,[18] and others are advocates of using an activated appliance pinned in place to which force is applied by turning a jackscrew to move the segments. Orthopedic maneuvers may also have some beneficial effects on the outcome of primary nasoplasty, as well. However, it is well documented that it does not have long-lasting effects on the final dental occlusion.[53]

However, orthopedic alignment of the segments is essential at the time of bone grafting. Although there is general agreement that restoration of the continuity of the alveolar segments via bone grafting is desirable, the timing is open to debate. Enthusiasm for early bone grafting with wide dissection of mucoperiosteal flaps waned when reports of growth disturbances began to appear.[24,25,50,56,57] However, rib bone grafting in infancy with minimal undermining

preceded by presurgical orthopedics may not disturb growth, as demonstrated by Rosenstein and Kernahan.[52] Most authors advocate secondary bone grafting in the period of mixed dentition.[1]

Reconstruction of the distorted nasal anatomy is the last in the evolution and *the seventh principle* of cleft lip repair. The anatomic effects of the cleft on the nasal structures have been well described by numerous authors and include (Figure 52-2):

1. Slumping of the alar dome on the cleft side
2. Lateral displacement and recurvatum of the lateral crus on the cleft side
3. Lateral displacement of the alar base on the cleft side
4. Shortening of the medial crus of the lower lateral cartilage on the cleft side
5. Loss of continuity of the piriform aperture and bony platform
6. Displacement of the septum and anterior nasal spine toward the normal side
7. Loss of the normal overlap of the upper and lower lateral cartilages with inferior displacement of the alar rim on the cleft side

The degree of nasal deformity is proportional to the severity of clefting but is always seen in even the most minor clefts. Earlier in the evolution of cleft lip surgery, surgeons recommended against primary nasal repair out of concern for damaging the delicate cartilages supporting the nasal tip. More recently, McCoomb,[35] Anderl,[2] Salyer,[55] and others have championed primary nasal tip plasty. Evidence is now sufficient to show that long-lasting improvements can be achieved without detrimental effects on the growth and development of the nasal tip cartilages. These authors all advocate wide undermining of the nasal tip cartilages to separate them from the skin envelope. They are repositioned and maintained in their new position with sutures tied over external bolsters. Although much has been achieved by these efforts, the complete correction of the cleft nasal deformity still remains an unsolved challenge for future generations of cleft surgeons.

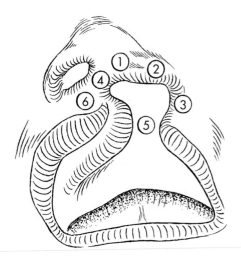

Figure 52-2. The cleft lip nasal deformity.

THE AUTHOR'S APPROACH

Primary Evaluation

The management of the child born with a cleft lip begins with a meeting with the affected child and his or her parents as soon as possible after the diagnosis is made. Now that prenatal diagnosis is possible in the second trimester, this may mean a prenatal consultation to answer the many questions raised by the usually unexpected news. Although cleft lip and palate occur relatively frequently, most parents have little or no personal experience with a person with a cleft and often have frequent misconceptions based on inadequate or incomplete information. Ultrasound diagnosis can be quite accurate in diagnosing cleft lip but usually not cleft palate, so often a discussion of both must be undertaken in broad terms. If the child is already born, attention to essentials of successful feeding, airway control, weight gain, and possible associated anomalies is of paramount importance, particularly in children with an associated cleft palate. Close communication with the child's pediatrician is essential. Photographs of successfully treated children and diagrams describing the steps needed to complete treatment may be helpful, depending on the parents' inquisitiveness and comfort with knowing details.

The surgeon must present an honest appraisal of the cleft condition and outline clearly the surgical steps needed to achieve a successful outcome, including potential risks and complications. Parents want to know how long surgery will take, whether general anesthesia is needed, how much pain is expected, and how it will be treated. The fact that there will be a permanent scar at the site of repair is sometimes a surprise and disappointment to parents. The probable need for touch-up procedures to maximize the appearance of the nose and lip and the long-term ongoing nature of treatment must be reviewed, even in minor clefts that are not likely to need bone grafting or much if any orthodontic care. Despite parents' sometime apparent fragility, a carefully outlined, realistic picture is usually well received and appreciated and can help solidify the surgeon-patient/parent relationship. Showing compassion and sensitivity and emphasizing of the positives goes a long way in preparing the parents for their child's care whether the diagnosis is made prenatally or postnatally. The use of parent support groups has been very valuable in helping parents through this difficult period. Directing the patients to the American Cleft Palate-Craniofacial Association through their CLEFTLINE phone number (800-24-CLEFT) can provide access to a great deal more written and spoken information and opens parents up to the resources of this nonprofit organization devoted to the education of patients and parents of children with these afflictions. There are also a number of sites on the Internet that can be accessed for information.

During this initial evaluation, the surgeon must decide about the timing of surgery. In the child of normal gestational age, I prefer to perform lip closure according to the long-accepted principles of pediatric surgery at approximately 10 to 12 weeks of age. Although some surgeons have enthusiasm for early repair, often before the child leaves the hospital because of the possible benefits of better wound healing in the more "fetal-like" tissue and the social benefits of having the mother bring home "normal" child, I have not embraced this philosophy. Although the scar may potentially be better, precise measurements are more difficult in a newborn, potentially increasing the need for secondary revision and obviating the potential beneficial effects on scarring from early repair. Additionally, the newborn will be subjected to an relatively long anesthetic at a time when he or she is not an ideal anesthetic risk. In the United States, with the advent of managed care and reduced lengths of hospital stay after a normal delivery (initially 24 hours and now 48 hours), surgery on the newborn would have to be within this window of time to conform to these guidelines. Finally, I have not seen published long-term results that would convince me to abandon the current practice.

In the child with a very wide cleft, some surgeons advocate the use of presurgical orthopedic appliances as described above. Others have advocated the use of adhesive taping.[45] This method requires close monitoring of the skin for irritation but can be successful. I have preferred the use of lip adhesion under these circumstances to mold the widely separated alveolar segments closer together and to convert the complete cleft into an incomplete one. There is general agreement that an incomplete cleft is easier to repair than a complete one.[47] Although some surgeons have done the adhesion under local anesthesia, I routinely use general anesthesia.

Management within the context of cleft palate team care is ideal because it provides a setting in which parents can recognize that there is a plan that will be carried out over a long term in a coordinated, interdisciplinary fashion by specialists who are interested, educated, and experienced in the care of children with clefts. Shaw et al[58] have proposed that the outcome of management of cleft lip and palate is better when those providing treatment are not occasional cleft lip and palate surgeons, based on outcomes of surgery performed in the United Kingdom compared with those achieved by teams in continental Europe. This concept has been promoted in the arena of cardiac surgery in the United States. The shortcoming of this approach, however, is the thwarting of the brilliant innovation by the individual who does only a small number of cleft repairs but has the insight to make a quantum leap discovery.

Design of Skin Incisions

The repair begins with a careful analysis of the defect and the configuration of the critical component elements of the lip and nose. Each cleft is unique and has varying degrees of distortion just as each individual's lip is not precisely the same as anyone else's. The basic elements are the same, but the details are different. It is incumbent on the surgeon to modify the design to duplicate the features of the noncleft side in an attempt to create a symmetric, normal-looking lip for that individual. One should not be wedded to a single procedure for all lip repairs. Depending on the degree of

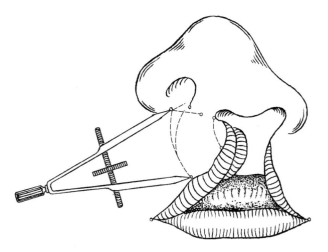

Figure 52-3. Using the normal anatomy as a guide to designing the incisions on the cleft side.

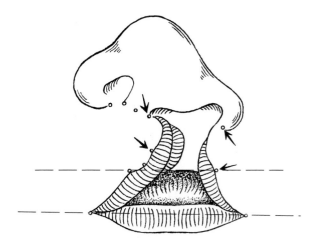

Figure 52-4. Outlining the key points on the cleft lip skin and vermilion.

clefting and the distortion that is present, one can choose to use a Millard type of repair or a Mohler design or even Rose and Thompson's. It is important for the surgeon to view these various repairs as principles of repair—a guideline to be followed, not a rigid design to which the surgeon must strictly adhere. The surgeon should use his or her creativity and basic knowledge of plastic surgical principles to modify and adjust the fundamental design to correct the distortions unique to each cleft lip that is treated. The surgeon can use the features of the normal side to help design the incisions on the cleft side. One should envision where the closed incisions would lie on the normal side, draw them on the skin of the normal side, and use them as a guide to the design of the proposed incisions on the cleft side. This exercise is very helpful in learning the principles of repair and as a guide to defining the length of incisions and the size of various flaps used in the repair (Figure 52-3).

First, the key points are identified on the normal and cleft side (Figure 52-4):

Midline and bases of the columella: It is not essential that the points at the bases be at any specific site, only that they be symmetrically placed.

Alar base: Place these symmetrically. Follow the alar crease as it joins the nasal floor in the vestibule as a guide to its placement. Roll the nostril medially with finger pressure to help define the eventual configuration

Peak of Cupid's bow and midpoint of Cupid's bow on the noncleft side: Use the frenulum as a guide to the midline. Place a series of dots along the vermilion-cutaneous border to help identify the key point. Duplicate the measurement between the peak on the noncleft side and the midpoint to identify the new Cupid's bow point. The proposed point can be moved slightly toward the midline because of the contraction and shortening of the skin away from the cleft.

Proposed point of Cupid's bow on the cleft side: Identify a point that is horizontal with the Cupid's bow point on the noncleft side. The vermilion-cutaneous roll should be

well developed at this point to provide for continuity of the roll in the repaired lip.

Next, analyze the configuration of the philtrum and the degree of displacement and distortion caused by the unrestrained lateral pull of the unrepaired orbicularis oris muscle. The muscle pulls the philtral column into a convex curve away from the midline on the medial side, as is the corresponding skin on the lateral lip element. The design of the skin incisions should mimic and reflect this and compensate for it. A series of dots drawn along the philtral ridge will elucidate this. A family of curves can be visualized on the philtrum and the proposed incision can parallel these (Figure 52-5, *A* and *B*). The shape of the philtrum will become evident—whether it is shield-shaped or rectangular. If it is shield-shaped, a Millard type of incision is used; if it is rectangular, a Mohler repair is chosen. With either design, the incision lines are curved to compensate for the displaced skin and philtral column (see Figure 52-5). In a very minor cleft, a Rose-Thompson repair can be used. A quill type of pen point and methylene blue dye are useful for marking. It permits one to draw fine, precise lines, and the key points can be tattooed into the skin with the pen's point.

To gain additional length, to maintain the continuity of the vermilion-cutaneous roll, and to restore the normal profile of the lip, a small triangular flap is developed at the vermilion-cutaneous junction on the lateral lip. It is the height of the vermilion-cutaneous roll and is introduced into a back-cut in the medial lip (Figure 52-6).

Lidocaine (Xylocaine) 1% with 1:100,000 epinephrine is used for hemostasis and injected after the planning and marking is complete. Marking is best done from the head of the table to help achieve symmetry.

Muscle Repair

The muscle bellies are dissected from within the skin and mucosal envelope. The skin dissection is more extensive and may extend as far as the nasolabial fold to obtain a smooth contour. However, a less extensive dissection is needed on the

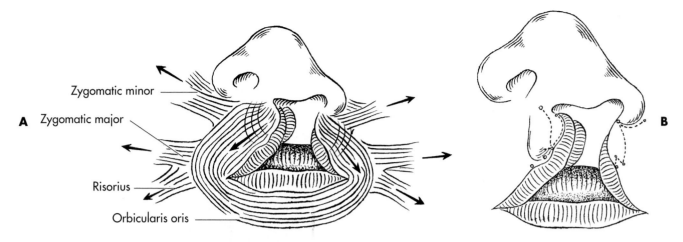

Figure 52-5. **A,** The unopposed pull of the discontinuous fibers of the orbicularis oris muscle pulls the philtral column into a convex curve away from the midline. Laterally, the muscle does the same to the skin of the lateral lip element. **B,** The skin incisions should parallel these curves so that in the scars will mimic the normal anatomy after repair.

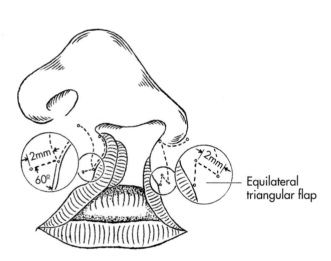

Figure 52-6. A small equilateral triangular flap is introduced into the lateral lip incision at the vermilion-cutaneous junction. It is the width of the vermilion-cutaneous roll (approximately 2 mm) and is inserted into a back-cut in the medial lip. Its purpose is to (l) restore continuity of the vermilion-cutaneous roll, (2) restore the normal profile of the lip, and (3) gain extra length if needed.

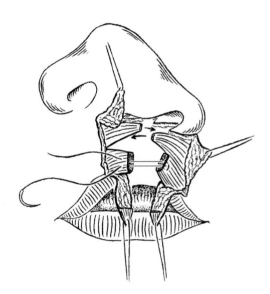

Figure 52-7. The muscle is exposed and divided into an upper triangular and lower rectangular flap. If sufficient muscle is available deep to the alar base and columella, additional slips can be developed in these regions.

mucosal surface and should be limited to the most superior aspect of the flap—that closest to the labial sulcus. This is done to reduce the risk of postoperative "draping" of the vermilion edge, as is often seen in lacerations of the mucosa of the lip. The muscle dissection is carried up into the floor of the nose on the medial and lateral side because these uppermost fibers can be used to improve the contour of the nasal floor and to help reposition the columella and alar base.

The triangle-shaped muscle is then split in the direction of its fibers at two or three sites, depending on the quantity of muscle and how far into the nasal floor it extends (Figures 52-7

and 52-8, *B*). This creates triangle-shaped slips at the level of nostril sill and in the more superior part of the lip. The inferior of the two incisions on the medial side ends deep to the philtral dimple, and on the lateral side it ends opposite this point. The tips of the most inferior of the triangles are resected to create rectangular flaps. Muscle above the level of the nostril sill and columellar crease, if present, forms additional muscle flaps that are useful in reconstruction of the nasal floor. The flaps are then interdigitated and approximated, as shown in the diagram. This configuration of the muscle fibers seems to reorient the majority of the fibers in the right direction and has been helpful in restoring a more normal motion to the reconstructed lip.

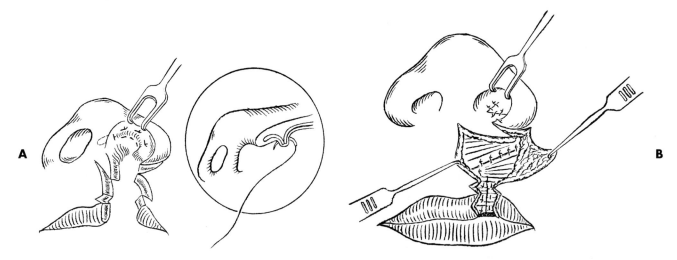

Figure 52-8.   A, After wide undermining of the nasal tip skin, polyglycolic acid sutures secure the overlapped upper and lower lateral cartilages along the nasal valve and across the medial crura. **B,** The completed nasal floor closure with V-Y advancement flaps and an alar base flap to rotate and advance the alar base. The muscle flaps help secure the position of the alar base and reinforce the philtral dimple while reorienting the muscle fibers.

The Cleft Lip Nose

I concur with the philosophy that primary nasal repair is beneficial and long lasting and does not interfere with the growth and development of the nose. McComb,[35] Anderl,[2] Salyer,[55] and others have emphasized the importance of separating the deformed lower lateral or alar cartilage from the overlying skin envelope, repositioning it, and allowing the skin to redrape over the newly positioned cartilage. They use sutures over external bolsters to maintain the position during the early healing phase. All of these authors have shown long-term benefit from this approach. I have incorporated these principles in a 5-step approach to the primary repair of the cleft lip nasal deformity[27] (see Figure 52-8).

1. Wide undermining of the external skin envelope on the normal and cleft side to release the medial and lateral crura of the alar cartilages
2. Intranasal polyglycolic acid sutures along the internal nasal valve and across the middle crura to overlap the upper and lower lateral cartilages and to adjust the domal height
3. Repair of the nasal floor with V-Y advancement flaps
4. Repositioning of the alar base with a V-Y alar base flap
5. Muscle repair of the paranasal muscles to help restore and maintain the position of the columella and alar base

The Alveolar Cleft

Restoration of the bony continuity of the cleft alveolus has obvious benefits:

1. Provides a bony matrix for the eruption of teeth bordering the cleft alveolus
2. Provides for the long-term maintenance of teeth bordering the cleft
3. Stabilizes the maxillary segments

4. Promotes oral hygiene by closure of fistulas and pits in the cleft area
5. Reduces the need for fixed dental appliances
6. Improves periodontal health of the teeth bordering the cleft[1]

We began bone grafting using iliac crest marrow and rib in 1974 following the principles elucidated by Boyne et al.[4] Cranial bone was introduced as a donor source for grafting the craniofacial skeleton with the emergence of craniofacial surgery. Wolfe et al[64] advocated its use in grafting of the cleft alveolus because it was easily harvested, left a well-hidden and relatively painless donor site, was bonelike, and resulted in graft take comparable with other bone graft donor sources. We embraced this approach and initially found it to be comparable with iliac bone in its rate of successful graft take. However, with time it appeared that the quality of bone graft take was not as good as with iliac crest marrow. In an evaluation of the long-term results, we noted a statistically significant superiority of iliac crest bone in the quantity and quality of bone at the grafted site.[26,64] This was particularly evident in more severe complete clefts of the lip and palate. We attributed this to the larger particle size and greater volume of spongy, cancellous bone in the iliac crest graft material. This promotes early revascularization of the cancellous matrix, survival of donor osteocytes, preservation of the donor architecture, and hence a greater volume of surviving bone graft. Wolfe[64] has pointed out that the small volume of cancellous bone in cranial grafts can be increased by using Aesculap Power Shovel (Aesculap, Tuttlingen, Germany). We feel that this diminishes the value of using the cranial site and would prefer to use the iliac site, where the graft material is virtually pure cancellous bone. We still, however, use cranial bone harvested from burr holes using a hand-held Hudson brace

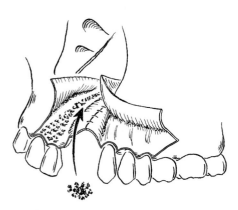

Figure 52-9. Superiorly based mucoperiosteal flaps are elevated from the buccal plate of the maxilla and into the cleft space. The oral and nasal mucosae are closed. Iliac or cranial bone is introduced into the cleft cavity.

for grafting of smaller defects of the alveolus in patients with clefts of the lip and alveolus only because the cranial donor site is less painful and recovery is more rapid. We use the hand-held device because Sadove[54] has shown that there is more graft loss when the bone is harvested using a power-driven bit. The scalp incision is made transversely in the parietal scalp because it is more easily camouflaged by the hair.

If the maxillary arches are malaligned, orthopedic repositioning is an essential part of the management. Their position is maintained with a heavy arch wire, fixed appliance, or night guard type of splint until the bone graft take is complete. Radiographs are taken 3 months after grafting to assess the quality of bone graft take. If grafting has been successful, orthodontic manipulation of teeth can be undertaken whenever it is believed to be appropriate by the orthodontist.

Most agree that bone grafting during the eruption of the mixed dentition is not detrimental to facial growth. Likewise, it is accepted by most that grafting should be done before the eruption of the canine teeth. Vig et al[63] have pointed out that the postgraft bone height is dependent on the pregraft level of the bone at the interdental septum on the teeth bordering the cleft. This position is fixed after eruption and cannot be elevated by simply placing graft material against the tooth surface above this point. The grafted bone will resorb back to this level. Furthermore, the erupting tooth brings bone with it into the site, augmenting the bone that survives the grafting procedure. This may help explain why alveolar cleft grafting has been found by most authors to be less successful when done at a later age. For these same reasons, I prefer to graft earlier, about the time of the eruption of the lateral incisor teeth bordering the cleft. Mayro et al[34] have emphasized that dental age rather than chronologic age should be used as a guide to grafting. The surgeon should rely on the orthodontist's recommendations regarding timing (Figure 52-9).

Revisional Surgery

The timing of revisional surgery is influenced by several variables:

1. The severity of the defect
2. The potential adverse effects on normal growth and development of the affected part
3. The psychosocial milieu
4. The possibility of avoiding an independent operative intervention and anesthetic by coupling the revision with another planned procedure

Several important events punctuate the child's (and parents') life during development from infancy through childhood and adolescence: the entrance into school, the evolution of self-image in later childhood transitions from one school to another, the onset of puberty, and transition into young adulthood. An appreciation of the psychosocial milieu during these periods is important to the timing of revisional surgery. For the early years, time is our ally because children do not have a well-established sense of self until after age 7. Many children seem to become most sensitive to appearance issues at about age 8 to 9. Surgical revisions of minor lip deformities can often be coupled with elective procedures, such as myringotomies and tube placement, often before a child enters regular school for both the parents' and child's sake. Moderate to severe distortions of the nasal tip can be treated at the time of bone grafting, which in my clinic is between 6½ years and 7½ years of age, coinciding nicely with the acquisition of self-image. Milder degrees of nasal deformity can be corrected, if necessary, either when the child expresses concern or when complete nasal growth has been achieved.

Minor degrees of unevenness of the vermilion-free border can be corrected with elliptical excisions of full-thickness vermilion down to underlying orbicularis. The excision is done in the moist mucosa to hide the scar. The parents should be counseled that the postoperative edema is slow to resolve in this area.

Irregularities of the vermilion-cutaneous border can be corrected by realignment, small triangular flaps, or Z-plasties, depending on the defect.

Correction of the cleft lip nasal deformity once again requires a careful analysis of the features of the deformity. Patients may have all or varying degrees of the following deviations:

1. Depression and slumping of the nasal dome on the cleft side
2. Deviation of the septum to the normal side
3. Lateral and possible superior or inferior displacement of the alar base
4. An intranasal web that is the caudal margin of the lateral crus of the alar cartilage that is shortened and tethered to the nasal floor
5. Shortage of vestibular lining
6. Bony asymmetries

Some of these features may be so minimal as to not require correction, whereas others will constitute the main focus of the revisional surgery.

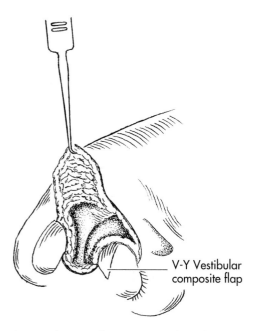

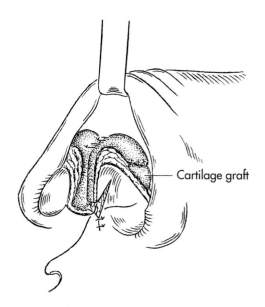

Figure 52-10. Incisions for an open tip rhinoplasty at the waist of the columella and bordering the caudal margin of the lower lateral cartilage. A composite V-Y advancement flap for elevating the nasal dome.[31] A V-Y of the lateral crus can be used, as well.[42]

Figure 52-11. The repositioned alar cartilages are secured with clear permanent sutures. A cartilage graft may be needed to replace deficient cartilage of the lateral crus.

I prefer an open-tip approach with the incision at the waist of the columella for correction of nasal tip deformities. It permits complete visualization of the anatomy of both alar cartilages, as well as access to the caudal septum, which frequently requires shifting back into the midline from its displaced position on the side opposite the cleft (Figures 52-10 and 52-11). The depressed dome on the cleft side can be released and repositioned into parity with the normal side. Permanent sutures of clear nylon or polypropylene are used to prevent relapse. A composite flap of medial or lateral crus and vestibular lining as described by Lewis[31] and Ortiz-Monasterio[43] can be used to make up for a shortage of lining should this be the case. Because of the posterior displacement of the maxillary platform, the lateral crus is tethered, and when released, there is frequently a shortage of cartilage. A cartilage graft is often needed to correct for this deficiency and to provide support for the internal valve. The cephalad portion of the lower lateral cartilage is a good donor source because this cartilage is readily available and may be discarded during a rhinoplasty. Onlay grafts can added under direct vision if needed. When necessary, the alar base can be moved medially with a V-Y advancement flap. A Z-plasty of the intranasal web is sometimes needed, as well. The surgeon can call on a variety of techniques used in primary and secondary rhinoplasty to correct the cleft lip nasal deformity. Achieving perfect symmetry is usually impossible, and patients and parents must be given a realistic appraisal of what might be possible.

Economic Issues in Treatment

The treatment of a cleft lip can extend over many years, involving several hospital encounters and more than one specialist. In the current milieu of cost containment and cost cutting, practitioners must be cognizant of these issues and seek strategies to contain cost without sacrificing the quality of care or outcome. Hospital stays have dramatically shortened for both primary and secondary treatment of cleft lip–related problems, and there is a mounting body of evidence demonstrating that surgery can be performed safely. Canady et al[9] showed no increase in complications if patients were admitted the day of surgery for primary palatoplasty and cleft lip/palate revision. Similar results were found by Eaton, Marsh, and Pilgrim[14] in their study of two comparable patients' groups, one in which the vast majority were admitted the day before and in the other admitted the day of surgery. In addition to similar morbidity, overall stay was reduced by 2 days and the cost saving in hospital days was the equivalent of $138,000 (1991 dollars). Cleft lip surgery can sometimes be done on an outpatient basis. Additional efforts have been made to reduce the number of "routine preoperative tests" to those that are essential for the safe performance of surgery.

Thus primary and secondary cleft surgery can be safely performed, presents no disadvantage to patients, and results in measurable cost savings. Less easily measured and still unreported is the possible cost savings (or losses) to the parents in terms of work time lost in additional trips for preoperative testing and in providing home care that would have otherwise been provided in a hospital setting.

Our protocol includes same day admission for all cleft-related procedures in the absence of special medical need. Unless indicated by specific medical conditions or history, patients having surgery for the first time have a hemoglobin/hematocrit, prothrombin time, and partial thromboplastin time. All patients are allowed to feed immediately postopera-

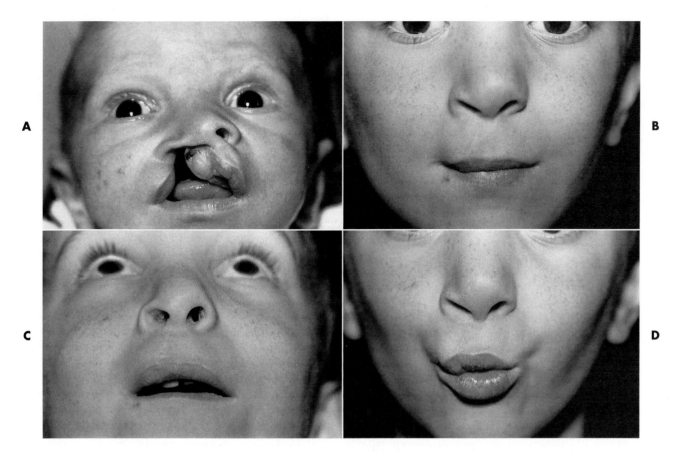

Figure 52-12. A patient example. **A,** Preoperative view with a complete cleft lip and palate. The philtrum has a rectangular configuration. **B,** Postoperative view after repair with a Mohler modification of a rotation-advancement technique. **C,** Worm's-eye view. **D,** With lips pursed.

tively. Infants are permitted to nurse or are bottle-fed after lip repair. Arm restraints are used routinely. All patients for cleft lip repair leave the following day, and some are discharged the day of operation if they are feeding well. Sutures are removed while infants are being bottle-fed to distract them 4 to 5 days postoperatively. Virtually all secondary procedures are done on a outpatient basis, except for alveolar bone grafting, which requires an overnight stay.

SUMMARY

The strides and advances in the evolution of cleft surgery have been dramatic and gratifying for the patients and their surgeons. Through a greater understanding of the normal and pathologic anatomy, innovative procedures are giving better, more predictable results through fewer surgeries. Care coordinated through multidisciplinary teams handling large patient volumes can be helpful in these endeavors. Challenges remain to be solved by future generations of surgeons in the achievement of normal lip motion and in the management of the cleft lip nasal deformity. The ultimate challenge is the prevention of the deformity through an understanding of the genetics of causation and appropriate intervention.

REFERENCES

1. Abyholm F, Bergland O, Semb G: Secondary bone grafting of alveolar clefts, *Scand J Plast Reconstr Surg* 15:127, 1981.

2. Anderl H: Simultaneous repair of lip and nose in the unilateral cleft (a long term report). In Jackson IT, Sommerland B, editors: *Recent advances in plastic surgery,* Edinburgh, 1985, Churchill Livingstone.

3. Blair VP, Brown JB: Mirault operation for single harelip, *Surg Gynecol Obstet* 51:81, 1930.

4. Boyne PT, Sands NR: Secondary bone grafting of residual alveolar and palatal clefts, *J Oral Surg* 30:87, 1972.

5. Brauer RO, Cronin TD: The Tennison lip repair revisited, *Plast Reconstr Surg* 71:633, 1983.

6. Brown JB, McDowell F: Surgical repair of cleft lips, *Arch Surg* 56:750, 1948.

7. Burdi AR: Section I. Epidemiology, etiology, and pathogenesis of cleft lip and palate, *Cleft Palate J* 14:469, 1971.

8. Burston WR: The early orthodontic treatment of cleft palate conditions, *Dental Practice (Bristol)* 9:41, 1958.

9. Canady JW, Glowacki R, Thompson SA, et al: Complication outcomes based on preoperative admission and length of stay for primary palatoplasty and cleft lip/palate revision in children aged 1 to 6 years, *Ann Plast Surg* 33:576-580, 1994.

10. Cardoso AD: A new technique for harelip, *Plast Reconstr Surg* 10:92, 1952.

11. Carolus J/MF: La Chirurgie de Maitre Jean Yperman, *F. and E. Gyselynck*, 1894, Gand.

12. Dado DO, Kernahan DA: Anatomy of the orbicularis oris muscle in incomplete cleft lip based on histological examination, *Ann Plast Surg* 15:90, 1985.

13. DeMey A, et al: Anatomy of the orbicularis oris muscle in cleft lip, *Br J Plast Surg* 42:710, 1989.

14. Eaton AC, Marsh JL, Pilgrim TK: Does reduced hospital stay affect morbidity and mortality rates following cleft lip and palate repair in infancy? *Plast Reconstr Surg* 94:911-915, 1994.

15. Fara M: The importance of folding down muscle stumps in the operation of unilateral clefts of the lip, *Acta Chir Plast* 13:162, 1971.

16. Fogh-Anderson P: *Inheritance of harelip and cleft palate,* Copenhagen, 1943, Ejuar Munksgaard Forlag.

17. Fraser GR, Calnan JS: Cleft lip and palate: seasonal incidence, birth weight, birth rank, sex, site, etc., *Arch Dis Child* 36:420, 1961.

18. Georgiade NG, Latham RA: Maxillary arch alignment in the bilateral cleft lip and palate infant, using the pinned coaxial screw appliance, *Plast Reconstr Surg* 56:52, 1975.

19. Habib Z: Factors determining occurrence of cleft lip and cleft palate, *Surg Gynecol Obstet* 146:105, 1978.

20. Habib Z: Genetic counselling and genetics of cleft lip and cleft palate, *Obstet Gynecol Surv* 33:441, 1978.

21. Hagedorn WH: A modification of the harelip operation, *Centralbl f Chirurgie* 11:756, 1884.

22. Hotz MM, Goinski WM: Effects of early maxillary orthopedics in coordination with delayed surgery for cleft lip and palate, *J Maxillofac Surg* 7:210, 1979.

23. Ivy RB: Modern concept of cleft lip and cleft palate management, *Plast Reconstr Surg* 9:121, 1952.

24. Johanson B: Secondary osteoplastic completion of maxilla and palate. In Schuchardt K, editor: Treatment of patients with clefts of the lip, alveolus and palate. Topic 10, *Second Hamburg International Symposium, 1964,* Stuttgart, 1966, Georg Theime Verlag.

25. Johanson B, Ohlsson A, Friede H, et al: A follow-up study of cleft lip and palate patients treated with orthodontics, secondary bone grafting and prosthetic rehabilitation, *Scand J Plast Reconstr Surg* 8:21, 1974.

26. LaRossa D, Buchman S, Rothkopf DM, et al: A comparison of iliac and cranial bone in secondary grafting of alveolar clefts, *Plast Reconstr Surg* 96:4, 789-797, 1995.

27. LaRossa D, Donath G: Primary nasoplasty in unilateral and bilateral cleft lip nasal deformity, *Clin Plast Surg* 20,4:781, 1993.

28. Latham RA: Orthodontic advancement of the cleft maxillary segment, *Cleft Palate J* 17:227, 1960.

29. Latham RA, Deaton TG: The structural basis of the philtrum and the contour of the vermilion border: a study of the musculature of the upper lip, *J Anat* 121:151, 1976.

30. LeMesurier AB: A method of cutting and suturing the lip in the treatment of complete unilateral clefts. *Plast Reconstr Surg* 4:1, 1949.

31. Lewis M: Personal communication.

32. Malgaigne JF: Du Bec-de-Lievre, *Journal De Chirurgie de Paris* 2:1-6, 1844.

33. Marcks KM, Travaskis AE, daCosta A: Further observations in cleft lip repair, *Plast Reconstr Surg* 12:392, 1953.

34. Mayro R, Minugh-Purvis, Malone P, et al: *Optimal age for secondary bone-grafting procedures: revisited.* Paper presented at the annual meeting of the American Cleft Palate-Craniofacial Association, San Diego, 1996.

35. McComb H: Primary correction of unilateral cleft lip nasal deformity. A 10-year review. *Plast Reconstr Surg* 75:791, 1985.

36. McNeil CK: *Oral and facial deformity,* London, 1954, Pitman.

37. Millard DR: A primary camouflage of the unilateral harelip. In *Transactions of the International Society of Plastic Surgeons, First Congress, 1955,* Baltimore, 1957, Williams & Wilkins.

38. Mirault G.: Lettre Sur L'Operation Du Bec-de-Lievre, *Journal de Chirurgie,* Par M. Malgaine, 2:257-265, 1884.

39. Mohler L: Unilateral cleft lip repair, *Plast Reconstr Surg* 80:511, 1987.

40. Mulliken JB, Pensler JM, Kozakewich HP: The anatomy of Cupid's bow in normal and cleft lip, *Plast Reconstr Surg* 92:395-403, 1993.

41. Nicolau JP: The orbicularis muscle: a functional approach to its repair in the cleft lip, *Br J Plast Surg* 36:141, 1983.

42. Noordhoff MS: Reconstruction of vermilion in unilateral and bilateral cleft lips, *Plast Reconstr Surg* 73:52, 1984.

43. Ortiz-Monasterio F: Personal communication.

44. Paré A: *Les Oeuvres de M. Ambroise Pare,* Paris, 1575, G. Buon.

45. Park CG, Ha B: The importance of accurate repair of the orbicularis oris muscle in the correction of unilateral cleft lip, *Plast Reconstr Surg* 96:780-788, 1995.

46. Pool R, Farnsworth TK: Preoperative lip taping in the cleft lip, *Ann Plast Surg* 32:3, 243, 1994.

47. Randall P: A lip adhesion operation in cleft lip surgery, *Plast Reconstr Surg* 38:444, 1965.

48. Randall P: A triangular flap operation for the primary repair of unilateral clefts of the lip, *Plast Reconstr Surg* 23:331, 1951.

49. Randall P, Whitaker LA, LaRossa D: The importance of muscle reconstruction in primary and secondary cleft lip repair, *Plast Reconstr Surg* 54:316, 1974.

50. Robertson NR, Jolleys A: An 11-year followup of the effects of early bone grafting in infants born with complete clefts of the lip and palate, *Br J Plast Surg* 36:438, 1983.

51. Rose W: *Harelip and cleft palate,* London, 1976, HK Lewis and Co.

52. Rosenstein SW, Monroe CW, Kernahan DA, et al: The case of early bone grafting in cleft lip and cleft palate, *Plast Reconstr Surg* 70:297, 1982.

53. Ross RB: Treatment variables affecting facial growth in unilateral cleft lip and palate. Part 2: presurgical orthopaedics, *Cleft Palate J* 24:24, 1987.

54. Sadove AM, Nelson CL, Eppley BL, et al: An evaluation of calvarial and iliac donor sites in alveolar bone grafting, *Cleft Palate J* 27:3, 225, 1990.

55. Salyer KF: Primary correction of the unilateral cleft lip nose: a 15-year experience, *Plast Reconstr Surg* 77:558, 1986.

56. Schmid E: Die Aufbauende Kieferkammplastik, *Ost Z Stomat* 51, 1954.

57. Schuchardt K, Pfeifer G: Erfahrungen uber primare knochentransplantaionen bei Lippen-Keifer-Gaumenspalten, *Langenbecks Arch Klin Chir* 295:881, 1960.

58. Shaw WC, Williams AC, Sandy JR, et al: Minimum standards for the management of cleft lip and palate: efforts to close the audit loop, *Ann R Coll Surg Engl* 78:110-114, 1996.

59. Skoog T: The cleft lip. In *Plastic surgery,* Stockholm, 1974, Almqvist & Wicksell International.

60. Tennison CW: The repair of the unilateral cleft lip by the Stencil Method, *Plast Reconstr Surg* 9:115, 1952.

61. Thompson JE: An artistic and mathematically accurate method of repairing the defect in cases of harelip, *Surg Gynecol Obstet* 14:498, 1912.

62. Trauner M: Results of cleft lip operations, *Plast Reconstr Surg* 40:209, 1967.

63. Vig KWL: Personal communication.

64. Wolfe SA, Berkowitz S: The use of cranial bone grafts in the closure of alveolar and anterior palatal clefts, *Plast Reconstr Surg* 72:5,659, 1983.

65. Wong KC, Wu LT: *History of Chinese medicine,* Tientsin, China, 1932, Tientsin Press.

66. Wynn AK: Lateral flap cleft lip surgery technique, *Plast Reconstr Surg* 25:509, 1960.

CHAPTER

Bilateral Cleft Lip

Ghada Y. Afifi
Robert A. Hardesty

INTRODUCTION

Despite the advancements in surgical technique and overall comprehension regarding bilateral cleft lip patients, the repair of this congenital anomaly remains one of the most challenging hurdles in the field of cleft surgery today. This probably accounts for the myriad of surgical approaches presented in the literature during the past 50 years. In 1947, John Barrett Brown asserted that "surgical repair of double cleft lips is about twice as difficult as in single clefts and the results about half as good."[7] He remarked that it presented a three-dimensional problem for a two-dimensional mind, referring to the associated nasal and maxillary distortions. Almost 40 years later, Mulliken further asserted that the bilateral deformity in fact presented a *four*-dimensional dilemma for a three-dimensional mind, alluding to the temporal variations exhibited with growth and tissue remodeling.[33]

The difficulties encountered in a bilateral cleft lip patient reflect the active and passive components of the anatomic distortion, which may be incomplete or complete with respect to its involvement from the nasolabial plane, through the alveolar process, and potentially involving the entire palate. Exhibiting a spectrum of presentations, the complete form presents two lateral components of lip-alveolar-palatal segments with an intervening segment composed of prolabium and premaxilla that varies in its degree of protrusion (Figure 53-1). The discrepancy of both bony and soft tissue elements, with resulting passive and active anatomic distortions, presents a reconstructive challenge even with today's advanced surgical comprehension.

The issues presented include (1) analysis and timing of repair; (2) single or staged reconstruction; (3) surgical techniques used; (4) nasal deformity management, including timing of columellar lengthening; (5) management of the premaxillary segment; and (6) the role of dentofacial orthopedic appliances. All have ramifications for surgical outcome, with subsequent impact on speech, orthodontia, facial expression, and, perhaps most importantly, the patient's own self-perception and social growth.

INDICATIONS

All patients with a cleft lip deformity should be evaluated for repair, whether the deformity is complete or incomplete. The repair goals include restoring functional and anatomic defects of the orbicularis oris muscle, nasal deformity, and palatal soft tissue and bony components. Optimally, the ultimate result would be to enable symmetric growth and development of the maxillary segments and hence midface and, not less importantly, normalize dentition and speech.

APPROACH

Analysis of Defect
The bilateral cleft lip may be either complete or incomplete. The complete cleft lip involves the entire upper lip, with the cleft transversing the alar base and potentially involving the primary and secondary palates.

Bilateral incomplete cleft lips may be repaired in one stage. If complete on one side and incomplete on another, the defect may be repaired in two stages, that is, with an interval lip adhesion on the complete side if the lip components are deemed too far apart for a one-stage definitive repair. Bilaterally complete cleft lips are performed either in one definitive stage or in two stages with a preceding bilateral lip adhesion before definitive reconstruction.

The other anatomic components of a bilateral cleft lip include (see Figure 53-1):
1. Widened alar bases, with laterally flared internal nasal valves
2. Appearance of a shortened columella, with malpositioned alar cartilages
3. Excessively obtuse nasolabial angle (versus normal range 90 to 120 degrees)
4. Hypoplastic prolabial lip segment
5. Vertically short upper lip, particularly centrally at prolabium
6. Premaxillary alveolar segment with variable degree of protrusion

769

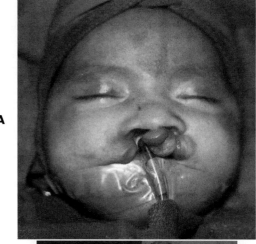

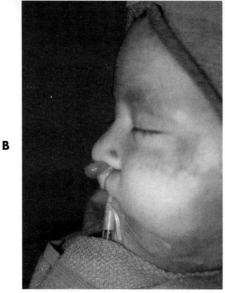

Figure 53-1. Child with complete bilateral cleft lip and palate: frontal view **(A)** and side view **(B)**.

7. Absence of normal labial-gingival sulcus in prolabial-premaxillary segment
8. Absence of orbicularis oris musculature in prolabial segment
9. Absence of a central philtral dimple, defined philtral columns, or philtral tubercle
10. Absence of Cupid's bow
11. Absence of white roll in prolabial lip segment
12. Aberrant insertion of lateral lip orbicularis oris musculature into alar-facial bases
13. Aberrant dry and moist vermilion on prolabial segment
14. Potential involvement of the primary and/or secondary palate
15. Potential presence of other craniofacial or noncraniofacial congenital anomalies

Classification of Defect

It is important to accurately analyze and report a cleft lip and/or palate deformity in a standardized manner. This would enable optimal analysis and perioperative planning, as well as improving multicenter reporting and analysis retrospectively and prospectively. Originally published in 1962, a classification system was presented by the Nomenclature Committee of the American Association for Cleft Palate Rehabilitation, which was later accepted by the Cleft Palate Association.[19]

However, because of its complexity, it was not uniformly used. In 1971, Kernahan[22] then introduced a simpler classification scheme that may be reported on a diagrammatic Y-shaped symbol, with the incisive foramen represented at the focal point (Figure 53-2). This was subsequently utilized by Millard, and other versions were later proposed. In 1993, Schwartz et al[42] proposed a modification of the Kernahan Y such that number 1 is assigned to the first limb positions 1-3, the number 2 assigned to left-sided positions 4-6, and the number 3 assigned to base positions 7-9. The modification was proposed to allow easier computerized entry for all anatomic cleft variants.

Epidemiology/Etiology

The incidence of bilateral cleft lip varies in different demographic groups. Racial heterogeneity has been demonstrated, with the mean incidence per 1000 live births being approximately 2.1 in Asians, 1 in Caucasians, and 0.41 in African-Americans.[9,15,34] Cleft lip defects are noted to occur in the ratio 6:3:1 for unilateral left, unilateral right, and bilateral locations, respectively.[49] Bilateral lip defects were associated with palate clefting in 86% of cases versus only 68% in unilateral cases.[18] Other epidemiologic factors noted are summarized in Box 53-1.

Although most patients have the deformity as a sporadic occurrence, with probable multifactorial components, subgroups of patients have the diagnosis as part of a malformation syndrome (Box 53-2), well elucidated by Jones[21] in 1993. Further chromosomal anomalies have been reported to be increased in this population, and the reader is referred to Jones' work for further details.

Environmental factors possibly involved in cleft lip pathogenesis include alcohol, anticonvulsants (e.g., phenytoin [Dilantin]), 13-*cis*-retinoic acid, tobacco, and folic acid/vitamin B_6 deficiency.

Given that a family has a cleft child, it is important to identify further risk in subsequent children, with Table 53-1 summarizing the accepted standard predisposition.

Timing of Repair

All patients diagnosed with a cleft lip or palate should be evaluated by a multidisciplinary cleft team. This enables assessment of the defect and its impact on feeding and development and evaluates for additional anomalies, either sporadic or syndromic, including cardiac anomalies. This helps improve overall health and perioperative care of the child. Counseling regarding future risks of genetic transmission for the family and child is also possible.

For those without contraindications delaying or prohibiting operative reconstruction, the age of repair varies between 8

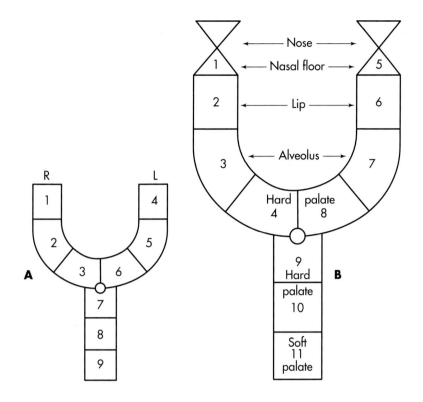

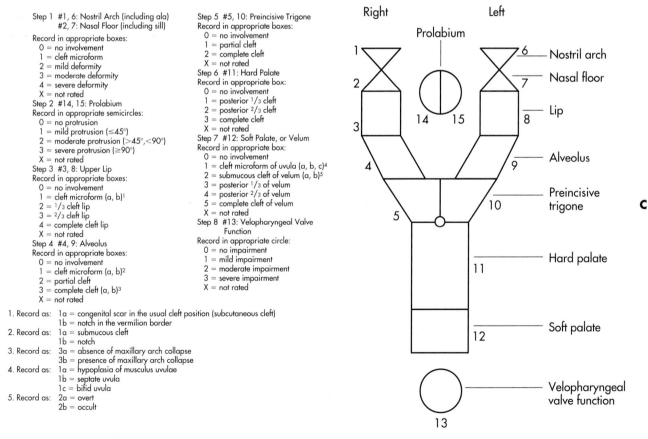

Coding Instructions

Step 1 #1, 6: Nostril Arch (including ala)
        #2, 7: Nasal Floor (including sill)
Record in appropriate boxes:
  0 = no involvement
  1 = cleft microform
  2 = mild deformity
  3 = moderate deformity
  4 = severe deformity
  X = not rated
Step 2 #14, 15: Prolabium
Record in appropriate semicircles:
  0 = no protrusion
  1 = mild protrusion ($\leq$45°)
  2 = moderate protrusion (>45°,<90°)
  3 = severe protrusion ($\geq$90°)
  X = not rated
Step 3 #3, 8: Upper Lip
Record in appropriate boxes:
  0 = no involvement
  1 = cleft microform (a, b)[1]
  2 = 1/3 cleft lip
  3 = 2/3 cleft lip
  4 = complete cleft lip
  X = not rated
Step 4 #4, 9: Alveolus
Record in appropriate boxes:
  0 = no involvement
  1 = cleft microform (a, b)[2]
  2 = partial cleft
  3 = complete cleft (a, b)[3]
  X = not rated

Step 5 #5, 10: Preincisive Trigone
Record in appropriate boxes:
  0 = no involvement
  1 = partial cleft
  2 = complete cleft
  X = not rated
Step 6 #11: Hard Palate
Record in appropriate box:
  0 = no involvement
  1 = posterior 1/3 cleft
  2 = posterior 2/3 cleft
  3 = complete cleft
  X = not rated
Step 7 #12: Soft Palate, or Velum
Record in appropriate box:
  0 = no involvement
  1 = cleft microform of uvula (a, b, c)[4]
  2 = submucous cleft of velum (a, b)[5]
  3 = posterior 1/3 of velum
  4 = posterior 2/3 of velum
  5 = complete cleft of velum
  X = not rated
Step 8 #13: Velopharyngeal Valve
        Function
Record in appropriate circle:
  0 = no impairment
  1 = mild impairment
  2 = moderate impairment
  3 = severe impairment
  X = not rated

1. Record as: 1a = congenital scar in the usual cleft position (subcutaneous cleft)
               1b = notch in the vermilion border
2. Record as: 1a = submucous cleft
               1b = notch
3. Record as: 3a = absence of maxillary arch collapse
               3b = presence of maxillary arch collapse
4. Record as: 1a = hypoplasia of musculus uvulae
               1b = septate uvula
               1c = bifid uvula
5. Record as: 2a = overt
               2b = occult

Figure 53-2. Symbolic representations of cleft lip and palate. **A,** Classic Kernahan "Y" (1971, 1973). **B,** Millard modification (1977). **C,** Schematic system of Friedman et al, proposed to be further inclusive. (**A** from Kernahan DA: *Plast Reconstr Surg* 47:469, 1971; **B** from Millard DR Jr: *Cleft craft,* vol 1, Boston, 1977, Little, Brown; **C** from Friedman HI, Sayetta RB, Coston GN, et al: *Cleft Palate Craniofac J* 28:252, 1991.)

Box 53-1.
Epidemiology of Cleft Lip Deformity

Race: Asian > Caucasian > Black
Left > right > bilateral lip involvement
Bilateral deformity: increased association with cleft palate
Increased with increased parental age
Seasonal variation: ? increase in January/February
Association with lower socioeconomic class: ? nutrition
Familial facies: parents may have maxillary underdevelopment
Associated congenital defects: club feet, CNS, cardiac, Pierre Robin syndrome, hemifacial microsomia, other

Box 53-2.
Associated Malformations

Down syndrome
Van der Woude's syndrome
Dysplasia-clefting syndrome
Opitz syndrome
Aarskog syndrome
Coffin-Siris syndrome
Distal arthrogryposis type 2
Fryns syndrome
Waardenburg's syndrome
Fetal alcohol syndrome
Maternal diabetes
CHARGE association
Craniofacial microsomia
Amnion rupture sequence

Modified from Jones MC: *Clin Plast Surg* 20:599, 1993.

Table 53-1.
Risk of Subsequent Child with Cleft Lip/Palate

FAMILY STATUS	PROBAND WITH CL ± CP (%)	PROBAND WITH CP (%)
General population frequency	0.1	0.04
PARENTS UNAFFECTED		
Child affected: risk that next child affected if:		
No affected relatives	4	2
Affected relative	4	7
Affected child with another malformation	2	2
Parents are related	4	—
Affected child has unilateral CL/P	4.2	—
Affected child has bilateral CL/P	5.7	—
Child affected: risk that next child has different type of malformation:	Same as general population risk	
Two affected children: risk that third child affected:	9	1
ONE PARENT AFFECTED		
No affected children: risk affected child	4	6
Child affected: risk next child affected	17	15

Modified from Fraser FC: Etiology of Cleft Lip and Palate. In Grabb WC, Rosenstein SW, Bzoch KR (eds): *Cleft lip and palate: surgical, dental, and speech aspects*, Boston, 1971, Little, Brown; and Habib Z: *Surg Gynecol Obstet* 146:105, 1978.

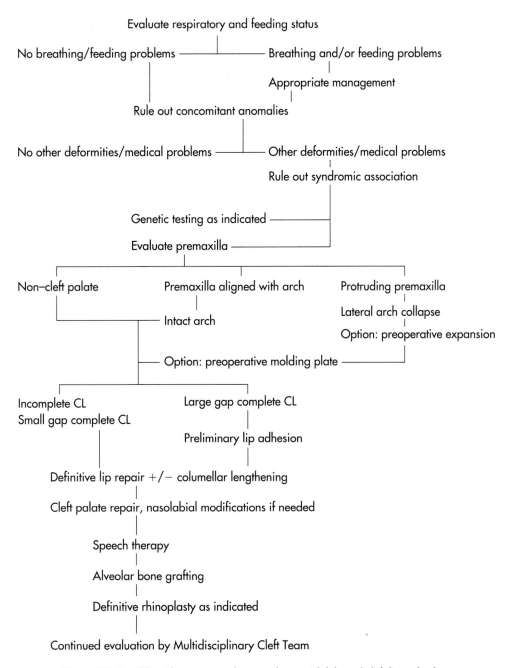

Figure 53-3. Algorithmic approach to newborn with bilateral cleft lip and palate.

weeks to 6 months at most centers. An algorithm for the evaluation of the newborn with bilateral cleft lip is presented in Figure 53-3, modified from Marsh's earlier rendition.[26]

At our institution, unless contraindicated, the general scheme is as follows (Table 53-2):

1. At 6 weeks to 3 months of age: lip adhesion, molding plate ± dental impression if indicated (e.g., wide gaps), passive or active molding appliance per defect

2. At 6 months of age: definitive lip repair
3. At 9 to 12 months of age: cleft palate repair if indicated
4. At 4 to 5 years of age (before school initiated): columellar lengthening
5. At 7 to 12 years of age: alveolar bone grafting if applicable
6. Early teenage years (sooner as needed per defect and patient): rhinoplasty

Table 53-2.
General Scheme for Cleft Lip and Palate Patients—Loma Linda University Protocol

	CLEFT TYPE			
	ISOLATED PRIMARY CLEFT		PRIMARY AND SECONDARY PALATE CLEFT	ISOLATED SECONDARY CLEFT
	MICROFORM INCOMPLETE LIP	COMPLETE LIP PRIMARY PALATE		
Age				
Birth	Complete multidisciplinary craniofacial team evaluation ⟶			
6 weeks		Lip adhesion	Lip adhesion, passive molding plates	
3 months	Lip repair			
6 months		Lip repair	Lip repair, dental impressions	
1 year			Palate repair ⟶	
			Dental impressions	
	Complete multidisciplinary craniofacial team evaluation ⟶			
2 years	Yearly multidisciplinary craniofacial team evaluation ⟶			
3 years			Yearly evaluation of velopharyngeal function and as needed Secondary management of velopharyngeal incompetence	
5-7 years	← Alveolar bone grafting to primary cleft →			
13-18 years	← Rhinoplasty +/- orthognathic surgery as needed →			

OPERATIONS

OVERALL MANAGEMENT ISSUES AND PRINCIPLES

The ultimate goal for cleft lip reconstruction is to completely reconstruct the labial-maxillary and nasal subunits such that complete symmetry, proportion, and function are restored in as few surgical stages as possible. We concur with Mulliken's advocation of following appropriate surgical principles rather than overly emphasizing any one technique.[30] Thus our institution's goals include:

1. Creating symmetry of nasolabial units during definitive repair.
2. Regaining optimal function by restoring orbicularis oris muscle continuity.
3. Avoiding skin tension during the final repair. Thus we prefer a two-stage reconstruction for wide complete defects: the lip adhesion reapproximates the labial segments while avoiding disruption of future important anatomic landmarks for the final repair. Subsequent repair is then performed tension free, minimizing tissue migration and scar widening.
4. Recreating important physical features of the upper lip, including Cupid's bow with its white roll, appropriately sized prolabial dimensions, and median tubercle fullness.
5. Symmetrically aligning the nasal subunits, including alar bases; positioning them at even horizontal levels; and attempting to ensure symmetric alignment with Cupid's bow (establishing the same distance from alar bases to lip high points bilaterally).
6. Avoiding unnecessary dissection over the maxillary processes and maintaining all necessary mobilization in the supraperiosteal plane, thus optimizing future bony growth and potentially minimizing maxillary retrusion.
7. Obtaining the absolutely best surgical result possible in minimal number of procedures. We concur that revisionary procedures usually do not obtain the best results because of less malleable, scarred tissue planes. Thus all landmarks are precisely measured intraoperatively to objectify symmetry and proportion.

BILATERAL SYNCHRONOUS VERSUS UNILATERAL ASYNCHRONOUS REPAIR

The current standard is to perform the reconstruction on both sides in a synchronous manner. This has evolved from earlier practices of repairing one side of a bilateral cleft lip at a time. The exception to this is a patient with a wide complete cleft defect on one side and an incomplete defect of the contralateral lip segment; we prefer to perform an initial adhesion procedure for the wide complete cleft lip anomaly, followed by a synchronous bilateral definite procedure to obtain symmetry without tension on the repair.

ONE-STAGE VERSUS TWO-STAGE REPAIR: ROLE OF LIP ADHESION

As previously alluded, our threshold is low for reconstructing complete cleft lips in two surgical stages if the lip segment gap is deemed too wide to repair the cleft without tension. A lip adhesion is done at 6 weeks to 3 months, with subsequent final repair 3 months later. Despite others' advocation for this approach for similar reasons, an objective algorithm to aid in this one-stage versus two-stage approach has never been fully elucidated. The decision ultimately rests on the surgeon's judgment, experience, and training. We assess "rather wide" distances between the prolabial and lateral lip segments as those greater than 1 cm, for whom we consider a preliminary adhesion.

MANAGEMENT OF PROLABIAL LIP SEGMENT

The prolabial segment is embryologically derived from the lip origins with histologic examinations demonstrating adnexal appendages and submucosa similar to the lateral lip.[25] Despite earlier use for columellar reconstruction, its current standard use is for midline vertical lip formation as originally advocated by Veau,[47] Cronin,[10] and others. Earlier use of medial approximation of lateral lip segment flaps, resulting in excessive vertical lip length, was abandoned. The prolabial segment not only provides the necessary dimensions of the central upper lip segment but also allows surgical scars to fall along respected natural anatomic lines: the philtral columns. It also expands vertically and horizontally as a result of traction from the attached lateral lip segments.

In complete bilateral cleft lips, the absence of orbicularis muscle in the prolabial lip segment necessitates bilateral muscle apposition. Authors differ in their use of edge-to-edge versus interlocking muscle flaps to restore orbicularis muscle continuity. First introduced by Schultz[41] in 1946, the latter concept was reintroduced and advocated by Randall.[38] Mohler[29] noted that philtral shape differed in individuals, proposing three main shapes: shieldlike, low shieldlike, and rectangular. To avoid the often widened prolabial segment later demonstrated in earlier techniques, Mulliken[30] advocated narrowing the prolabial flap to 2 mm rather than the previously advocated 6 to 8 mm to create a more natural resulting philtral contour.

There are different surgical options proposed on the surgical management of the prolabial segment that are further elaborated in the Operations section. Most surgeons find that a much bigger dilemma arises in the management of the protruding premaxilla often associated with a bilateral cleft lip deformity.

MANAGEMENT OF PREMAXILLARY SEGMENT

Evaluation of Premaxilla

Embryologically, cleft lip and palate results from failure of mesenchymal fusion between the nasofrontal and lateral facial components of the fetus at 4 to 7 weeks gestation.[44] The spectrum of clefting varies from the subtle philtral marking of the *form fruste* to the complete bilateral clefting of the palatal-alveolar-lip-nasal structures. The latter, involving the palate and lip, often results with an overly projecting premaxillary process. Atherton,[2] asserting that this protrusion is unique to the human model, attributed this to the normal absence of a premaxillary-maxillary growth suture with resulting normal restriction of premaxillary anterior growth. In affected patients, the cleft may act as the normally absent suture, resulting in abnormal forward projection. This results in a vertically long maxilla, absent anterior nasal spine, apparently short columella, and blunted nasal tip.

The evaluation of the premaxilla should include its relationship to overall facial skeletal growth; the overlying soft tissue, such as the prolabial-columellar and lateral lip segments; and the accompanying lateral alveolar bony segments. Most surgeons would concur that it is the *degree of anterior premaxillary protrusion* that presents the biggest challenge to a satisfactory reconstruction.

Control of Premaxillary Segment Protrusion

Management of premaxillary protrusion may be categorized as either nonoperative or operative. For the vast majority of cases requiring preoperative molding of an overly protruding premaxillary segment, *nonoperative* control is used. Such options have included: (1) a head cap and elastic band for traction, (2) preoperative taping of the premaxillary segment posteriorly, and (3) the use of intraoral acrylic plates.

Operative measures to correct premaxillary malalignment include: (1) orthodontic manipulation, such as via a controlled fixed-pin traction device, most notably of Georgiade or Latham; (2) preliminarily performed lip adhesion procedures to encourage alveolar segment alignment, or for unusual refractory cases; and (3) surgical setback of the premaxilla, a least favored option.

Generally, bilateral cleft lips with intersegmental gaps deemed wide (which may be arbitrarily defined as greater than 1 cm or deemed such per surgeon's judgment) often accompany the malpositioned premaxilla so that both anomalies are corrected in concert.

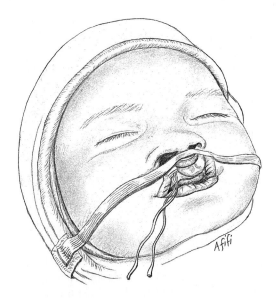

Figure 53-4. Elastic traction of protruding premaxilla with position adjusted by moving band in relation to head cap. Note palatal obturator with attached safety string.

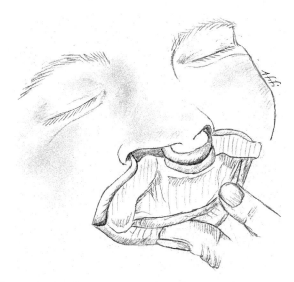

Figure 53-5. Preoperative orthopedic manipulation: creating alginate impression.

The decision regarding which treatment option is used is dependent on multiple factors, including degree of protrusion and alveolar arch malalignment; patient age; availability of orthodontic treatment, particularly in this of managed care with accompanying option restriction; and the training and experience of the multidisciplinary cleft team, particularly the plastic surgeon and/or orthodontist.

PREOPERATIVE TAPING. Pool[36] began to uniformly utilize preoperative taping across complete unilateral cleft lips after dehiscence of lip adhesions resulted from very wide clefts. He noted that the soft tissue and bony mobilization was so effective that he no longer performed lip adhesions. The alveolar remodeling narrowed average gaps of 12.4 mm to 5.8 mm in a 6-week interval, although the exact number of patients followed was uncited and the experience with bilateral cleft lip patients unknown. Our institution uses this technique soon after birth for all complete unilateral and bilateral cleft lip patients. With growth, for those still exhibiting wide lip segment gaps, an adhesion procedure is performed.

ELASTIC TRACTION VIA HEAD CAP. Alternatively, others use elastic traction via attachment to a head cap (Figure 53-4), a method first utilized in the sixteenth century.[14] The goal would be to reverse premaxillary protrusion while allowing maxillary segment growth. However, lateral pressure from the elastic may prevent the lateral segments' outward expansion, a phenomenon that may be avoided via a concomitant intraoral acrylic splint and intraoral screw plate.[39]

Results are usually obtained in several weeks to a few months. Major disadvantages of both above presented nonsurgical methods include variable times eliciting such effects and requirement of conscientious cooperation by the parents of the patient.

PREOPERATIVE ORTHOPEDIC MANIPULATION. In occasional cases of lateral maxillary segment collapse, preoperative prosthetic expansion is used (Figure 53-5). The goal is to obtain uniform alignment of the lateral maxillary and premaxillary segments before a single-stage cleft palate repair.

Known as the original proponents of this preoperative modality, Georgiade and Latham[17] utilized a pinned coaxial system to enable external traction, with subsequent advocation by Georgiade[16] of pinned intraoral devices to allow controlled premaxillary retraction and lateral maxillary expansion. Rutrick[40] recently asserted that this regimen enabled his institution to perform a single-stage lip repair and precluded medial collapse of the maxilla, although his study only involved unilateral cases.

Although our own institution utilizes preoperative alveolar molding for rare exceptions in which the premaxillary-lateral alveolar arch malalignment precludes *any* successful lip apposition, we have noted that a preliminary lip adhesion was extremely successful not only to allow the same purpose of alignment but also to ultimately allow optimal definitive repair in a *consistent* manner for wide cleft lips.

PRELIMINARY LIP ADHESION. We concur with Randall[37] and others in their recent readvocation of the lip adhesion procedure as the primary modality for those patients with very wide clefts prohibiting a facile and tension-free primary repair. The exact definition of "small" versus "large" distances between the lip segments has been disputed by different surgeons and institutions. At our institution, those complete cleft lip patients with interlip gaps of at least 1 cm undergo preoperative taping as demonstrated to the parents. At 6 weeks to 3 months of age, if the gaps are still deemed wide, a lip adhesion is performed. Incomplete cleft lips are repaired at the same time of definitive repair, which is done at 6 months of age. Alternatively, for excessively wide bilateral complete cleft lips, sequential lip adhesions may be performed one side at a time, although we have rarely encountered this need.

Certainly, this approach may also be used for those failing nonoperative premaxillary segment management. Additionally, as with other large craniofacial centers, our institution evaluates patients from a large referral base. Patient age at presentation and degree of parental compliance with instructions is not uniform: sole use of preoperative taping may be inadequate and has reinforced our more consistent results with the lip adhesion for wide clefts. Occasionally, custom-designed intraoral obturators to guide segmental remodeling during this surgical extraoral traction are used for select cases.

The following describes our method of performing a lip adhesion, which differs from that classically delineated by Randall, which apposes small labial-mucosal flaps from the cleft sides. We fully mobilize the soft tissue tethering of the labial-cheek soft tissue via a supraperiosteal plane, create the labial gingival sulcus, and inset a vermilion-mucosal flap into an intercartilaginous incision at the internal nasal valve. The method described is identical for each side of the complete cleft lip.

Preoperative Considerations. A baseline complete blood count (CBC), with prothrombin time and partial thromboplastin time (PT/PTT) as dictated by the bleeding history, is obtained. Blood type and cross is not routinely obtained unless mitigated by particular comorbid conditions. Although most institutions routinely administer a first-generation cephalosporin, such as cefazolin (Kefzol), our institution actually noted no difference in infection rate when no antibiotics were administered in the healthy patient.[50] However, appropriate antibiotics are administered in those with certain conditions, for example, cardiac disease or with prosthetic devices. General anesthesia is administered via an endotracheal tube secured at the chin midline: an oral RAE tube may optimize visualization.

At our institution, the flexible laryngeal mask airway (fLMA) is being used more frequently, although the diameter is relatively larger in the younger infant. It rests in the hypopharynx, protecting it from upper airway secretions, blood, and surgical debris. The fLMA is advocated by our anesthesia colleagues for certain advantages: an excellent airway for lip repairs with decreased vocal cord and tracheal trauma, prevention of secretions being aspirated around the noncuffed endotracheal tube in infants, simple insertion (laryngoscope not required), and a relatively large bore and low resistance. Disadvantages include possible anterior protrusion of the more flexible tube and risk of gastric regurgitation and aspiration in unknown nonfasting patients. Ongoing studies are still in progress at our institution.[48]

Surgical Technique of Lip Adhesion. Because each millimeter of tissue should be correctly aligned, we mark the landmarks for a cleft lip repair before local anesthesia injection to avoid tissue disturbance and possible distention causing an inexact repair. The landmarks are those used in the definitive repair; this is to ascertain that they are undisturbed during the adhesion procedure.

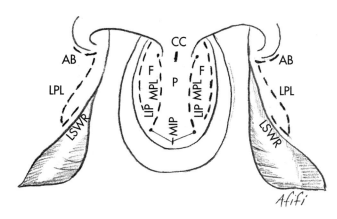

Figure 53-6. Bilateral cleft lip repair: skin landmarks. Prolabial segment markings: *CC,* central columella; *MIP,* midline of inferior prolabium; *LIP,* lateral point of inferior prolabium; *MPL,* medial philtral lines; *P,* philtral flap; *F,* fork flaps (bilateral). Lateral lip segment markings: *AB,* alar base; *LSWR,* lateral segment white roll; *LPL,* lateral philtral line.

The following points are marked and referred to in the definitive repair section. They are shown in Figure 53-6. The procedure is described for *each complete cleft side requiring an adhesion procedure.*

The *skin* markings are:

1. Midline or central point of columellar base (CC)
2. Either side of columellar base
3. Alar bases laterally (AB): a curvilinear mark
4. Midline of inferior prolabium (MIP): about 1 mm above vermilion border
5. Lateral points to inferior prolabial midline (LIP): we designate 2 mm from the inferior prolabial midline (IPM), at a more superolateral level; lines are drawn from the MIP to each LIP, and this outlines the *philtral flap*
6. Anticipated philtral columns or *medial philtral lines* (MPL): marking is made in hourglass configuration, as advocated by Mulliken, from either side of the columellar base to each LIP point
7. Lateral to the outlined philtral flap, the *bilateral fork flaps* are marked by connecting the posteroinferior columellar base points to the LIP, with the line curved in a convex shape including only the anterior lip skin medial to the vermilion
8. The lateral lip segment white roll is identified on either side; just above the white roll, a 2-mm line parallel to the vermilion border is marked: the *lateral segment white roll* (LSWR)
9. A gently curving line is marked from the medial AB to the lateral point of the LSWR: each side's line is the *lateral philtral line* (LPL); the ultimate goal is to have equally long LPLs with closure

The *vermilion* markings are (Figure 53-7):

1. The *prolabial vermilion flap*: the curved rectangular flap will be turned down, debulked as indicated, then resutured to the nasal spine to create the upper labial sulcus.

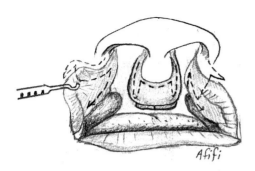

Figure 53-7. Bilateral cleft lip adhesion: vermilion-mucosal marking.

2. Lateral segment vermilion is marked by creating a curvilinear line from medial point of LSWR, around the lip posteriorly, widening it medially to increase the bulk of the future tubercle, then ascending on the mucosal side (parallel to the LPL), and stopping just proximal to the lingual mucosal-maxillary junction, before creating a backcut line laterally. The most lateral limit of the outlined backcut needs to be several millimeters medial to the parotid duct orifice to avoid injury. The subsequent incision would then enable supraperiosteal release of the labial soft tissue tethering from the underlying maxillary complexes.

Markings may be intraoperatively tattooed with methylene blue or brilliant green via a 25-gauge needle tip to avoid distortion with the anesthetic injection. We use equal halves of 2% lidocaine with 1:100,000 epinephrine and 0.5% bupivacaine (Marcaine) with 1:100,000 epinephrine (resulting in 1% lidocaine and 0.25% bupivacaine). The entire anticipated surgical field is infiltrated, including the anterior maxillary surface for subsequent dissection of lateral labial-cheek soft tissue mobilization. While reviewing the sequential instrumentation needed with other operating staff, a minimum of 7 minutes is allowed to elapse to allow epinephrine-induced vasoconstriction, thus optimizing hemostasis.

The cleft lip adhesion is performed on each wide-gaped complete cleft side (Figure 53-8). Retracting the nasal tip up and lateral lip segment out, the ipsilateral internal nasal valve is marked from just distal to the dome to the base of the lip segment, short of the maxillary component. The L flap is designed by continuing the marking anteroinferiorly onto the lateral lip segment's wet-dry vermilion junction, all within the mucosa. A superiorly based triangular flap is thus delineated by marking back to the maxillary segment, a few millimeters short of the lingual-gingival sulcus, then designing a backcut posterolaterally. The backcut's lateral limit is the parotid duct orifice. The above flap is thus L-shaped, or lateral shaped, hence its name.

After injection of local anesthesia as described above, the incision is made as outlined, increasing the thickness of the L flap at its base for optimal perfusion. After the backcut is made, supraperiosteal dissection over the underlying maxilla releases all tethering of the overlying lateral lip segment. The surgeon's

thumb or digit is gently placed over the infraorbital canal site, avoiding superficial dissection and possible globe or nerve iatrogenic injury. Dissection is complete once the mobilized lip segment freely and without undue tension approximates to the prolabium. The L flap is rotated and inset in the internal nasal valve incision already created.

Well within the mucosa and away from the future ipsilateral Cupid's high point site, an M flap is designed in the prolabial-premaxillary segment. The flap leaflets are turned outwards, like pages of a book. The lateral lip segment is mobilized medially to appose the M flap's components, suturing the corresponding 3 layers sequentially (see Figure 53-8, *E-G*): inner mucosal (A to A'), intervening maloriented orbicularis oris muscle via two overlapping horizontal mattress sutures, and outer mucosal layers (B to B'). Absorbable sutures are used. Bacitracin is applied to the wound, with the postoperative care analogous to that after definitive lip repair (later section).

PREMAXILLARY SURGICAL SETBACK. The least favored option for the surgical management of a overly prominent premaxilla is a surgical setback procedure, currently condemned by most. The indication would be an overly projecting premaxilla causing inability by any other means to close the bilateral cleft lip deformity. This is extremely rare and not encountered at our institution.

As noted by Cronin,[11] this procedure may be reserved for those older patients with procumbent segments despite adequate lip repair. A vomer section posterior to the vomer-prevomerine suture site is resected 4 to 5 mm less anteroposteriorly than the protrusion amount. A horizontal resection of the corresponding septal cartilage is then removed to allow posterior transfer of the premaxilla. Although mentioned for possible unusual cases encountered abroad, we reiterate that this method has never been required at most institutions, and in fact, it is the maxillary *retrusion* encountered with facial growth that often requires correction in these patients.

SURGICAL TECHNIQUES OF LIP REPAIR

Overview

Throughout the years, there have been numerous proposed surgical techniques advocated for bilateral cleft lip repairs, attesting to the difficulty in obtaining consistently optimal results by any one method. The majority used today utilize the prolabium for reconstruction of the central upper lip. The absence of orbicularis muscle fibers in the prolabium of complete cleft lips, with its resulting absence of white roll, has resulted in the use of the white roll of the lateral lip segments to be incorporated into the philtral base in most current common techniques.

Variations in specific repairs include incision location and method of reconstructing orbicularis oris muscle continuity. As noted by Byrd,[8] most repairs use either closures via a straight line or Z-plasty technique. Table 53-3 summarizes the most well-known methods and their proponent surgeon. The

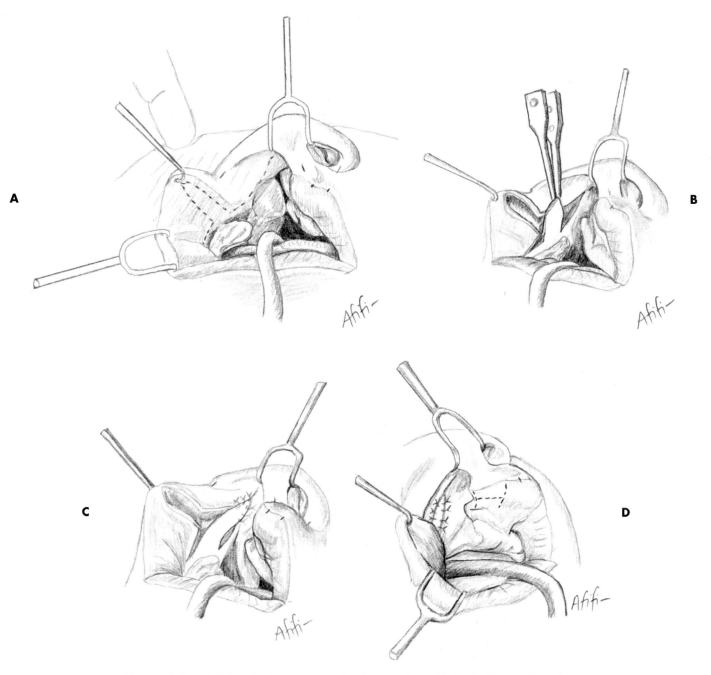

Figure 53-8. Cleft lip adhesion procedure (as shown unilaterally). **A,** Incision markings. L flap design is along internal nasal valve onto lateral lip segment, then backwards superior and parallel to lateral maxillary segment. Oblique hatched area indicates supraperiosteal undermining of lower ipsilateral maxillary segment, thus releasing tethering of lateral lip segment for medial mobilization. Surgeon's digit is on inferior alveolar nerve site for protection and enforcing superior extent of dissection. **B,** Elevation and rotation of L flap. **C,** L flap inserting. **D,** Design of medial lip. Prolabial M flap (dashed lines) outlined well lateral to future definitive repair landmarks. *Continued*

following are brief mentions of bilateral cleft lip repairs with expansion of the more common repairs used today, including our preferred technique.

Straight Line Closure

Veau II Repair (1931); Barsky Repair (1950). Mentioned for historical reasons, the prolabium underwent vertical incisions from the lateral columellar bases connected transversely across, proximal to the vermilion junction. The lateral lip segments were incised from the medial alar bases out laterally, incorporating portions of the white upper lip and vermilion for medial closure inferior to the prolabial segment (Figure 53-9, *A*). No longer used because of its unnatural appearance, specific disadvantages include vertical excess, inferior horizontal central lip deficiency, abnormal prolabial bulge, and lack of Cupid's bow definition.

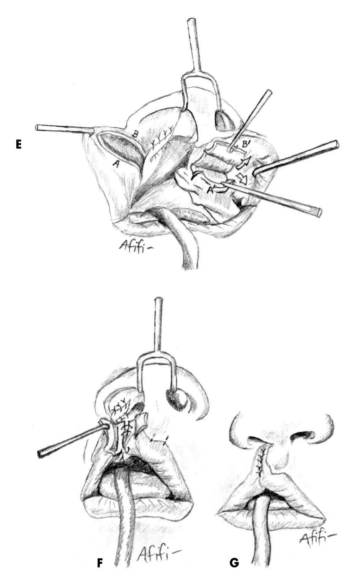

Figure 53-8, cont'd. E, Elevation of M flap leaflets. Three-layered closure is performed with inner mucosal (A to A'), middle muscular (via two overlapping horizontal mattress sutures), and outer mucosal (B to B') layers. **F,** Closure of posterior mucosal layer, which is followed by approximation of muscle layers via horizontal mattress sutures. **G,** Closure of final layer, the outer mucosa and vermilion. (From Afifi GY, Hardesty RA: Unilateral cleft lip repair. In *Operative plastic surgery*, St Paul, Minn, 2000, Clarinda Publications.)

Table 53-3.
Bilateral Cleft Lip Repair Methods

METHOD	YEAR
STRAIGHT LINE CLOSURE	
Barsky repair	1950
Veau II repair	1931
Veau III repair	1938
Cronin	1957
Manchester	1965
Black	1984, 1985
Z-PLASTY	
Lower Lip Z-plasty	
Bauer, Trusler, Tondra	1959
Berkeley	1961
Modified Tennison repair	1966
Upper Lip Z-plasty	
Millard	1960
Modified Manchester	
Wynn	1960
Mulliken repair (Millard variant)	1985
Noordhoff repair (Millard variant)	1986
Combined Upper and Lower Lip Z-plasty	
Skoog	1965
PRIMARY ABBE FLAP REPAIR	
Clarkson	1954

Veau III Repair (1938). Considered one of the more direct closures, this repair nevertheless results in some scar contracture symmetrically concentrated at Cupid's bow peaks. This may result from any straight line method. The prolabial incision starts from the columellar bases, with the philtral width approximately 6 mm in the infant (Figure 53-9, *B*). The prolabial vermilion is completely excised. Vertical incisions in the lateral lip segments start from the medial alar bases to above the anticipated lateral lip white roll. The lateral flaps are turned down to meet together and form the philtral tubercle. Volume may be increased via flap cross-lapping. Extra-wide prolabial tissue may be banked as forked flaps in the nasal floor for future columellar reconstruction. Contraindications for this repair include a relatively small prolabium, for which a Millard or Wynn type of repair may be used.

Manchester (1965). Manchester[24] was an early advocate of preoperative orthopedic alveolar-premaxillary segment alignment via splints with a head cap and band before surgical repair of bilateral cleft lip and palate. Anteriorly based prolabial vermilion is elevated along with laterally based vermilion from the lateral lip segments (Figure 53-9, *C*). The lateral segment mucosal edges are sutured together in the midline, forming the premaxillary anterior labial sulcus. Lateral vermilion deepithelialization is performed before folding the flaps together to form the tubercle. The midline is then covered with the prolabial vermilion flap. Of note, the orbicularis muscle is not approximated because of Manchester's belief that this would produce an overly tight closure and possible maxillary retrusion. Main disadvantages

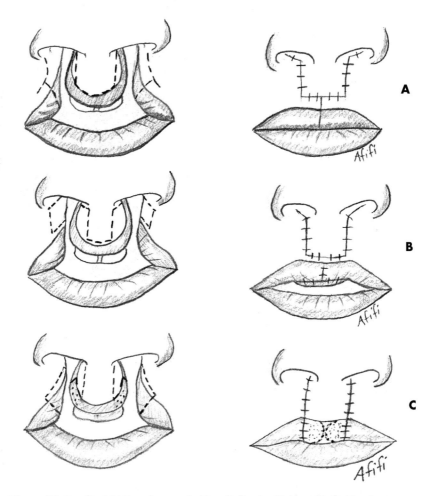

Figure 53-9. Straight line closure. **A,** Veau II, Barsky. **B,** Veau III. **C,** Manchester.

include the now-visible prolabial-lateral vermilion color mismatch, straight line scar contracture, and absence of a defined prolabial white roll.

Black Repair (1984, 1985). Black[6] also utilized preoperative orthopedic alignment before repair at 2 to 3 months of age. Similar to above, prolabial incisions create a superiorly based rectangular flap (Figure 53-10). Lateral to the prolabial flap, triangular flaps are raised for eventual insertion into the medial alar base. The remaining lateral prolabial lip tissue is sutured medially together, forming the premaxillary side of the labial sulcus. After alar base backcuts, laterally based rectangular flaps are turned down and sutured together to form the anterior labial sulcus. Aberrantly inserted orbicularis muscle is released and reoriented transversely before bilateral apposition at the midline. The prolabial flap is then reset downward to recreate the central upper lip and Cupid's bow.

Disadvantages are identical to those of the Manchester repair. These have decreased the use of the straight line repair method. Incorporating some of the above mucosal-muscle apposition and avoiding the straight line skin sequelae, the Z-plasty was then utilized in an attempt to improve surgical results.

Z-plasty
LOWER LIP Z-PLASTY

Tennison (1952). Originally introduced by Tennison[45] for unilateral cleft lip repair, the "stencil" method has been modified for use in the bilateral lip reconstruction. The triangular flap repair was then developed. The markings and eventual closure are depicted in Figure 53-11, *A*. On each side, a laterally based vermilion-muscle flap is turned down, interdigitating with the prolabial flap such that a Z-plasty closure is performed at the lower lip. However, because of the risk of impaired circulation to the inferior prolabium with bilateral medially oblique incisions, it was advocated that one side be repaired at a time. Obvious disadvantages include a two-stage repair, nonalignment of the incisions with the usual philtral columns, and an oblique, possibly notable scar across the central tubercle.

Bauer, Trusler, and Tondra (1959). Likewise proposing a two-stage and Z-plasty repair of the bilateral cleft lip, Bauer, Trusler, and Tondra[4] proposed a variation of the modified Tennison repair. Partial prolabial elevation and apposition to the ipsilateral lateral lip segment was performed via a Z-plasty closure (Figure 53-11, *B*). A laterally based mucosal flap with orbicularis fibers is sutured to the inferiorly rotated prolabial

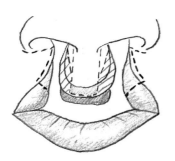
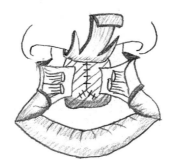
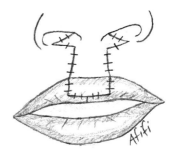

Figure 53-10. Straight line closure: Black's repair.

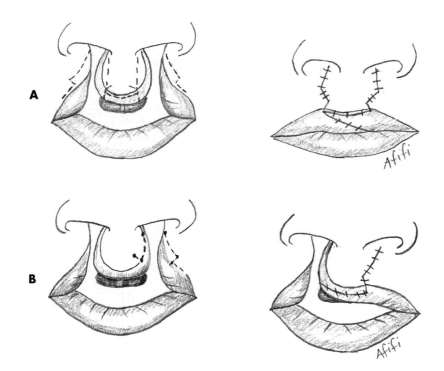

Figure 53-11. Lower lip Z-plasty. **A,** Modified Tennison. **B,** Bauer, Trusler, and Tondra (first stage).

vermilion flap. The alar cartilage lateral crus is rotated upward, slightly augmenting columellar length and improving alar contour.

Although the proposed advantage was for a Z-plasty to minimize scar contracture, obvious disadvantages included non–anatomically placed scars as with the previous method, lack of orbicularis continuity, staged method, and risk of the medial scars disrupting distal prolabial vascularity and causing an abnormal central lip bulge, hence its obvious disfavor.

Berkeley (1961). Also proposing a variant of the Tennison adaptation, Berkeley[5] stressed the importance of not incising the prolabial flap too high on the columellar base; this would risk an overly short columella in future reconstruction. Although the risk of iatrogenic shortening would be decreased, most assert that the majority of patients will need a separate columellar lengthening procedure.

UPPER LIP Z-PLASTY

Wynn (1960). Wynn[51] created a Z-plasty in the lateral upper lip–columellar complex for consecutively repairing each cleft lip side. Superiorly based, a narrow triangular flap is turned superomedially from the lateral lip and inset into the incised columellar-prolabial junction (Figure 53-12, *A*). This would lengthen the prolabium and columella. Purported advantages include decreased scar contracture, treatment of smaller prolabial segments, and minimal sacrifice of transverse lip dimensions. Disadvantages include vertical lip excess for larger prolabial segments, tubercle vermilion undercorrection, and two-stage method because of the risk of compromising prolabial vascularity if the upper transverse scars are too close together.

Millard (1960): Incomplete Bilateral Cleft Lip. Originally proposed for unilateral cleft lips, Millard adapted his rotation-

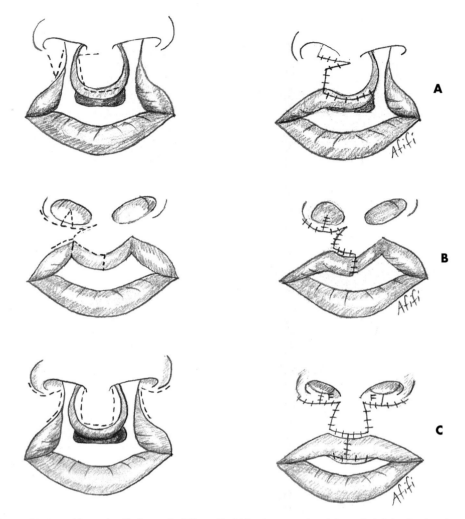

Figure 53-12.   Upper lip Z-plasty. **A,** Wynn. **B,** Millard: incomplete bilateral cleft lip (each side repaired at separate stage). **C,** Millard: complete bilateral cleft lip (forked flaps banked in nasal floor for future columellar lengthening).

advancement technique for bilateral deformities.[28] Bilateral incomplete cleft lip patients usually have adequate columellar length despite a possibly decreased prolabial size. Bilaterally complete deformities have an apparently short columella, usually requiring reconstruction. The Millard repair is classically performed one side at a time.

A curvilinear incision is made from the Cupid's trough midline, upward and halfway across the columellar base (Figure 53-12, *B*). The subsequent triangular defect is filled by the advancement of a triangular flap produced by a backcut around the alar base. The incised lateral prolabium is simultaneously rotated downward. For complete clefts, the aberrantly inserted orbicularis muscle is released from the alar base, reoriented transversely with the mucosa, and sutured posterior to the prolabial midline, thus creating the labial sulcus. A vertically oriented triangular skin wedge is removed from the nasal floor for usual cases of excess alar width. The lateral-based vermilion flap recreates the Cupid's bow peak and vermilion ridge or white roll.

In a second stage, the contralateral cleft lip is repaired likewise. Of note, the prolabial curvilinear incision apex is stopped several millimeters short of the previously placed mirror image scar to avoid producing vertical excess of the lip. The complete side of a bilateral deformity is repaired before the incomplete side so that the latter's prolabial vascularity is maintained.

The lateral aspect of the incised prolabium, known as the **C** flap in the unilateral repair, may be banked in the nostril sill for future columellar lengthening.

Millard (1971): Complete Bilateral Cleft Lip. Thus Millard proposed raising the lateral prolabial flaps, known as forked flaps, concomitantly with a single-stage lip repair, and then banking the flaps in the nostril base (Figure 53-12, *C*). An adequate prolabial size was required; otherwise, the standard rotation-advancement or Veau III straight line method was used to increase prolabial dimensions via traction.

The prolabial incisions start on either side of the columellar base, across the prolabial base, just proximal to the vermilion junction. After elevation of the philtral flap, the vermilion is turned down and sutured toward the nasal spine, thus creating the posterior labial sulcus wall. Lateral to the philtral flap, the white prolabial flaps are elevated as forked flaps described above.

The lateral lip segments are incised as described in the previous section, with the lateral oblique incision made just above the white roll. Alar base backcuts are made and the vermilion flaps carrying the mucocutaneous junction–white roll are turned down. Their mucosal-muscle edges are brought together in the midline, forming the anterior labial sulcus wall, with their vermilion–white roll creating the tubercle and its superoanterior white roll, respectively. The philtral flap is then turned down and sutured to the lateral lip segments and inferior white roll–vermilion complex. After medial advancement of the alar bases, the forked flaps are inset into the circumalar incision sites.

Mulliken Repair (1985) (Millard Variant). Mulliken[33] preoperatively used orthopedic appliances to align the alveolar-premaxillary segments for correction of any lateral segment collapse and premaxillary protrusion. The repair is similar to that proposed by Millard with some modifications, notably of the prolabial flap dimensions and the nasal reconstruction performed during lip repair.

Performed at 3 to 5 months of age, the *first* stage was the lip repair. The philtral flap is biconcave with peaks of Cupid's bow approximately 4 mm apart, with the flap base 2 mm at the columellar-labial junction (Figure 53-13, *A*). Fork flaps and central vermilion flap are created as previously described.

Alar base incisions are made, and intercartilaginous incisions are used to superiorly advance the lateral alar cartilages before suturing them overlapped with the upper lateral cartilages. The lateral lip segments' aberrant orbicularis and mucosal insertions are freed and reoriented transversely to recreate the anterior labial sulcus and muscular continuity. The most superior suture is secured to the anterior nasal spine. The alar base flaps are then medially transposed.

The lateral segment white roll–vermilion–mucosal flaps are then sutured together at the midline to form the tubercle unit. The philtral flap's posterior side may be incised to increase its concave contour. The forked flaps are then rotated laterally and banked in the nasal floor.

Performed at 8 to 9 months of age, Mulliken's *second* stage reconstructed the cleft nasal deformity via three incision types (Figure 53-13, *B*). Bilateral alar base incisions liberate the forked flaps and continue around the alar complex via the membranous septum into the intercartilaginous lines. The forked flaps are then rotated superoanteriorly and inset along the membranous septal portion of the columella into the medial intercartilaginous incision site. The second incision is at the vertical midline of the nasal dome and exposes the inferiorly displaced alar cartilages for resuspension to the upper lateral cartilages. The cleft bifid tip is corrected by suturing the alar cartilage domes and the medial crura together. The third incision is made along the nasal rim, exposing the alar cartilages for the above reconstruction and enabling direct excision of the overhanging rim. Post-operative fixation may be provided by a stent, worn for 2 to 3 months.

According to Mulliken's series, at 2 years of age, the prolabial increased width was 2.5-fold at the columellar junction and twofold at Cupid's bow.

Noordhoff Repair (1986) (Millard Variant). Also proposing modifications to Millard's repair, Noordhoff[35] incorporated nasal reconstruction with his bilateral lip repair. Originating on either side of the columellar base, vertical lines are

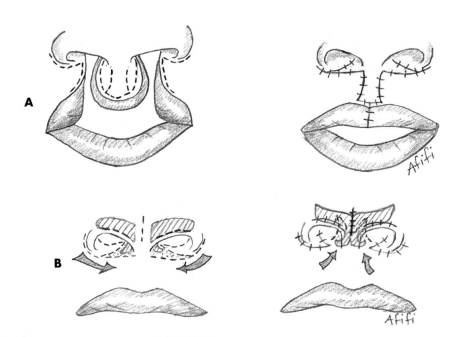

Figure 53-13. Mulliken staged lip-nasal reconstruction. **A,** First stage lip repair. **B,** Second stage nasal repair.

marked ending in a triangular base such that Cupid's bow is 6 to 8 mm wide (Figure 53-14). Lateral forked flaps are also outlined before then elevating all philtral-based flaps from the surrounding vermilion. The prolabial mucosal-vermilion complex is thinned before being sutured together, creating the midline posterior labial sulcus.

The lateral lip segments are incised vertically down from the medial alar base, analogous to the originally made prolabial incisions. Medially based buccal mucosal flaps, along with the orbicularis muscle–mucosal flaps, are rotated from the alar base to a horizontal direction. The alar cartilages are freed via an intercartilaginous incision, originating from the piriform aperture, and secured together at the domes and to the upper lateral cartilages. The buccal mucosal flaps are then sutured into the inferior intercartilaginous incision to increase length for the nasal floor reconstruction.

As with the Millard repair, mucosal-orbicularis flaps are sutured together to create the anterior labial sulcus, with the most superior suture secured to the nasal spine to prevent inferior displacement. The lateral segment may donate a forked flap to rotate medially and insert in the posterior columellar apex incision. The inferior white roll–vermilion–mucosal flaps are apposed to create Cupid's bow and tubercle complex.

COMBINED UPPER AND LOWER LIP Z-PLASTY

Skoog Repair (1965). Only mentioned for historical reasons, the Skoog[43] repair entailed a two-stage, combined upper and lower lip Z-plasty, with each side reconstructed sequentially. Two Z-plasty incisions are made in the inferior prolabium and superior lateral lip segment, enabling the insertion of superior and inferior triangular flaps from the lateral segment into the apexes of the columellar and inferior prolabial incisions. The two-stage lip repair, potential vascular compromise to the columellar-prolabial junction, and non-anatomically placed philtral scars has made this repair of historical interest only.

Abbe Flap Repair —Clarkson (1954)

The cross lip, or Abbe, flap is usually reserved as a secondary surgical treatment for tight or overly scarred, deformed bilateral cleft lip repairs. However, it is also a possible last option for primary reconstruction. In 1954, Clarkson[20] utilized the primary Abbe flap for 1-month-old patients with wide bilateral clefts, suturing one side 7 to 10 days before the contralateral side to avoid airway compromise. The pedicle was divided at 3 weeks. A decade later, Honig[20] utilized the flap in an infant, followed by Antia[1] years later, who used it for 10 patients, the majority older than 1 year of age. Thus

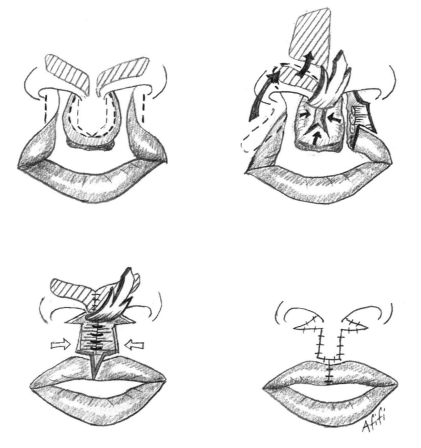

Figure 53-14. Noordhoff repair.

the Abbe flap may occasionally be used for difficult primary and certainly secondary cases, refractory to the usual repair modalities.

AUTHORS' PREFERRED TECHNIQUE

Recognizing that each patient mandates an individualized approach, our institution nevertheless does favor a modification of the Millard repair as our most commonly used bilateral cleft lip reconstruction technique. Attempting to incorporate the best of all repair methods proposed, some features are also analogous to those presented by Veau, Manchester, Black, Randall, Mulliken, and Noordhoff. As discussed previously, a single definitive lip repair is performed on those with incomplete cleft lips, with a small intervening gap between lip segments, or those who previously underwent an initial lip adhesion procedure. This is performed between 3 and 6 months of age.

The perioperative considerations are identical to those mentioned in an earlier section on the adhesion technique, as are the markings of the anatomic landmarks (see Figure 53-6). The prolabium is first incised. As previously described, the *skin* landmarks include CC; either side of columellar base; bilateral AB; MIP, which is about 1 mm above vermilion border; and the LIPs, which are 2 mm from the IPM, at a more superolateral level. A wide double-pronged skin hook is placed on either side of the columella, gently retracting the nasal tip upward to optimize visualization. Incisions are made from the MIP to each LIP and the hourglass-outlined philtral columns or MPLs. This creates the *philtral flap*. The *bilateral fork flaps* are then elevated from either side, being careful to stay medial to the vermilion (Figure 53-15).

On the lateral lip segments and just above the white roll, a 2-mm incision is made parallel to the vermilion border: the LSWR. A gently curved incision is made from the medial AB to the lateral point of the LSWR: the LPL. The ultimate goal is to have equally long LPLs with closure.

As depicted in Figures 53-7 and 53-15, the *vermilion* markings are made and then incised. The curved rectangular *prolabial vermilion flap* is turned down, debulked, and sutured to the nasal spine to create the posterior labial sulcus. The lateral segment vermilion is incised in a curvilinear manner from the medial point of LSWR, posteriorly around the lip, and widened medially to increase the bulk of the future tubercle. The incision then ascends on the mucosal side (parallel to the LPL) and stops just proximal to the lingual mucosal-maxillary junction before creating a backcut line laterally. The backcut's most lateral limit is several millimeters medial to the parotid duct orifice. A supraperiosteal dissection releases the labial soft tissue from the underlying maxillary complexes.

After the medial AB, LPL, LSWR, and delineated vermilion incisions are made, the intervening lip skin-vermilion segment (alternatively, the lip adhesion scar) is discarded. Full mobilization of the lateral soft tissue segments

is reassessed with manual tension. It is believed that the supraperiosteal dissection is superior to that at the subperiosteal plane because there is less bleeding and potentially decreased risk of delayed maxillary growth. The aberrantly inserted orbicularis oris muscle is liberated from the alar base and rotated along with its underlying mucosa to a more normal transverse orientation. The LSWR attached flaps are also rotated horizontally, maintaining excess mucosal-submucosal tissue at the midline such that a full philtral tubercle is reconstructed.

After completing the above dissection, the closure commences from the mucosal layer, which creates the anterior labial sulcus. The bilateral lateral lip segment tissue is first opposed via chromic sutures to reconstruct the *mucosal layer* in the midline. As noted above, the most superior suture had been placed to the anterior nasal spine to avoid future lip descent.

The orbicularis oris *muscle layer* is then closed. Complete muscular continuity is achieved via overlapping horizontal sutures. As proposed by Randall, we occasionally interdigitate the muscle fibers to achieve this goal. The LSWR flaps are then opposed, occasionally freeing the dermal ends to create everted fullness for the tubercle.

The *skin layer* closure commences by insetting the philtral flap into the skin gap between the lateral lip segments. To decrease tension on this flap, a horizontal mattress suture is placed from one lateral segment dermal layer to the contralateral side, thus avoiding excess lateral traction on the intervening philtral flap and hence possible scar widening. If the philtral flap is of adequate thickness, a suture may be placed at its inferior midline to enhance the anatomic trough present at the base of a normal philtral unit.

Before placement of all the dermal sutures, the AB-to-Cupid's bow peak distance is measured on either side. If one side has an increased distance, a triangular skin wedge may be removed from the ipsilateral alar base such that both lengths are equidistant (Figure 53-16). AB to CC is also assessed: a vertical triangle is removed from the medial nostril floor to achieve symmetry while maintaining the scar in a relatively hidden site in those cases with a widened alar width on one side. Each side's alar base width and Cupid's bow peak distances are also measured to ensure symmetry. During the insetting of the forked flaps into the nasal floor, the flap may need to be trimmed to naturalize the closure. In individual cases, we occasionally remove the forked flaps and close the alar floor directly if another option will be utilized for future columellar lengthening.

After the dermal layer is closed with 4-0 Vicryl suture, final skin closure is done via 5-0 Prolene. Nonabsorbable suture is used because we believe that upon its removal, the resulting scar would be superior to that closed via absorbable suture resulting from the lack of foreign body-induced inflammation. The dermal closure should completely tension-free so that skin layer closure is achieved only for cosmesis. This running fine suture layer ensures exact tissue edge alignment.

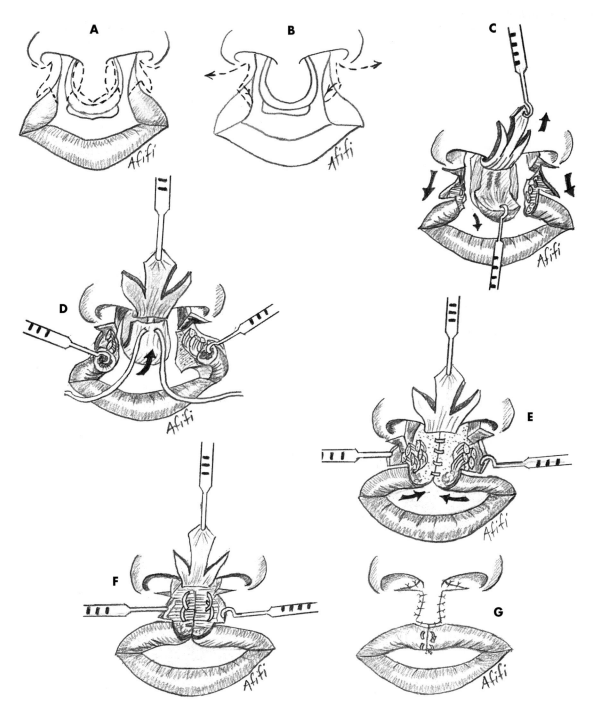

Figure 53-15. Authors' definitive bilateral cleft lip repair. Note the incorporation of multiple aspects of previously described methods. **A,** Skin markings for prolabial philtral flap with bilateral fork flaps, prolabial vermilion flap, and alar base-lateral lip segment flaps (see Figure 53-6). Each side of prolabial philtral flap apex is approximately 2 mm (total 4 mm) in infant. Each corresponding future horizontal lateral lip flap incision likewise 2 mm long, made just above discernable white roll (lateral segment white roll [LSWR]—see text). **B,** Vermilion and buccal mucosal flap markings of lateral lip segments. These are made analogous and parallel to skin markings. Lateral limit of buccal mucosal backcuts on either side is parotid orifice. Sufficient supraperiostal dissection of lateral lip segments is performed to enable ease in approximation at midline. **C,** Prolabial philtral and fork flaps thinned and retracted superiorly. Prolabial vermilion flap unfurled inferiorly. Alar base *(AB)*-lateral philtral line *(LPL)* lateral point of LSWR incision is then made on either side. The orbicularis oris muscle fibers are detached from their aberrant insertions to AB and rotated with attached mucosa to more normal transverse plane. **D,** Prolabial vermilion flap after debulking is sutured to inferior nasal spine, creating posterior labial sulcus. **E,** Approximation of both lateral lip segments via initial closure of mucosal layer (thus bringing together muscular layers). The most superior suture is secured to the anterior nasal spine, thus decreasing risk of future upper lip descent. **F,** Closure of orbicularis oris muscle layer. Complete muscular continuity is achieved either by overlapping horizontal mattress sutures (above) or by muscle bundle interdigitation per Randalll (see text). **G,** Closure of skin layer via insetting of philtral flap and appropriate placement of forked flaps into nasal floor. Care is taken to optimize vermilion bulk, recreating fullness of philtral tubercle.

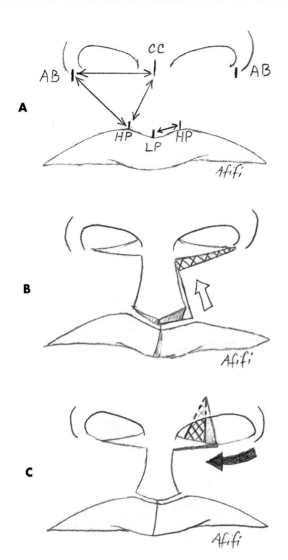

Figure 53-16. Achieving symmetry in lip-nasal repair: alar base excisions. **A,** Anatomic measurements: alar base *(AB)*, central columella *(CC)*, high point of Cupid's bow *(HP)*, low point of Cupid's bow *(LP)*. AB to CC, AB to HP, CC to HP, LP to HP. **B,** Alar base excision for ipsilateral vertical height excess. **C,** Superomedial nasal floor excision for ipsilateral horizontal length excess.

Examples of clinical cases are shown in Figures 53-17 to 53-19.

POSTOPERATIVE CARE

As noted above, anatomic landmark symmetry is objectively ensured via intraoperative and postoperative measurement. Occasionally, we use rolled Xeroform gauze as nasal stents after reorientation of the lateral alar cartilages to maintain the new form in the immediate postoperative period. Bacitracin is applied to the wound. Alternatively, for occasionally snug closures or to minimize patient self-manipulation, Steri-Strips may be applied across the repair.

Care and attention is maintained during extubation and postoperatively to avoid iatrogenic injury to the repair. The child is placed comfortably and upright in a crib or infant car seat with the arms placed in restraints. This prevents the child's self-injury by rolling onto the wound or disrupting it with his or her hands. The restraints are continued for a period of about 4 to 6 weeks postoperatively, at least when the child is unsupervised.

The diet is slowly resumed as tolerated, instructing the parents to be careful with bottle nipple feeding. At 1 week, the sutures are removed, either by distracting the child while bottle feeding (as done by LaRossa[23]) or using a mild analgesic before the office visit (as done by our institution). The next visit is at 3 weeks to ensure no immediate postoperative complication, followed by routine interval plastic surgery and craniofacial team visits.

MANAGEMENT OF NASAL DEFECT

Analysis of Defect

It is impossible to evaluate a bilateral cleft lip without concomitantly assessing its associated nasal components, alluded to in previous sections. Patients present with a spectrum of nasal deformities, the degree of which reflects that of the primary cleft severity. The spectrum starts with an essentially normal nasal structure with the form fruste to the slightly widened alar base of the incomplete cleft lip and continues to the significant nasal deformity associated with complete clefts involving the palate, lip, and facial structures. There are many variants along this spectrum. A so-called *simian band* may connect the columella to the ipsilateral alar base, with resulting less lateral alar displacement than in classic complete cleft lip defects. Alternatively, one side may be complete with the other incomplete.

In either case, the associated nasal deformities may include the following features:

1. Laterally flared or displaced alar bases
2. Flattened nasal tip
3. Apparently shortened columella
4. Inferiorly oriented alar cartilage domes
5. Indistinct columellar bases
6. Obtuse nasolabial angles
7. Recessed alar base resulting from absent piriform rims

The degree of nasal symmetry is also dependent on that of the lip defect. Unequal lip involvement produces greater nasal asymmetry. Underlying maxillary involvement further varies the anterior-posterior plane disparities, including torqued columellar bases, malpositioned alar wings, and anteriorly displaced columellar bases from overprojecting premaxillary platforms (see Figure 53-1).

Alar Base Reconstruction

Although many surgeons may vary in their overall approach and timing of cleft nasal repair, most will agree that there are specific goals for alar base reconstruction that should be con-

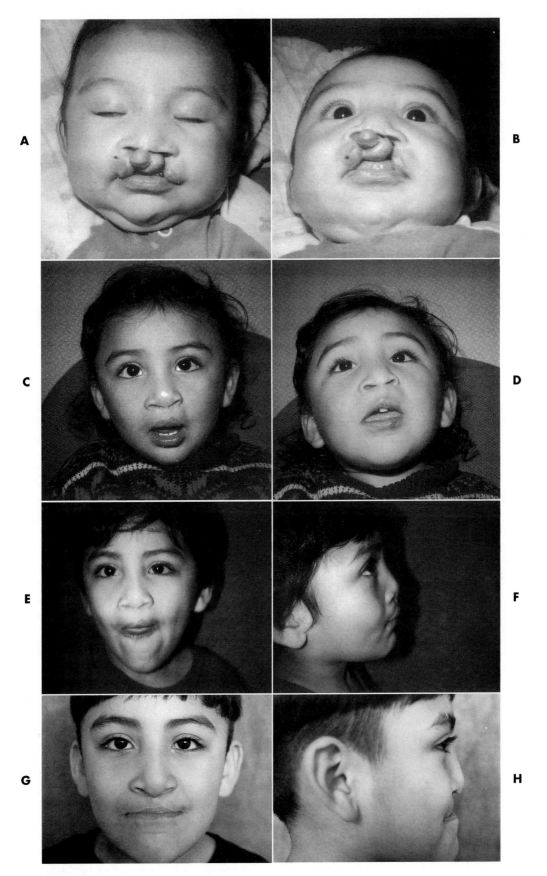

Figure 53-17. **A** and **B,** Patient at 2 months of age, with bilateral complete cleft lip and palate; underwent lip adhesion, Latham device application, followed by definite repair. **C** and **D,** Two years after repair. **E** and **F,** Frontal and lateral views 4 years after repair. **G** and **H,** Frontal and lateral views 7 years after repair. Note increasing maxillary retrusion.

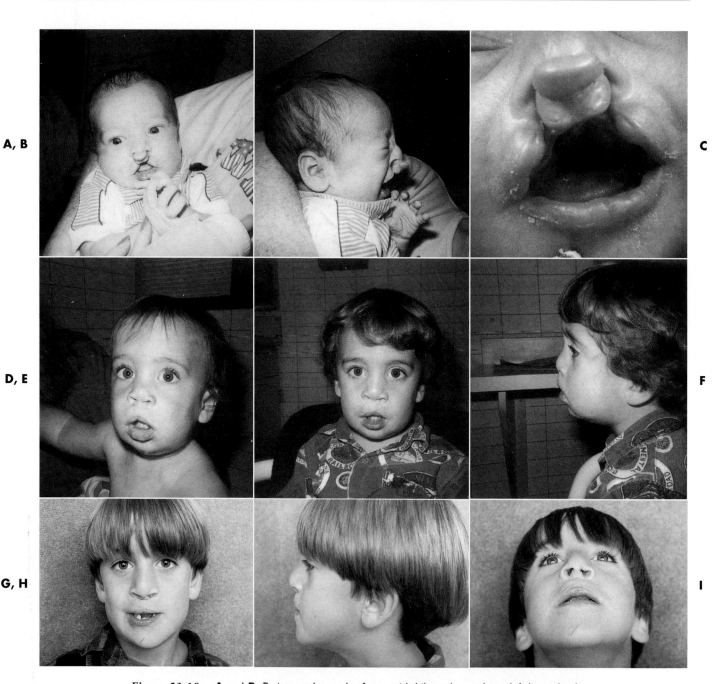

Figure 53-18. **A** and **B,** Patient at 1 month of age, with bilateral complete cleft lip and palate. Note degree of premaxillary segment protrusion. **C,** Close-up frontal view of protruding premaxillary segment. **D,** One year after staged repair of bilateral cleft lip. **E** and **F,** Frontal and lateral views 2 years postoperatively. **G** and **H,** Frontal and lateral views 7 years postoperatively; has undergone earlier columellar lengthening. **I,** Basal view 7 years postoperatively; will require rhinoplasty to improve tip correction (see prior lateral view) and reposition alar margins.

comitantly obtained during lip repair. At our institution, we advocate the following during the definitive lip reconstruction:

1. Obtaining symmetry of alar base widths
2. Aligning alar bases at the same transverse level
3. Symmetrically reconstructing the internal and external nasal valves
4. Simultaneous assurance of nasal airway patency

These steps are delineated in the Authors' Preferred Technique section.

Columellar Reconstruction/Lengthening

The columellar structure appears shortened in complete bilateral cleft lip defects, although Mulliken[30] stresses that all anatomic structures are present but simply overly splayed out.

The most common method used to lengthen the columella is probably an adaptation of one originally proposed by *Cronin*[10] in 1958. In 1990, he noted the average age at surgery was 6 years rather than, as previously done, at 2 to 3 years.[11] He performed a V-Y advancement of previously banked nasal

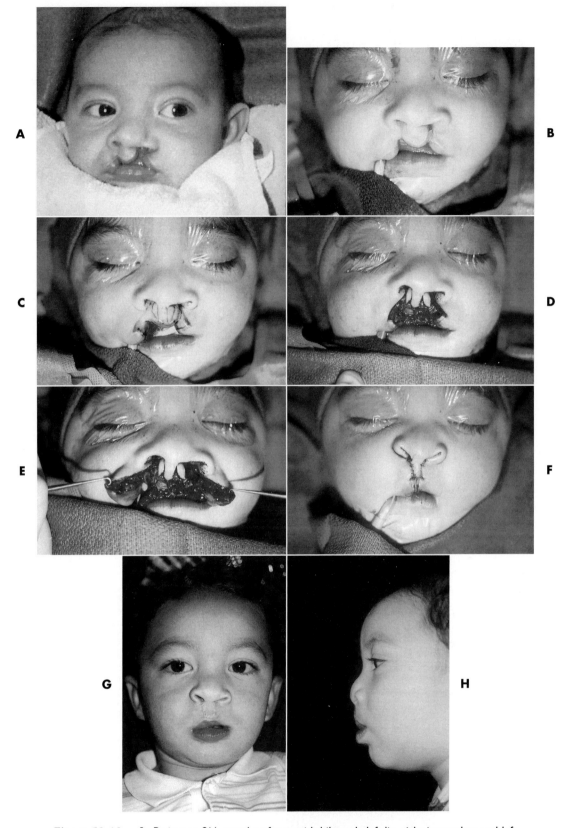

Figure 53-19. **A,** Patient at 2½ months of age, with bilateral cleft lip, right incomplete and left complete. **B,** Age five months, after lip adhesion. **C,** Incisions marked, followed by infiltration of local anesthetic with vasoconstrictor. Note increased vertical length on right side. **D,** Incisions made, creating philtral flap with adjacent bilateral fork flaps, prolabial vermilion turndown flap, and lateral lip segment flaps (maintaining white roll). **E,** Lateral lip segment incisions on vermilion side vertically up and laterally out for segment mobilization (see text). **F,** After closure with philtral flap replaced, over lateral segment mucosal-muscle-vermilion/white roll apposition. A triangular segment was excised from right alar base to equalize lateral lip vertical height. **G,** Frontal view 1 year after lip repair. Some lip volume deficiency on left apparent. **H,** Lateral view 1 year after lip repair. Columellar lengthening is next planned procedure.

floor flaps into the columella while medially rotating the laterally splayed alar bases (Figure 53-20). The lateral flaps had increased thickness to recreate the pyramidal columellar base. Alar width was decreased by the removal of triangular skin segments from either inferior to the alar base or from the base itself. The alar complexes are mobilized medially while the

columellar apex and nasal tip is retracted upwards via a skin hook.

After appropriate mobilization, the underlying maxillary soft tissue may be sutured together via a buried, nonabsorbable crossing suture to maintain a more narrowed nasal base. Tip projection may be ensured via intercrural and/or interdomal

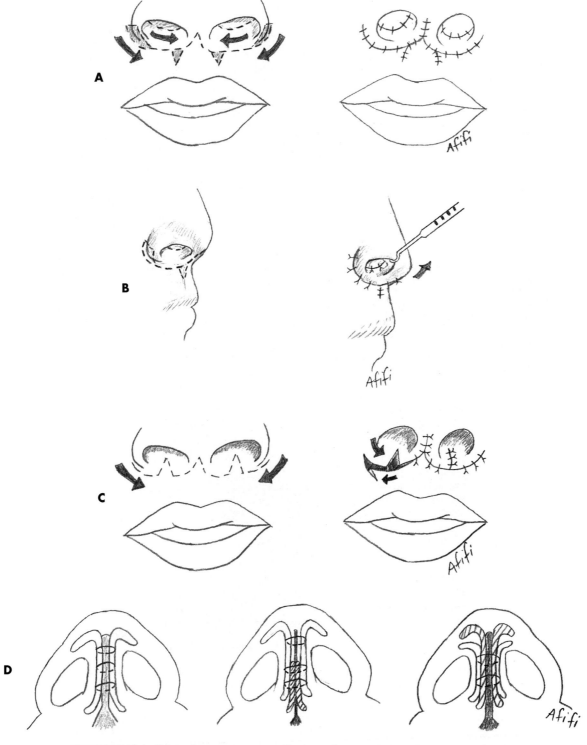

Figure 53-20. Columellar reconstruction: Cronin techniques. **A,** Lengthening columella, vertical triangle excised from superior philtral scars. **B,** Lateral views. **C,** Variation utilizing Z-plasty based on nasal floor and alar base. **D,** Variations of cartilage manipulation for increasing tip support. Crosshatched cartilage represent autologous grafts (e.g., septal, auricular).

cartilage suturing along with columellar strut or tip grafts as indicated. Graft donor sites include septal and auricular sources. Our technique is a modification of the Cronin with greater tip elevation via cartilaginous fixation, performed at preschool years.

Millard[28] originally proposed that columellar lengthening be performed 1 to 3 months after lip repair, then revised it for the preschool period. For incomplete clefts, he occasionally performed a lengthening procedure within the year although cautioned about the increased risk of vertically long lips slipping over the premaxillary segment. His secondary forked flap procedure used excess prolabial width as the donor site for tissue advanced superomedially onto the columella while advancing the nasal tip upward (Figure 53-21).

Also utilizing the prolabial's excess width as a donor source, *Bardach*[3] proposed a central V-Y procedure of the superior central lip. The alar cartilages are mobilized and sutured together to increase tip projection, while the V-Y closure elongates the columella and narrows the central lip (Figure 53-22).

Multiple methods have been proposed that incorporate a more formal nasal reconstruction along with the cleft lip repair. *Mulliken*[31,32] utilizes a vertical incision in the nasal tip midline

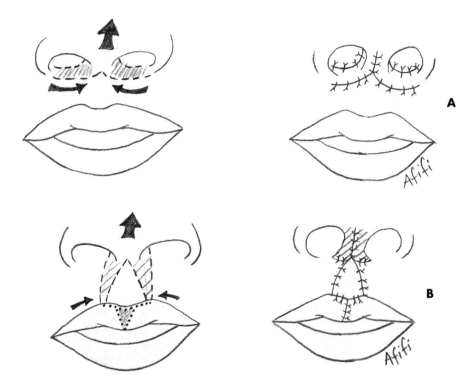

Figure 53-21. Columellar reconstruction: Millard's forked flap procedures. **A,** Utilizing forked flaps previously banked at medial alar bases (shaded). Bipedicled flaps are mobilized via alar base and membranous septum incisions. **B,** Secondary forked flap procedure utilizing tissue from excessively wide prolabium (if present), which is mobilized superiorly into columella (shaded). Any excess width of prolabial vermilion is excised as triangular wedge with vermilion readvancement and closure.

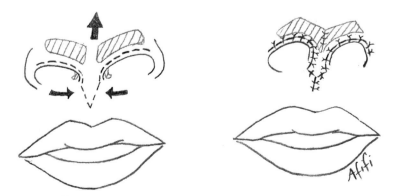

Figure 53-22. Columellar reconstruction: Bardach's central V-to-Y technique. Superiorly based V flap is harvested from excess superior prolabial width and mobilized superiorly to elongate the columella. After suturing the medially mobilized alar cartilages together to increase tip projection, the V-to-Y advancement is sutured along with the bilateral rim incisions.

and bilateral apical incisions to medialize and secure the alar cartilages in the midline, thus reconstructing the columella and creating tip projection. The advantage is the simultaneous nasal and lip correction along with improved vascularity of the prolabial-columellar site; the disadvantage is the apical tip scar.

McComb[27] similarly described a nasal rim incision done at the time of lip adhesion: a V-Y "gull wing" incision enables medial alar cartilage mobilization and suturing, columellar reconstruction, and alar width reduction (Figure 53-23).

Other simultaneous nasal-lip reconstruction methods were made by *Trott*[46] and *Cutting*.[13] Their techniques involve dissecting the prolabial flap superiorly enough to enable retrograde dissection and medial suturing of the alar cartilages. Although no incisions are needed in the tip or columellar-lip junction, the vascularity of the prolabial tip may be more precarious. Cutting[12] advocates presurgical columellar elongation with molding appliances used to align the alveolar segments, retract the premaxilla, and reposition the nasal dome (Figure 53-24). By

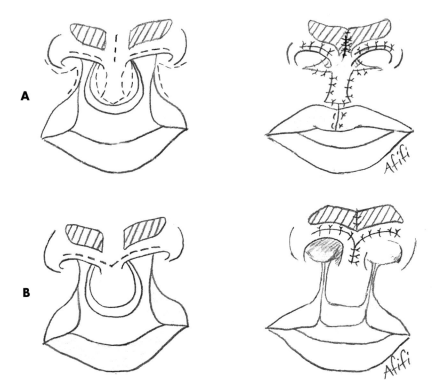

Figure 53-23. Columellar reconstruction contiguous with lip repair: **A,** Mulliken's technique. **B,** McComb's technique.

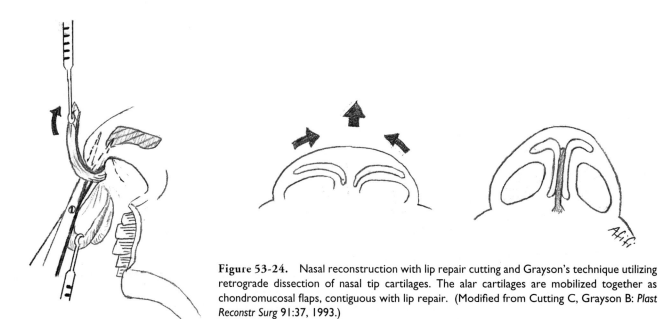

Figure 53-24. Nasal reconstruction with lip repair cutting and Grayson's technique utilizing retrograde dissection of nasal tip cartilages. The alar cartilages are mobilized together as chondromucosal flaps, contiguous with lip repair. (Modified from Cutting C, Grayson B: *Plast Reconstr Surg* 91:37, 1993.)

correcting the alar cartilage position, Cutting asserts that a one-stage nasal-lip reconstruction results in normalized columellar length. A simultaneous gingivoperiosteoplasty is performed. Although contending that the subsequent need for bone grafting has decreased, he admits that the principle disadvantage is the requirement for much presurgical nasoalveolar molding by the orthodontist. Parental commitment to this process is also mandated. Many institutions may find these requirements difficult to fulfill.

Bone Grafting

Nasal base and columellar reconstruction would not be complete without correction of the skeletal platform of the piriform base. For clefting involving the alveolus, after lip and palatal reconstruction and optimal alveolar arch alignment, bone grafting is performed in conjunction with the orthodontic team. This is usually performed at 5 to 12 years of age, classically before the eruption of the permanent canines. The cleft piriform platform is reconstructed; this elevates the depressed alar base and completes the alveolar arch such that future dental alignment is allowed.

Thus the piriform base should be corrected as necessary before any complex tip rhinoplasty. For example, apparent tip projection deficits may simply reflect recessed alar bases resulting from underlying skeletal deficiencies. Further discussion of alveolar bone grafting and subsequent evaluation for possible orthognathic surgery or osteogenic distraction to correct maxillary retrusion is deferred to the appropriate chapter.

OUTCOMES

The postoperative evaluation of patients who have undergone a bilateral cleft lip repair is probably most valuable once multiple institutions join in a combined effort to report, in a standardized format, preoperative diagnoses of the deformity, perioperative anatomic measurements, uniform definitions of associated complications, and length of followup. Combined in a centralized database, the evaluation would be more valuable than reporting each institution's retrospective evaluation. This would avoid results reflecting the institution's own approach and technique, both of which mirror individual training and experience.

Our experience in cleft-related procedures at Loma Linda University Medical Center and Children's Hospital, Loma Linda, California, was reviewed for the last 22 years. A total of 1745 operations were performed on 812 patients, 589 of which were cleft lip procedures. Of these, 189 were lip adhesions, with the remaining 400 being formal repairs. The major complication rate (defined as an unexpected outcome resulting in either a prolonged hospitalization, i.e., more than overnight, or requiring another procedure) was 10.8% when the cases were critically evaluated. Postoperative sequelae included an overall incidence of 3.7% dehiscence (including cases accidentally induced posttrauma by the child after discharge to home),

2.2% fever, and less than 1% infection. With further critical appraisal, the minor complication rate was 9%, but as defined, no clinical sequelae resulted.

The complication rate was not affected by outpatient versus inpatient status, antibiotic usage, or whether the procedure was performed by a supervised resident or an attending surgeon. More importantly, anatomic landmark symmetry was very satisfactory to both the surgeon objectively and patient's family subjectively. Long-term objective assessment is currently underway.

COMPLICATIONS

The following are brief overviews of possible complications of bilateral cleft lip repair, including our institution's utilized prevention protocol.

Wound dehiscence is most likely due to excessive tension on the repair and would explain our slightly higher incidence after an adhesion procedure. Underlying infection or other wound healing inhibiting factors need to be ruled out. Preoperative correction of any premaxillary protrusion is the best prevention, hence our institution's use of primary adhesion procedures. Once present, however, conservative wound care is initiated until all inflammation resolves. After optimizing all preoperative factors, such as nutrition, and correcting any causative factors, re-repair may be attempted.

Wound expansion also results from excess tension, which is likewise best treated by prevention. Once present, we favor allowing the child to develop until the next stage of cleft reconstruction, at which time a scar revision may be performed without requiring a separate anesthetic. As always, exceptions are dictated by individual cases.

Wound infection, relatively less common because of the face's excellent blood supply, may occur as a result of contamination of the site, inadvertent trauma from an active infant whose postoperative lip sensation may be decreased, and any local inflammation that may be induced from buried sutures. We avoid overvigorous wound cleansing, which may disrupt the delicately sutured area. This may be particularly true when hydrogen peroxide is used repeatedly on chromic suture closures. Occasional gentle cleaning is done, after which bacitracin may be applied. When present, local wound infections are treated by removal of any offending suture and by conservative local care. Unless mitigated by rare occurrences of cellulitis, systemic antibiotics are usually not indicated.

Premaxillary malposition, such as tilting or retrusion, may result after repair. Again, prevention of excessive tension is a critical deterrent. If premaxillary protrusion is anticipated and being corrected, concomitant acrylic expansion plates or splints may be used to offset possible overly restrictive anterior forces on the premaxilla. Certainly, recognized maxillary retrusion resulting from aberrant growth associated with these cleft deformities may be corrected by Le Fort I advancement osteotomy or osteogenic distraction when age appropriate, usually during the early teenage period.

Whistle deformity refers to vermilion deficiency and possible associated retraction along the line of the lip repair. It may be avoided by the full use of the lateral segment's orbicularis muscle–vermilion mucosal flap in its midline apposition to the contralateral side. A secure closure is critical lest a muscle dehiscence occur underneath the vermilion-mucosal closure, resulting in this deformity. This would also result in an absent or deficient philtral tubercle, often a tell-tale indication of a cleft lip repair. The correction involves surgical reapproximation of the vermilion-muscle-mucosal subunits. We close the vermilion–wet roll junction with mattress sutures to ensure wound edge eversion.

Lip length abnormality or asymmetry is best avoided by precise intraoperative measurement of important anatomic distances, such as Cupid's bow low point to high point or alar base-Cupid's bow high point distances. It may also result from lack of adequate tissue fixation. For example, excess ipsilateral traction from inadequate mobilization may produce asymmetry. An excessively vertically long lip may result from inadequate midline tissue fixation to the anterior nasal spine, enabling tissue prolapse over the premaxilla. At the procedure's end, all measurements should be as desired; no allowance should be made for the healing process to contract or relax a scar to enable its alignment or symmetry.

Lateral maxillary segment collapse medially and posterior to the premaxilla may result if premaxillary protrusion is not correctly treated along with the lip repair. Prevention and/or treatment with orthopedic manipulation, such as via acrylic plates or other palatal shelf expanders, are options as discussed. For those with a great disparity between the alveolar segments, traction on the lip elements should be accompanied by simultaneous intraoral protheses to counteract the soft tissue envelope restriction and better control alveolar alignment.

Nasal deformity evaluation should be concomitant with cleft lip assessment. Recognizing that the degree and timing of reconstruction varies with surgeon and institution, the ultimate goals should still be similar: symmetry of anatomic distances, adequate tip projection, adequate bony platform, and normalization of soft tissue–cartilaginous framework. Any surgical plan not optimizing such parameters is inadequate. Dependent on deformity and patient, any resultant irregularities should be repaired either with the next procedure or more formally in the teenage years.

SUMMARY

The optimal repair of a bilateral cleft lip deformity presents a challenging and fascinating dilemma to the plastic surgeon because of the multiple involved components and their presentation both passively and dynamically. The ultimate result depends on the surgeon's understanding of the defect itself and the options by which to repair it. Each surgeon may then best choose the methods to reconstruct the anomaly and optimize the outcome. Thus the *individualized approach* is more important than repetitively

duplicating a methodology, thus the beauty and evolution of this field.

The surgical techniques usually involve either a straight line closure or incorporate a Z-plasty. Straight line closure has been advocated by Barsky, Veau, Cronin, Manchester, and Black. The Z-plasty method has been utilized in the lower lip (by Bauer, Trusler, Tondra, Berkeley, and those using Tennison modifications), or in the upper lip (by Wynn, Millard, and variants by Mullliken and Noordhoff). A combined upper and lower lip Z-plasty was proposed by Skoog, now rarely used. For rare cases of near-absent prolabial segments, a primary Abbe flap is an option, although with limited application for primary repair.

Our institution attempts to combine the best features of previously proposed repair methods, recognizing that each surgeon evolves a technique based on the successes of his or her colleagues and that alterations are used for individual circumstances. Thus some features are analogous to those presented by Veau, Millard, Manchester, Black, Mulliken, Randall, and Noordhoff. Our goal is to symmetrically reconstruct the lip, ensuring *objective precision* by intraoperative measurements, and simultaneously correct the associated nasal deformity's basic components. As with other authors, we perform columellar lengthening, alveolar bone grafting, and a more formal cleft rhinoplasty, as indicated, in subsequent procedures.

We are currently recording our method's preoperative and postoperative anthropometric measurements to more precisely follow and report the long-term static and dynamic results of our technique. Along with many others, our aim is to continue the legacy of building on the surgical feats of our forebears in the ongoing evolution of bilateral cleft lip management.

ACKNOWLEDGMENTS

The first author is indebted to my mentors at the Hospital of the University of Pennsylvania: Drs. Scott Bartlett, Don LaRossa, David Low, Peter Randall, and Linton Whitaker, in propagating my love of craniofacial surgery. I am grateful to the friendship and support of Dr. Robert Hardesty in enabling me to pursue this love and Dr. Don LaRossa for being a model teacher, surgeon, and deeply caring friend.

REFERENCES

1. Antia NH: Primary Abbe flap in bilateral cleft lip, *Br J Plast Surg* 12:215, 1973.
2. Atherton JD: The natural history of the bilateral cleft, *Angle Orthod* 44:269, 1974.
3. Bardach J, Salyer K (eds): *Surgical techniques in cleft lip and palate,* St Louis, 1991, Mosby.
4. Bauer TB, Trusler HM, Tondra JM: Bauer, Trusler, and Tondra's method of cheilorrhaphy in bilateral lip. In *Cleft lip and palate,* Boston, 1971, Little, Brown.

5. Berkeley WT: The concepts of unilateral repair applied to bilateral clefts of the lip and nose, *Plast Reconstr Surg* 27:505, 1961.

6. Black PW, Scheflan M: Bilateral cleft lip repair: putting it all together, *Ann Plast Surg* 12:118, 1984.

7. Brown JB: Double clefts of the lip, *Surg Gynecol Obstet* 85:20, 1947.

8. Byrd SH: Cleft lip I: Primary deformities, *Selected Readings in Plastic Surgery* 8:1-37, 1997.

9. Chung CS, Myriathoppoulos NC: Racial and prenatal factors in major congenital malformations, *Am J Hum Genet* 20:44, 1968.

10. Cronin TD: Surgery of the double cleft lip and protruding premaxilla, *Plast Reconstr Surg* 19:389, 1957.

11. Cronin TD, Cronin ED, Roper P, et al: Bilateral clefts. In McCarthy JG (ed): *Plastic surgery,* Philadelphia, 1990, WB Saunders.

12. Cutting CB: Primary cleft lip and nose repair. In Aston SJ, Beasley RW, Thorne CM (eds): *Grabb and Smith's plastic surgery,* ed 5, Philadelphia, 1997, Lippincott-Raven.

13. Cutting C, Grayson B: The prolabial unwinding flap method for one-stage repair of bilateral cleft lip, nose, and alveolus, *Plast Reconstr Surg* 91:37, 1993.

14. Franco P: *Traite des hernies,* Lyon, France, 1561, Thiebaud Payen.

15. Fraser FC: The genetics of cleft lip and palate, *Am J Hum Genet* 22:336, 1970.

16. Georgiade NG, Mason R, Riefkohl R, et al: Preoperative positioning of the protruding premaxilla in the bilateral cleft lip patient, *Plast Reconstr Surg* 83:32, 1989.

17. Georgiade NG, Latham RA: Maxillary arch alignment in the bilateral cleft lip and palate infant, using the pinned coaxial screw appliance, *Plast Reconstr Surg* 56:52, 1975.

18. Habib Z: Genetic counselling and genetics of cleft lip and cleft palate, *Obstet Gynecol Surv* 33:441, 1978.

19. Harkins CS, Berlin A, Harding RL, et al: A classification of cleft lip and cleft palate, *Plast Reconstr Surg* 29:31, 1962.

20. Honig CA: The operative treatment of bilateral complete clefts of the primary and secondary palate in the first year of life. *Early treatment of cleft lip and palate,* International Symposium, University of Zurich Dental Institute, Berne, Switzerland, 1964, Hans Huber.

21. Jones MC: Facial clefting: etiology and developmental pathogenesis, *Clin Plast Surg* 20:599, 1993.

22. Kernahan DA: On cleft lip and palate classification, *Plast Reconstr Surg* 51:578, 1973.

23. LaRossa D: Personal communication, Plastic Surgery Division, Hospital of the University of Pennsylvania, 1997-1999.

24. Manchester WM: The repair of double cleft lip as part of an integrated program, *Plast Reconstr Surg* 45:205, 1970.

25. Marcks KM, Trevaskis AE, Payne MJ: Bilateral cleft lip repair, *Plast Reconstr Surg* 19:401, 1957.

26. Marsh JL, Martin DS: Bilateral cleft lip: an unorthodox management, *Clin Plast Surg* 20:661, 1993.

27. McComb H: Primary repair of the bilateral cleft lip nose: a 15 year review and a new treatment plan, *Plast Reconstr Surg* 86:882, 1990.

28. Millard DR Jr: *Cleft craft,* vols 1-3, Boston, 1976, 1977, 1980, Little, Brown.

29. Mohler LR: Unilateral cleft lip repair, *Plast Reconstr Surg* 80:511, 1987.

30. Mulliken JB: Primary repair of the bilateral cleft lip and nasal deformity. In Georgiade GS, Riefkohl R, Levin LS (eds): *Plastic, maxillofacial and reconstructive surgery,* ed 3, Philadelphia, 1997, Williams & Wilkins.

31. Mulliken JB: Bilateral complete cleft lip and nasal deformity: an anthropometric analysis of staged versus synchronous repair, *Plast Reconstr Surg* 96:9, 1995.

32. Mulliken JB: Correction of the bilateral cleft lip nasal deformity: evolution of a surgical concept, *Cleft Palate Craniofac J* 29:540, 1992.

33. Mulliken JB: Principles and techniques of bilateral complete cleft lip repair, *Plast Reconstr Surg* 75:477, 1985.

34. Neel JV: A study of major congenital defects in Japanese infants, *Am J Hum Genet* 10:398, 1958.

35. Noordhoff MS: Bilateral cleft lip. In Cohen M (ed): *Mastery of plastic and reconstructive surgery,* Boston, 1994, Little, Brown.

36. Pool R: Tissue mobilization with preoperative lip taping, *Oper Tech Plast Reconstr Surg* 2:155, 1995.

37. Randall P: Lip adhesion, *Oper Tech Plast Reconstr Surg* 2:164, 1995.

38. Randall P, Whitaker LA, LaRossa D: The importance of muscle reconstruction in primary and secondary cleft lip repair, *Plast Reconstr Surg* 54:316, 1974.

39. Rutrick R, Black PW, Jurkiewicz MJ: Bilateral cleft lip and palate: presurgical treatment, *Ann Plast Surg* 12:105, 1984.

40. Rutrick RE, Cohen SR, Black PW, et al: Presurgical orthopedic management of the unilateral cleft lip and palate newborn patient, *Oper Tech Plast Reconstr Surg* 2:159, 1995.

41. Schultz LW: Bilateral cleft lips, *Plast Reconstr Surg* 1:338, 1946.

42. Schwartz S, Kapala JT, Rajchgot H, et al: Accurate and systematic numerical recording system for the identification of various types of lip and maxillary clefts (RPL system), *Cleft Palate Craniofac J* 30:330, 1993.

43. Skoog T: The management of the bilateral cleft of the primary palate, *Plast Reconstr Surg* 35:34, 1965.

44. Stark RB: The pathogenesis of harelip and cleft palate, *Plast Reconstr Surg* 13:20, 1954.

45. Tennison CW: The repair of the unilateral cleft lip by stencil method, *Plast Reconstr Surg* 9:115, 1952.

46. Trott JA, Mohan N: A preliminary report on one stage open tip rhinoplasty at the time of lip repair in bilateral cleft lip and palate: the Alor Setar experience, *Br J Plast Surg* 46:215, 1993.

47. Veau V: *Bec-de-Lievre.* Paris, 1938, Masson.

48. Wat L: Personal communication, Department of Anesthesiology, Loma Linda University Medical Center, 1999.

49. Wilson MEAC: A 10 year survey of cleft lip and cleft palate in the southwestern region, *Br J Plast Surg* 25:224, 1972.

50. Witt PD, Moon W, Hardesty RA, et al: *Infectious complications in the cleft lip and palate population.* Presented at American College of Surgeons annual meeting, Santa Barbara, Calif, 1993 (abstract).

51. Wynn SK: Lateral flap cleft surgery technique, *Plast Reconstr Surg* 26:509, 1960.

Cleft Palate

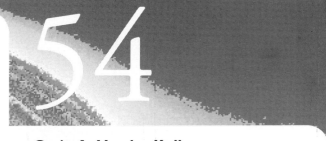

Craig A. Vander Kolk

INTRODUCTION

Cleft palate is a relatively common facial disorder characterized by a separation of the palatal segments with a resultant open communication of the mouth to the nose. The separation of the palate results in difficulty eating, speaking, hearing, and with the development of the teeth. Treatment of the cleft palate seeks to correct the deformity and normalize function. The purpose of this chapter is to define this deformity, outline goals of treatment, review techniques for repair, and examine outcomes in accomplishing the goals of therapy.

Cleft palate can occur as an isolated cleft palate or as a cleft lip and cleft palate. Although the patient often is diagnosed as having a cleft palate, the isolated cleft palate is genetically and morphologically different from a cleft lip with a cleft palate. The former has an incidence of 1:2000 and is equal cross all ethnic backgrounds. Cleft lip with cleft palate has an incidence of 1:1000 in Caucasians; is relatively infrequent in African-Americans, at 1:2000; and is more frequent in Asians, occurring almost once in 500 births. An additional difference between the two is that isolated cleft palate generally has a much higher incidence of associated anomalies, resulting in a diagnosis of a syndrome in almost one third to one half of patients. This is distinctly dissimilar to cleft lip with cleft palate, in which it is unusual to have other associated anomalies or an identifiable syndrome.

Cleft palate alone can be further classified as cleft of the soft palate or cleft of the entire soft and hard palates. Between each of these, there are various degrees of the deformity. A complete cleft palate includes the hard and soft palates and extends from the incisive foramen posteriorly. Soft palate clefts can be of the entire soft palate or a portion of the soft palate, and in some instances, a submucous cleft can also occur. In a submucous cleft the oral and nasal mucosa are intact but there is a cleft of the muscles as they insert into the back of the either side of the palate, which is typical of all clefts of the palate. Typically, these patients have a bifid uvula and a notch at the back of the hard palate.

Cleft lip with cleft palate is traditionally separated into right, left, and bilateral cleft lip with cleft palate. This chapter does not focus on the alveolar cleft, or primary palatal cleft, because this is covered in Chapter 55. Rarely patients have an isolated cleft lip or cleft lip and primary palate clefts have an associated partial cleft of the palate, such as the cleft of a soft palate.

INDICATIONS

Children born with a cleft palate and/or cleft lip and cleft palate need to be initially evaluated with a full history and physical examination to rule out associated anomalies. They frequently have difficulty feeding because they are not able to generate negative pressure in sucking. Formula must be delivered to the mouth, which they can subsequently swallow. Initially regurgitation is common; however, this usually improves with time. Options for feeding include everything from special nipples to enlargement of the nipple to a squeeze bottle to a Haberman Feeder, all the way to nasogastric tube feeding and a gastrostomy. The latter two are reserved for those patients who typically demonstrate neuromuscular abnormalities in addition to the cleft palate because most infants with cleft palate are able to feed when the formula is delivered to them for swallowing.

The most common associated anomaly with cleft palate would be the Pierre Robin sequence. This is defined as a patient who exhibits a small mandible, glossoptosis, and a cleft palate. Typically the palatal cleft is U-shaped as opposed to a more V-shaped cleft in a nonsyndromic or nonassociated patient. These Robin children often have difficulty with breathing and maintaining an adequate airway. Initial treatment for problems with breathing is to place the patient in the prone position. Usually the neuromuscular control improves within a few days to weeks, and airway maintenance becomes stable enough to prevent the need for adjunctive techniques (nasogastric tube or gastrostomy tube) and, as a last resort, a tracheostomy. Occasionally, further intervention is necessary. More recently, I have utilized distraction osteogenesis to

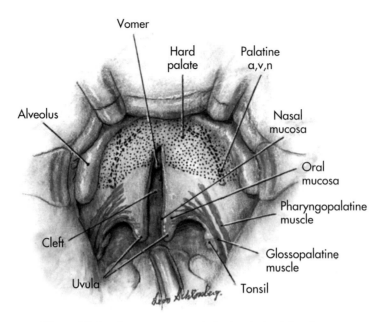

Figure 54-1. Important anatomic landmarks in cleft palate.

advance the mandible and prevent a tracheostomy or remove one placed at a young age. This procedure has been performed in seven patients under the age of 4 months and has been highly successful.

The goal of cleft palate treatment is to separate the oral and nasal cavities. Although this is not absolutely necessary for feeding, it is advantageous to normalize feeding and decrease regurgitation and nasal irritation. More important than repairing the oral and nasal mucosa is the repositioning of the soft palate musculature to anatomically recreate the palate so that normal speech can be established (Figure 54-1). The goal of separating the oral and nasal mucosa is sometimes, if not always, completely achieved. When incompletely closed, fistula formation occurs, which can lead to regurgitation and nasal irritation with sinusitis. Rarely, a large fistula can result in speech abnormalities.

While striving to separate the oral and nasal cavities and promote normal speech, another goal of palate repair is to minimize restriction of growth of the maxilla and in both sagittal and transverse dimensions. Although limitations in growth can be corrected orthodontically and surgically, every effort should be made to minimize this as much as possible.

It is believed that palate repair with repositioning of the palatal musculature is advantageous to eustachian tube function and ultimately to hearing. Because the levator veli palatini and tensor veli palatini have their origin along the eustachian tube,[22] repositioning improves function of these muscles; improves ventilation of the middle ear; and decreases serous otitis, which further decreases the incidence of hearing abnormality. Palate repair alone does not usually completely correct this dysfunction, and additional therapy frequently

includes antibiotics and placement of pneumonostomy tubes as necessary.

OPERATIONS

There are a multitude of techniques to close a cleft palate and promote normal function.[14,29,40] However, generally speaking, techniques can be divided into the types of flaps that are used. The flaps can be bipedicle flaps, as in a von Langenbeck's repair,[42] or the flaps can be divided anteriorly based on a single pedicle of the greater palatine vessels (as proposed by Bardach). A Veau-Wardill-Kilner type of repair often uses four flaps to accomplish the palatal closure.[20,41,43] Two anterior palatal flaps close off the region of the incisive foramen while the posterior palatal flaps are pushed back to lengthen the palate. Finally, the most recent advance in palate repair has been the Furlow's or double-opposing Z-plasty, in which Z-plasty principles are utilized to lengthen the palate.[16]

Each of the techniques attempts to recreate normal anatomic reconstruction, including the nasal layer, oral layer, and muscle layer. The latter occurs after division of the abnormal insertion of the muscles from the back of the hard palate and repositioning to recreate the levator sling across the midline.[8] Vomer flaps may be required to assist in closure of the nasal lining in wide and bilateral clefts. My preferred technique is traditionally a von Langenbeck's procedure[42] with extensive

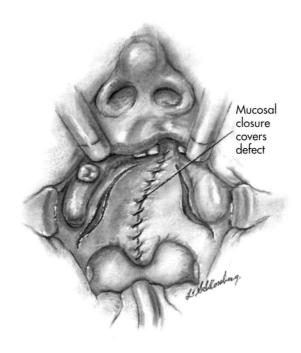

Figure 54-2. Appearance of closure with von Langenbeck's repair of a unilateral cleft lip and palate.

dissection and reconstruction of the muscle layer (Figure 54-2). Occasionally, one flap needs to be completely detached anteriorly to allow adequate rotation for complete anterior closure. This is most common in wide unilateral clefts. Bilateral clefts almost always need vomer flaps for nasal closure to obtain anatomic oral and nasal mucosal reconstruction. In wide bilateral clefts, a two-flap technique is needed to complete the anterior closure.

Furlow's double-opposing Z-plasty appears to lengthen the palate at the time of surgery.[15] There has been some recent suggestion that there has been improvement in speech utilizing this technique[32]; however, several authors have also reported that extensive dissection of the muscle with an intravelar veloplasty results in similar speech outcomes. Difficulty with Furlow's repair can be fistula formation secondary to a tight anterior closure because the width of the flap closure is sacrificed for additional length.

AUTHOR'S TECHNIQUE

Timing of repair is determined by the extent of the cleft, with an overall goal of performing the repair as early as possible. Although several reports have suggested an advantage with cleft palate repair in patients younger than 6 month of age, it appears to be too early to make this a routine part of cleft palate care.[13,44] Complete clefts are traditionally repaired at 9 months of age, and incomplete clefts at 6 months of age, unless they are associated with a Pierre Robin sequence. Mild Pierre Robin sequence patients have clefts repaired at 9 months, and those with a more severe deformity at 12 months.

The patient is evaluated by the multidisciplinary cleft team because these are the patients that benefit most from this interdisciplinary approach. At the time of the multidisciplinary team evaluation, the ears are evaluated with a complete audiogram. If there are significant hearing abnormalities, flat tympanograms, or history and physical findings of chronic fluid, then the otolaryngologist usually recommends placement of pressure equalization (PE) tubes at the time of cleft palate repair. Dental and orthodontic services inform the family of the need for good oral hygiene because orthodontic intervention may be necessary in the future. Genetic evaluation is accomplished to rule out any other associated syndromes or associated anomalies. Informed consent is achieved by drawing out the operation so that the family understands the type of procedure being performed, along with the risks and complications.

The patient is admitted to the same-day care center after appropriate preoperative testing has been completed and anesthesia has seen the patient. Typically these patients can undergo preoperative sedation unless there is history of difficulty with the airway. The patient is taken into the operating room and placed under anesthesia. PE tubes are traditionally placed before the endotracheal intubation. A Reye tube is used for tracheal intubation because it can be positioned out of the field of view for the repair. Once the patient is appropriately under anesthesia, antibiotics are given. Typically this consists of cefazolin (Kefzol) or penicillin.

The table is turned 90 degrees, and the patient is positioned at the end of the operating table with the adjustable headrest. A roll is placed beneath the shoulders. Using the anesthesiologist's laryngoscope, the initial areas of incision are injected with 1% lidocaine with epinephrine 1:100,000. The patient undergoes a standard preparation with povidone iodine (Betadine) solution and is appropriately draped.

A Dingman mouth gag is carefully inserted, with care taken to preserve the position of the endotracheal tube and not overly compress the tongue. Without having to wait (because the previous injection had already been accomplished), the margins of the cleft can be incised. This typically begins at the junction of the hard and soft palates and extends posteriorly to the uvula (Figure 54-3, *A*). Care is taken to extend the incision anteriorly throughout the entire margin of the cleft, leaving a small cuff nasal mucosa to facilitate nasal lining repair. The relaxing incisions are then performed from approximately 1 cm behind the greater tuberosity of the alveolus. The incision is brought up toward the greater tuberosity, deviating toward the midline so that the attached gingiva is not incised. The incision then comes forward to within 1.5 cm of the alveolus in a complete cleft lip and cleft palate. In cleft palate alone, the incision is brought to approximately 1 cm in front of the anterior extent of the cleft. Mucoperiosteal flaps are then elevated on the hard palate (Figure 54-3, *B*), and the dissection is then extended posteriorly, with care taken to preserve the greater palatine vessel at the back of the hard palate. With elevation of the mucoperiosteum, the posterior palate can be easily visualized and the muscle incised and dissected free (Figure 54-3, *C*). Dissection in the space of Ernst is carefully accomplished and only the

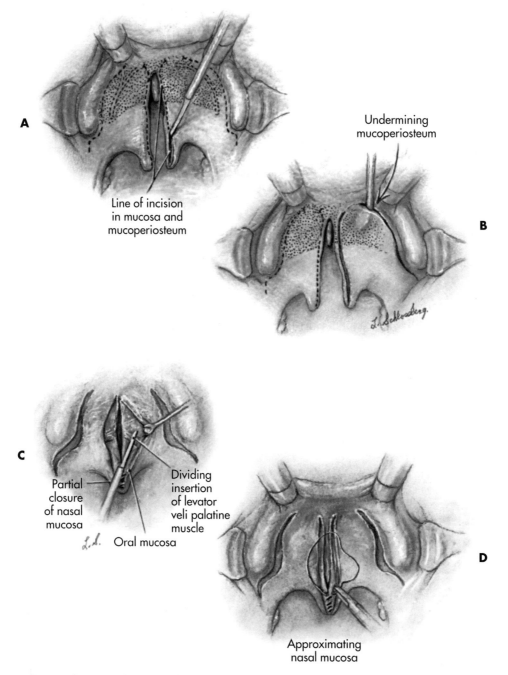

Figure 54-3. von Langenbeck's repair. **A,** Proposed incisions at the margins of the cleft and for lateral relaxing incisions. **B,** Undermining mucoperiosteum begins anteriorly, away from the neurovascular bundle. **C,** Division of the abnormally inserting levator veli palatini muscle. **D,** Nasal mucosal closure with 4-0 or 5-0 Chromic.

Continued

minimum amount performed to prevent injury to the muscles. The posterior-lateral hard palate can then be identified. The oral mucosa and submucosa are dissected off of the muscle in the region of the soft palate. The nasal mucosa is closely adherent to the underlying uvula muscle and is only dissected for approximately 2 mm.[17,18]

A vomer flap can be used to assist in closure of the nasal layer or to rotate anteriorly for alveolar closure. Most commonly it is incised in the midline in bilateral clefts, elevated bilaterally, and then reflected laterally to allow repair to the cuff of nasal mucosa.

Repair begins with the nasal mucosa (Figure 54-3, *D*).

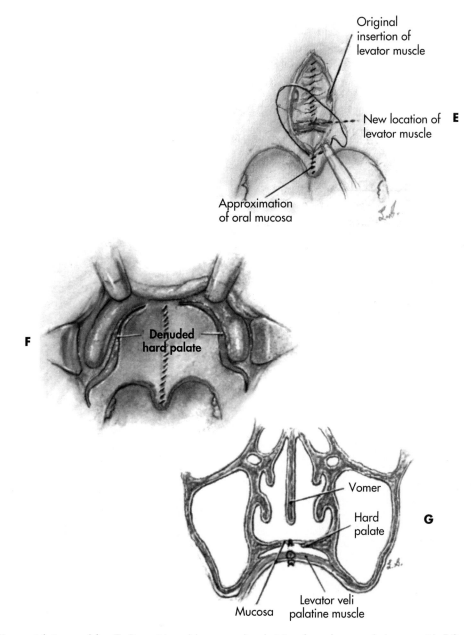

Figure 54-3, cont'd. **E,** Repositioned levator veli palatini and nasal mucosal closure with 5-0 PDS. **F,** Oral mucosal closure (ideally this should be horizontal or vertical mattress suture) with 4-0 or 5-0 Vicryl. Oral mucoperiosteal flaps are advanced medially, leaving a lateral defect that closes in 7 to 10 days. **G,** As the oral mucoperiosteal flaps fall caudally during the repair, less medial advancement is required.

Chromic can be used because it is easy to tie and lasts for a sufficient period of time to allow healing. 4-0 Chromic on a G-2 needle (Ethicon, Inc., Somerville, NJ) allows mucosal closure in the narrow spaces of the anterior palatal cleft defect. A Castroviejo needle driver helps to delicately manipulate the tissues in such a confined operative field. The nasal mucosal repair begins anteriorly and precedes posteriorly to the back of the hard palate, with a running type of suture. The soft palate portion of the closure begins posteriorly and proceeds anteriorly and incorporates a portion of the muscle in the anterior portion of the repair. The muscle layer is repaired in a reoriented position with 5-0 PDS using a simple or sometimes a horizontal mattress suture (Figure 54-3, *E*). In wide clefts the oral mucosa and the muscle are approximated with a horizontal, tension-reducing suture just behind the hard palate. Finally, the oral mucosa is repaired with horizontal or preferably vertical mattress sutures (Figure 54-3, *F*). The keys to successful closure are well-vascularized tissue and flaps and a tension-free closure with broad apposition of surface area. Careful planning and dissection of the flaps provide good vascularity.[28] Adequate mobilization of the flaps decreases tension. In addition, the change in orientation of the palatal mucoperiosteal flaps from vertical to horizontal brings the flaps closer together and decreases tension (Figure 54-3, *G*). Finally, mattress sutures on the oral side make for a watertight closure with good surface approximation.

Very wide clefts can be difficult to close. Clefts that are 1.8 to 2.0 cm wide at the junction of the hard and soft palates need an alternative approach for repair. The first goal is to get the soft palate closed. The nasal lining can be released from the back of the hard palate to help with closure. This is followed by using one of the mucoperiosteal flaps (modified Bardach's technique) and pushing it back to support the soft palate closure. The anterior palatal defect can then be closed at a later date, usually when the alveolar segments have medialized. With these wide clefts, careful approximation and eversion of the mucosa is necessary because the nasal mucosa cannot be closed and a watertight closure decreases the incidence of fistula formation.

Furlow's double-opposing Z-plasty is an important alternative to the extended or modified intravelar veloplasty highlighted above (Figure 54-4, *A* to *C*). I have performed this technique on a number of occasions and found it to lengthen the palate and provide good speech. It is more time consuming and difficult in wider clefts and younger patients. There appears to be a learning curve to the technique because slight modifications have been reported that are helpful for closing a wide variety of clefts.[16,21]

OUTCOMES

The goals of cleft palate repair are usually accomplished with a well-executed surgical repair. This is particularly true for separation of the oral and nasal cavity and limiting fistula formation. Cohen[10] reported that fistula formation was surgeon dependent and to a lesser extent dependent on technique and type of cleft. The incidence of fistula formation has been reported to be between 0% and 34%.[1] The author's

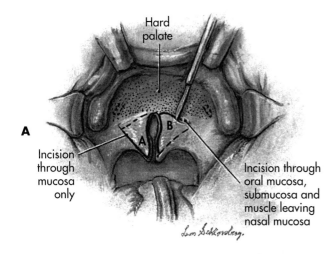

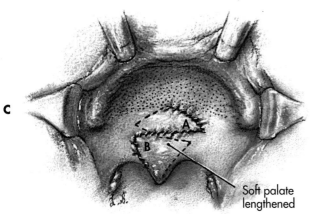

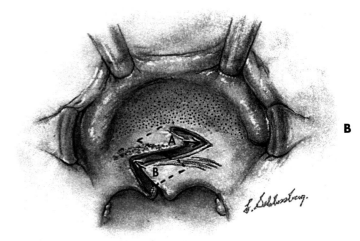

Figure 54-4. Furlow's double-opposing Z-plasty cleft palate repair. **A,** Incisions for Furlow's double-opposing Z-plasty cleft palate repair (dotted lines demonstrate nasal mucosal incisions). Muscle is carried with oral and nasal flap that is incised from back of hard palate. **B,** Repositioned oral mucosal flaps and nasal flaps lengthen the soft palate as a function of the 60-degree Z-plasty. **C,** Closure of oral mucosal can be a running 4-0 or 5-0 Vicryl after flaps are tacked into position with interrupted sutures. Muscle is repositioned with the reoriented oral and nasal flaps.

review of 100 consecutive cleft palate repairs following the protocol described demonstrated a fistula rate of 4% and a partial dehiscence (small separation of the repair at the uvula) of 3%. Most of the fistulas were small and were easily repaired during subsequent surgical procedures. Ease of secondary repair is a consequence of my preferred technique, which limits the creation of flaps and preserves tissue on either side of the midline repair where the fistula occurs. Local rotation flaps that are not extensively scarred and are well vascularized can be used in the fistula repair. Small anterior fistulas or areas near the alveolus that open up are not repaired because they are rarely symptomatic and are addressed at the time of bone grafting.[7,9,31,35]

The most important outcomes in cleft palate repair are the establishment of normal speech and hearing. This is best accomplished for each individual patient by the frequent monitoring of the patient's development through a multidisciplinary team clinic.[4-6] Once the palate repair has been performed and PE tubes placed, frequent evaluation is necessary so that adjunctive measures can be undertaken when speech abnormalities are identified. Early speech intervention is advantageous for all cleft palate patients because almost all of them demonstrate some language delays and articulation errors on careful evaluation.

Despite a well-executed palatoplasty, careful speech follow-up, and early intervention, 10% to 15% of patients will develop velopharyngeal dysfunction. As reported by Witt,[46] this appears to be independent of the type of repair performed. It may, however, be dependent on the underlying diagnosis of the patient because syndromic patients, such as those with Pierre Robin sequence, have a higher incidence. The indications, techniques, and outcomes of treatment for velopharyngeal insufficiency are discussed at length in Chapter 56.

Maturation and development of the cleft palate patient confounds the determination of outcomes in palate surgery. This is particularly true in regards to growth of the palate and maxilla. Although the pressures associated with a tight cleft lip repair probably affect midface growth more than palate repair, this must still be considered in palatoplasty. Most complete cleft lip and palate patients will have some alveolar collapse, resulting in a crossbite that will require orthodontic intervention. The use of a vomer flap in closure of the anterior palate has been implicated in causing growth disturbances. Although this has been challenged in long-term studies, such as those by the Oslo Cleft Lip and Palate Team,[36,37] I prefer not to use it in closing the anterior palate based on anecdotal experience reviewing multiple patients treated with this technique. The anterior opening that frequently results from the technique listed above is symptomatic for only a short period of time, and parents rarely report that it is of major consequence for the child.[11]

Complications related to cleft palate repair are generally infrequent. Bleeding requiring reoperation occurred in only one patient in the 100 consecutive palate repairs that I reviewed. Infection was never noted despite operating in the mouth and probably in spite of the perioperative antibiotics given to all patients. Airway compromise occurred in one

patient in my experience of 250 palatoplasties. This occurred in a moderately severe Pierre Robin sequence child repaired at the age of 12 months. Although careful monitoring is recommended in these patients and a tongue stitch of 2-0 silk is placed if anesthesia reports that the intubation was extremely difficult, the timing of repair is not drastically altered.

Definitive outcomes in cleft treatment are important but have been difficult to obtain for a multitude of reasons.[3,24,30,38,39] It is important to keep in mind all of the goals listed above for the treating physician to provide an environment that promotes successful outcome. With this in mind, the most controversial and important aspect of cleft palate repair is obtaining normal speech. This is where the most work has been done to answer the question of which is the best technique for palate repair.[19,23,25] McWilliams[26] reported that success rates ranged from 21% to 95%, with an average of 29%. The fact that there are so many articles on this subject implies that there is no perfect answer. This may be because there are some inherent abnormalities that are beyond the control of the treating physician. This would include patients with syndromes and the type of cleft being repaired. In addition, it is important to keep in mind that postoperative therapy plays a role in obtaining good speech.

The recent article by the surgeons from the Children's Hospital of Philadelphia highlight this issue.[21] In this study, the authors' extensive experience (390 patients) with Furlow's double-opposing Z-plasty is summarized. They have 181 patients who are available for speech analysis after 209 patients are separated out for a multitude of reasons. The modifications that the authors describe are helpful, and it is interesting to note that they utilize lateral relaxing incisions to assist in hard palate closure in addition to their use of the double-opposing Z-plasty for the soft palate.

The results they report are excellent because they perform or recommend secondary surgery of a posterior pharyngeal flap in only 7.2% of the patients. In addition, they report that, although there was a trend toward better results with earlier surgery (before 6 months) and poorer results depending on the cleft type (Veau classes I and II—clefts of the secondary palate), these findings where not statistically significant. Most importantly, a significant number of patients had borderline speech. Furlow[16] in his discussion points out that 18% of patients have "close but not quite" and "sometimes but not always" normal speech. It is this group of patients that highlights the difficulty of determining outcomes in surgery. Although the authors attempt to further elucidate the issue by using the Pittsburgh Weighted Values for Speech Symptoms Associated with VPI and separate out nasal emission and articulation errors as a component of abnormal speech, it still provides an unclear picture. Are these (18%) patients the same ones upon whom other surgeons over the years have performed secondary surgery and therefore have reported a higher incidence of a need for pharyngoplasty? Are these a part of the same subset of patients in whom the Philadelphia group previously reported a decrease of velopharyngeal dysfunction from 50% to 20% in their first report on the outcome of the use of the double-opposing Z-plasty in contrast to previous techniques? McWilliams[27] reports that the group from Philadelphia in their early series performed pharyngeal flaps for patients with mild hypernasality. It is difficult to tell definitively, but it appears that they have found a significant improvement in their care of patients with cleft palate. However, any reference to other procedures of the past must be carefully done. In fact, the authors themselves have in the past pointed out the importance of doing a randomized prospective study.

In the same issue of the journal *Plastic and Reconstructive Surgery,* Schendel[34] reports a success rate of 90.8% with Delaire's palatoplasty, a modified intravelar veloplasty.[12] Although the follow-up time for this paper is short compared with that of the Philadelphia paper, it echoes the report of several surgeons at the Plastic Surgery Educational Foundation Symposium on the long-term results of cleft treatment in 1997 that extensive surgical reorientation of the soft palate musculature is the key to a successful palate repair. Only a well-controlled prospective outcome study will finally answer this question.

Although outcomes in cleft surgery are difficult to obtain for the reasons noted above, they are important for the future of these patients.[33] When insurance companies are universally questioning care practices of health care providers and surgeons, the only way to counteract their control is to be proactive and search for answers that will establish the best treatment. This will then ensure patients access to multidisciplinary team and the established treatments that maximize the outcome. The future in this regard is bright, with the current multiinstitutional outcome study supported by the National Institutes of Health and fostered by the American Cleft Palate Association.[2]

SUMMARY

Cleft palate is a complex problem that requires meticulous attention to detail to obtain the best possible result. Cleft palate teams must provide multidisciplinary care and monitor the functional outcomes of the surgery to achieve all of the goals of repair. Although a well-controlled randomized prospective study is important to advance our understanding of treatment, each surgeon needs to be cognizant of the needs and results of treatment to help cleft children become successful, well-adjusted adults.[45]

REFERENCES

1. Abyholm RE, Borchgrevink HHC, Eskeland G: Palatal fistulae following cleft palate surgery, *Scand J Plast Reconstr Surg* 13:295, 1979.

2. American Cleft Palate-Craniofacial Association: Parameters for the evaluation and treatment of patients with cleft lip/palate or other craniofacial anomalies, *Cleft Palate Craniofac J* 30: (suppl 1):S1, 1993.

3. Asher-McDade C, Brattstrom V, Dahl E, et al: A six-center international study of treatment outcome in patients with clefts of the lip and palate: Part 4. Assessment of nasolabial appearance, *Cleft Palate Craniofac J* 29:409, 1992.

4. Bardach J, Morris H, Olin W, et al: Late results of multidisciplinary management of unilateral cleft lip and palate, *Ann Plast Surg* 12:235, 1984.

5. Bardach J, Morris HL, Olin WH: Late results of primary veloplasty: the Marburg Project, *Plast Reconstr Surg* 73:207, 1984.

6. Bardach J, Morris HL, Olin WH, et al: Results of multidisciplinary management of bilateral cleft lip and palate at the Iowa Cleft Palate Center, *Plast Reconstr Surg* 89:419, 1992.

7. Bergland O, Semb G, Abyholm FE: Elimination of the residual alveolar cleft by secondary bone grafting and subsequent orthodontic treatment, *Cleft Palate J* 23:175, 1986.

8. Braithwaite F, Maurice DG: The importance of levator veli palati muscle in cleft palate closure, *Br J Plast Surg* 21:60, 1968.

9. Clark DE, D'Antonio L, Liu JR, et al: Radiographic demonstration of oronasal fistulas in patients with cleft palate with use of barium sulfate contrast, *Oral Surg Oral Med Oral Pathol* 74:661, 1992.

10. Cohen SR, Kalinowski J, La Rossa D, et al: Cleft palate fistulas: a multivariate statistical analysis of prevalence, etiology, and surgical management, *Plast Reconstr Surg* 87:1041, 1991.

11. D'Antonio L, Barlow S, Warren D: *Studies of oronasal fistulae: implications for speech motor control,* paper presented at the Annual Meeting of Speech-Language-Hearing Association, San Antonio, November 20-23, 1992.

12. Delaire J: Reconstruction of the uvula and posterior parts of the congenital cleft palates, *Ann Chir Plast* 17:99, 1972.

13. Denk MJ, Magee WP Jr: Cleft palate closure in the neonate: preliminary report, *Cleft Palate Craniofac J* 33:57, 1996.

14. Dorrance GM: Lengthening the soft palate in cleft palate operations, *Ann Surg* 82:208, 1925.

15. Furlow LT Jr: Cleft palate repair by double opposing Z-plasty, *Plast Reconstr Surg* 78:724, 1986.

16. Furlow LT Jr: Discussion: cleft-palate repair by modified Furlow double-opposing Z-plasty: the Children's Hospital of Philadelphia experience, *Plast Reconstr Surg* 104:2011, 1999.

17. Huang MJ, Lee ST, Ranjendran K: Anatomic basis of cleft palate and velopharyngeal surgery: implications from a fresh cadaveric study, *Plast Reconstr Surg* 101:613, 1998.

18. Huang MJ, Lee ST, Ranjendran K: Structure of the musculus uvulus: functional surgical implications of an anatomic study, *Cleft Palate Craniofac J* 34:466, 1997.

19. Holtmann B, Wray RC, Weeks PM: A comparison of three techniques of palatorrhaphy: early speech results, *Ann Plast Surg* 12:514, 1984.

20. Kilner TP: Cleft lip and palate repair technique, *St Thomas Hosp Rep* 2:127, 1937.

21. Kirschner RE, Wang PW, Jawad AF, et al: Cleft-palate repair by modified Furlow double-opposing Z-plasty: the Children's Hospital of Philadelphia experience, *Plast Reconstr Surg* 104:1998, 1999.

22. Kriens OB: An anatomical approach to veloplasty, *Plast Reconstr Surg* 43:29, 1969.

23. Lindsay WK: The end results of cleft palate surgery and management. In Goldwyn RM (ed): *Long term results in plastic and reconstructive surgery,* Boston, 1980, Little, Brown.

24. Mars M, Asher-McDade C, Brattstrom V, et al: A six-center international study of treatment outcome in patients with clefts of the lip and palate: Part 3. Dental arch relationship, *Cleft Palate Craniofac J* 29:405, 1992.

25. Marsh JL, Grames LM, Holtman B: Intravelar veloplasty: a prospective study, *Cleft Palate J* 26:46, 1989.

26. McWilliams BJ, Morris HL, Shelton RL: *Cleft palate speech,* ed 2, Philadelphia, 1990, BC Decker.

27. McWilliams BJ, Randall P, La Rossa D, et al: Speech characteristics associated with the Furlow palatoplasty as compared with other surgical techniques, *Plast Reconstr Surg* 98:610, 1996.

28. Mercer NSG, MacCarthy P: The arterial supply of the palate: implications for closure of cleft palates, *Plast Reconstr Surg* 96:1038, 1995.

29. Millard DR, Jr: *Cleft craft,* vol 3, Boston, 1980, Little, Brown.

30. Molsted K, Ashner-McDade C, Brattstrom V, et al: A six-center international study of treatment outcome in patients with clefts of the lip and palate: Part 2. Craniofacial form and soft tissue profile, *Cleft Palate Craniofac J* 29:398, 1992.

31. Randall P: Management and timing of cleft palate fistulas repair (discussion), *Plast Reconstr Surg* 78:746, 1986.

32. Randall P, La Rossa D, Solomon M, et al: Experience with the Furlow double reversing Z-plasty for cleft palate repair, *Plast Reconstr Surg* 77:569, 1986.

33. Roberts CT, Semb G, Shaw WC: Strategies for the advancement of surgical methods in cleft lip and palate, *Cleft Palate Craniofac J* 28:141, 1991.

34. Schendel SA, Lorenz HP, Dagenais D, et al: A single surgeon's experience with the Delaire palatoplasty, *Plast Reconstr Surg* 104:1993, 1999.

35. Schultz RC: Management and timing of cleft palate fistula repair, *Plast Reconstr Surg* 78:739, 1986.

36. Semb G: A study of facial growth in patients with unilateral cleft lip and palate treated by the Oslo Cleft Lip and Palate Team, *Cleft Palate Craniofac J* 28:1, 1991.

37. Semb G: A study of facial growth in patients with bilateral cleft lip and palate treated by the Oslo Cleft Lip and Palate Team, *Cleft Palate Craniofac J* 28:22, 1991.

38. Shaw WC, Asher-McDade C, Brattstrom V, et al: A six-center international study of treatment outcome in patients with clefts of the lip and palate: Part 1. Principles and study design, *Cleft Palate Craniofac J* 29:393, 1992.

39. Spriesterbach DC, Dickson DR, Fraser FC, et al: Clinical research in cleft lip and cleft palate: the state of the art, *Cleft Palate J* 10:113, 1973.

40. Trier WC: Primary palatoplasty, *Clin Plast Surg* 12:659, 1985.

41. Veau V: *Division Palatine,* Paris, 1931, Masson.

42. von Langenbeck B: Operation der angeborenen totalen Spaltung des harten Gaumens nach einer neuen Methode, *Dtsch Klin* 8:231, 1861.

43. Wardill WEM: The technique of operation for cleft palate, *Br J Surg* 25:117, 1937.

44. Witt PD: Cleft closure in the neonate: a preliminary report (discussion), *Cleft Palate Craniofac J* 33:62, 1996.

45. Witt PD, Berry L, Marsh JL, et al: Speech outcome following palatoplasty in primary school children: do lay peer observers agree with speech pathologists? *Plast Reconstr Surg* 98:958, 1996.

46. Witt PD, D'Antonio L: Velopharyngeal insufficiency and secondary palatal management, a new look at an old problem, *Clin Plast Surg* 20:707, 1993.

CHAPTER

Alveolar Cleft Management

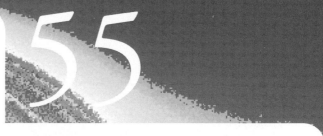

Barry L. Eppley
A. Michael Sadove

INTRODUCTION

Bone grafting of the alveolus has become an essential part of the contemporary surgical management of many orofacial cleft deformities. Although the concept of grafting of the cleft maxilla was introduced in the early 1900s, it was not widely recognized until a half-century later.[9] Beginning in 1955, reports from several European centers espoused the successful cortical grafting of maxillary clefts in both infancy and later childhood.[12,24] Since that time, alveolar cleft grafting has continued to grow in both popularity and success and is now generally acknowledged to be as integral to the management of the cleft patient as that of the primary lip or palate repair.

As the procedure has grown in its use, numerous controversies have arisen in regards to both the timing of the surgery and the selection of graft material. As such, a variety of differing alveolar cleft procedures have been described that can be confusing in both surgical technique and in assessing their long-term outcomes.

INDICATIONS

Any patient born with a complete orofacial cleft is a potential candidate for alveolar cleft bone grafting. The benefits and goals of this procedure are well recognized and include (1) stabilization of the maxillary arch, (2) elimination of oronasal fistula, (3) odontogenic bony support, and (4) nasal bony support.

STABILIZATION OF MAXILLARY ARCH

The creation of a one-piece U-shaped maxilla (minus the hard palate in the cleft patient) prevents collapse of the lesser segment behind the greater segment in unilateral clefts and the greater segments behind the premaxilla in bilateral clefts. This

not only improves occlusal interdigitation and masticatory efficiency but also prevents transverse collapse of the orthopedically expanded maxilla (Figure 55-1).

ELIMINATION OF ORONASAL FISTULA

Separating the oral and nasal cavities prevents liquid and food particle regurgitation through the nose, improves oral hygiene of teeth adjacent to the cleft, and eliminates an oral source for halitosis (Figure 55-2).

ODONTOGENIC BONY SUPPORT

Creation of an intact alveolus provides osseous tissue to support tooth eruption into its proper position into the maxillary arch, with or without orthodontic traction and guidance. In addition, adequate alveolar bone height to the tooth root prevents periodontal pockets and better ensures long-term stability and retention of the erupted teeth.

NASAL BONY SUPPORT

Augmenting the hypoplastic piriform aperture and maxilla improves the hard tissue support of the depressed alar base. This raises the cleft alar base to a symmetric level with the normal side, which complements rhinoplastic correction.

NOMENCLATURE

An important issue in alveolar cleft management, albeit not without considerable controversy, is the timing of bone graft placement. To avoid confusion in discussing this concept, the chronologic nomenclature used in alveolar bone grafting must be precisely defined. Conventionally, the terms *primary* (younger than 2 years of age), *early secondary* (between 2 and 5 years of age), *secondary* or *intermediate* (between 5 and 12 years of age), and *late secondary* (older than 12 years of age)

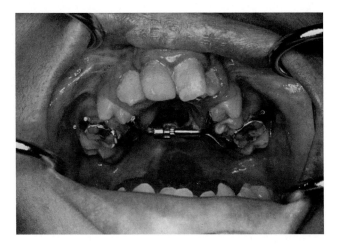

Figure 55-1. The cleft maxilla is prone to transverse collapse of the arches, which frequently require expansion through palatal expanders, lateral maxillary corticotomies, or both.

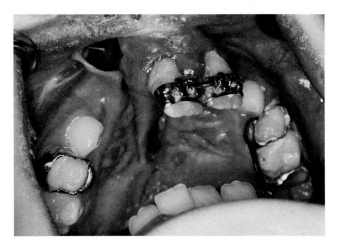

Figure 55-2. The persistence of oronasal fistula through the alveolar cleft site is a source of not only liquid escape into the nose but also instability between the maxillary segments.

are used.[2,4,5] These terms are based almost exclusively on patient age and dental development. From the perspective of postoperative facial growth, however, it may be better to relate the timing of cleft alveolar bone grafting in relation to repair of the cleft palate. Surgical closure of the cleft palate is well known to have a significant adverse effect on midfacial growth, particularly in the transverse maxillary dimension.[27] Therefore we prefer to categorize alveolar grafting *before* palatal repair as primary and alveolar grafting *after* palatal repair as secondary.

OPERATIONS

Currently, the operations of primary and secondary alveolar cleft grafting represent two methods with similar objectives but vastly different surgical techniques. Although secondary grafting remains by far the most common approach, primary grafting has a smaller but growing number of advocates.[6]

PRIMARY BONE GRAFTING

The principal aim in primary alveolar grafting is to prevent significant transverse maxillary collapse and occlusal distortions between the upper and lower arches. Ideally, this early stabilization decreases the time period of orthodontic treatment in the transitional and adult dentition periods, as well as the eventual need for orthognathic surgery. In addition, the early obliteration of the alveolar oronasal fistula eliminates nasal liquid escape and improves oral hygiene in the preschool and early school periods.

Within the first month of life, all patients with complete clefts are fitted with a maxillary obturator appliance. Incomplete clefts in which the hard palate is not completely segmentalized are not at risk for maxillary collapse and do not need an obturator unless it is warranted for feeding purposes.

The obturator's dynamic purpose is to orthopedically align the maxillary segments before surgery. This occurs through the passive palatal position of the obturator and the active process of external molding achieved through the primary lip closure. Rotation of the greater maxillary segment in unilateral clefts and posterior repositioning of the premaxilla in bilateral clefts is needed so that end-to-end abutment of the arch segments across the cleft is obtained. This process may occasionally be supplemented by an active obturator in which an expansion screw is incorporated into the midportion of the palatal plate.

It is extremely important that optimal maxillary segmental alignment be obtained before proceeding with the placement of the bone graft. Even in direct end-to-end abutment, a 5-to 7-mm gap between the bone ends will exist once the mucosa is peeled back. Therefore, if larger mucosal gaps exist at the time of grafting, the bone discrepancy can be quite large. This leaves an increasing space beneath an overlying onlay graft, which limits maxillary bone-to-graft contact and decreases the potential for successful bony consolidation. Furthermore, a large intersegmental gap requires increased tension on the mucosal closure over the bone graft, and the risk of postoperative wound dehiscence and graft exposure is more likely. Typically, good segmental alignment occurs between 9 and 12 months of age, depending on the original cleft width.

The surgical technique for primary bone grafting is relatively simple. Under general anesthesia and mucosal infiltration with a vasoconstrictor, a trapezoidal mucosal flap is raised into the vestibule of the upper lip. This dissection will expose the posterior surface of the orbicularis muscle from the previous lip repair. Leaflets of mucosa along the cleft margins are raised, turned back, and sutured to create a palatal lining. Anterior subperiosteal elevation is limited to the labial surfaces of the alveolus on both sides of the cleft without extensions onto the palate or around the piriform aperture onto the face of the maxilla. A small rib graft (sixth, seventh, or eighth rib) is taken from the lateral chest wall (2.5 cm length for unilateral clefts and 3.5 cm length for bilateral clefts) through a small incision placed below and lateral to the inframammary fold. The rib is then sectioned longitudinally with an intact outer

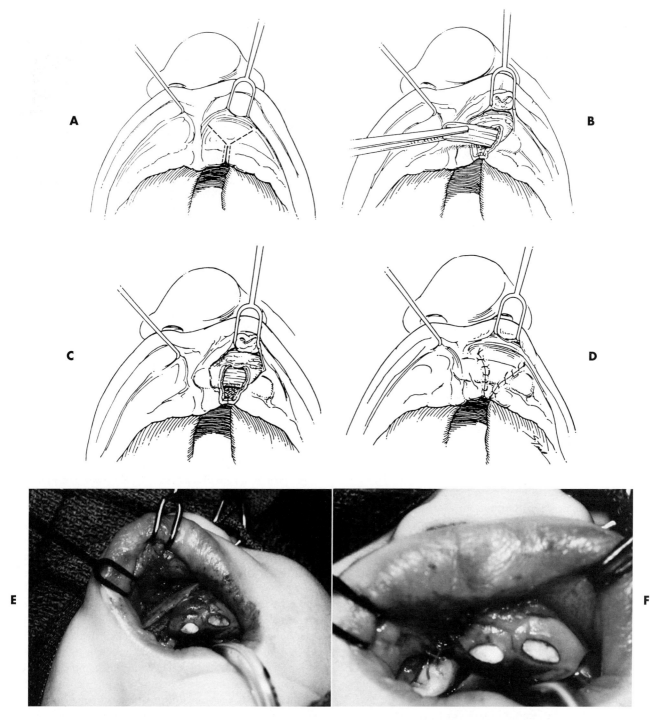

Figure 55-3. Primary alveolar bone grafting technique. **A,** Mucosal flap design. **B,** Subperiosteal rib graft placement. **C,** Labial cortical onlay rib graft spanning the alveolar cleft. **D,** Advancement of mucosal flap for closure. **E,** Outer portion of rib graft is split and needs contouring to underlying maxilla before placement. **F,** Mucosal closure temporarily shortens the maxillary vestibule.

cortical half onlayed over the labial surface and the inner half particulated and packed into the underlying space between the onlay graft and palatal flaps. The trapezoidal mucosal flap is then advanced over the graft for closure. This grafting technique is a procedure of limited dissection that steers clear of the important midfacial growth region of the premaxillary-vomerine suture (Figure 55-3).

SECONDARY BONE GRAFTING

The principal aim in secondary bone grafting is to unify the maxilla and create an osseous environment that will support tooth eruption into the arch. Typically, this procedure is undertaken at the stage of the transitional dentition (when the canine root is still incompletely formed) and in conjunction

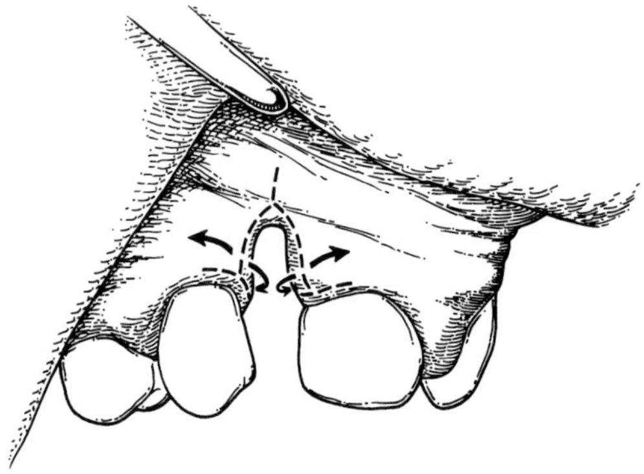

Figure 55-4. Typical illustration of flap design for secondary alveolar grafting, which misses two key points about flap design. A gingival cuff should not be left when raising the mucoperiosteal flaps and the posterior incision must extend along several teeth (often with a back-cut into the sulcus) to provide adequate mobilization (usually 1 to 1½ tooth widths) to close over the graft.

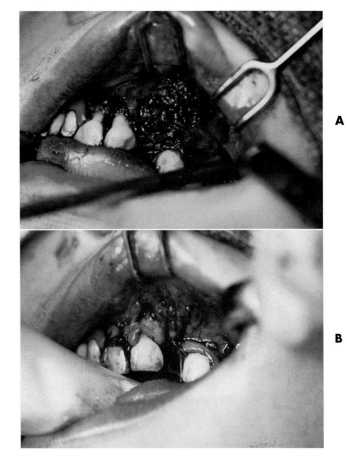

Figure 55-5. Secondary alveolar grafting technique. **A,** Thorough filling of the alveolar defect up to the lower crown level of the adjacent teeth is needed. **B,** Mucosal advancement and closure over the graft.

with orthodontic therapy. Although small amounts of maxillary segmental alignment can be done postoperatively, it is best to attempt to optimize maxillary arch alignment before graft placement. This will usually involve varying degrees of transverse maxillary expansion that occasionally may need to be assisted surgically through lateral maxillary corticotomies.

One of the most crucial surgical issues in secondary grafting, albeit often overlooked, is the flap design. It is necessary to appreciate the importance of gingival mucoperiosteal flaps for the success of this procedure. This type of mucosal flap provides similar tissue characteristics, both in texture and histology, to that of the adjacent alveolus. Unlike labial-based flaps, it can support tooth eruption and provide the proper periodontal qualities to sustain their longevity once in proper position in the arch.

Under general anesthesia and mucosal infiltration of a vasoconstrictor, gingival mucoperiosteal flaps are outlined on both sides of the cleft. They are raised on the labial surface of the maxilla from the gingival sulcus of the teeth both anteriorly and posteriorly from the cleft. Whereas small flaps are raised over the greater segment of the maxilla in unilateral clefts and on the premaxilla in bilateral clefts, larger posterior flaps are needed because the translocation of this tissue anteriorly provides the majority of the soft tissue closure over the graft. The anterior flaps do nothing more than cover the medial aspect of the bony cleft (Figure 55-4). To acquire adequate mobility of the posterior flap, it must be extended to the first or second molar and back-cut up into the sulcus. These flaps are raised up to and around the piriform aperture and separated from the nasal mucosa. The palatal mucosa along the margins of the cleft is then elevated onto the palatal bone, which produces complete exposure of all bony margins of the cleft and the extent of the defect at the level of the nasal floor. The nasal floor defect is repaired by either direct suturing or further elevation and closure of surrounding nasal lining. Gentle probing from the intranasal surface should be done to ensure competency of this important inner lining. The palatal

mucoperiosteum is then turned back and sutured to separate the palatal oral cavity from the alveolar graft site.

Grafting of the cleft defect is accomplished with cancellous tissue from the ilium or tibia or corticocancellous particulate from the calvaria or mandibular symphysis. Most commonly, cancellous marrow grafts from the ilium are used and currently serve as the gold standard by which all other donor sites are compared.[3] The graft material should be compressed before placement into the defect to optimize the number of osteocompetent cells and osteoid material per graft volume. Graft placement around the piriform aperture and onto the face the maxilla may be needed if alar base support is significantly lacking (Figure 55-5).

Closure is obtained by medial advancement of the previously raised posterior flaps to the more immobile anteriorly based flaps (Figure 55-6). This usually results in an anterior movement of the dental papillae one full tooth distance. The posterior back-cut above the molars is left open to heal secondarily. If the patient was in orthodontics before surgery, the arch wire may be replaced across the cleft site if the orthodontist is in attendance. In bilateral clefts, the replacement of this arch wire may be critical to provide stabilization of an otherwise mobile premaxilla (Figure 55-7).

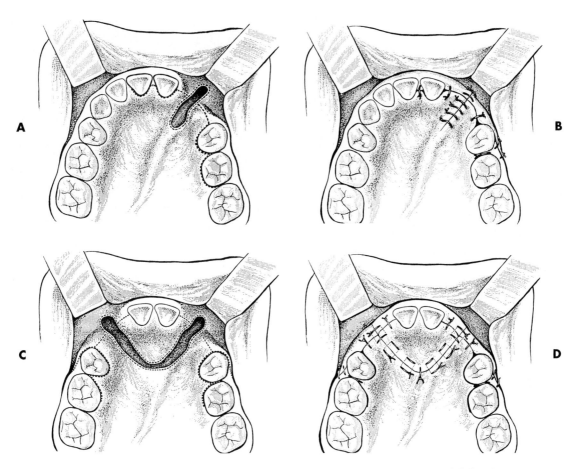

Figure 55-6. Secondary alveolar grafting flap design and closure. **A,** Unilateral cleft flap design. **B,** Unilateral cleft closure. **C,** Bilateral cleft flap design. **D,** Bilateral cleft closure.

There are two secondary alveolar cleft situations that deserve special mention. Bilateral clefts frequently pose unique problems because of the greater soft tissue deficiency and potential difficulty with preoperative positioning of the premaxilla (Figure 55-8, *A*). When the premaxilla is unable to be orthodontically moved into the arch, repositioning with bone grafting must be done. In this situation, vascularity to the premaxilla must be maintained by keeping maximal labial attachments with essentially no mucosal undermining. The premaxilla is separated posteriorly from its septal support being pedicled only on this labial soft tissue. Bone grafts are placed after the premaxilla is mobilized and stabilized into the arch by a maxillary occlusal splint.[7] Premaxillary fixation is usually needed for 6 to 8 weeks (Figure 55-8, *B* and *C*). Occasionally, advancement of the premaxilla may create or open an anterior palatal fistula that only a tongue flap can adequately close (Figure 55-9).

A more difficult alveolar cleft problem is when both orthognathic surgery and alveolar grafting are needed simultaneously. In these patients the presence of a constricted and hypoplastic maxilla combined with oronasal and palatal fistula results in an extreme case of hard tissue dysplasia. The incisional approach in this patient must be carefully planned to

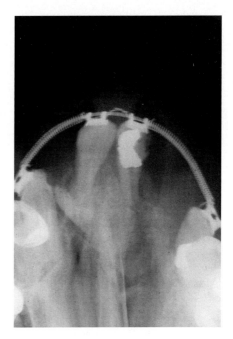

Figure 55-7. In bilateral cleft grafting, stabilization of the premaxilla is essential for success. This is usually obtained with a cross-arch orthodontic wire.

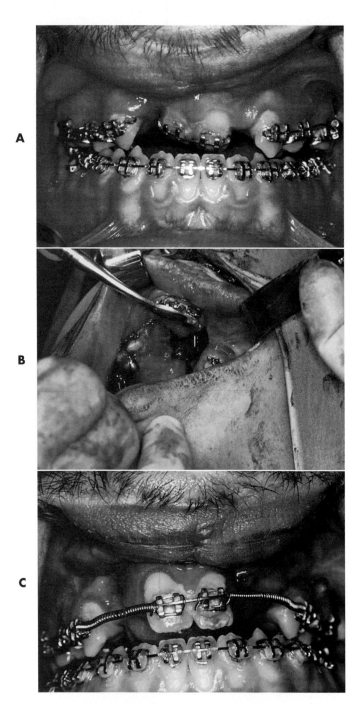

Figure 55-8. Repositioning of the premaxilla in bilateral clefts frequently unmasks soft tissue deficiencies of the anterior palate. **A,** Preoperative premaxillary position. **B,** Premaxilla freed and advanced through an osteotomy. **C,** Final premaxillary position after advancement, alveolar bone grafting, and tongue flap closure of the palatal defect.

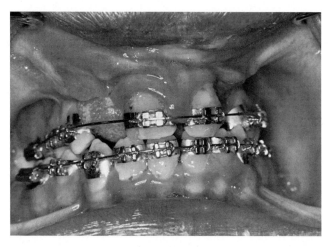

Figure 55-9. Tongue flaps are frequently needed for providing palatal closure in cases of surgical correction of retropositioning of the premaxilla in bilateral clefts.

ensure blood supply to all maxillary segments.[15] A high vestibular incision combined with marginal incisions around the alveolar cleft as previously described is used with maximal preservation of the palatal mucoperiosteal attachments. Often the alveolar cleft size is reduced by maxillary segmental advancement, which decreases the amount of graft material needed and lessens tension on the soft tissue closure. A more conservative and less risky approach is to stage the procedure with preoperative orthodontics, premaxillary osteotomy if needed, and an initial alveolar graft to unify the maxilla. A one-piece maxillary osteotomy is then performed secondarily.

OUTCOMES

PRIMARY GRAFTING

Bone grafting at this early age has historically been disappointing with the frequent reporting of subsequent midfacial growth retrusion, poor arch forms, and inadequate alveolar bone.[8,14,16,17] In these early attempts, however, extensive hard palatal dissection around and across the vomerine-premaxillary suture and an inlayed bone graft were performed. The recent resurgence of primary grafting, as is evident by the previous description of the surgical technique, differs considerably. Therefore this modified approach should be judged on the results of its own postoperative orofacial effects.

Recent reports of primary grafting have failed to show any long-term midfacial growth problems. Rosenstein,[18,21] in two separate clinical series that evaluated unilateral and bilateral cleft patients, showed no differences in facial growth from unoperated patients by cephalometry. Further results from Indiana University, where over 200 primary grafts have been placed over the past 15 years, have shown that, although the primary grafted group was proportionately smaller than noncleft controls, no significant differences were seen in standard lateral cephalometric measurements.[11,22] In addition, Rosenstein[19] has also reported that primary bone graft patients, when followed through adolescence, do not experience an increased need for maxillary skeletal surgery.

The successful take and consolidation of an onlayed rib graft to the maxilla is quite good, approximating 90% in a large series.[22] With graft take comes a concomitant elimination of the oronasal fistulas, which may still stay closed even if the graft

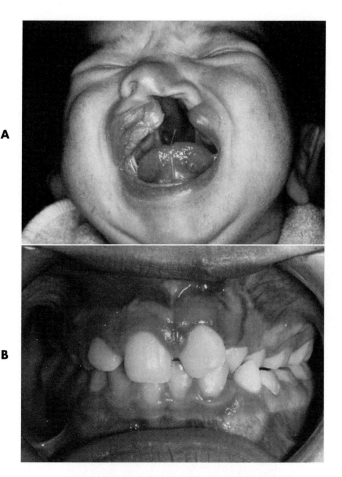

Figure 55-10. Primary alveolar bone grafting is effective at preventing significant long-term maxillary segmental collapse. **A,** Wide unilateral cleft lip and palate deformity. **B,** Four-year occlusal result after primary lip, alveolar, and palate repairs.

does not result in a radiographic bridge of bone across the cleft. Graft failure seems to occur mainly by breakdown of the overlying tissue flaps with subsequent graft extrusion. When contrasted with a near-negligible rate of donor site morbidity other than a small scar on the infant chest[6] (in comparison with the risks of pleural tears and postoperative pain when harvesting a rib in an adult), the procedure offers considerable appeal.

However, the primary bone graft procedure must also be judged on its effects on maxillary arch form and creation of adequate alveolar bone (i.e., need for secondary grafting). Unfortunately, adequate and convincing data in both these regards are currently lacking. It is our impression that the subsequent development of severe maxillary arch collapse in both unilateral and, in particular, bilateral clefts is prevented by early bone grafting. Maxillary arch collapse, however, is not completely prevented by the primary graft. The trends in unilateral clefts at the mixed dentition stage show minimal narrowing at the maxillary molars and an increased crossbite tendency at the incisor and canine positions[20,25] (Figure 55-10). This would indicate that most of the arch constriction is dental rather than skeletal in origin. This is clearly less than

that seen in nongrafted clefts and suggests that decreased orthodontic efforts will subsequently be needed. These trends are even more apparent in bilateral clefts. Further multicenter efforts, however, are needed to verify the orthodontic and orthognathic needs of these patients.[18,19,21]

Currently, the need for secondary augmentation of the primarily grafted alveolus is required in a relatively small number of patients. Average root support as determined by periapical and occlusal radiographs has been reported to be greater than 75% for both lateral incisors and cuspids, which compares favorably to that achieved with secondary grafting.[20] When an additional grafting procedure is indicated, the volume of bone required is significantly less than that associated with the traditional secondary alveolar bone graft.

SECONDARY GRAFTING

Delayed grafting and repair of the cleft alveolus with cancellous tissue has widespread acceptance because of the predictable production of an ample stock of viable bone with adequate cross-sectional width for tooth eruption, orthodontic tooth movement, or endosteal implant placement.[13] Secondary graft failures are uncommon (<5%) and are manifest as loss of the graft and/or reopening of the oronasal fistula. Infrequently, a small fistula reopens even though the bone graft itself has been successful. This seems to occur most often at the apex of the palatal closure in bilateral cleft cases. If the patient has liquid nasal escape, an additional procedure is needed to close the fistula. Poor tissue quality is the most common reason for compromised results and failures. Tissue adjacent to the cleft is often chronically inflamed as a result of inherent problems of hygiene. If extreme care is taken preoperatively to improve oral hygiene, the failure rate becomes negligible.[4]

The choice of donor site for graft material is overwhelmingly the ilium, where ample amounts of cancellous tissue can be easily obtained.[3] Particulate bone grafts are superior to block cortical or corticocancellous grafts because they are more readily incorporated into the alveolus with the capacity for postoperative remodeling. Occasionally, small particles of the cancellous graft may exfoliate through the incision, but this does not usually affect the overall take of the graft. Historically, the use of the ilium was associated with significant postoperative pain and morbidity and prompted surgeons to seek other donor sites. The favorable experience with calvarial bone in a variety of craniomaxillofacial sites logically led to its application in alveolar clefts.[28] This donor source has been reported to offer high rates of success, but the method of its harvest has been shown to significantly affect its transplanted osteonic capability.[23] Other donor sources have included the tibia (in adults) and the mandibular symphysis. With improved methods of graft harvesting, however, the ilium remains the gold standard for secondary alveolar bone grafting.[1]

The restoration of alveolar bone height is one of the best benefits of the secondarily grafted alveolus. This procedure typically provides greater than 80% root coverage of incisors and cuspids adjacent to the cleft.[10] With such bony coverage,

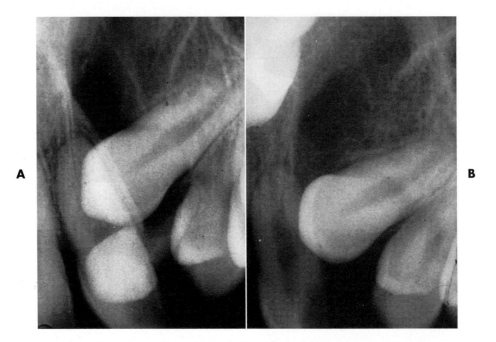

Figure 55-11. Secondary grafting of the cleft alveolus consistently produces good alveolar bone. **A,** Preoperative unilateral alveolar cleft defect. **B,** Postoperative alveolar fill with trabecular bone.

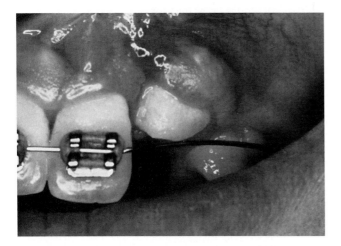

Figure 55-12. Secondary grafting provides a good stock of bone to support tooth eruption.

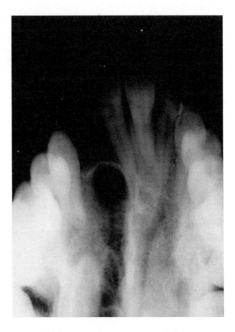

Figure 55-13. When teeth are not available to erupt through an alveolar graft, the retained alveolar height after grafting may not be as substantial as desired (maxillary occlusal radiograph 1 year after grafting).

the incidence of periodontal defects and fistulas are decreased and long-term tooth retention is markedly improved[26] (Figure 55-11). The amount of retained alveolar bone height, however, appears to be related to whether teeth erupt through the graft site. When teeth are present and erupt into the grafted alveolus, usually with the aid of surgical exposure and orthodontic assistance, alveolar bone height is retained (Figure 55-12). When teeth are not present to erupt through the graft, partial resorption of the graft occurs even when intraoperatively overfilled[4] (Figure 55-13). This suggests that alternative bone filler materials, such as hydroxyapatite, may be useful in the more mature patient when no unerupted teeth are present and the placement of endosteal implants is not anticipated.

SUMMARY

Bone grafting of the alveolus is an essential step in the reconstruction of the orofacial cleft deformity. Secondary grafting with particulate material from the ilium consistently produces trabecular bone to unify the maxilla and provide odontogenic support. It requires preoperative maxillary segmental alignment, well-designed mucoperiosteal flaps, and good oral hygiene to be most successful. Its high success rates makes it the preferred approach at the present time.

Primary grafting with rib tissue results in a bridge of bone across the alveolus without adversely affecting midfacial growth. It prevents significant maxillary segmental collapse, particularly in the bilateral cleft patient. It is simple to perform, has no real morbidity, and offers considerable appeal because of its execution in infancy. Whether it can consistently produce an adequate stock of alveolar bone to support long-term odontogenic needs, however, awaits further clinical documentation.

REFERENCES

1. Boustrad AM, Fernandes D, van Zyl AE: Minimally invasive iliac cancellous bone graft harvesting, *Plast Reconstr Surg* 99:1760-1761, 1997.

2. Boyne PJ: Correction of dentofacial deformities associated with residual alveolar and palatal clefts. In Bell WH, editor: *Surgical correction of dentofacial deformities,* vol 3, Philadelphia, 1985, WB Saunders.

3. Boyne PJ, Sands NR: Secondary bone grafting of residual alveolar and palatal clefts, *J Oral Maxillofac Surg* 30:87-92, 1972.

4. Cohen M, Polley JW, Figueroa AA: Secondary (intermediate) alveolar bone grafting, *Clin Plast Surg* 4:691-705, 1993.

5. Dado DV: Primary (early) alveolar bone grafting, *Clin Plast Surg* 4:683-689, 1993.

6. Eppley BL: Alveolar cleft bone grafting. (Part I) Primary bone grafting, *J Oral Maxillofac Surg* 54:74-82, 1996.

7. Eppley BL, Sclaroff A, Delfino JJ: Secondary management and reconstruction of the premaxilla in bilateral cleft patients, *J Oral Maxillofac Surg* 44:987-996, 1986.

8. Friede H, Johanson B: Adolescent facial morphology of early bone-grafted cleft lip and palate patients, *Scand J Plast Reconstr Surg* 16:41-53, 1982.

9. Lexer E: Die Verwendung der frien Knochenplastic nebst Versuchen uber Gelenkversteifung und Gelenktransplantation, *Arch Klin Chir* 86:939-943, 1908.

10. Long RE Jr, Paterno M, Vinson B: The effect of cuspid positioning in the cleft at the time of secondary alveolar bone grafting on eventual graft success, *Cleft Palate Craniofac J* 33:225-230, 1996.

11. Nelson CL, Chemello PD, Jones JE, et al: The effect of primary alveolar bone grafting on facial growth, *J Oral Maxillofac Surg* 46:M33, 1988.

12. Nordin KE, Johnason B: Frei Knochentransplantation bei Defektem in Alveolar Kamm nach Kiefer-orthopadischen Einstellung der Maxilla bei Lippen-Gaumenspalten. In *Fortschritten der Kiefer und Gesichts-Kirurspalten,* vol 1, Stuttgart, 1955, Thieme.

13. Ochs MW: Alveolar cleft bone grafting (Part II): secondary bone grafting, *J Oral Maxillofac Surg* 54:83-88, 1996.

14. Pickerell K, Quinn G, Massengill R: Primary bone grafting of the maxilla in clefts of the lip and palate, *Plast Reconstr Surg* 41:438-445, 1968.

15. Posnick JC, Dagys AP: Skeletal stability and relapse patterns after Le Fort I maxillary osteotomy fixed with miniplates: the unilateral cleft lip and palate deformity, *Plast Reconstr Surg* 94:924-931, 1994.

16. Rehrmann AH, Koberg WR, Koch H: Long-term postoperative results of primary and secondary bone grafting in complete clefts of the lip and palate, *Cleft Palate J* 7:206-212, 1969.

17. Robertson NRE, Jolleys A: Effects of early bone grafting in complete clefts of the lip and palate, *Plast Reconstr Surg* 42:414-420, 1968.

18. Rosenstein SW, Dado DV, Kernahan DA, et al: The case for early bone grafting in cleft lip and palate: a second report, *Plast Reconstr Surg* 87:644-654, 1991.

19. Rosenstein SW, Kernahan D, Dado D, et al: Orthognathic surgery in cleft patients treated by early bone grafting, *Plast Reconstr Surg* 87:835-842, 1991.

20. Rosenstein SW, Long RE Jr, Dado DV, et al: Comparison of 2-D calculations from periapical and occlusal radiographs versus 3-D calculations from CAT scans in determining bone support for cleft-adjacent teeth following early alveolar bone grafts, *Cleft Palate Craniofac J* 34:199-205, 1997.

21. Rosenstein SW, Munroe CW, Kernahan DA, et al: The case for early bone grafting in cleft lip and cleft palate, *Plast Reconstr Surg* 70:297-307, 1982.

22. Sadove AM, Eppley BL: Timing of alveolar bone grafting: a surgeon's viewpoint, *Probl Plast Reconstr Surg* 2:39-48, 1992.

23. Sadove AM, Nelson CL, Eppley BL, et al: An evaluation of calvarial and iliac donor sites in alveolar cleft grafting, *Cleft Palate J* 27:225-228, 1990.

24. Schmid E: Die Annaherung der Kiefer-Stumpfe bei Lippen-Kiefer-Gaumenspalten; ihre schadlichen Folgen und Vermeidung. In *Fortschritten der Kiefer und Gesichts-Kirurspalten,* vol 1, Stuttgart, 1955, Thieme.

25. Tanamura L: *Long-term follow-up of maxillary growth in cleft patients treated with primary alveolar bone grafting,* master's thesis, Indianapolis, 1992, Indiana University School of Dentistry.

26. Turvey TA, Vig K, Moriarty J, et al: Delayed bone grafting in the cleft maxilla and palate: a retrospective multidisciplinary analysis, *Am J Orthod* 86:244-251, 1984.

27. Viteporn S, Enemark H, Melsen B: Postnatal craniofacial skeletal development following a push back operations of patients with cleft palate, *Cleft Palate Craniofac J* 28:392-399, 1991.

28. Wolfe SA, Berkowitz S: The use of cranial bone grafts in the closure of alveolar and palatal clefts, *Plast Reconstr Surg* 72:659-666, 1983.

Velopharyngeal Insufficiency

Peter D. Witt

INDICATIONS

VELOPHARYNGEAL FUNCTION AFTER PALATOPLASTY

About 20% of children who undergo cleft palate repair develop speech production disorders, most commonly velopharyngeal dysfunction, that require additional intervention.[62] This percentage seems independent of the type of palatoplasty. Velopharyngeal dysfunction is diagnosed clinically by a constellation of symptoms that include pathologically incurred nasal resonance (hypernasality), misarticulation, escape of air through the nose (nasal emissions), and aberrant facial movements (grimacing).

NOSOLOGY

Although the terms velopharyngeal *incompetence, inadequacy,* and *insufficiency* historically have been used interchangeably, they do not necessarily mean the same thing. Trost-Cardamone[57] has proposed a taxonomy for velopharyngeal disorders, based on causative factors. The all-encompassing term *velopharyngeal dysfunction* does not assume or exclude any possible cause of the perceived speech symptoms or management approach. Velopharyngeal dysfunction includes any structural and/or neuromuscular disorder of the velum and/or pharyngeal walls at the level of the nasopharynx in which there is interference with normal sphincteric closure. Velopharyngeal dysfunction may result from anatomic, myoneural, behavioral, or combination disorders. In this chapter, the term *velopharyngeal insufficiency* is reserved specifically to refer to speech and resonance symptoms related to a known structural deficit that has been determined by perceptual and instrumental differential diagnosis.

OPERATIONS

EVOLUTION OF SURGICAL SOLUTIONS TO VELOPHARYNGEAL DYSFUNCTION

Differential Management

Although it is now possible to separate various causes of velopharyngeal dysfunction using instrumental evaluations, contemporary treatments for velopharyngeal dysfunction were developed irrespective of its etiology. The efforts of an international working group to standardize fluoroscopic and endoscopic velopharyngeal functional evaluations[18] may permit development of differential treatment based on differential diagnosis.

Partial obstruction, either temporary or permanent, of the velopharyngeal port is the unifying feature of most surgical treatments for velopharyngeal dysfunction. Two classes of operations are currently used to manage velopharyngeal dysfunction: (1) attempts to lengthen the palate by repositioning of the velum (e.g., V-Y pushback, intravelar veloplasty, double-opposing Z-plasty) and (2) reductions of the static opening between the nasal and oral pharynges. The latter may be accomplished by creating a subtotal central obstruction of the velopharyngeal port (pharyngeal flap[46]), by posterolateral diminution of the central cross-sectional area of the port (sphincter pharyngoplasty[25]), or by posterior port diminution (posterior pharyngeal wall augmentation[66]). All of these procedures are capable of producing iatrogenic perioperative airway morbidity. They should be used very cautiously in patients who are at risk for airway complications because of syndromic conditions, or in patients who have upper airway disturbances.

Pharyngeal Flap

The pharyngeal flap has been the most common method for secondary management of velopharyngeal insufficiency over the past three decades. Tissue from the posterior pharyngeal wall is attached to the soft palate, creating a midline subtotal obstruction of the oral and nasal cavities with two small, lateral openings or ports that, ideally, remain patent during respiration and nasal consonant production and close for oral consonants. The pharyngeal flap originally was described by Schoenborn[46] in 1876, which underscores the long-standing interest of surgeons in the problem of velopharyngeal insufficiency. The procedure came into more common use during the 1950s and subsequently.[36,39] Through the years, several problems with and complications of the pharyngeal flap have been identified. As a result, it has undergone several modifications. The problems include construction of the appropriate width of flap, the use of a superiorly or inferiorly based flap, and whether the flap should be lined (in an attempt to address postoperative flap contraction).

Both the width and proper level of insertion of the pharyngeal flap are crucial in its construction to allow closure of the two lateral ports during speech by the action of the lateral pharyngeal walls. The flap must not be so wide that the lateral ports are occluded at rest nor too small for effective nasal respiration. If the flap is too wide, the patient will develop mouth breathing, hyponasality, and possibly sleep disturbances ranging from snoring to sleep apnea.[33] If the flap is too narrow, persistent hypernasality is a result of inability of the lateral pharyngeal walls to close the portals.

Historically, surgeons have relied on intraoral inspection at the time of surgery to determine flap width. Most surgeons, recognizing the problem of postoperative contraction and the vagaries of wound healing, have created fairly wide flaps (i.e., as wide as the field would allow). An unlined flap leaves a raw surface of exposed pharyngeal tissue after elevation. The flap is developed from a relatively wide portion of tissue, but the healing process brings about marked contraction and thus reduction of the width of the flap. Therefore initially, symptoms of velopharyngeal insufficiency may be improved; however, with healing, they may return. Consequently, to combat the problem of contraction, surgeons have modified the procedure to add lining, chiefly by way of turnover flaps, with the intent of maintaining the original flap width as much as possible.

Recognition of the importance of the position of flap inset has helped solve the problem of flap contraction; that is, distal insertion of a wide, short flap along the free margin of the soft palate can lessen the problem of contraction for unlined flaps.[2] The theoretic goal of these modifications is to narrow the apertures left between the base of the flap and the adjacent tonsillar folds where they merge with the pharyngeal wall. However, the theory behind the modifications does not account for what we know about velopharyngeal function; that the activity of the remaining components of the velopharynx (lateral and posterior pharyngeal walls) may contribute actively to the closure process.

During the 1970s the concept of "lateral port control" was introduced by Hogan[22] as a means of controlling the size of the lateral ports. Using indirect information about the size of the velopharyngeal port from differential nasal and oral

airflow, studies by Warren,[59] Warren and Devereau,[60] and Isshiki et al[26] proposed that port size correlated with perceptual evaluation of nasal resonance. Based on these findings, Hogan devised a surgical technique to account for port size. Catheters measuring 10 mm^2 total cross-sectional area were the crucial variable for anticipated normal resonance. Although design of a flap in which the intraoperative port openings meet this specification theoretically is attractive, uncontrolled variables, such as scarring and postoperative flap migration, make the control of the lateral port size unreliable at best. Furthermore, the original data and variables did not consider the presurgical pattern of velopharyngeal closure.

Shprintzen et al[51] suggested that the effectiveness of pharyngeal flap surgery can be markedly improved when the flap width and inset are prescribed or "tailored" according to the degree of lateral pharyngeal wall motion and gap size seen preoperatively with multi-view videofluoroscopy and nasendoscopy. Shprintzen and colleagues assigned a group of 60 patients to one of three surgeons on the basis of preoperative findings about the mechanism of closure seen with instrumental assessment. Each surgeon was known to perform pharyngeal flaps consistently of different widths. The surgeons did not know that patients were being assigned to them for any specified flap width other than their customary procedure. The surgical outcome for these patients was then compared with a control population. The control group consisted of another 60 patients who were assigned to surgeons at random regardless of the preoperative pattern of closure. Results obtained when a surgical procedure was assigned to specific surgeons, based on the preoperative closure pattern, were shown to be superior to the results for patients assigned to surgeons at random without regard for the individual pattern of velopharyngeal function.

Although these results clearly indicate that a higher surgical success rate can be achieved by taking into account an individual patient's pattern of velopharyngeal function, this study did not assess the ability of the surgeon to tailor the flap intraoperatively. That is, essentially, each surgeon performed his or her routine procedure while the patients were assigned to the procedure based on their specific need. Pilot data from D'Antonio et al[11] suggested that, more frequently than not, the surgeon's intraoperative perception of pharyngeal flap width may not coincide with the desired flap width. It remains to be shown whether or not tailoring of pharyngeal flaps really is technically possible on a consistent basis.

Surgeons have debated the merits of the superiorly based pharyngeal flap over the inferiorly based pharyngeal flap, although Whitaker et al[61] and others were unable to show a difference. However, as Trier[56] points out, there are compelling reasons why the superiorly based flap is used more frequently. The inferiorly based flap has severe length limitations and also has the disadvantage of tethering the flap in an inferior direction, away from the palatal plane[39] and in the opposite direction of necessary motion for affecting velopharyngeal closure.

We may ask for whom the pharyngeal flap is an appropriate operation. Certainly, differential diagnostic data may help to answer this question. Shprintzen et al[51] and Argamaso et al[3] have clarified the importance of the contribution of lateral wall motion to effective postoperative valving in a pharyngeal flap operation. Therefore, from fluoroscopic and endoscopic visualization of velopharyngeal function, it appears that the pharyngeal flap procedure is most effective in managing patients with satisfactory lateral pharyngeal wall motion with sagittal or circular closure patterns.

Sphincter Pharyngoplasty

In addition to the pharyngeal flap, other procedures have been devised to manage velopharyngeal insufficiency. Sphincter pharyngoplasty is an alternative designed to tighten the central orifice and occlude the lateral ports. The original concept of sphincter pharyngoplasty was described by Hynes[25] and has been modified by others, including Orticochea.[38] Jackson[27] described the sphincter pharyngoplasty that is in common use today. The sphincter pharyngoplasty involves construction of palatopharyngeus myomucosal flaps from the posterior tonsillar pillars, which are sutured to the posterior pharyngeal wall and to each other (Figure 56-1).

Several recent publications have advocated sphincter pharyngoplasties for management of velopharyngeal insufficiency.[54] Many of the reports that promote the various sphincter pharyngoplasties have not been validated consensually by large numbers of patients, nor have the surgical results been subjected to critical analysis. Most reports lack clear delineation of the anatomic, physiologic, and perceptual factors used for the diagnosis of velopharyngeal insufficiency and identification of the need for surgical intervention. Few studies have included sufficient data regarding the criteria or methods for assessing surgical outcome.[13]

The literature is confounded further by the fact that there are several different types of surgical procedures that have been referred to as "sphincter pharyngoplasties" and have been grouped together as one procedure. Although theoretically similar, these procedures are different in terms of muscle tissue used for transposition, level of insertion, and whether an additional pharyngeal flap is incorporated into the operation. However, in many reports, these different operations have been discussed as if they represented a single operation.

Recently, several attempts to analyze the surgical outcome of sphincter pharyngoplasty have appeared in the literature. Riski et al[44] documented the necessity for proper anatomic placement of the myomucosal flaps that comprised the neo-sphincter, and the improvement in velopharyngeal function following attention to anatomic placement over a 6-year experience. The height of insertion of the lateral flaps appears to be the critical variable for success. In a followup report, Riski et al[43] commented on results of sphincter pharyngoplasty over a 15-year period. The results showed a statistically significant relationship between severity of preoperative resonance symptoms and elimination of hypernasality. Patients with mild hypernasality were more likely to improve than were patients with severe resonance symptoms. Additionally, results showed that patients with a circular velopharyngeal closure pattern were more likely to be successfully managed with sphincter

pharyngoplasty than were those with other closure patterns. Children under 6 years of age also were more likely to have successful surgical outcomes than were older patients.

Witt et al[63] separated preoperative speech and instrumental assessments to give perceptual information and physiologic/anatomic correlates. Only 18% of patients showed complete resolution of hypernasality and nasal emission. Additionally, 30% of patients in the study population were judged to be hyponasal or obstructed postoperatively or both, whereas none had been preoperatively. The high "success rates" reported in previous papers were not found in this experimental study. These results do not negate the value and usefulness of the sphincter pharyngoplasty, but they do point out the need for prospective studies to document its strengths and weaknesses. They also call for an objective definition of "success," which requires more than one evaluation method judged by more than one observer.

Although sphincter pharyngoplasty was first described more than 70 years ago, it has only recently gained enthusiasm among many clinicians. Thus, unlike the pharyngeal flap procedure, in which studies detailing its benefits and risks appeared in the literature with increasing frequency as it became more widely adopted, many of the pitfalls and complications of the various sphincter pharyngoplasties remain to be delineated. The sphincter pharyngoplasty procedure has theoretic advantages and, undoubtedly, is an effective means of management for velopharyngeal insufficiency for some patients. However, further studies on sphincter pharyngoplasty are needed to determine for which patients it is the procedure of choice, and how the "success" of the procedure can be improved.

Palatal Lengthening

The notion of "palatal lengthening" has been used in attempts to eliminate small gaps.[15] This concept has significant theoretic appeal for use in secondary palatal management because the technique attempts to lengthen the palate without violating the remainder of the dynamic function of the velopharyngeal mechanism, and it would appear to be more "physiologically normal" than the pharyngeal flap or various sphincter pharyngoplasties. Historically, the V-Y pushback procedure was designed to create a retrodisplacement of the palatal mucoperiosteum and velar musculature in the setting of primary palatoplasty. The primary goal of this procedure is to lengthen the palate during initial palatoplasty and thereby lower the occurrence of postoperative velopharyngeal insufficiency.

Most reports regarding palatal lengthening are derived from studies of its use at primary palatoplasty and not as a form of secondary management. Although the pushback procedure offers several purported advantages, the efficacy of this maneuver in secondary management for velopharyngeal insufficiency has never been established in prospective studies. Dreyer and Trier[15] point out that no global clinical conclusions about speech status can be made based on palatal lengthening independent of concurrent procedures. The operation is theoretically attractive because it would not be

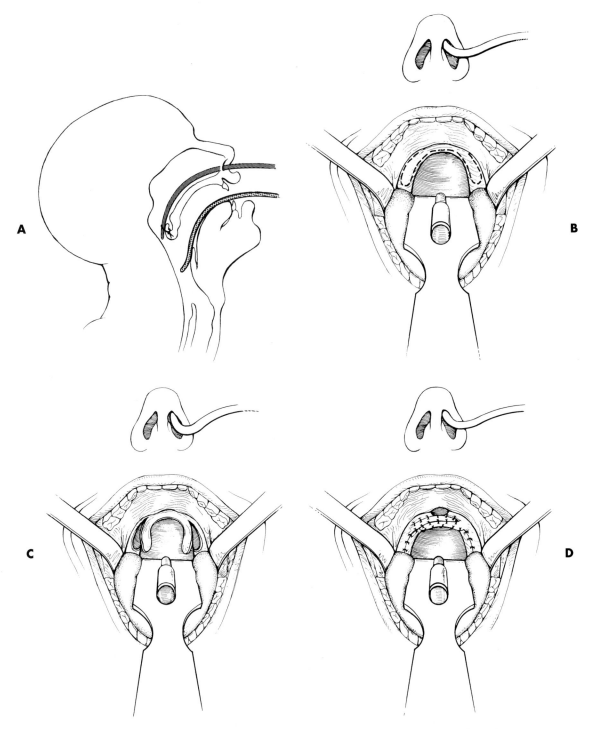

Figure 56-1. **A,** Catheter has been passed transnasally and attached to the uvula. The velum has been elevated, exposing the posterior pharyngeal wall. **B,** Oropharynx with the donor sites outlined *(dashed lines)*. The orotracheal tube is in place. The posterior pillars are exposed by retraction of the tonsils. **C,** The posterior tonsillar pillars are raised as myomucosal flaps-based cephalad. The posterior pharyngeal wall is incised transversely at the proposed area of insertion in conjunction with the cephalad extent of the elevation of the flaps. **D,** The superior mucosa of the left flap is attached to the mucosa of the superior incision of the posterior pharyngeal wall. The caudal mucosa of the left flap is attached to the superior mucosa of the right flap. The caudal mucosa of the right flap is attached to the inferior mucosa of the posterior pharyngeal wall. (From Witt PD, Marsh JL, Muntz HR, et al: *Cleft Palate Craniofac J* 33:183-189, 1996.)

expected to obstruct the nasal airway so that velopharyngeal valving integrity might be achieved without untoward respiratory deficits, such as chronic mouth breathing, snoring, or obstructive sleep apnea.

The combination of the pushback procedure and pharyngeal flap may be advantageous for some patients in the setting of primary palatoplasty. In 1979, Shprintzen et al[51] compared results achieved with (1) the pushback procedure combined with the pharyngeal flap, (2) the sandwich pharyngeal flap, and (3) the split-return with the flap. In this series, pushback combined with pharyngeal flap was more likely to result in less hypernasality without hyponasality. However, a number of problems may be associated with the use of lengthening procedures at primary palatoplasty. For example, Kremenak et al[28] have objected to the extensive mucoperiosteal stripping involved in the technique, arguing that it has deleterious effects on long-term facial growth. Additionally, high rates of fistulization have been reported[56] owing to the fact that three or four suture lines converge at one point, commonly occurring at the junction of the hard and soft palates. The vagaries of wound healing, postoperative contraction and scarring, and so on have made it impossible to predict the ultimate length gained with this surgical maneuver. Whether these problems are relevant to the use of palatal lengthening in secondary management has not been studied.

During the last decade, the Furlow[17] double-opposing Z-plasty procedure has become accepted as a means of gaining palatal length and restoring the velar musculature anatomically. Reports concerning its efficacy have been documented both at primary palatoplasty and as a secondary management procedure.[9,42] This procedure appears to benefit patients with unrepaired submucous cleft palate with small, residual, central velopharyngeal gaps. Its use as a secondary procedure is currently under investigation. In two separate reports on large series of patients, Chen et al[8,9] have demonstrated that the Furlow procedure may be effective for patients with a specific velopharyngeal closure pattern, namely, patients with a small, central velopharyngeal gap associated with unrepaired submucous cleft palate, or symptomatic patients with previously repaired cleft palate who demonstrate a midline "trough," or muscular diastasis. Because the double-opposing Z-plasty does not interfere with sphincteric function, it may be the procedure of choice when the gap between the posterior pharyngeal wall and the velum is quite small and centrally based, particularly owing to a central "trough." Once again, differential diagnostic information obtained from extensive evaluation of speech and velopharyngeal function is crucial to identify the population subset for whom this procedure may be beneficial because its application may be narrowly defined for a small group of patients.

Posterior Wall Augmentation

Surgeons may be reluctant to perform pharyngeal surgery on patients with mild symptoms of velopharyngeal insufficiency. The risk-to-benefit ratio must be thoroughly considered in arriving at the treatment recommendations in these cases. For some patients, posterior wall augmentation would have several advantages. The goal is to achieve velopharyngeal closure without altering the function of the velum or lateral walls.

Many nonautogenous materials have been used for providing anterior displacement of the posterior pharyngeal wall, including petroleum jelly, paraffin, Silastic, Teflon, and Proplast. Many of these techniques have been abandoned because of unpredictable results or restrictions imposed by the U.S. Food and Drug Administration. Silastic, Teflon, and Proplast implants are examples of the latter. The potential problems include tissue incompatibility and migration of the implant. Injectable forms of these substances can create problems with respect to embolism or transport of the prosthetic matter to regional lymph nodes.

The putative advantages and disadvantages of autogenous materials (e.g., cartilage, adjacent soft tissue, fat) have been documented in other publications.[4a,5b-5d,14a,16a-18a,28a,42a,55a] Usually, utilization of these procedures has been restricted to patients with small velopharyngeal gaps. Advantages of pharyngeal augmentation appear to include the following: (1) there is no alteration of the nasal airway, (2) the procedure is safe in children who are at risk for airway complications because of syndromic conditions or who have respiratory disturbances, (3) the procedure seems to be relatively simple and can be performed with shorter anesthesia and hospitalization times, and (4) it is potentially reversible.

Witt et al[66] conducted a retrospective concurrent study to evaluate the efficacy of autogenous posterior pharyngeal wall augmentation. Using a rolled superiorly based pharyngeal myomucosal flap, 14 patients who fulfilled two criteria were treated between November 1989 and June 1992. All subjects had velopharyngeal dysfunction unresponsive to speech therapy and small (<20%) coronal gap on velopharyngeal nasendoscopy. Of these, three had prior prosthetic velopharyngeal management, including two patients with Pierre Robin sequence. All patients were evaluated preoperatively and 3 months postoperatively with recorded (audio-video tape) perceptual, nasendoscopic, and fluoroscopic standardized speech and airway evaluations. The tapes were used for construction of a randomized master tape, which was presented in blinded fashion and random order to three skilled raters for independent assessment of numerous perceptual and instrumental parameters of speech. The raters were uninvolved in the care of the patients or this study, and their intra-observer and inter-observer reliabilities were known.

Preoperatively, the majority of patients had nasal turbulence. All patients had variable degrees of hypernasality ranging from intermittent to pervasive. Parameters rated included: (1) resonance (hypernasality, hyponasality, mixed), (2) auditory nasal emission (including nasal turbulence), and (3) visual characteristics regarding velopharyngeal closure. The visual parameters consisted of questions about whether a pharyngeal bulge was present or absent, descriptions of posterior pharyngeal wall movements with speech, level of closure, completeness of velopharyngeal closure, and quantitative descriptions about the percentage of velopharyngeal closure postoperatively. Examiners were instructed to evaluate a static and/or dynamic projection, or bulge (i.e., Passavant's ridge), and if present, whether the level of velopharyngeal closure was on the same plane as the neoposterior pharyngeal bulge.

Results of the extramural judgments of those parameters showed that there was no statistically significant tendency for patients' speech to be rated as more normal after the augmentation procedure than before it. These results suggested that autogenous posterior pharyngeal wall augmentation does not result in speech improvement and that it does not impair the nasal airway.

NONOPERATIVE ALTERNATIVES: PROSTHETIC MANAGEMENT

A palatal prosthesis, a velar lift, or a velopharyngeal obturator may be used as an alternative to surgical velopharyngeal management. A comparison of speech outcomes using prosthetic versus surgical management showed no difference for patients who complied with the prostheses.[31] However, because nearly 30% of patients referred for prostheses did not comply, surgery was more efficacious overall.

Prosthetic appliances are used as a nonsurgical intervention for velopharyngeal dysfunction. These include the speech bulb and the palatal lift prostheses. This modality of treatment has been available for many decades. The speech bulb is an acrylic mass that is used for obturating residual velopharyngeal gaps when there is inadequate tissue to effect closure. The palatal lift generally is reserved for patients in whom there is adequate tissue but poor control of coordination and timing of velopharyngeal movements. The speech bulb often is used for the patient with overt velopharyngeal insufficiency when there is some contraindication for surgical intervention. It also is appropriate as a trial management method for patients with variable velopharyngeal closure in whom it is unclear whether surgical management of the velopharynx alone will provide a noticeable or significant improvement in speech quality. In these patients, a trial of prosthetic management may provide the diagnostic information needed to help establish an appropriate management plan. In this situation, a prosthesis is a "reversible" test of the effect of velopharyngeal management.[12]

In another diagnostic capacity, a prosthesis may be used to determine whether dynamic velopharyngeal activity can be stimulated or improved. Some reports have indicated that prosthetic management may improve or facilitate motion of the velum, posterior pharyngeal wall, or lateral walls in some patients.[32] A trial of prosthetic management may be appropriate for those patients in whom little or no velopharyngeal movement is observed, and surgical intervention therefore would require near or complete obstruction of the nasopharyngeal airway. If improved muscle or structural function can be demonstrated, this information might be useful in altering an existing diagnosis or management plan.

Witt et al[67] conducted a retrospective concurrent evaluation of a palatal lift prosthesis to stimulate the neuromuscular

activity of the velopharynx. Nasendoscopic evaluations were audio-videotaped preprosthetic and postprosthetic management for 25 patients who underwent placement of a palatal lift prosthesis for velopharyngeal dysfunction. These audio-videotapes were presented in blinded fashion and random order to three speech pathologists experienced in assessment of patients with velopharyngeal dysfunction. They rated the tapes on the following parameters: velopharyngeal gap size, closure pattern, orifice estimate, direction and magnitude of change, and qualitative descriptions of the adequacy of velopharyngeal closure during speech.

Results of that study showed that velopharyngeal closure for speech was unchanged in 69% of patients and the number of patients rated as improved and deteriorated was nearly identical at about 15%. Postintervention, gap shape remained unchanged in 70% of patients. The extent of velopharyngeal orifice closure during speech remained unchanged in 57% of patients. Articulations that could impair velopharyngeal function improved in 30% of patients while deteriorating in only 4%. Results of this study neither supported the concept that palatal lift prostheses alter the neuromuscular patterning of the velopharynx nor provided objective documentation of the feasibility of prosthetic reduction for weaning. This study could be a model for others evaluating different types of velopharyngeal management.

PREFERRED METHOD: SPHINCTER PHARYNGOPLASTY

Conceptually, the goal of the sphincter pharyngoplasty procedure is to narrow the central velopharyngeal orifice, thereby diminishing air flow through the nose during phonation. The putative advantages of this procedure include technical ease of execution, lack of violation of the velum, and the possibility of dynamic sphincteric closure as a result of retained neuromuscular innervation. These advantages make it an attractive surgical alternative to the pharyngeal flap for management of velopharyngeal dysfunction, particularly in those patients at risk for airway obstruction.

Preoperative Management: Technology to Assist Surgeon

SPEECH AND VELOPHARYNGEAL ASSESSMENT. Patients having symptoms of velopharyngeal dysfunction (i.e., hypernasality, nasal emission, facial grimacing, and/or compensatory misarticulations) on perceptual speech screen are referred to the velopharyngeal diagnostic center for video-recorded standard perceptual, nasendoscopic,[11] and fluoroscopic[52,53] speech evaluations. The videos and patient records are reviewed by the interdisciplinary velopharyngeal dysfunction team (speech/language pathology, otolaryngology, prosthodontics, and plastic surgery), and a consensus is reached for recommended management.

Candidates for sphincter pharyngoplasty fulfill both of the following criteria: (1) velopharyngeal dysfunction resulting from an anatomic, myoneural, or combined deficiency of the velopharyngeal sphincter that would not be expected to be managed by speech therapy alone, and (2) preoperative nasendoscopic indications for surgery that include patients with large-gap coronal, circular, or bow-tie closure patterns, or velopharyngeal hypodynamism.[71] In addition, patients requiring surgical velopharyngeal management who have risk factors for upper airway obstruction are preferentially recommended for sphincter pharyngoplasty based on reports of its minimal effect on the airway.[27,54]

AIRWAY EVALUATION. Prevelopharyngeal management tonsillectomy and/or adenoidectomy are advised if the initial airway evaluation anticipates that the lymphoid mass would compromise performance of the operation or patency of the ports. The friability of the adenoid pad may preclude placement of sutures or flap inset at the most favorable position. Normally, this position correlates with the level of the first cervical vertebra as seen on lateral videofluoroscopic examination. Tonsillectomy and/or adenoidectomy is performed 3 months before sphincter pharyngoplasty as needed to facilitate technical execution of the procedure.

We assume that clinical manifestations of velopharyngeal dysfunction (i.e., hypernasality, nasal emission, nasal grimacing) worsen after tonsillectomy and adenoidectomy, and it is wise to counsel patients and parents accordingly. Repeat videonasendoscopy and speech videofluoroscopy evaluations are performed 3 months after tonsillectomy and adenoidectomy because of potential changes in velopharyngeal closure patterns that might alter the treatment plan as a result of such surgery.

SUBSPECIALTY EVALUATIONS. Preoperative consultations from appropriate subspecialties are recommended as needed by the interdisciplinary velopharyngeal team. Information provided by specialists in medical genetics, cardiology, ophthalmology, and psychology may be relevant for patients with multiple malformation syndromes (i.e., Stickler syndrome, velocardiofacial syndrome, Treacher Collins syndrome, and possibly submucous cleft palate).

OPERATIVE TECHNIQUE. The detailed operative technique for sphincter pharyngoplasty has been described in previous publications[25] and is beyond the scope of this chapter.

Postoperative Management

After velopharyngeal surgery, patients are routinely hospitalized for 1 night to observe for immediate airway compromise. Some children with syndromic conditions may require longer hospitalizations. Tongue stitches and arm splints are not used. Recommendations for postoperative feeding include a soft or liquid diet for 3 weeks or until the first office visit. At that time, if intraoral inspection shows satisfactory wound healing, a normal age-appropriate diet is resumed.

Posttreatment velopharyngeal assessment is performed at 3 and 12 months postoperatively and consists of the same perceptual, nasendoscopic, fluoroscopic, and airway evalua-

tions performed preoperatively. Treatment is considered "successful" if perceptual oral resonance is acceptable, there is adequate velopharyngeal closure on endoscopy and/or fluoroscopy, there is no subjective evidence of upper airway obstruction, and there is no sleep apnea. Velopharyngeal function is documented. Primary management resulting in hyponasality without other morbidity is considered a successful outcome.

All patients undergoing surgical intervention for velopharyngeal dysfunction should receive a comprehensive postsurgical evaluation.[62] The velopharyngeal symptoms may be diminished by surgery, but residual articulation errors and learned habits might persist and therefore must be addressed through behavioral therapy. Other patients might demonstrate that surgery was an appropriate management decision, but it may not have provided an adequate closure mechanism. Certainly, some patients may demonstrate no noticeable change in velopharyngeal function after surgery.

The postsurgical evaluation, especially with direct observation of velopharyngeal function, provides the surgeon with necessary feedback regarding successes and failures, thus serving as an internal quality control mechanism. This information is essential if one strives for continued improvement in operative technique. Without it, there is little to prevent one from continuing to make the same mistakes or, worse, to disseminate inappropriate knowledge within our specialty. Postsurgical speech therapy, if indicated, should be based on the same comprehensive evaluation process suggested for the unoperated patient. It should never be assumed that the patient has been given an adequate velopharyngeal mechanism that he or she must simply learn to use effectively.

Complications

ACUTE OBSTRUCTIVE SLEEP APNEA. Attempts have been made to define the reasons for morbidity and failure after sphincter pharyngoplasty. It seems warranted to ask which patients are at risk for development of obstructive sleep apnea after sphincter pharyngoplasty. The frequency of obstructive sleep apnea after sphincter pharyngoplasty appears to be substantial, occurring in about 13% of the 58 patients included in a preliminary report by Witt et al.[69] The outcome measures reviewed were patient demographic factors (e.g., age, etc.), associated medical problems, genetics evaluations, nasendoscopic characteristics of velopharyngeal closure, anesthetic evaluation of the patients, and the incidence and severity of perioperative complications. This experience suggested that risk factors may include microretrognathia and/or identifiable syndromes; a history of perinatal respiratory dysfunction; early age at sphincter pharyngoplasty surgery; and, possibly, upper respiratory tract infections.

Occasionally, sleep apnea may be severe enough to precipitate hospitalization and treatment with continuous positive airway pressure. Thus far, all patients so managed were weaned from treatment successfully, without requiring surgical take-down of the pharyngoplasty flaps. There appears to be an adaptation period during which one or more of the following may occur: (1) the patient becomes accustomed to the diminished patency of the velopharyngeal sphincter; (2) the sphincter area at rest increases with resolution of perioperative edema and progression of postoperative wound contraction; or (3) unidentified factors. Parental instruction, clinical nurse telephonic home monitoring, and frequent surgeon's office visits make home use of and weaning from continuous positive airway pressure possible.

Another common theme among patients affected by obstructive sleep apnea is early age at treatment. The four patients who developed clinically significant and prolonged postoperative airway compromise after sphincter pharyngoplasty at our center were 5 years old or younger.[64] We suspect that the low pulmonary functional residual capacity in small children may place them at greater risk for hypoxia at shorter durations of apnea than adults.

MICRORETROGNATHIA. The predisposition of patients with microretrognathia, with or without the Pierre Robin malformation sequence, to develop frank obstructive sleep apnea after velopharyngeal narrowing procedures, including sphincter pharyngoplasty, supports the hypothesis that their upper airways remain compromised well after birth.[29] Thus infants displaying significant improvement or resolution of symptoms shortly after birth may still have a compromised but well-compensated airway. Overt obstructive sleep apnea may not manifest itself until the time of palatoplasty or velopharyngeal management, even in some children who lack the anatomic characteristics of Pierre Robin malformation sequence. Such children maintain a patent airway when awake but, with the diminution of pharyngeal muscular support during sleep, develop obstructive sleep apnea. They may demonstrate varying degrees of noisy awake breathing, or mild feeding difficulties, and still maintain adequate ventilation when awake. Nevertheless, these patients may be at risk for airway obstruction at the time of sphincter pharyngoplasty surgery.

Examination of an infant's immediate postnatal period and recognition of the presence of congenital anomalies may provide important predictive information regarding the potential for airway complications after velopharyngeal management. Patients with the Pierre Robin sequence and histories of complications in the early months of life, as well as those having identifiable congenital syndromes, can be expected to demonstrate airway complications at the time of velopharyngeal management in a significant number of cases.

DEHISCENCE. There are several theoretic anatomic and technical reasons for pharyngoplasty flap dehiscence that deserve comment. First, surgeons can expect to follow a learning curve phenomenon as experience is gained with sphincter pharyngoplasty. The majority of dehiscences (80%) in our experience occurred during early experience with the procedure.

Second, dehiscence may relate to previous performance of tonsillectomy and/or adenoidectomy. A frequent obstacle to positioning the palatopharyngeus flaps high enough is a large adenoid pad. If needed, one should do not hesitate to perform tonsillectomy and/or adenoidectomy in preparation for definitive velopharyngeal management. This is done to obviate the possibility of lymphoid port obstruction and the technical difficulties associated with placement of stitches in friable adenoid tissue. Flap dehiscence may be caused by increased tension on the flaps as height is maximized. Tonsillectomy performed at a previous setting may result in atrophy and scarring of the palatopharyngeus muscle, which can undermine the integrity of the pharyngoplasty. This assertion remains unproved and must be viewed in light of the finding that 35% of patients undergoing successful initial sphincter pharyngoplasty at our center have also undergone previous tonsillectomy and/or adenoidectomy.

Third, dehiscence may relate to the palatal configuration and microretrognathia of the Pierre Robin sequence. The wide U-shaped cleft often results in a short and immobile velum after primary palatoplasty. Patients with Pierre Robin malformation sequence are often lacking in sufficient posterior tonsillar pillar tissue with which to construct the sphincter with a tension-free inset. Clearly, excessive tension can jeopardize the integrity of the pharyngoplasty.

Fourth, the reduced oral opening and narrowed pharynx of patients with Pierre Robin malformation sequence compromises surgical access with respect to both visualization and manipulation. Adequate exposure of the surgical field is considered essential to successful execution of the procedure in these circumstances.

TONSILLECTOMY AND ADENOIDECTOMY. Performance of tonsillectomy and/or adenoidectomy does not appear to correlate overtly with sphincter pharyngoplasty failure or need for subsequent revisional surgery.[64] Tonsillectomy performed at a previous setting may result in atrophy and scarring of the palatopharyngeus muscles, which may jeopardize a tension-free inset of the flaps. Under such circumstances, the resulting velopharyngeal port would of necessity be tight, owing to the relative paucity of tonsillar pillar tissue. Presumably, the tighter the sphincter pharyngoplasty port, the greater the potential for postoperative airway morbidity. We do not understand the influence of tonsillectomy on intervention outcome of sphincter pharyngoplasty, particularly as it relates to the possible development of postoperative obstructive sleep apnea. Because the tonsils and adenoids are often important components of the velopharyngeal closure mechanism, tonsillectomy and particularly adenoidectomy should be avoided in any child with symptoms of velopharyngeal dysfunction until a differential diagnosis is established[12] and a management plan formulated by the providers and accepted by the patient and family.

ANOMALOUS INTERNAL CAROTID ARTERIES. Nearly all cases of velocardiofacial syndrome reported to date have had cleft palate and hypernasal speech. Therefore the majority have required surgical management of velopharyngeal dysfunction, most often with pharyngeal flap surgery. Anomalous internal carotid arteries have been shown to be a frequent feature of velocardiofacial syndrome. Whether observed pulsations in the posterior pharyngeal wall should preclude pharyngeal flap surgery if they occur near the donor site is a subject of current debate.[72] The question is, in centers where nasopharyngoscopy is not performed routinely on patients, should the diagnosis of velocardiofacial syndrome be a sufficient deterrent to the application of pharyngeal flap surgery? Because these ectopically located vessels pose a potential risk for hemorrhage during pharyngeal flap surgery, some surgeons advocate sphincter pharyngoplasty instead of pharyngeal flap surgery when preoperative vascular imaging studies (magnetic resonance angiography or videonasendoscopy) demonstrate observable pulsations in the posterior pharyngeal wall.

Contraindications

Sphincter pharyngoplasty may be contraindicated in the following circumstances[38]: (1) management of children for whom surgery is contraindicated because of risk or patient choice; (2) there is a known or suspected neurologic history with potential for airway compromise; (3) there is inconsistent, intermittent closure that is responsive to stimulation or speech therapy; and (4) cases in which further diagnostic information is necessary (e.g., situations with minimal lateral wall movement). Patients who have undergone preoperative tonsillectomy may have insufficient tissue and/or excessive scarring in the region of the proposed pharyngoplasty. Absence of suitable donor palatopharyngeus myomucosal tissue generally mandates pharyngeal flap rather than sphincter pharyngoplasty surgery.

SECONDARY PROCEDURES

Palatal Fistulas

A palatal fistula may occur anywhere along the site of the original cleft as a complication of palatoplasty. The reported incidence of fistulization varies widely, ranging from 0% to 34% of all patients with repaired clefts.[7] A palatal fistula may result in audible nasal air escape during speech, hypernasality, resonance, nasal regurgitation during drinking and eating, and production of socially undesirable sounds.

There is controversy concerning accurate identification of a symptomatic fistula, the extent of its effects on speech, and decisions regarding surgical management. However, many speech pathologists feel that a symptomatic fistula may cause a deterioration in speech quality and intelligibility, thereby leading to significant communication impairment. Surgical repair of palatal fistulas can be technically difficult, owing to a paucity of virgin local tissue for closure or excessive scarring. Therefore many surgeons repair only those fistulas that they believe are likely to be symptomatic.

Many opinions have been expressed in the surgical literature concerning which fistulas are likely to be symptomatic.[1,7,16,41,47] The most common variables discussed are size and position of the fistula. An intraoral view of a palatal fistula, however, is not necessarily representative of its functional aperture into the nasal passage or of its inferior-to-superior course. Oneal[37] presents a conservative opinion, suggesting

that the functional significance of a palatal fistula must be determined for each patient individually. This is the opinion expressed in most of the current speech literature.[33,50]

D'Antonio et al[10] showed a significant relationship between fistula size and speech symptoms but no relationship between fistula size and change in symptoms when the fistula was temporarily occluded. That is, larger fistulas may be associated with more significant hypernasality and nasal emission, but the size of a fistula alone does not relate to the amount of change in speech symptoms when a fistula is temporarily obturated or repaired. This finding supports the data reported by Henningsson and Isberg,[19,20] that improvement in speech associated with occlusion of a fistula is not due solely to the reduction in air flow through the fistula alone. Using videofluoroscopy, they demonstrated that the occlusion of a fistula can cause concomitant improvement in velopharyngeal valving.

In some cases, it is wise to repair a symptomatic palatal fistula before further evaluation and management of velopharyngeal function. Admittedly, this approach theoretically may require a patient to undergo two separate operations: one for the repair of the palatal fistula and the other for the management of the velopharynx. However, such a management algorithm is rational in view of the fact that some patients show complete elimination of velopharyngeal symptoms after fistula repair alone.

Rarely, the entire cleft palate repair will dehisce or, more commonly, the velum alone will. In these cases, surgical rerepair is performed after waiting for the inflammatory reaction to subside. Whether such re-repair negatively affects palatal function for speech is unknown.

OUTCOMES

METHODOLOGY AND SHORTCOMINGS OF PREVIOUS CLEFT LIP AND PALATE OUTCOME RESEARCH

Regarding diversity of management of patients with cleft anomalies, few areas of surgery have generated such a wide array of surgical methods. State-of-the-art reviews consistently indicate that few, if any, centers conform to the same approach in surgical technique, timing, or sequence, not to mention the variety of ancillary interventions: presurgical orthopedics, orthodontics, speech therapy, secondary operations, etc.[55] At one recent meeting, 34 teams presented their programs of treatment and produced 34 different programs.[24] As with all surgery, individual levels of skill and practice idiosyncrasies between surgeons further cloud the picture.

The contemporary keystone of cleft management is the multidisciplinary cleft care team.[40] Although most cleft care providers believe in team care, surprisingly little information exists on the long-term results of multidisciplinary management of patients with cleft lip and palate. Minimal information is available on the total number of surgeries and the cost necessary to habilitate the patient with a cleft lip and palate. Review of a major section of the cleft lip and palate literature over the last 25 years reveals a general lack of rigorously executed studies that adhere to contemporary standards of clinical trial design.[45]

Much of the cleft literature is descriptive and focuses on anatomic integrity and aesthetic result. More recently, comparative studies have been reported that assess functional outcome with respect to speech,[23] dentoskeletal development and growth, psychosocial issues, and airway. A survey of papers in *Cleft Palate Craniofacial Journal* since its inception in 1964 identified 200 reports on some aspect of treatment outcome.[45] These can be broken into three broad categories: descriptive, procedural, and evaluative. The first group consists of descriptive studies that document some aspect of the treated cleft lip and palate population without reference to a specific treatment method. These studies often involve comparison with noncleft subjects or between cleft lip and palate subtypes as a means of exploring the morphology or social morbidity of treated cleft subjects. A second group is procedural, examining methods of diagnosis, assessment, or prediction of outcome. A third group, the main interest of this chapter and corresponding to just over half the reports, attempts to evaluate specific treatment methods and outcomes, including primary or secondary surgery, speech therapy, orthodontics, or audiology.

Why is it that critical information on long-term outcomes in cleft care is so hard to come by? The time lapse between surgery (primary surgery within the first 18 months of life in particular) and measurement of outcome (at craniofacial growth maturity in mid to late adolescence) creates major difficulties for clinical researchers. Retrospective study requires information on primary management practices 5, 10, and 15 years previously and presupposes clearly described treatment protocols. Even when this exists, such practices may have little relevance to the research questions of current interest. Where treatments have been described with insufficient detail, treatment-related variation and outcome may remain undetectable. Similarly, if the results of prospective studies are to be timely and relevant, it is important that they be completed within a reasonable length of time. Unfortunately, the measurement of some aspects of outcome, for example, dentoskeletal development, are best deferred until the patient reaches maturity.

The location of the cleft palate anomaly leads to possible impairments of breathing, hearing, speech, dental relationships, craniofacial growth, and facial appearance with possible consequent social-psychologic impairment. Thus comprehensive examination of the outcome of treatment should be multifaceted, especially as trade-off in outcome may occur. For example, delayed closure of the hard palate may reduce growth disturbance but increase speech impairment.[4] Evidence that adequate palatal closure has a salutary effect on the ubiquitous problem of middle ear pathology, the possible benefits of avoiding disuse atrophy in the levator veli palatini musculature, and the early establishment of swallowing and crying all indicate that closure might provide a number of benefits if done much earlier. None of these factors has been clarified by objective studies. Prospective, longitudinal investigations of the clinical management of cleft lip and palate are necessary to answer the three central problems of that management: the best time to treat, the techniques of treatment most appropriate in a particular case, and the effects of treatment.

WHY OUTCOME STUDIES? WHY NOW?

There is a need for rigorous evaluation of competing therapies for managing patients with facial clefts because patients and payers are expecting ever-higher standards for clinical outcomes while policy makers and insurers are demanding more and more stringent cost containment. The American health care system lacks a coherent mechanism for assembling and analyzing the data needed to meet these goals. This is the challenge for cleft lip and palate researchers at the turn of the century.

The following section is a critical review of results published in the cleft palate literature with a focus on the important epidemiologic parameters of length of follow-up, reproducibility and validity of outcome measures, diversity of management, and sample sizes. Attention will also be paid to common patient descriptors that tend to influence process or outcomes such as demographics (age, gender, education); health factors (diagnosis, severity of primary diagnosis, comorbidity); and other factors, such as lifestyle and patient expectations for treatment and results valued by the patients. A successful outcomes measurement system should do the following:

1. Document change in clinical conditions as a result of medical intervention.
2. Collect data in a common format.
3. Maintain data collected from multiple clinical sites in a single site to facilitate comparison of outcomes.
4. Incorporate standardized and validated methods of accounting for a health care organization's effect on health and quality of life.
5. Enable physicians to assess and select medical treatments based on actual results and cost of a treatment to enable accurate prediction of resources needed for care.
6. Provide data to establish standards or guidelines for treatment.
7. Provide patients with specific facts to help them make medical decisions, including treatment cost, efficacy, and impact on quality of life.

LONG-TERM OUTCOMES

Given that initial palate surgery is preferentially performed within the first 18 months of life on physically and functionally immature tissues, the growth and function of those tissues must be followed into maturity to assess the assets and liabilities of the interventions. The multidimensionality of cleft outcomes include the effects of the anomaly and its repair on respiration, nutrition, speech, hearing, appearance, dental occlusion, craniofacial growth, and psychosocial function. Modification of surgical techniques and/or timing to optimize one of these variables may induce untoward consequences in another; for example, delayed closure of the hard palate, recommended to minimize maxillary growth disturbance resulting from palatoplasty, has been shown to increase speech impairment.[4] Key studies addressing long-term outcomes in cleft surgery are discussed below.

Euro Cleft Intercenter Comparison Study

A six-center study has identified clinically important differences in the outcome of treatment of children with repaired clefts of the lip and palate.[30,48,49] The participating cleft-craniofacial centers included Amsterdam, Copenhagen, London, Manchester, Stockholm, and Oslo. One of the protocols defined a cohort of consecutively treated children with complete unilateral cleft lip and palate, born in the years 1976-1979, and treated at the respective centers. A multidimensional comparison of outcome on these patients at age 8 to 10 years identified clinically important and statistically significant differences between the centers.

The Euro Cleft study included the Speech Project, which was established in 1989 to investigate the speech performance of the children from the six centers involved with the Euro Cleft Orthodontic Study.[30] The project investigated the speech skills of 131 subjects aged 11 to 14 years with cleft lip and palate. A sampling procedure and an analytic framework were devised for the study, which enabled comparisons to be made between the speech results for five European languages. The analytic framework identified characteristic error patterns in cleft palate speech and focused on the "vulnerable" consonants that are common in the five languages. The overall resonance characteristics of the subjects' speech were also evaluated. The results indicated good outcomes with regard to accuracy in consonant articulation across the whole population with common minor (sub phonemic) errors in all languages for a minority of subjects. The results for resonance characteristics were somewhat less positive, with slight hypernasality in 20% of subjects. Nonetheless, there were few indications of seriously disordered speech. There were no significant differences between centers. However, the detectable differences matched the findings of the Orthodontic Study, especially in regard to the performance ranking of the centers.

Oslo Cleft Lip and Palate Growth Archive

Two examples of outcome research in cleft lip and palate were drawn from the Oslo Cleft Lip and Palate Growth Archive, which represents a good example of current databases in the field: pharyngoplasty and primary palatoplasty.[5a] The Oslo Cleft Lip and Palate team formed during the 1940s. From the early 1950s, for the majority of Norwegian infants with cleft lip and palate, it has provided surgery and all subsequent treatment, including orthodontics and speech therapy. Reasonable uniformity of primary surgical management has been maintained over the years, with relatively minor changes in

techniques and timing. Cephalometric recording of all patients has been standardized and adheres well to a regular protocol of collection. Nonetheless, the database contains substantial treatment-related variation.

RETROSPECTIVE MATCHING— PHARYNGOPLASTY

Some patients will be unable to satisfactorily close their velopharyngeal sphincter for appropriate speech tasks after uncomplicated cleft palate repair. These patients require secondary velopharyngeal management. An example of such selective secondary intervention is present within the Oslo Cleft Lip and Palate Growth Archive with respect to pharyngeal flap operations. Approximately 20% of patients with complete clefts of the palate were judged to require this operation to reduce nasopharyngeal incompetence in speech. Growth data were available on each subject before the operation and 5 years later. Cases could be matched to gender, cleft subtype, and ages at which records were obtained. Patients requiring the procedure were shown to have some preexisting differences in their preoperative craniofacial form. When account was taken of these, no growth disturbance attributable to pharyngoplasty could be discerned. Because this procedure significantly benefits speech, its denial to a control group for several years could not have been justified. Nonetheless, it was desirable to perform this comparison to obtain reassurance that secondary growth disturbance was not induced.

HISTORICAL CONTROLS—PRIMARY CLEFT PALATE SURGERY

Using a restricted number of standard cephalometric radiographic measurements, an attempt was made to assess the effect on facial growth of differences in age at surgery, type of lip repair, and surgeon seniority by selecting historical controls within the database. Using multivariate statistical methods, an attempt was made to discern effect associated with primary surgery in a series of patients with complete cleft lip and palate. Examination of the database, however, demonstrated a series of associations between treatment parameters, such as changes in the technique of lip repair and reductions in age of both cleft lip and palate repair. With surgeons active at different time periods and with each patient having two operations, any effect of surgeon seniority was confounded with changes in surgery and age at operation.

Inevitably, the strong association of such factors creates problems in attempting to analyze them independently of each other. After adjustment for multiple comparison effects, no statistically significant factors associated with primary surgery could be discerned. Had significant differences emerged, the multiplicity of confounding effects would still have made interpretation unclear because in observing the effect of any difference in a specific factor one must recognize that this may be the outcome of several factors acting simultaneously or even acting to cancel one another. We believe that such short-comings related to historical control studies will generally confound this approach when evaluating primary surgery.

PATIENT SATISFACTION

What is a successful outcome? Delineation of success may depend on what criteria are used and who assesses the data. Historically, many outcome studies failed to define unambiguous criteria and often had caregivers evaluate their own patients. The need for rigorous reliable assessment tools and the use of extramural professional and lay raters is increasingly appreciated. An example of such is the recent concern that cleft professionals might be recommending velopharyngeal management for mild velopharyngeal dysfunction that was discernible to the professionals but not of psychosocial significance to the patient.[70] The aim of this study was twofold: (1) to test the ability of normal children to discriminate the speech of children with repaired cleft palate from the speech of unaffected peers, and (2) to compare these naive assessments of speech acceptability with the sophisticated assessments of speech pathologists.

The study group (subjects) was composed of 21 children of school age (ages 8 to 12) who had undergone palatoplasty at a single cleft center, and 16 matched controls. The listening team (student raters) was composed of 20 children who were matched to subjects for age, gender, and other variables. Randomized master audiotape recordings of the children who had undergone palatoplasty were presented in blinded fashion and random order to student raters who were inexperienced in the evaluation of patients with speech dysfunction. The same sound recordings were evaluated by an experienced panel of extramural speech pathologists whose intrarater and interrater reliabilities were known; they were not direct care providers. Additionally, the master tape was presented in blinded fashion and random order to the velopharyngeal staff at the cleft center for intramural assessment. Comparison of these assessment methodologies formed the basis of this report.

Naive raters were insensitive to speech differences in the control and cleft palate groups. Differences in the mean scores for the groups never approached statistical significance, and there was adequate power to discern a difference of 0.75 on a 7-point scale. Expert raters were sensitive to differences in resonance and intelligibility in the control and cleft palate groups but not to other aspects of speech. The expert raters recommended further evaluation of cleft palate patients more often than control patients.

These data suggested that speech pathologists discern differences that the laity does not. Consideration should be given to the utilization of untrained listeners to add real-life significance to clinical speech assessments. Peer group evaluations of speech acceptability may define the morbidity of cleft palate speech in terms that are most relevant to the patients themselves and may safeguard against the possibility of offering treatment that may be unnecessary.

Results of this study raised many questions concerning the perception of speech after palatoplasty. Is there a developmental trajectory such that a cohort of unaffected individuals, older than the school-age cohort, would detect the speech abnormalities among their affected peers? If so, when does the transition to "awareness" occur chronologically? Is the morbidity of speech associated with cleft palate defined by the affected school-age child; his or her peers, teachers, or parents; uninvolved lay adults; or tertiary care providers? What factors should determine the need for intervention? Who should serve as raters: patients, parents, peers, or professionals? These questions deserve overt answers, and outcome research pertaining to such questions is underway at our institution.[65]

FUTURE DIRECTIONS IN OUTCOMES RESEARCH

How Do Outcome Studies Relate to Cleft Lip and Palate Surgery, and Why Are Outcomes Studies Necessary?

Today's national emphasis on cost and quality issues in health care will continue to drive the movement toward developing outcomes measurement systems. These instruments have the potential to help physicians and other providers improve the quality and effectiveness of patient care. Much work is necessary to develop an expert consensus on a gold standard for outcomes measurement in cleft care.

Goals for clinical research in cleft lip and palate include reduction of the prevalence of the disorder, achievement of more effective functional results, amelioration of the psychologic problems of affected persons and their families, and reduction of the financial cost of treatment. Research should be conducted to develop standards by which cleft lip and palate operations can be evaluated reliably at various times between birth and maturity in late adolescence. In addition, it needs to be determined whether successes and failures can be identified before the completion of growth and development to facilitate the emotional and economic adaptation of the affected individual and his or her family to the need, if any, for future care.

Prospective randomized series and multi-institutional collaborative studies are necessary so that one contemporary operation can be compared objectively with another. Although sophisticated cadaveric studies of the components of the velopharyngeal sphincter have been published,[34,35] additional information is needed regarding the functional in vivo anatomy of the velopharynx in individuals with a cleft palate. It would be useful if objective criteria could be established to accurately predict adequacy of the velopharyngeal sphincter at the time of the primary palatal repair. If the predicted result is an inadequate velopharynx, an additional pharyngeal procedure could be added to the routine palate closure in an attempt to obviate the need for that procedure secondarily.

There are theoretic arguments favoring closure of a cleft palate much earlier than is currently practiced by most surgeons. Although it may be safe to perform early palatoplasty,[14] the efficacy of such surgery remains to be documented.[68]

Longitudinal studies can be performed best at a limited number of regional cleft centers. Some of the important criteria for the selection of such centers are: larger and controlled case flow available from birth, availability of adequate treatment personnel and facilities to provide interdisciplinary resources for habilitation, close association of the clinical treatment staff and research members of the unit, maximum assured utilization of staff and facilities, standardized regular documentation, willingness to conduct regular continuing training programs in clinical management, and the facilities and climate conductive to research. Such centers should, in addition, be capable of developing consortia of affiliated satellite institutions to ensure maximum utilization of the expertise of both the center and the affiliated hospitals and clinics. The Euro Cleft Group is a paradigm for imitation.

Prospective, longitudinal investigations have a practical application in the clinical management of children with cleft lip and palate because only by collecting reliable data can one deal with the three central problems of management: the best time to treat, the most appropriate techniques of treatment, and the anticipated effects of treatment in an individual case. In addition, there is an opportunity to enrich the training of health care professionals from a wide variety of disciplines by using these data to demonstrate the continuum of morphologic variations that may be expected.

SUMMARY

Cleft palate research during the past 25 years has been largely descriptive. The findings of this research has substantially improved the appearance, speech, hearing, eating, and dental health in patients with clefts while reducing the number of interventions while improving their efficacy. However, for further progress to be made, new directions and methodologies of research must be developed. The future demands projects that are not only well defined but that also seek to discover the ways in which many variables act together to influence the clinical result. Projects must be designed to produce data that can be appropriately interpreted, generalized, and applied.[10] Although such research is difficult, with suitable planning, collaborations of surgical teams supported by competent ancillary researchers will be able to break new ground in advancing the management of patients with cleft lip and palate.

REFERENCES

1. Abyholm FE, Borchgrevink HHC, Eskeland G: Palatal fistulae following cleft palate surgery, *Scand J Plast Reconstr Surg* 13:295, 1979.

2. Argamoso R: Post palatoplasty velopharyngeal incompetency. In Marsh JL, editor: *Current therapy in plastic and reconstructive surgery*, Philadelphia, 1989, BC Decker.

3. Argamoso RV, Shprintzen RJ, Strauch B, et al: The role of lateral pharyngeal wall movement in pharyngeal flap surgery, *Plast Reconstr Surg* 66:214, 1980.

4. Bardach J, Morris HL, Olin WH: Late results of primary veloplasty: the Marburg Project, *Plast Reconstr Surg* 73:207-215, 1984.

4a. Bardenhauser D, Vorschlage ZU: Plastischen Operationen bei chirurgischen Eingriffen in der Mundhohle, *Arch Klin Chir* 43:32, 1892.

5. Bentley FH: Speech after repair of cleft palate, *Lancet* 2:862, 1947.

5a. Bergland O, Semb G, Abyholm FE: Elimination of the residual alveolar cleft by secondary bone grafting and subsequent orthodontic treatment, *Cleft Palate J* 23:175, 1986.

5b. Bluestone CD, Musgrave RH, McWilliams BJ: Teflon injection pharyngoplasty: status 1968, *Laryngoscope* 78:558, 1968.

5c. Bluestone CD, Musgrave RH, McWilliams BJ, et al: Teflon injection pharyngoplasty, *Cleft Palate J* 5:19, 1968.

5d. Braur RO: Retropharyngeal implantation of silicone gel pillows for velopharyngeal incompetence, *Plast Reconstr Surg* 51:254, 1973.

6. Calnan JS: Congenital large pharynx, *Br J Plast Surg* 24:263, 1971.

7. Cohen SR, Kalinowski J, LaRossa D, et al: Cleft palate fistulas: a multivariate statistical analysis of prevalence, etiology, and surgical management, *Plast Reconstr Surg* 87:1041, 1991.

8. Chen PKT, Wu J, Hung KF, et al: Surgical correction of submucous cleft palate with Furlow palatoplasty, *Plast Reconstr Surg* 97:1136-1145, 1996.

9. Chen PKT, Wu JTH, Chen YR, et al: Correction of secondary velopharyngeal insufficiency in cleft palate patients with Furlow palatoplasty, *Plast Reconstr Surg* 94:933, 1994.

10. D'Antonio L, Barlow S, Warren D: Studies of speech motor control. Presented at the annual meeting of Speech-Language-Hearing Association, San Antonio, Nov. 20-23, 1992, *ASHA* 34:28A, 1993.

11. D'Antonio L, Muntz HR, Marsh JL, et al: Practical application of flexible fiberoptic nasopharyngoscopy for evaluating velopharyngeal function, *Plast Reconstr Surg* 82:611, 1988.

12. D'Antonio LL: Evaluation and management of velopharyngeal dysfunction: a speech pathologist's viewpoint. In Lehman JA, editor: *Cleft palate surgery*, Philadelphia, 1992, JB Lippincott.

13. Dalston RM, Marsh JL, Vig KW, et al: Minimal standards for reporting the results of surgery on patients with cleft lip, cleft palate or both: a proposal, *Cleft Palate J* 25:3, 1988.

14. Denk MJ, Magee WP Jr: Cleft palate closure in the neonate: preliminary report, *Cleft Palate Craniofac J* 33:57-61, 1996.

14a. Denny AD, Marks SM, Oliff-Carneol S: Correction of velopharyngeal insufficiency by pharyngeal augmentation using autologous cartilage: a preliminary report, *Cleft Palate Craniofac J* 30:46, 1993.

15. Dreyer TM, Trier WC: Comparison of palatoplasty techniques, *Cleft Palate J* 21:251, 1984.

16. Dufresne CR: Oronasal and nasolabial fistulas. In Bardach J, Morris HL (eds): *Multidisciplinary management of cleft lip and palate,* Philadelphia, 1990, WB Saunders.

16a. Eckstein H: Demonstration of a paraffin prosthesis in defects of the face and palate, *Dermatology* 11:772, 1904.

17. Furlow L: Cleft palate repair by double reversing Z-plasty, *Plast Reconstr Surg* 78:724, 1986.

17a. Gersuny R: About a subcutaneous prosthesis, *Z Heilk* 21:199, 1900.

18. Golding-Kushner KJ, Argamoso RV, Cotton RT, et al: Standardization for the reporting of nasopharyngoscopy and multiview video fluoroscopy: a report from an international working group, *Cleft Palate J* 27:337, 1990.

18a. Hagerty RF, Hill MJ: Cartilage pharyngoplasty in cleft palate patients, *Surg Gynecol Obstet* 112:350, 1961.

19. Henningson G, Isberg A: Oronasal fistulas and speech production. In Bardach J, Morris HL (eds): *Multidisciplinary management of cleft lip and palate,* Philadelphia, 1990, WB Saunders.

20. Henningson G, Isberg A: Influence of palatal fistulae on speech and resonance, *Folia Phoniatr (Basel)* 39:183, 1987.

21. Hess DA, Hagerty RF, Mylin WK: Velar mobility, velopharyngeal closure and speech proficiency in cartilage pharyngoplasty: an eight year study, *Cleft Palate J* 5:153, 1968.

22. Hogan MV: Clarification of the surgical goals in cleft palate speech and the introduction of lateral port control (LPC) pharyngeal flap, *Cleft Palate J* 10:331, 1973.

23. Holtmann B, Wray RC, Weeks PM: A comparison of three techniques of palatorrhaphy: early speech results, *Ann Plast Surg* 12:514-518, 1984.

24. Hotz M, Gnoinski W, Perko H, et al: *Early treatment of cleft lip and palate,* Toronto, 1986, Hans Huber Publishers.

25. Hynes W: Pharyngoplasty by muscle transplantation, *Br J Plast Surg* 3:128, 1950.

26. Isshiki N, Honjow I, Morimoto M: Effects of velopharyngeal incompetence upon speech, *Cleft Palate J* 5:297, 1968.

27. Jackson IT: Sphincter pharyngoplasty, *Clin Plast Surg* 12:711, 1985.

28. Kremenak CR, Huffman WC, Olin WH: Maxillary growth inhibition by mucoperiosteal denudation of palate shelf bone in non-cleft beagles, *Cleft Palate J* 7:817, 1970.

28a. Kuehn DP, Van Demark DR: Assessment of velopharyngeal competency following teflon pharyngoplasty, *Cleft Palate J* 15:145, 1978.

29. Lehman JA, Fishman JRA, Neiman GS: Treatment of cleft palate associated with Robin sequence: appraisal of risk factors, *Cleft Palate Craniofac J* 32:25-29, 1995.

30. Mars M, Asher-McDade C, Brattstrom V, et al: A six-center international study of treatment outcome in patients with clefts of the lip and palate: Part 3. Dental arch relationship, *Cleft Palate Craniofac J* 29:405-408, 1992.

31. Marsh JL, Wray RC: Speech prosthesis versus pharyngeal flap: a randomized evaluation of the management of velopharyngeal incompetency, *Plast Reconstr Surg* 65:592-594, 1980.

32. McGrath CO, Anderson MW: Prosthetic treatment of velopharyngeal incompetence. In *Multidisciplinary management of cleft lip and palate,* Philadelphia, 1990, WB Saunders.

33. McWilliams BJ, Morris HL, Shelton RF: *Cleft palate speech,* Philadelphia, 1990, BC Decker.

34. Mercer NSG, MacCarthy P: The arterial basis of pharyngeal flaps, *Plast Reconstr Surg* 96:1026-1037, 1995.

35. Mercer NSG, MacCarthy P: The arterial supply of the palate: implications for closure of cleft palates, *Plast Reconstr Surg* 96:1038-1044, 1995.

36. Moran RE: The pharyngeal flap operation as a speech aid, *Plast Reconstr Surg* 7:202, 1951.

37. Oneal RM: Oronasal fistulas. In Rosenstein SW, Bzoch KR (eds): *Cleft lip and palate,* Boston, 1971, Little, Brown.

38. Orticochea M: Construction of a dynamic muscle sphincter in cleft palates, *Plast Reconstr Surg* 41:323, 1968.

39. Owsley JQ, Lawson LI, Miller ER, et al: Experience with high attached pharyngeal flap, *Plast Reconstr Surg* 38:232, 1966.

40. Parameters for the evaluation and treatment of patients with cleft lip/palate or other craniofacial anomalies, *Cleft Palate Craniofac J* 30(suppl 1), 1993.

41. Randall P: A commentary on: Management and timing of cleft palate fistula repair, *Plast Reconstr Surg* 78:746, 1986.

42. Randall P, LaRossa D, Solomon M, et al: Experience with the Furlow double reversing Z-plasty for cleft palate repair, *Plast Reconstr Surg* 77:569, 1986.

42a. Remacle M, Bertrand B, Eloy P, et al: The use of injectable collagen to correct velopharyngeal insufficiency, *Laryngoscope* 100:269, 1990.

43. Riski JE, Ruff GL, Georgiade GG, et al: Evaluation of the sphincter pharyngoplasty, *Cleft Palate Craniofac J* 29:254, 1992.

44. Riski JE, Serafin D, Riefkohl R, et al: A rationale for modifying the site of insertion of the Orticochea pharyngoplasty, *Plast Reconstr Surg* 73:882, 1984.

45. Roberts CT, Semb G, Shaw WC: Strategies for the advancement of surgical methods in cleft lip and palate, *Cleft Palate Craniofac J* 28:141-149, 1991.

46. Schoenborn D: Uber eine neue methode der staphylorraphies, *Arch F Klin Chir* 19:528-531, 1876.

47. Schultz RC: Management and timing of cleft palate fistula repair, *Plast Reconstr Surg* 78:739, 1986.

48. Shaw WC, Asher-McDade C, Brattstrom V, et al: A six-center international study of treatment outcome in patients with clefts of the lip and palate: Part 1. Principles and study design, *Cleft Palate Craniofac J* 29:393-397, 1992.

49. Shaw WC, Dahl E, Asher-McDade C, et al: A six-center international study of treatment outcome in patients with clefts of the lip and palate: Part 5. General discussion and conclusions, *Cleft Palate Craniofac J* 29:413-418, 1992.

50. Shelton RL, Blank JL: Oronasal fistulas, intraoral air pressure, and nasal air flow during speech, *Cleft Palate J* 21:91, 1984.

51. Shprintzen RJ, Lewin ML, Croft CB, et al: A comprehensive study of pharyngeal flap surgery: tailor made flaps, *Cleft Palate J* 16:46, 1979.

52. Skolnick ML, McCall GN: Velopharyngeal competence and incompetence following pharyngeal flap surgery: video fluoroscopic study in multiple projections, *Cleft Palate J* 9:1, 1972.

53. Skolnick ML, McCall GN: A radiographic technique for demonstrating the causes of persistent nasality in patients with pharyngeal flaps, *Br J Plast Surg* 26:12, 1973.

54. Sloan GM, Reinisch JR, Nichter LS, et al: Surgical treatment of velopharyngeal insufficiency: pharyngoplasty vs. pharyngeal flap, *Plast Surg Forum* 13:128, 1990.

55. Spriesterbach DC, Dickson DR, Fraser FC, et al: Clinical research in cleft lip and palate: the state of the art, *Cleft Palate J* 10:113-165, 1973.

55a. Sturim HS, Jacob CT Jr: Teflon pharyngoplasty, *Plast Reconstr Surg* 49:180, 1972.

56. Trier WC: Primary palatoplasty, *Clin Plast Surg* 12:663, 1985.

57. Trost-Cardamone JE: Coming to terms with velopharyngeal insufficiency: a response to Loney and Bloem, *Cleft Palate J* 26:68, 1989.

58. Wardill WE: Results of operation for cleft palate, *Br J Surg* 16:127, 1928.

59. Warren DW: Velopharyngeal orifice size and upper pharyngeal pressure flow patterns in normal speech, *Plast Reconstr Surg* 33:148, 1964.

60. Warren DW, Devereau JL: An analog study of cleft palate speech, *Cleft Palate J* 3:103, 1966.

61. Whitaker LA, Randall P, Graham WP, et al: A prospective and randomized series comparing superiorly and inferiorly based posterior pharyngeal flaps, *Cleft Palate J* 9:304, 1972.

62. Witt PD, D'Antonio LL: Velopharyngeal insufficiency and secondary palatal management, a new look at an old problem, *Clin Plast Surg* 20(4):707-721, 1993.

63. Witt PD, D'Antonio LL, Zimmerman GJ, et al: Sphincter pharyngoplasty: a preoperative and postoperative analysis of perceptual speech characteristics and endoscopic studies of velopharyngeal function, *Plast Reconstr Surg* 93:1154-1168, 1994.

64. Witt PD, Marsh JL, Grames LM, et al: Revision of the failed sphincter pharyngoplasty: an outcome assessment, *Plast Reconstr Surg* 96:126-138, 1995.

65. Witt PD, Miller DC, Marsh J, et al: Perception of postpalatoplasty speech differences in school-age children by parents, teachers, and professional speech pathologists, *Plast Reconstr Surg* 100:1655-1663, 1997.

66. Witt PD, O'Daniel TG, Marsh JL, et al: Surgical management of velopharyngeal dysfunction: outcome analysis of autogenous posterior pharyngeal wall augmentation, *Plast Reconstr Surg* 99:1287-1296, 1997.

67. Witt PD, Rozzelle, A, Marsh JL, et al: Do palatal lift appliances stimulate velopharyngeal neuromuscular activity? *Cleft Palate Craniofac J* 32:469-475, 1995.

68. Witt PD: Invited commentary on Denk MJ and Magee WP, Cleft closure in the neonate: a preliminary report, *Cleft Palate Craniofac J* 33:62-64, 1996.

69. Witt PD, Marsh JL, Muntz HR, et al: Nasal airway obstruction as a complication of sphincter pharyngoplasty, *Cleft Palate Craniofac J* 33:183-189, 1996.

70. Witt PD, Marsh JL, Muntz HR, et al: Speech outcome following palatoplasty in primary school children: do lay peer observers agree with speech pathologists? *Plast Reconstr Surg* 98:958, 1996.

71. Witt PD, Marsh JL, Grames LM, et al: Management of the hypodynamic velopharynx, *Cleft Palate Craniofac J* 32:179-187, 1995.

72. Witt PD, Miller DC, Marsh JL, et al: Limited value of preoperative cervical vascular imaging in patients with velocardiofacial syndrome, *Plast Reconstr Surg* 101:1184-1195, 1998.

Secondary Cleft Lip and Cleft Nasal Deformities

Eric H. Hubli
Kenneth E. Salyer
David G. Genecov

INDICATIONS

Management of the cleft lip and palate patient has improved over the past two decades. Advances in surgical technique combined with a comprehensive team approach have yielded gratifying results. However, despite these advances, secondary cleft lip and nose deformities remain. The factors that may lead to a secondary deformity vary, but they can be distilled down to three primary causes: severity of the initial cleft deformity, errors in surgical planning or technique, and the biologic vagaries of wound healing.[2] The extent of the resultant deformities are varied, as well. Secondary deformities may be minimal, consisting of subtle vermilion mismatches, or they may be severe, reflecting a composite osseous–soft tissue disharmony. Regardless of the cause, a carefully planned, anatomically based, individualized treatment plan is essential if consistently excellent outcomes are to be achieved.

In the initial assessment of the patient presenting with a secondary cleft lip/nasal deformity, a careful history and physical examination are a must. The history should include a review of the type of initial cleft and the timing, type, and extent of primary repair. Any untoward events that may have contributed to the unacceptable outcome should be documented and accounted for to minimize their risk of recurrence. Preoperative photographs are helpful guides, if available. After the history, a careful physical examination is required. The examination should focus on all levels of the deformity, including the "unseen" osseous anatomy, which plays such a vital role in determining soft tissue placement.

We routinely begin our examination with the nose. The nasal bones are evaluated for symmetry, and any canting of the structures is noted. Next, the upper lateral cartilages, the domal elements, and the alar cartilages are assessed. In the unilateral cleft deformity, the upper lateral cartilage on the affected side is laterally displaced and is longer than the corresponding structures on the noncleft side. We also note that the tip is asymmetric, with the cleft domal elements assuming a depressed position, thus creating an obtuse angle at the vestibular genu. The alar cartilage on the cleft side is lateralized and widened because of its initial position at the time of presentation. This creates an overall widening of the cleft nares compared with the normal side. In some secondary cleft patients the cleft side nares may be small as a result of poor surgical technique. Evaluation of the internal nasal structures reveals a deviation of the septum toward the noncleft side and bilateral turbinate hypertrophy caused by the turbulent air flow generated across the basically abnormal nasal anatomy. Nasal air flow should be evaluated and is usually found to be compromised in both nasal pathways. This nasal airway obstruction may reduce nasal air escape and as such mask an underlying velopharyngeal incompetence. A full speech assessment should be made before any nasal surgery to document the presence or absence of velopharyngeal incompetence.

Continuation of a systematic examination leads to the vomer and the underlying osseous anatomy. In this area, one notes a mild to moderate hypoplasia of the maxillary structures on the cleft side and an associated canting of the vomer toward the noncleft side. The orientation of the palatal shelves is noted because any deviation from the normal alveolar arch pattern will adversely affect the positioning of the nasal and labial elements and must be accounted for during the planning stages of the repair. It is imprudent to generate a "normal" reconstruction over abnormal osseous anatomy that, when corrected, will cause undesired shifting of the overlying soft tissue.[2,3,15,25]

Once these factors are accounted for, a careful evaluation of the lip at rest and during dynamic function is carried out. Resting assessment focuses on lip symmetry, highlighting the vertical and horizontal lip components. Any lip length discrepancies are noted, and plans for a correction are made. The structure of the Cupid's bow is assessed; and the alignment of the white roll, vermilion, and red line are evaluated to discern any horizontal linear discrepancies. Next, dynamic lip function is examined by asking the patient to purse his or her lips. In the appropriately repaired lip, one will see a normal function of the orbicularis oris musculature. The incomplete repair will demonstrate two distinct muscle bulges at the edge of the cleft repair. Dynamic examination may prove challenging in the very young child in that patient compliance is not optimal. It is our experience that careful observation of facial expression during play will usually allow for an adequate assessment of muscular function.

The bilateral cleft patient presents with a unique set of anatomic challenges. Although the overall pattern of assessment is the same as that for the unilateral cleft patient, the findings can be dramatically different. The severity of the secondary deformity in the bilateral cleft patient is due to the tissue deficiency and the anatomic malalignments inherent in the cleft itself. The resultant secondary lip defect is most dramatically affected by the initial size, shape, and positioning of the premaxillary and prolabial segments. Generally the premaxillary and prolabial segments are hypoplastic, anteriorly displaced, axially rotated, and skewed to one side of the arch. At the time of initial repair, attempts to rectify these anomalies can lead to significant lip asymmetries that may not be easily correctable because of soft tissue deficiencies. We also note that a shortened columella and an underdeveloped premaxillary gingival-buccal sulcus is the rule rather than the exception.[27]

When assessing the nose in the secondary bilateral cleft patient, the most striking feature is the flattening of the nasal tip resulting from domal separation and columellar tethering. The alar cartilages tend to be broad, flattened, and enlarged. They assume a horizontal orientation in which they are inferiorly rotated and posterolaterally displaced. In many cases, the maxillary and nasal bones are hypoplastic yet symmetric. Internal nasal examination reveals a small nasal vestibule with septal deviation and the associated turbinate hypertrophy.[2]

Once the clinical assessment is complete, a thorough review of the findings should be given to the patient or the parents of the patient. Anomalous anatomic structures should be pointed out and the methods of repair described. During this period, we believe that it is very important to highlight the relevant soft tissue deficiencies and to point out any underlying osseous anomalies that may not be addressed at the time of early secondary repair. We also highlight the presence or absence of cicatrix and indicate how it will affect tissue mobility, blood supply, and future healing. Finally, we emphasize that cleft care is a growth-dependent, progressive challenge that will reach its terminus in the late teenage years. We try to have the patient and the parents understand that there is a timing and sequence to cleft care that must be followed to achieve optimal results.

In general, we feel that in both the unilateral and the bilateral cleft deformity the greater the degree of the initial deformity, the greater the possibility for a significant secondary deformity.

OPERATIONS

SECONDARY UNILATERAL CLEFT LIP REPAIR

Asymmetry of the Vermilion

Vermilion irregularities are one of the most frequently occurring and readily identifiable secondary lip deformities. These deformities may arise because of postoperative scar contracture, inadequate approximation of the orbicularis oris musculature, vermilion mismatching at the time of initial suturing, or any combination of the preceding causative agents. Meticulous attention to detail, with precise approximation of the white roll, vermilion, and red line during the initial operative procedure, can prevent many of these deformities. However, even in the best of hands, discrepancies may arise.[9]

Most vermilion deformities can be treated using local tissue transposition procedures. White roll mismatches represent one of the smaller yet more noticeable vermilion asymmetries. These deformities can be treated by small Z-plasties (Figure 57-1) or direct excision using an elliptical or diamond pattern. Either technique will generate an excellent result. Notching of the vermilion may be limited, involving only the mucosal layer. In this setting, a simple V-Y advancement will usually correct the deformity. In more severe situations, in which mucosa and vermilion show inadequate fullness and associated

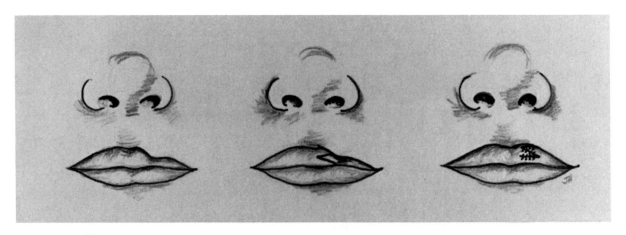

Figure 57-1. Small white roll/vermilion mismatches can be addressed using Z-plasties. The Z is drawn so as to increase vermilion fullness while maintaining integrity of white roll.

scarring, a series of Z-plasties may be needed to correct the deformities found in each respective area. We make a point of differentiating our treatment areas (mucosa and vermilion) because we believe strongly that mucosa should never be used to substitute for vermilion. When substituted for vermilion, mucosa will dry and crack, making the difference in tissue readily apparent.[2,9,27]

Vermilion asymmetry may be caused by excessive or deficient vermilion on one of the cleft segments. This tissue mismatch can be corrected by augmenting the deficient side or by reducing the side that is more full. In some instances, a combination of approaches is required. To fill out a deficient segment, one may use a series of equal or unequal Z-plasties.

Another technique involves a multilayered V-Y advancement in which the mucosal and muscle layers are freed up to the vermilion and advanced under the vermilion to increase its bulk and projection (Figures 57-2 and 57-3). Lip reduction procedures are self-explanatory and usually are accomplished by taking a horizontal ellipse of vermilion out of the segment that exhibits unwanted fullness (Figures 57-4 and 57-5). In the most severe cases of vermilion asymmetry, small local flaps may not provide adequate tissue repositioning. In these cases, we advocate reoperation with the re-creation and readjustment of the initial flaps. In this manner, tissue imbalances in each layer may be addressed independently and soft tissue harmony obtained.

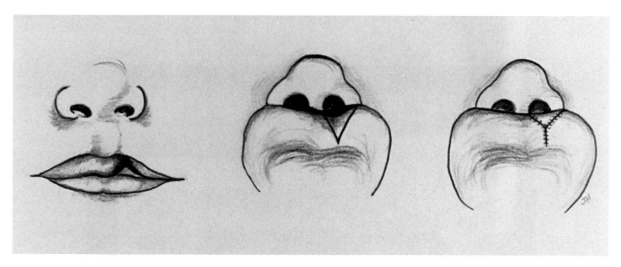

Figure 57-2. V-Y advancement of mucosa and vermilion to correct notching in a unilateral cleft.

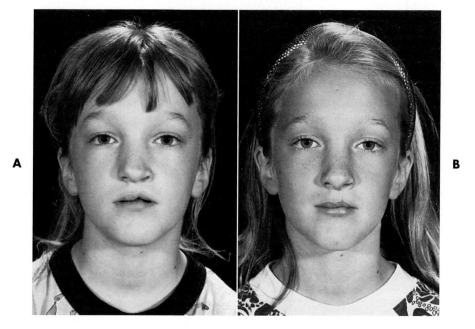

A, **B,**

Figure 57-3. **A,** Preoperative view demonstrating vermilion notching. **B,** Postoperative view demonstrating an increased fullness of vermilion after V-Y advance.

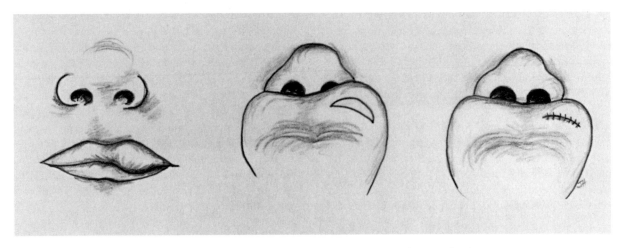

Figure 57-4. Correction of vermilion excess using elliptical mucosal reduction.

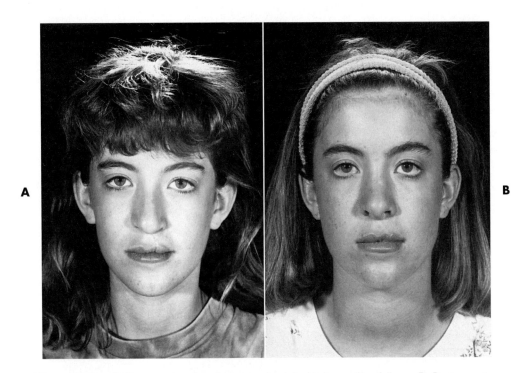

Figure 57-5. **A,** Preoperative view demonstrating left-sided vermilion fullness. **B,** Postoperative view demonstrating vermilion symmetry.

Short Upper Lip

The short upper lip deformity involves all layers of the reconstructed lip and is manifest by an asymmetry in the vertical lengths of the repaired cleft lip segments. This deformity arises from one of two distinct causes. The first and most common cause is poor planning and/or execution of the primary repair. In this setting, the initial measurements of the vertical cleft dimensions at the time of primary repair are inaccurate and thus of insufficient length. This creates short vertical arms at the cleft margin, which in turn causes lip shortening resulting from underrotation of the noncleft segment. The second factor that may lead to a short upper lip is dense scar contracture. This eventuality is uncontrollable and

may shorten even the most expertly performed primary cheiloplasty. In either situation, our preferred method of repair is a recreation of the initial defect with complete reoperation and multilayered reconstruction of the asymmetric segments. Careful preoperative measurements confirm the appropriate vertical lip lengths, after which we use a rotation advancement technique to readapt the cleft lip margins. In cases in which extra length is needed, we sometimes use a Z-plasty in either the nasal sill or just above the white roll to achieve the maximum aesthetic result.

Patients who present with hypertrophic scarring are a unique subset who require special consideration. Although the surgical approach remains the same, these patients also will receive injections of triamcinolone at the time of secondary repair. We also advocate 3 months of continuous lip taping and vigorous postoperative massage once complete wound healing has been accomplished. At times, we will recommend the utilization of a silicon dressing to take advantage of every available treatment modality. In this manner, we attempt to maximize our outcome by minimizing scar formation.

Constricted Upper Lip

The constricted lip deformity represents a variant of the short upper lip deformity in which both a vertical and a horizontal deficiency soft tissue is present. In the unilateral cleft, this deficiency is usually secondary to an overzealous soft tissue resection at the primary cheiloplasty. However, tissue hypoplasia and osseous cleft width may also contribute to the deformity. Regardless of the cause, repair must focus on augmenting the area of soft tissue deficiency. Some authors have advocated the use of the Abbe flap[1] as a primary means of treatment, but we think that this procedure is infrequently indicated in the unilateral cleft patient. Generally we find that a "reoperative" approach will be sufficient to restore lip symmetry. In this setting, the primary incision is reopened and tissue reorientation is addressed in a layered fashion. To date, this approach has yielded excellent results and alleviated the need for an Abbe flap.

Long Upper Lip

The long upper lip deformity represents the opposite extreme of the short upper lip. This problem is almost always due to an error in surgical planning or technique. If the primary repair consisted of a rotation advancement technique, the deformity results from overrotation of the affected lip segment. If the Le Mesurier technique was used, the deformity arises because of the action of the underlying muscular forces.[14] In either instance, our primary approach to repair mirrors that of the short upper lip. First, careful measurements are made to define the correct vertical lip lengths. If the discrepancy is mild or moderate, we use a reoperative technique in which the entire lip is taken down, the segments and structures are defined, and the lip is completely reconstructed, balancing all layers in the process.

If the lip length discrepancy is severe, a full-thickness elliptical lip reduction is added to the aforementioned procedure to correct any residual fullness.[2] The ellipse is placed at the nasal sill and may be skewed to one side or the other if the long lip discrepancy is asymmetric. As in the short upper lip repair, we advocate postoperative lip massage in association with 3 months of lip taping to minimize the effects of postoperative scar formation.

Muscular Diastasis

Muscular diastasis may be partial or complete. This deformity is not generally evident at rest unless there is an associated cutaneous component. Usually the diagnosis is made during dynamic examination of the labial structures. When the patient is asked to whistle or to purse his or her lips, an obvious bulge is noted at the edges of the cleft margins. These bulges represent the ends of the orbicularis oris muscle and by their presence confirm the lack of muscular continuity that defines this entity. The defect may be small and limited to the marginalis portion of the orbicularis oris muscle, or it may be complete, involving the full length of the muscle belly.

Although muscular diastasis may be due to postoperative trauma or infection, the most common causative factors lie in the hands of the surgeon. Incomplete muscular dissection, postoperative hematoma, or a high-tension closure resulting from inadequate tissue mobilization are the most frequent etiologic contributors. Meticulous dissection with tension-free closure will prevent the vast majority of these deformities.

When present, there is only one means of managing muscular diastasis: reoperation with careful muscular dissection and accurate muscular apposition. Postoperatively, we do not routinely use Steri-Strip bandages or a Logan bow for lip protection. The reason for this is that at the time of surgery, great care is taken to adequately mobilize the soft tissue envelope. If necessary, we do not hesitate to undermine the maxillary soft tissue in a preperiosteal plane. This comprehensive dissection ensures full tissue mobility and a tension-free closure. Recurrence rates for this deformity should be zero.

Mucosal Anomalies and Nasolabial Fistula

Nasolabial fistula is the most frequently occurring mucosal anomaly present in the cleft lip and palate patient. Although scarring and tethering of the labial mucosa does occur, it is usually not problematic. Simple release with a Z-plasty or fish-mouth closure will generally resolve any mucosal banding. Nasolabial fistula, however, requires a more advanced approach. If the patient is exhibiting no speech or feeding difficulties associated with the fistula, we do not feel pressed to correct the deformity at an early age. Generally, we wait until the patient is between 7 and 9 years of age and combine fistula repair with our procedure for alveolar bone grafting.[2,27] The exact timing of repair depends on dental development. The patient is scheduled for repair just before the eruption of the canine that is adjacent to the cleft site. At this operation, an incision is made in the gingivobuccal sulcus along the anterior border of the alveolar cleft. Care is taken to leave sufficient tissue within the cleft so as to allow for the creation of oral mucoperiosteal flaps. Dissection then proceeds cephalad with an incision along the mucosal line of the nasolabial fistula. These mucosal flaps are then separated from the overlying nasal skin so that a two-layered closure can be obtained. We then close the vestibular nasal skin and nasal mucosa with interrupted dissolvable suture. This effectively closes the nasal portion of the fistula. Next, the alveolar cleft is packed with iliac cancellous bone, after which the gingival and mucoperiosteal flaps are closed around the grafted material. If arch instability exists, an occlusal wafer is wired to the dentition, via orthodontic brackets, thus stabilizing the mobile segments.

Postoperative care consists of a liquid or blenderized diet for 3 months combined with assiduous oral care consisting of water pick lavage after every meal and 3-times-a-day oral antibiotic rinse. If the procedure requires an occlusal wafer, this is removed at 3 months.

Fistula recurrence is uncommon. However, if a fistula does recur, the standard approach to repair involves readvancement and inset of the previously raised flaps. If the problem persists, buccal mucosal and/or myomucosal flaps may be required to deal with this recalcitrant problem.

SECONDARY UNILATERAL CLEFT NOSE REPAIR

Throughout the ages, primary cleft care has focused on the repair of the lip deformity while ignoring the glaring nasal deformity. Many thought that it was taboo to manipulate the nasal structures during infancy and childhood because the possible adverse effects that this might have on future nasal growth and development. As such, many surgeons eschew early nasal surgery, preferring to approach this problem in the teenage years. We strongly disagree with this approach and advocate aggressive nasal recontouring at the time of primary cleft lip repair.[22,26,28] When performed with care, this approach greatly reduces the frequency and severity of our secondary nasal deformities without causing any noticeable growth disturbances.

Even with the beneficial affects of primary nasal repair at the time of primary cheiloplasty, we have not obviated the occurrence of, or the need for, secondary nasal surgery. Severely distorted nasal anatomy combined with abnormal skeletal growth and turbulent nasal air flow all contribute to subsequent functional and aesthetic deformities in up to 35% of our patients. The goal of the secondary nasal repair is to correct those anatomic discrepancies that contribute to functional impairment, such as septal deviation and turbinate hypertrophy, while restoring the symmetry between the cleft and noncleft sides.

This is accomplished by a multifaceted surgical approach. We start by infiltrating both the internal and external nasal structures with lidocaine 1% with epinephrine 1:100,000. This not only minimizes postoperative discomfort but also serves to reduce intraoperative and postoperative bleeding. Once the vasoactive effect of the infiltrate has taken effect, we begin the operative procedure by performing bilateral inferior turbinectomies. Attention is then turned to the septum, where an anterior septal incision is made and standard submucous dissection is accomplished with the aid of a Cottle dissector. The area of septal cartilage curvature is then resected using angled cartilage scissors or a swivel knife. Any vomerine spurs or osseous anomalies are reduced using a rongeur. We save the septal cartilage in a moist sponge because it will usually assist during the reconstructive phase of the operation. Once the septum is straight and centralized, we close the mucosa and turn our attention to the overlying cartilaginous structures. This dissection is begun with a rim incision, after which we may use an open or semiopen technique. In either instance, the medial middle and lateral crura are dissected free from the dorsal skin envelope and the underlying mucosa (Figure 57-6, A and B). Once free, the structures are delivered into the operative field, after which they are assessed for shape, size, and symmetry. The standard situation reveals a lateral alar cartilage

that is hypoplastic and of poor quality. This hypoplasia affects the medial crura and domal elements, as well. We find that these structures tend to be fragile, with the medial crura and footplate being susceptible to distortion from the surrounding soft tissue. Because of these factors, we generally use a vertical septal cartilage strut graft to help support the medial crura and to increase tip projection. If septal cartilage is unavailable, conchal cartilage will serve as an adequate substitute. Next, the intercrural ligament is released and the lateral alar cartilages are advanced medially. They are then sewn together at the genu, thus creating a more defined nasal tip and adding to nasal projection (Figure 57-6, C). In some cases these maneuvers are not enough to accomplish adequate tip projection. As such, a small shield-shaped tip graft is used to further refine tip anatomy. The last maneuver in the reconstruction consists of nasal bone osteotomies using a 2-mm osteotome. When appropriate shape and symmetry have been achieved, closure is accomplished in the standard fashion (Figure 57-6, D). Gentle nasal packing is used to help maintain nasal tip projection and to minimize postoperative bleeding. A dorsal nasal splint is also applied to support the nasal bones and to prevent posterior displacement of the anterior cartilaginous structures.

As a point of technical refinement, we find that many times it is advantageous to remove the paired alar cartilages from the nasal vestibule and to reconstruct the entire nasal tip unit on a side table. The elements are then carefully replaced in their appropriate positions and held in place by bolster sutures. If, at the time of closure, projection is compromised by the skin envelope, then a V-Y columellar advance and an intranasal mucosal advance may be necessary to obtain the desired aesthetic result.

Postoperatively, we see the patient in 3 days to remove the nasal packing. The patient is kept in the dorsal nasal splint for 2 to 3 weeks, after which he or she is instructed to tape the nasal dorsum for another 3 weeks.

Limited surgical approaches have their place in secondary cleft nasal reconstruction when the secondary nasal defect is truly minimal. We believe, however, that most cleft patients require a complete reconstitution of the deformed nasal anatomy. As such, we believe that a comprehensive approach that addresses all of the anatomic considerations in a single procedure is the optimal means of obtaining both an aesthetic and a functional result (Figure 57-7).

SECONDARY BILATERAL CLEFT LIP REPAIR

Whistle Deformity of the Lip

The whistle deformity is manifest by a soft tissue deficiency in the central portion of the lip vermilion. In this setting the cutaneous lip structures, such as the prolabium and the lateral lip elements, should be of appropriate size and in the proper position. This differentiates this deformity from the short upper lip deformity in which both the vermilion and the prolabial segment are insufficient. It is very important to differentiate between these two entities before surgery because

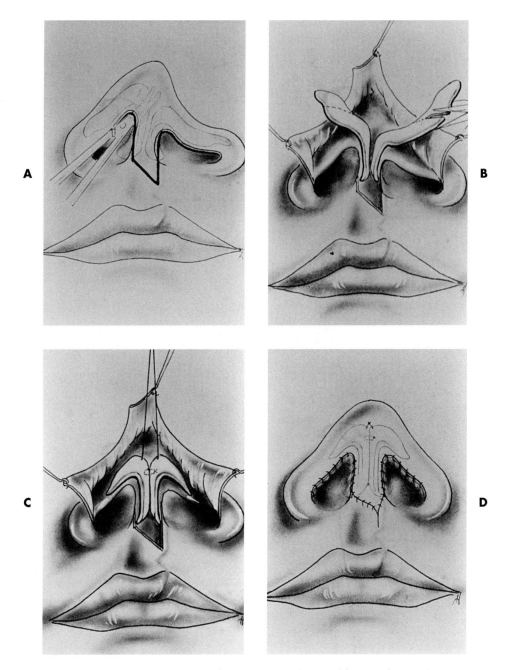

Figure 57-6. A, Nasal reconstruction via an open technique. After initial incisions, tenotomy scissors are insinuated at the soft triangle and subcutaneous dissection is accomplished. **B,** Once the alar cartilages are delivered, they are assessed for size, shape, and symmetry and are trimmed in the appropriate fashion. **C,** Medial advancement of lateral alar cartilages increases nasal projection. The reconstruction is maintained via plication sutures at the genu. **D,** Closure may involve a small V-Y advance at the columellar base to maintain maximal tip projection by minimizing downward soft tissue forces.

it is inappropriate to substitute a "vermilion" procedure for a cutaneous deficiency. If this is done, a tertiary deformity, in which excess vermilion is substituted for skin, is created. The whistle deformity arises because of an inadequate supply of vermilion at the time of primary repair. This occurs when the prolabial segment is extremely small (thus there is little central vermilion) or from a generalized vermilion deficiency at the time of initial cleft repair. In either case, there is not enough

tissue to fill the corresponding cleft and a V-shaped defect is made in the upper lip. Scar contracture and incomplete muscular transposition under the vermilion may also contribute to the deformity.

The type of repair required for correction of the whistle deformity of the lip is dependent on the extent of the defect. Small defects are approached in much the same way as vermilion notching in the unilateral cleft patient. In this

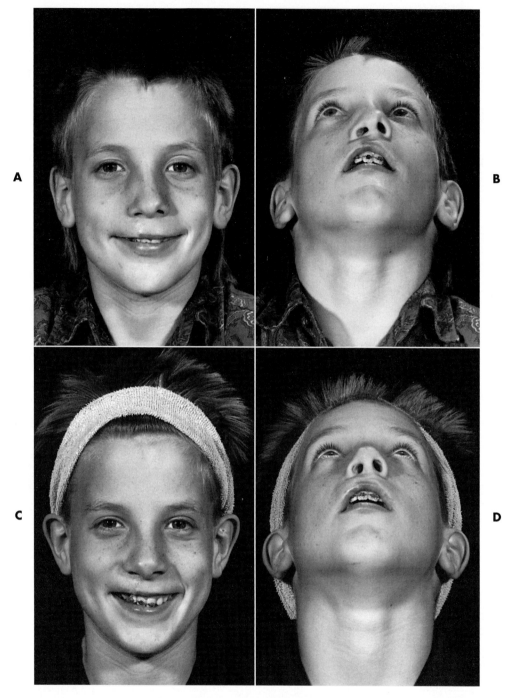

Figure 57-7. **A** and **B,** Preoperative view demonstrating nasal asymmetry associated with the unilateral cleft nasal deformity. **C** and **D,** Postoperative view demonstrating improved tip projection and alar symmetry.

setting, local mucosal or myomucosal V-Y advancement flaps (Figures 57-8 and 57-9) or cutaneous Z-plasties may transpose sufficient tissue to rectify the deformity.

In small to moderate deformities, bilateral, horizontally oriented, V-Y vermilion flaps (Kapetansky flaps) may be an adequate means of repair. This technique actually raises four flaps to correct the whistle deformity. The V-Y flaps are mobilized medially to augment the central vermilion, while a centrally placed upside-down W creates a space into which the lateral flaps will advance. The opening of the W allows for widening of the central lip element in the anteroposterior (AP) dimension. Thus the Kapetansky flap fills the central defect in all dimensions[8-11,24,30] (Figure 57-10).

Moderate to severe whistle deformities of the lip require more aggressive means of repair. In these cases, we will either reoperate and take the entire repair down so that all of the lip structures can be reoriented, or we may use a vermilion switch flap from the lower lip as a means of bringing new tissue into the upper lip defect. Both of these techniques have proven to be very effective.

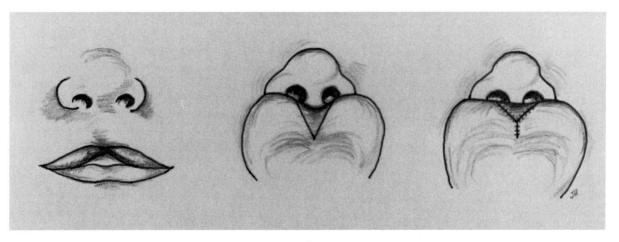

Figure 57-8. V-Y advancement for correction of whistle deformity associated with bilateral cleft lip.

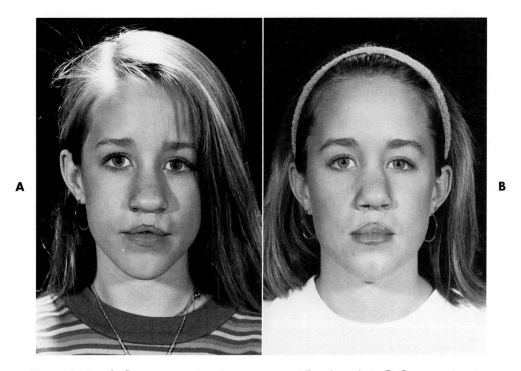

Figure 57-9. **A,** Preoperative view demonstrating midline hypoplasia. **B,** Postoperative view demonstrating increased lip fullness and symmetry.

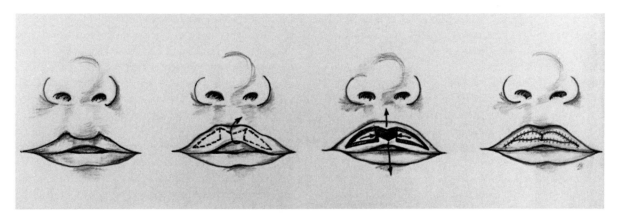

Figure 57-10. Kapetansky vermilion flaps. Triangular lateral vermilion swing flaps are advanced medially to reduce lateral lip fullness while augmenting the central lip element. A variant of this technique using mucosal swing flaps gives excellent results while minimizing vermilion scarring.

Short Upper Lip

The short upper lip or short prolabial deformity reflects a composite central lip deficiency. On examination, both the vermilion and the cutaneous prolabial segments are found to be of insufficient volume. As such, plans for repair must account for both deficiencies. Once again, the primary cause of the defect is the soft tissue hypoplasia present at the time of initial lip repair. The prolabial segment is, by definition, very short and inadequate for appropriate volumetric reconstruction at the time of primary cheiloplasty. The lateral lip elements are also hypoplastic and do not offer sufficient tissue to compensate for the size of the central defect. One way to minimize the potential of this deformity is to perform a staged primary repair. It is our experience that this will increase prolabial development and as such naturally augment the central lip structures.

Our preferred approach to the short lip deformity entails complete reoperation with readjustment of the muscular, cutaneous, and vermilion components of the lip.[2,27] At times, this can be accomplished using a unilateral rotation advancement technique; however, we believe that total reoperation, following the lines of previous repair, gives better overall results. This is because total reoperation allows for shaping of the prolabium (many times it is too wide) at the time of initial scar excision and allows for complete reorientation of all the soft tissue layers. The reoperative procedure is fairly straightforward in that the lines of incision are already present. The width and shape of the neoprolabium is measured and marked, after which L-shaped back-cuts are marked on the vermilion-cutaneous junction. Once diagrammed, the lip is incised and the mucosal, muscular, and cutaneous lip elements are dissected free. Horizontal back-cuts are made in the gingivobuccal sulcus to effectively release the entire lip. As in the primary cleft lip repair, further dissection up onto the maxilla may be necessary to obtain the appropriate tension-free advancement. Closure is begun with a deep muscular stitch. It is crucial to orient the muscular layer in exactly the desired fashion if an aesthetic correction is to be obtained. This is because the orbicularis oris muscle serves as the reconstructive cornerstone of the entire lip. As such, if the muscle layer is out of position, every subsequent layer will assume an anomalous position. The rest of the repair consists of lateral vermilion advancement and prolabial insetting. Postoperative care is analogous to the that of the secondary unilateral cleft lip repair.

Bardach[2] has designed multiple procedures for lengthening the short prolabium while simultaneously narrowing the alar base width. These procedures involve V-shaped incisions along the columella and within the nasal sill. A linear incision is then made down the central portion of the philtrum. All segments are then advanced medially and rotated caudally. In this fashion, two secondary bilateral cleft defects can be rectified with one procedure.

Constricted Upper Lip

The constricted upper lip deformity has many causative factors, ranging from anomalous osseous anatomy to soft tissue hypoplasia. If the premaxillary segment is protruding or malpositioned, it may place undue tension on the lip repair.

Conversely, if the prolabial segment is too deficient, the repair will be tighter than desired. Both problems become clinically manifest in the profile view of the patient. Upon examination of the lateral facial profile, the surgeon will note flattening of the upper lip and a relative protrusion of the lower lip. Obviously, the lower lip is normal and the defect is caused by the lack of upper lip projection. Preoperative planning must be thorough. Cephalometric analysis is essential and may reveal that the underlying deficiency stems from maxillary retrusion. If this is the case, operative intervention must incorporate an orthognathic component. If the maxillary and mandibular orientations are appropriate, however, soft tissue surgery alone may be sufficient to correct the deformity.

The constricted lip deformity is an extreme variant of the short upper lip deformity. In this setting, the profound hypoplasia associated with the primary cleft creates a soft tissue deficiency of such magnitude that there exists both a vertical and horizontal discrepancy in the corrected lip.

The flattened appearance of the upper lip is made more noticeable by the perceived fullness of the lower lip whose contrasting normalcy draws attention to the defect. Reoperation with reorientation of the lip segments is not an adequate means of correction because the inherent problem is not one of technique but rather of tissue deficiency. As such, the reconstructive plan must allow for the addition of well-vascularized, "like" soft tissue to the upper lip to obtain the desired lip symmetry. Our preferred reconstructive method is the staged Abbe flap.[1]

The Abbe flap is a full-thickness, triangularly designed, axial pattern lip flap based on the labial artery (Figures 57-11 and 57-12). Operatively, the flap is cut and maintained on one branch of the labial artery. Next it is inset into the area of soft tissue deficiency in the upper lip. The pedicled flap is left in place for 14 to 17 days, after which the vascular pedicle is transected and final flap inset is accomplished. Postoperatively, the patient is asked to minimize oral motion, pursue a liquid diet, and maintain good oral hygiene using an antibiotic oral rinse.

The success of this flap is dependent on patient compliance. Although we advocate the use of this approach on children and adults, we find that it is not well tolerated by the very young.

In the constricted lip deformity the Abbe flap is derived from the lower lip. The flap can yield spectacular results in this deformity because it addresses the problem on two levels. First, it brings new tissue to the upper lip and helps correct the inherent tissue deficiency. Second, by harvesting the flap from the lower lip, the volume of the lower lip is reduced. In this way, the size discrepancy between the upper and lower lip is minimized, thus making the deficient upper lip volume less noticeable. The renewed tissue balance enhances the overall aesthetic result.

Maxillary hypoplasia with associated retrusion and resultant Class III malocclusion can also give the appearance of a tight lip deformity. The osseous origin of the deformity, however, requires complex orthognathic assessment.

Consideration must be given to the positioning of the premaxilla and the status of the alveolar arch. Questions concerning dental positioning and arch stability must be

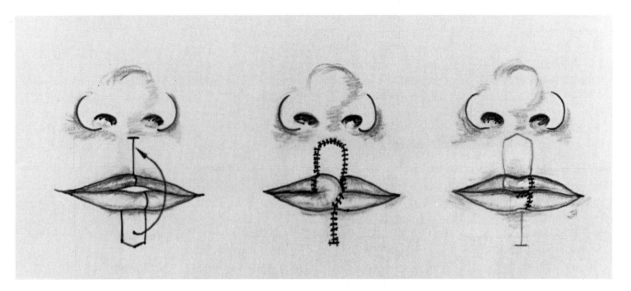

Figure 57-11. The Abbe flap is a full-thickness axial pattern lower lip flap based on the labial artery. The first stage involves the raising and insetting of the flap into the hypoplastic upper lip. Final insetting occurs 14 to 17 days after the initial procedure.

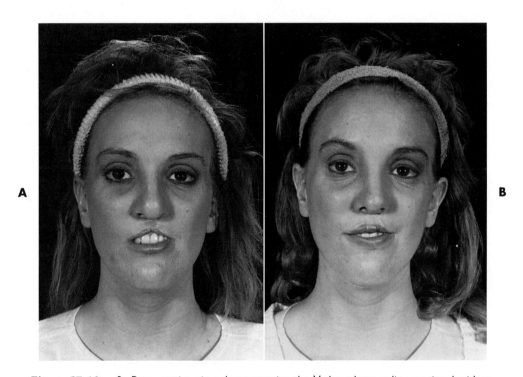

Figure 57-12. **A,** Preoperative view demonstrating the V-shaped upper lip associated with an extremely hypoplastic central lip element. **B,** Postoperative view demonstrating central lip fullness after final insetting of the Abbe flap.

addressed. Has the defect been previously bone grafted? Once these factors have been accounted for, the surgeon must decide if one-or two-jaw surgery is indicated. It is our experience that most bilateral cleft patients will require both maxillary and mandibular readjustment if dental and facial harmony is to be obtained. The operative planning and surgical techniques involved in this process are beyond the scope of the chapter; however, the details can be found in Chapter 58. One technical point that needs to be emphasized in the bilateral

cleft patient is relative to the initial approach to the maxilla. The premaxillary segment has a limited and temperamental blood supply. As such, the initial incision should never cut across the premaxillary mucosa or the segment may be devascularized and lost.

Long Upper Lip

The previous secondary cleft lip deformities come about because of the tissue deficiency associated with the presenting cleft deformity. The long upper lip deformity, however, arises as a result of a technical error in surgical planning and/or execution. In the long lip deformity, the central portion of the repaired lip is actually too long for the aesthetic norm of the patient's facial structures. This arises because the primary surgeon either overrotated the rotation advancement flaps or used the lateral lip elements to reconstruct the lower and midportion of the upper lip. Some techniques, like the Le Mesurier and the Barsky-Hagedorn procedures, by their

designs tend to create a longer than average central lip element.[2,14]

Aesthetic correction of the long upper lip can be extremely difficult to accomplish. Our standard approach consists of a curved elliptical excision just underneath the nasal sill (Figures 57-13 and 57-14). The excision ranges from one ala to the other and on rare occasions may be extended into the nasolabial fold. In all instances the excision includes all layers of the lip and requires that the underlying muscular layer be

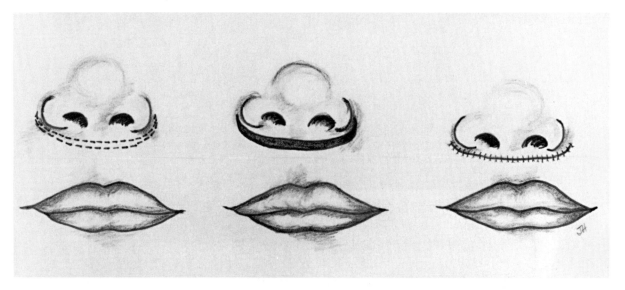

Figure 57-13. Correction of the long lip deformity using a full-thickness, curved, elliptical incision.

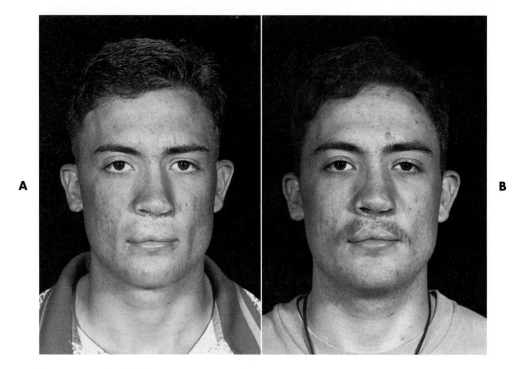

Figure 57-14. A, Preoperative view demonstrating increased columellar-to-labial distance. **B,** Postoperative view demonstrating restoration of the columellar-to-labial distance to a more normal proportion.

isolated and repositioned. Generally the muscle reorientation is accomplished by tacking the orbicularis oris to the nasal spine and/or the cartilaginous columella. Postoperative care is much the same as that of the previous lip repairs. Sutures are removed between postoperative days 5 and 7, and lip taping and massage begin shortly thereafter.

Muscular Diastasis

As in the unilateral cleft lip repair, muscular diastasis may lead to lateral subcutaneous bulging during dynamic lip function. Causative factors include muscular separation resulting from infection, hematoma, and/or poor surgical technique. In the primary bilateral cleft, the orbicularis oris muscle inserts into the alar base. Muscle bulging arises because the vertically oriented insertion has not been completely released and redirected into a horizontal plane. This in turn inappropriately directs the muscular pull of the orbicularis oris toward the alar base instead of across the lip. The one caveat related to this deformity in the bilateral cleft patient is that at the time of initial cleft repair, the surgeon may intentionally choose not to approximate the muscle bellies. This situation arises when it becomes evident that joining the muscle bellies over the premaxilla will create undue tension on the repair. As such, the surgeon may choose to suture the cut ends of the muscle to the lateral periosteum of the premaxilla. We have found that this approach has consistently yielded excellent lip function without creating the unsightly muscular bulges described above.

Once the extent of the defect is defined, complete reoperation is the only known means of affecting repair. As previously described, we use the primary lip incisions as our means of access to the underlying musculature. The orbicularis oris is completely released from the alar base, after which we analyze the mobility of the independent muscle bundles. If possible, we will approximate the cut ends in the midline. If attempted closure creates significant soft tissue tension, we will suture the muscular units to the premaxilla. In either case, a good result is expected. Postoperative care follows our standard cleft lip protocol.

SECONDARY BILATERAL CLEFT NOSE REPAIR

The primary cause of secondary nasal deformities stems from the prolabial tissue deficiency, which, by its presence, creates the short columella and tethered tip that is so characteristic of the bilateral cleft nose. These anatomic arrangements place undue stress on the domal and alar cartilaginous elements, causing the domal elements to be splayed laterally and the alar cartilages to lie in a horizontal orientation. Thus the three primary objectives of secondary nasal reconstruction in the bilateral cleft nasal repair are to increase columellar length, augment tip projection, and narrow the alar base while shifting the alar cartilages from an horizontal to an oblique position.[3,15,16,18,29] We believe that these changes should be accomplished in two stages.

The first nasal repair occurs when the patient is between 1 and 1½ years of age. At this time, the lip has been repaired and

the nasal tip is extremely flat because of the short columella. We employ the Salyer modification of the Cronin columellar lengthening procedure to achieve the aforementioned goals.[6] The nose is injected with 1% lidocaine with epinephrine. The operation begins with a gull wing incision cut along the line of the scar that is present at the base of the nasal sill. The incision starts at one alar base and then runs medially to the columella. Here it rises slightly as an inverted V up into the columella before proceeding on across to the contralateral alar base. Scissor dissection is then used to elevate the floor of the nose, after which the mucosal attachments at the piriform aperture are released. The lateral crura and alar cartilages are then completely dissected from the skin and underlying nasal mucosa. These maneuvers will allow the mucosa and cartilage to rotate and advance freely at the time of reconstruction.

Attention is next turned to the medial domal elements. Using the tenotomy scissors, the dorsal nasal skin above the dome is freed. This dissection is carried laterally to meet the previous dissection and will allow for delivery of the domal elements themselves. The mucosa of the soft triangle is not dissected.

Reconstruction begins with the suturing of the domal cartilages at the genu. A 5.0 nonabsorbable suture is used to advance and narrow the crural cartilages. This effectively narrows the tip while increasing tip projection. Next, an absorbable 3.0 suture is placed through both lateral alar bases and cinched so as to pull the alar bases symmetrically to the midline. This reorients the nares from an horizontal to an oblique position while concomitantly adding to columellar length. If the rotation is not facile and tension free, the nasal lining may be incised and released to accommodate the new nares position. Skin, cartilage, and mucosa are then readapted and reshaped using through-and-through bolster sutures.

Postoperatively, the patient is seen in 7 days. At this time, the nasal stents and the cutaneous sutures are removed. A nasal obturator may be used to minimize vestibular stenosis and to support the reconstruction. If used, the obturator is left in place for 3 to 6 months.

The second stage of the secondary bilateral cleft nose repair is performed after the patient reaches the mixed dentition stage. If possible, we prefer to deal with a stable premaxilla that is within the alveolar arch. Careful assessment of all underlying osseous anatomy is critical because these hidden anomalies can have a profound negative affect on the final aesthetic outcome. Our overall operative approach mimics that described in the unilateral cleft nose repair. The hallmarks in this instance are tip projection and refinement. Septal and conchal cartilage grafts are the norm rather than the exception because the compressed nature of the underlying cartilage scaffold is always in need of added structural support. One of the key differences in the bilateral versus the unilateral cleft nose repair lies in the columella. The secondary bilateral nose will always have a midline soft tissue deficiency. As such, any approach to repair will need to add to the substance of the columella. We usually approach the bilateral nose through an open technique, making the midline incision in the form of a V. In this fashion, columellar skin lengthening can be achieved via a V-Y advance.

Postoperative follow-up is as previously described, the caveat being that the bilateral cleft nose patient may need a nasal obturator to maintain shape and vestibular patency. As stated, these measures can be used for 3 to 6 months.

OUTCOMES

In cleft surgery, as in life, the old adage "an ounce of prevention is worth a pound of cure" still holds true. For this reason, we believe that the optimal time for correction of a secondary cleft deformity is at the time of primary cleft repair. It is our belief that cleft surgery is not a field to be "dabbled" in. Rather, it requires the immense experience that only comes with daily patient interaction. In this way, the practitioner will develop the skills required to expertly plan and execute the primary cleft repair. This high level of competence will minimize the need for secondary cleft surgery and as a result decrease the negative financial impact that repetitive surgical interventions can create. Unfortunately, even in the hands of the most skilled surgeon, secondary deformities do occur. Once again, experience is essential if one is to make the correct diagnosis and formulate a successful treatment protocol. Imprudent surgical decisions may lead to recurrent surgeries, and every subsequent attempt at correction of a deformity will only create a more difficult surgical challenge. As such, a lesser functional and aesthetic result can be expected because of the increased scar formation and decreased tissue pliability associated with repeated surgical assaults.

Assessment of cleft results must be reviewed through the microscope of years because normal growth and development are the only true measures of a successful outcome. The senior author has been a pioneer in cleft surgery for more than 25 years, and the following statistics reflect his ongoing desire to perfect his craft. Overall patient satisfaction in the secondary unilateral cleft lip/nose repair group has been outstanding, reaching the high 90th percentile. Satisfaction with the results of secondary bilateral cleft defects are high but not quite so gratifying at 75%. This lower satisfaction rate reflects our continued struggle to design the ideal primary bilateral cleft repair. Deficiencies inherent to the primary bilateral repair increase the possibility of a secondary deformity and greatly restrict the success of the subsequent operations. Secondary cleft results are destined to improve as new techniques for primary repair become available.

REFERENCES

1. Abbe R: A new plastic operation for the relief of deformity due to double harelip, *Med Rec* 53:477, 1898.
2. Bardach J, Salyer KE: *Surgical techniques in cleft lip and palate,* ed 2, St Louis, 1991, osby.
3. Berkeley WT: Correction of secondary cleft lip nasal deformities, *J Plast Reconstr Surg* 44:234-241, 1968.
4. Brauer RO: A comparison of the Tennison and Le Mesurier lip repairs, *J Plast Reconstr Surg* 23:249-259, 1959.
5. Cohen SR, Kawamoto HK: The free tongue graft for the correction of secondary deformities of the vermilion in patients with cleft lip, *J Plast Reconstr Surg* 88:613-619, 1991.
6. Cronin TD, Upton J: Lengthening of the short columella associated with bilateral cleft lip, *Ann Plast Surg* 1:75-94, 1978.
7. Cronin TD, Denkler KA: Correction of the unilateral cleft lip nose, *J Plast Reconstr Surg* 82:419-431, 1988.
8. Juri J, Juri C, DeAntueno J: A modification of the Kapetansky technique for repair of whistling deformities of the upper lip, *J Plast Reconstr Surg* 57:70-73, 1976.
9. Kawamoto HK: Correction of major defects of the vermilion with a cross lip vermilion flap, *J Plast Reconstr Surg* 64:315-318, 1979.
10. Kapetansky DI: Double pendulum flaps for whistling deformities in bilateral cleft lips, *J Plast Reconstr Surg* 47:321, 1971.
11. Kai S, Ohishi M: Secondary correction of the cleft lip and nose deformity: a new technique for revision of whistling deformity, *Cleft Palate J* 22:290-295, 1985.
12. Kernahar DA, Bauer BS, Harris GD: Experience with the Tajima Procedure in primary and secondary repair in unilateral cleft lip nasal deformity, *J Plast Reconstr Surg* 66:46-53, 1980.
13. Kirschbaum JD, Kirschbaum CA: The chondromucosal sleeve for the secondary correction of the unilateral cleft lip nasal deformity, *Ann Plast Surg* 29:402-406, 1992.
14. Le Mesurier AB: A method of cutting and suturing the lip in the treatment of complete unilateral clefts, *J Plast Reconstr Surg* 4, 1949.
15. McIndoe A, Rees TD: Synchronous repair of secondary deformities in cleft lip and nose, *J Plast Reconstr Surg* 24:150-161, 1959.
16. Matsuo K, Hirose T: A rotational method of bilateral cleft lip nose repair, *J Plast Reconstr Surg* 6:1034-1040, 1991.
17. Millard DR: The unilateral cleft lip, *J Plast Reconstr Surg* 34:169-175, 1964.
18. Millard DR: Closure of bilateral cleft lip and elongation of columella by two operations in infancy, *J Plast Reconstr Surg* 47:324-331, 1971.
19. Millard DR: Earlier correction of the unilateral cleft lip nose, *J Plast Reconstr Surg* 70:64-73, 1982.
20. Musgrave RH: Surgery of nasal deformities associated with cleft lip, *J Plast Reconstr Surg* 28:262-273, 1991.
21. Musgrave RH, Dupertus SM: Revision of the unilateral cleft lip nostril, *J Plast Reconstr Surg* 25:223-233, 1960.
22. Oriz Monasterio F, Olmedo A: Corrective surgery before puberty: a long term followup, *J Plast Reconstr Surg* 68:381-390, 1984.
23. Peterson RA, Ellenberg AH, Carroll DB: Vermillion flap reconstruction of bilateral cleft lip deformities (a modification of the Abbe procedure), *J Plast Reconstr Surg* 38:109-115, 1966.
24. Robinson DW, Ketchum LD, Masters FW: Double V-Y procedure for whistling deformity in repaired cleft lips, *J Plast Reconstr Surg* 46:241-244, 1970.

25. Salyer KE: Early and late treatment of unilateral cleft nasal deformity, *Cleft Lip Craniofac J* 29:556-569, 1992.

26. Salyer KE: New concepts in primary unilateral cleft lip and nose repair, *Worldplast* 1:83-97, 1995.

27. Salyer KE, Bardach J: *Atlas of craniofacial and cleft lip and palate surgical techniques,* Philadelphia, 1997, Lippincott-Raven.

28. Salyer KE: Primary correction of the unilateral cleft lip nose: a fifteen year experience, *J Plast Reconstr Surg* 77:558-566, 1986.

29. Van der Meulen IC: Columellar elongation in bilateral cleft lip repair: early results, *J Plast Reconstr Surg* 89:1060-1067, 1992.

30. Wagner JD, Newman MH: Bipedical axial cross-lip flap for correction of major Vermillion deficiency after cleft lip repair, *Cleft Lip Craniofac J* 31:148-151, 1994.

CHAPTER

Cleft-Orthognathic Surgery

58

Jeffrey C. Posnick

INDICATIONS

The optimal management of a child born with cleft lip and palate continues to challenge the health care delivery system.[22] The primary lip and palate repair performed during infancy and early childhood provides the foundation for normal speech, occlusion, facial appearance, and psychosocial development. One long-term negative effect of these early interventions is the occurrence of maxillary growth restriction that produces secondary deformities of the jaws that also negatively affects occlusion, speech, and self-esteem. Ross[28] documented that in approximately 25% of adults with a repaired unilateral cleft lip and palate, orthognathic surgery is necessary to permit an adequate functional relationship of the jaws and teeth. The cephalometric criteria he applied are traditional ones that underestimate the actual number of adolescents born with a cleft who would benefit from orthognathic surgery.[11]

The prevalence and extent of residual maxillofacial deformities in the adolescent born with a cleft vary widely, depending on the philosophy of the clinicians involved in the individual's care and on available technical expertise. In addition, despite a cleft team's preferred method of managing this deformity during infancy and childhood, there is a subgroup of patients who in adolescence have multiple neglected or residual cleft-related problems.

The generally accepted concepts of managing the cleft-related bony defects through the alveolus and the residual perialveolar oronasal fistula are to fill the skeletal gaps with autogenous iliac (hip) bone graft and to close all oronasal fistulas at each cleft site and throughout the palate in the mixed dentition before eruption of the permanent canine tooth through the cleft.[1,5,11,23,27] This procedure is preceded by a short phase of interceptive orthodontic treatment to expand the arch width to a normal range and then followed by orthodontic closure of the cleft-dental gap (in the region of the congenitally absent lateral incisor tooth) whenever feasible. If this approach is followed successfully, the adolescent with a cleft who has maxillary hypoplasia may undergo a standard Le Fort I osteotomy for correction.[2]

Unfortunately, there remains a subgroup of adolescents with a cleft-jaw deformity who have residual skeletal (alveolar) clefts and perforated (oronasal fistula) maxilla. Recognition of the unique circulation requirements of the (clefted) upper jaw at the time of osteotomy has allowed us to suggest an effective one-stage approach to manage these residual deformities (see next section).[11-21,24-26,30]

OPERATIONS

The literature warns of the possible complications of maxillary osteotomy in the cleft patient but until recently has provided only limited descriptions of techniques to guide the maxillofacial surgeon in the performance of safe, reliable osteotomies to solve these problems.[36] Surgical attempts to correct cleft lip and palate skeletal problems date back to Steinkamm's description in 1938 of a maxillary Le Fort I osteotomy in a bilateral cleft patient.[29] Around that time, Gillies[4] also reported completed jaw surgery in a bilateral cleft patient, stabilizing the result with autogenous bone graft. In 1974, Willmar[35] reported on the complications of maxillary surgery, in which 17 unilateral and 8 bilateral cleft lip and palate patients underwent Le Fort I osteotomy. One of the patients died, but details of the technique were not mentioned. One patient had aseptic necrosis and partial loss of the lesser segment of the maxilla. In 1974, Georgiade[3] suggested that a camouflage approach with mandibular osteotomy and setback was often preferred to direct maxillary surgery. Kiehn, Desprez, and Brown[8] warned of blood supply problems that might occur with maxillary surgery in cleft patients. In 1975, Henderson and Jackson[6] reported combining lip-scar revision, oronasal fistula closure, and maxillary osteotomy as a one-stage procedure. Their concept was innovative, but they did not specify the details of the operative technique. In 1978, Jackson further described a Le Fort I procedure as it applied to the cleft patient, stating that if a large fistula was present requiring extensive flap mobilization for closure, the maxillary blood supply might be in danger. In general, surgeons have been leery about flap necrosis with loss of maxillary bone and teeth. Ward-Booth, Bhatia, and Moos[32] later described an approach with the Le Fort II osteotomy designed to protect circulation to the jaw segments when maxillary hypoplasia exists in the cleft patient.

In 1980, Tideman, Stoelinga, and Gallia[31] further defined the maxillary Le Fort I osteotomy in cleft patients with a segmental posterior osteotomy. They stressed the importance of preserving a vertical soft tissue pedicle to protect circulation to the dentoalveolar segments. Unfortunately, the osteotomies were to be completed through tunnels rather than under direct vision. James[7] expressed concern that a more direct downfracture of the maxilla would risk vascular compromise to the segments. In 1985, Poole[10] proposed an additional modification but continued to use small vertical incisions on the labial aspect, requiring tunneling and lacking direct exposure for osteotomies, disimpaction, fistula closure, bone graft placement, or plate-and-screw fixation. He used a halo craniomaxillofacial fixation device for stabilization. Westbrook, West, and McNeil[33,34] described a simultaneous maxillary advancement and closure of bilateral clefts and oronasal fistulas. They used limited incisions to maintain circulation to the lateral maxillary segments, which unfortunately prevented direct exposure of the maxillary walls.

Posnick et al[11-21] described an operative technique that modifies the standard maxillary Le Fort I osteotomy to accommodate the unique deformities and circulation requirement that the unilateral or bilateral cleft lip and palate patient may present with (Figures 58-1 and 58-2). The principal modification consists of placement of soft tissue incisions allowing direct exposure for dissection, osteotomies, disimpaction, fistula closure, bone grafting, and application of plate-and-screw fixation that do not risk circulation injury to the dentoosseous-musculomucosal flaps. The routine surgical closure of residual cleft-dental gaps through differential maxillary segmental repositioning is also incorporated. For patients with unilateral cleft lip and palate or bilateral cleft lip and palate, approximation of the maxillary segments for closure of the cleft-dental gaps also close the dead space of the clefted alveolus and approximate the labial and palatal flaps to allow for efficient and effective closure of the recalcitrant oronasal fistula without tension, while providing keratinized mucosa to surround the cleft site(s) and adjacent teeth.

In anticipation of a degree of postoperative skeletal relapse, surgical overcorrection of several millimeters is generally planned in the horizontal and transverse dimensions. The exact amount varies with the interdigitation of the teeth. Autogenous corticocancellous iliac bone graft is generally placed and used to fill all residual palatal and floor-of-the-nose defects. After fixation of the maxilla with four miniplates, additional corticocancellous grafts are generally wedged between the zygomatic buttress and piriform aperture on each side and secured with microplates and screws.

Prefabricated interocclusal splints are used intraoperatively to facilitate correct placement of the jaws; the final splint is wired to the maxillary arch wire. The prefabricated splint generally remains secured to the maxillary orthodontic arch wire for a total of 6 to 8 weeks to be certain that the relationship of the maxillary teeth to one another and to the mandibular teeth remains unchanged. Guiding elastics are used intermittently during the initial healing period.

ORTHODONTIC OBJECTIVES

The unilateral and bilateral cleft lip and palate adolescent often presents with maxillary hypoplasia and residual fistula that have not been bone grafted effectively in the mixed dentition. For these patients, there will be two (for unilateral) or three (for bilateral) separate maxillary segments, each with a varied degree of dysplasia in all three planes. Each maxillary segment is evaluated and treated (orthodontically) individually in anticipation of segmental surgical repositioning for three-dimensional alignment. Radiographic assessment is essential before any orthodontic movement of the teeth adjacent to the bone-deficient cleft site(s). The Panorex radiograph is primarily useful for assessing tooth angulation. Occlusal and periapical radiographs through the cleft site(s) can help assess the amount and height of alveolar crestal bone of the adjacent teeth.

Both the number of permanent incisors and the amount of dentoalveolar bone in the anterior aspects of the maxilla will differ widely. Lateral incisor-like teeth frequently are found along the edges of the cleft site(s) in either in the premaxilla (bilateral cleft lip and palate) or in the lateral segment(s). These generally are rudimentary with limited root support. When a poorly formed lateral incisor is present, it is prudent to extract it in the interest of long-term function, aesthetics, and dental rehabilitation. Unerupted supernumerary teeth are also extracted, either at the time of bone grafting in the mixed dentition or at the time of orthognathic surgery.

The decision to extract fully erupted, normally formed teeth within the lateral segment(s) depends on the volume and height of the bone covering the dental roots and adjacent to the cleft(s) and the degree of crowding within each segment.[9] Bicuspid extraction(s) are often necessary to ensure that there is adequate bone for the leveling and aligning of all retained teeth without irreversibly weakening the periodontal support of the teeth adjacent to the cleft(s). The final occlusal result after orthodontic alignment and surgical repositioning of the lateral segment(s) will determine whether the maxillary third molars are required for opposing contact with the lower arch.

Planning for extractions in the mandibular arch depends on space requirements and on tooth movements needed to position the incisors ideally over basal bone. As may be used in the noncleft patient, an orthodontic trial setup of the teeth is helpful in establishing the most appropriate extraction pattern. This is especially important when, after surgery, the mandibular arch will occlude with the maxillary arch, where cuspids and bicuspids are advanced to the lateral incisor in cuspid positions. Incorporation of all erupted long-term teeth in each maxillary segment within the orthodontic mechanics

Text continued on p. 858.

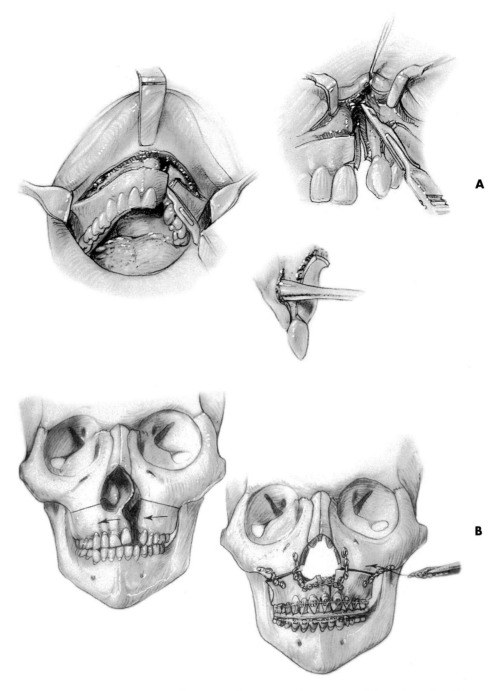

Figure 58-1.   Illustrations of modified Le Fort I osteotomy (two segments) in a unilateral cleft lip and palate patient. **A,** Illustration of direct incisions for completion of osteotomies and fistula closure. **B,** Frontal view of bony skeleton before and just after fixation of Le Fort I osteotomy in two segments. The inferior turbinates have been reduced, and a submucous resection of the deviated septum has been performed. Iliac, cancellous bone graft has been placed along the nasal floor. A miniplate is placed vertically along each zygomatic buttress and piriform aperture region, and a microplate is placed horizontally across the segmental osteotomy site. (From Posnick JC: Orthognathic surgery in the cleft patient. In Russell RC, editor: *Instructional courses, Plastic Surgery Education Foundation,* vol 4, St Louis, 1991, Mosby.)   *Continued*

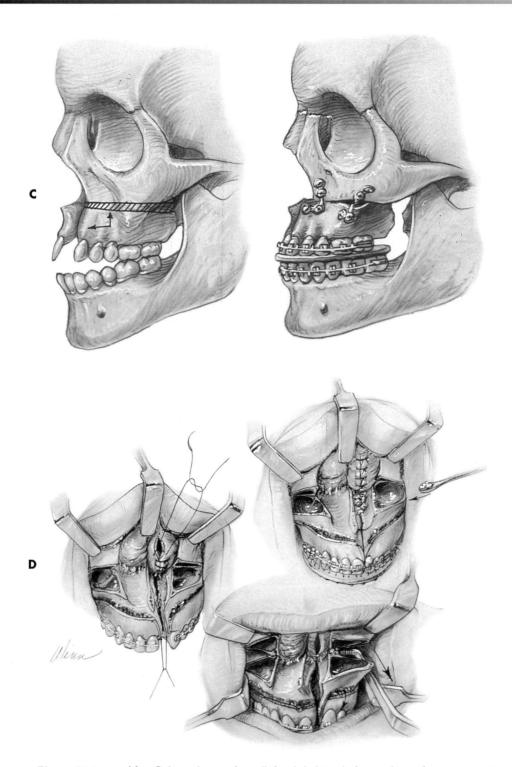

Figure 58-1, cont'd. **C,** Lateral view of maxillofacial skeleton before and just after osteotomies and fixation of modified Le Fort I osteotomy. **D,** Illustration of downfractured Le Fort I in two segments after submucous resection of septum and reduction of inferior turbinate along the nasal mucosa opening, followed by water-tight nasal side closure. (From Posnick JC: Orthognathic surgery in the cleft patient. In Russell RC, editor: *Instructional courses, Plastic Surgery Education Foundation,* vol 4, St Louis, 1991, Mosby.) *Continued*

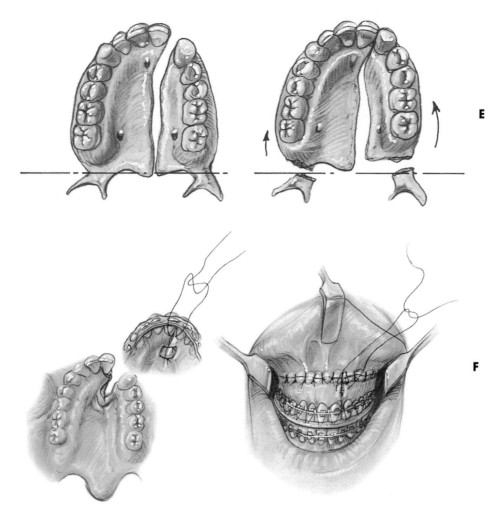

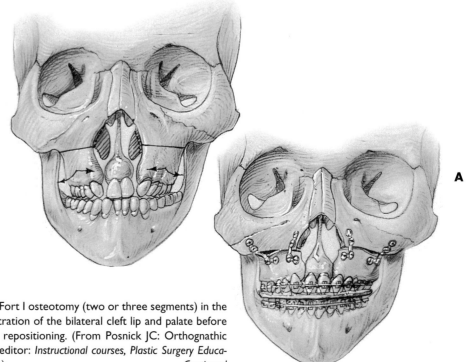

Figure 58-1, cont'd. E, Palatal view of bony segment before and after repositioning. **F,** Illustration indicated oral-side wound closure of both labial and palatal aspects after differential segmental repositioning.

Figure 58-2. Illustrations of modified Le Fort I osteotomy (two or three segments) in the bilateral cleft lip and palate patient. **A,** Illustration of the bilateral cleft lip and palate before and after lateral segment osteotomies and repositioning. (From Posnick JC: Orthognathic surgery in the cleft patient. In Russell RC, editor: *Instructional courses, Plastic Surgery Education Foundation,* vol 4, St Louis, 1991, Mosby.) *Continued*

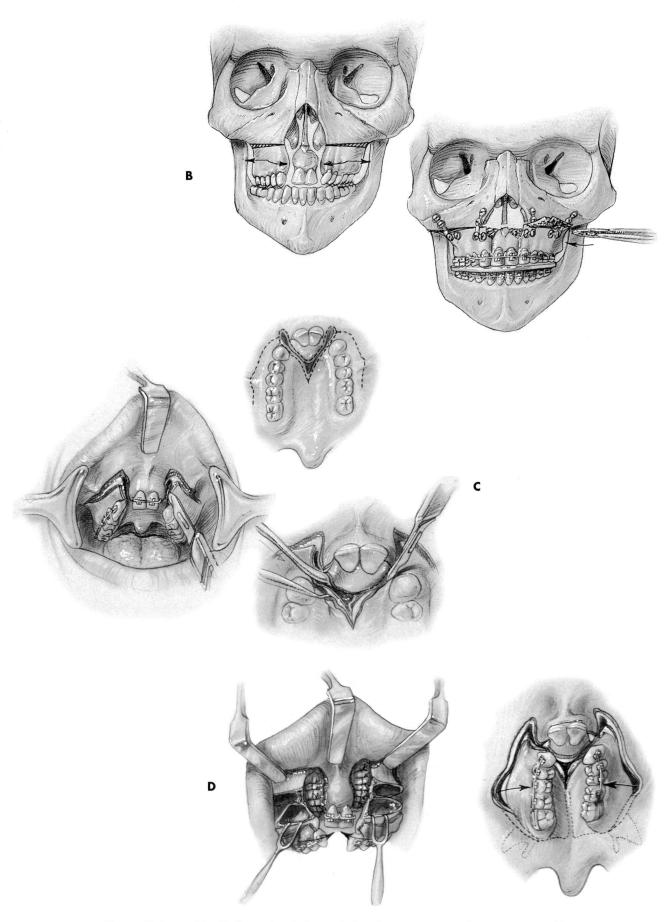

Figure 58-2, cont'd. B, Illustrations before and after three segment maxillary osteotomy with repositioning of the segments. **C,** Illustrations of incisions of modified Le Fort I in three segments. **D,** Illustration of downfractured lateral segments showing exposure of oronasal fistula and additional view of oral mucosa incisions. (From Posnick JC: Orthognathic surgery in the cleft patient. In Russell RC, editor: *Instructional courses, Plastic Surgery Education Foundation,* vol 4, St Louis, 1991, Mosby.)

Continued

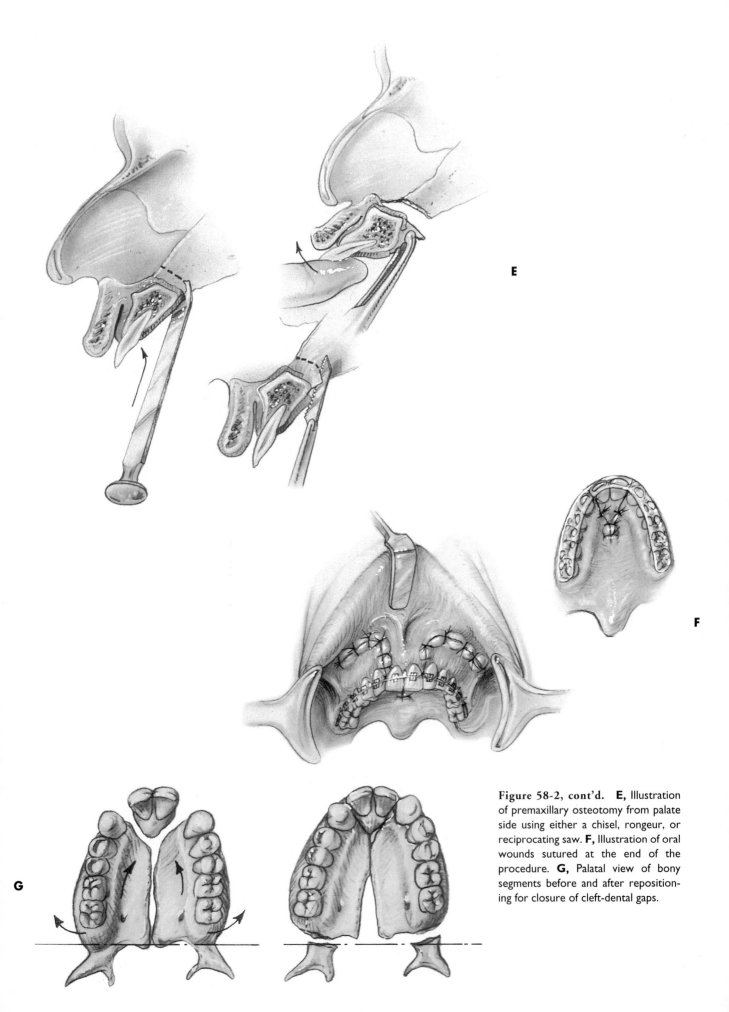

Figure 58-2, cont'd. **E,** Illustration of premaxillary osteotomy from palate side using either a chisel, rongeur, or reciprocating saw. **F,** Illustration of oral wounds sutured at the end of the procedure. **G,** Palatal view of bony segments before and after repositioning for closure of cleft-dental gaps.

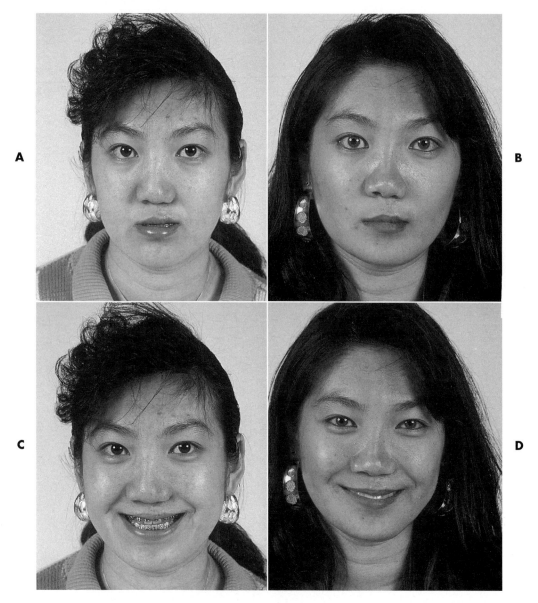

Figure 58-3. A 16-year-old girl with unilateral cleft lip and palate who underwent a modified Le Fort I osteotomy in two segments, bilateral sagittal split osteotomies of the mandible, and an osteoplastic genioplasty is shown before and 2 years after surgery. **A,** Preoperative frontal view in repose. **B,** Frontal view in repose 2 years later. **C,** Preoperative frontal view with smile. **D,** Frontal view with smile 2 years later. (From Posnick JC, Thompson B: *Plast Reconstr Surg* 96:255, 1995.) *Continued*

will facilitate arch leveling and development of the desired arch form.

OUTCOMES

Posnick et al[18] reported long-term results of 116 adolescents (67 males, 49 females; age range 15-25 years; mean age 18 years) born with either unilateral cleft lip and palate (N = 66) (Figure 58-3), bilateral cleft lip and palate (N = 33) (Figure 58-4), or isolated cleft palate (N = 17) (Figure 58-5) who underwent orthognathic surgery by one surgeon (Posnick) over a 6-year period using consistent surgical techniques.

All but one patient underwent perioperative orthodontic treatment. All were judged to be skeletally mature at the time of surgery, either by serial cephalometric radiographs or by epiphyseal plate closure on hand radiograph. A clinical follow-up ranged from 1 to 7 years (mean 40 months) at the close of the study.

The patient's primary surgeons (earlier in life) varied, as did the previous cleft-related procedures that they performed. All

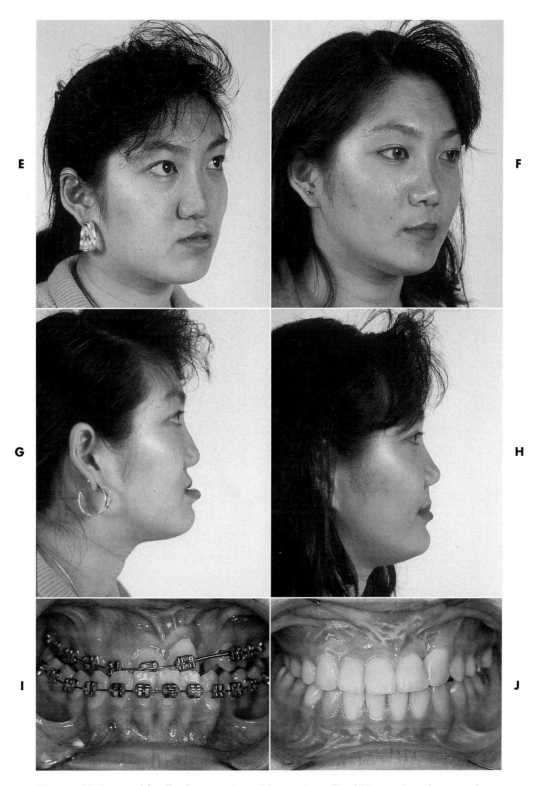

Figure 58-3, cont'd. **E,** Preoperative oblique view. **F,** Oblique view 2 years later. **G,** Preoperative profile view. **H,** Profile view 2 years later. **I,** Preoperative occlusal view. **J,** Occlusal view 2 years later. *Continued*

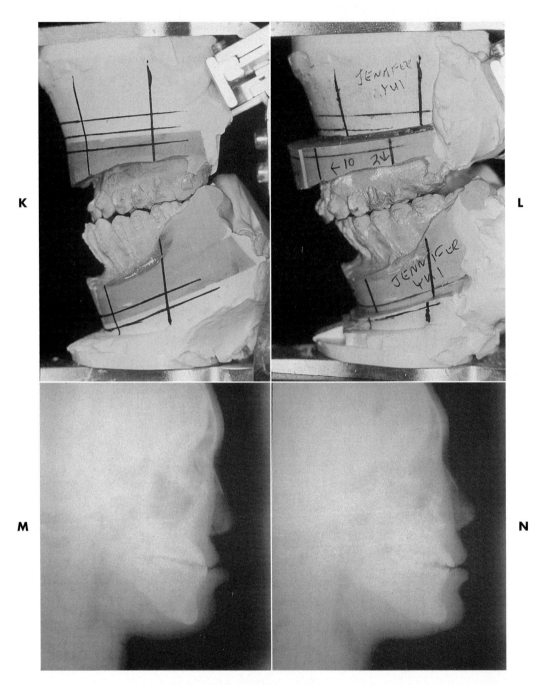

Figure 58-3, cont'd. K, Preoperative articulated dental casts. **L,** Articulated dental casts after model surgery. **M** and **N,** Cephalometric radiographs before and 1 year after surgery. (From Posnick JC, Thompson B: *Plast Reconstr Surg* 96:255, 1995.)

patients had undergone primary lip and palate repair in infancy and early childhood. The number and extent of previous revisional soft tissue lip, nose, and palatal procedures varied greatly (from 0 to 10 procedures). Most patients had undergone additional attempts to close the residual oronasal fistula; 20 patients underwent bone grafting to fill the alveolar cleft. Seven of 66 unilateral cleft lip and palate patients had previously undergone orthognathic surgery by another surgeon.

The basic orthognathic procedure performed in each of the patients (N = 116) included a Le Fort I osteotomy. Thirty-two of the patients also underwent simultaneous sagittal split osteotomies of the mandible; 87 underwent a vertical reduction and horizontal advancement genioplasty of varied degrees.

Postoperative variables reviewed by Posnick[18] in his published study related to: (1) the condition of the clefted dentoalveolar region, including the presence of residual

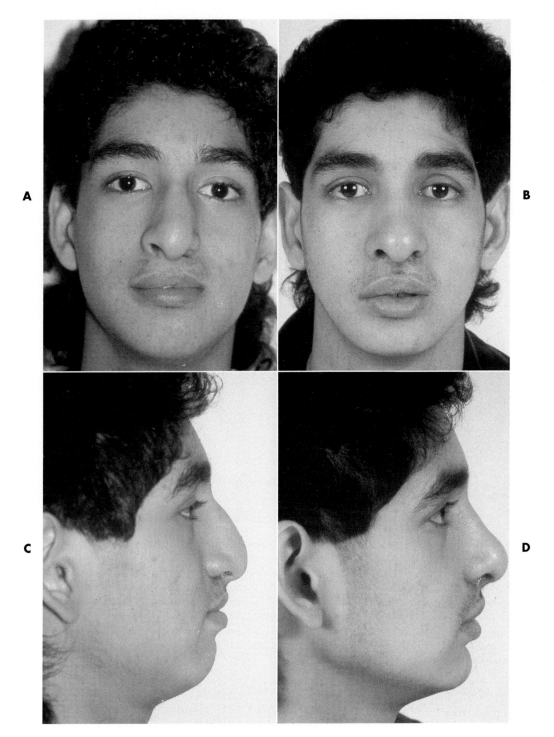

Figure 58-4. A 17-year-old patient with repaired bilateral cleft lip and palate. He initially presented in childhood with an elongated premaxilla, which eventually showed hypoplasia at skeletal maturity. His residual clefting problems were managed with a combined orthodontic and orthognathic surgical approach using a modified Le Fort I osteotomy in three segments. **A,** Preoperative frontal view. **B,** Postoperative frontal view. **C,** Preoperative lateral view. **D,** Postoperative lateral view. (From Posnick JC, Witzel MA, Dagys AP: Management of jaw deformities in the cleft patient. In Bardach J, Morris HL, editors: *Multidisciplinary management of the cleft lip and palate,* Philadelphia, 1990, WB Saunders.) *Continued*

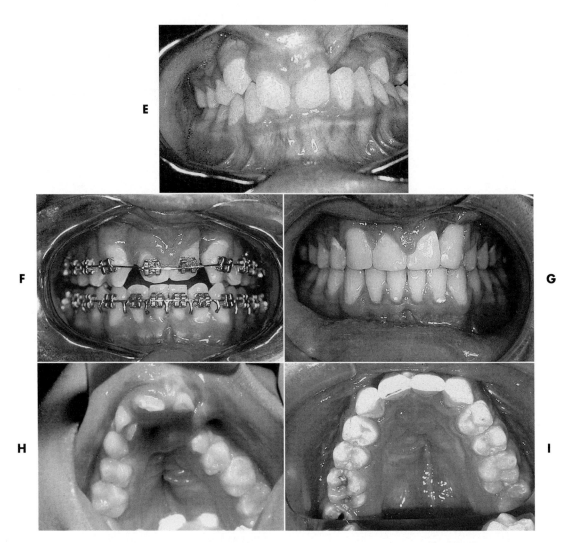

Figure 58-4, cont'd. E, Preoperative occlusal view at 13 years of age. Note that the premaxilla appears to be vertically long. **F,** After preoperative orthodontic treatment in preparation for jaw surgery at 17 years of age. **G,** At 18 months after surgery, completion of orthodontics and dental restorations with resin buildups of anterior teeth. **H,** Occlusal view in mixed dentition phase. Note cheek rotation flap use for fistula closure had decreased the vestibular depth and placed nonkeratinized mucosa over the tooth-bearing surface. A sliding mucogingival rotation flap would have been preferable. **I,** Dental arch forum after modified Le Fort I osteotomy with differential repositioning of the three segments to close fistulas and cleft-dental gaps in the regions of the congenitally absent lateral incisors.

oronasal fistula, mobility of the premaxilla (in bilateral cleft lip and palate patients), adequacy of the bone bridge across the alveolus, any increase in gingival recession and root exposure of cleft adjacent teeth, success of closure of the residual cleft dental gap(s), presence of keratinized mucosa along the labial aspect of cleft-adjacent teeth, and the need for a prosthetic appliance to complete dental rehabilitation; (2) perioperative complications; and (3) the long-term maintenance of a positive overjet and overbite as determined from the late, postoperative cephalometric radiographs.

Overall, 89% of residual fistulas underwent successful closures as part of the orthognathic surgical procedure.[18] Surgical cleft-dental gap closure was achieved and maintained to the extent planned in 92% of the cleft sites. A fixed (prosthetic) bridge was used successfully for dental rehabilita-

tion to close the gap(s) in all other patients in each cleft site (N = 9). All patients with alveolar clefts (N = 99) maintained keratinized mucosa along the labial surface of the cleft-adjacent teeth (N = 264 teeth).

Complications were few and generally not serious. There was no segmental bone loss or loss of teeth because of aseptic necrosis, infection, or other reasons. Only 5% of cleft-adjacent teeth underwent a degree of gingival recession or root exposure as a result of the maxillary osteotomy procedure; all were retained long term. The long-term maintenance of overjet and overbite measured directly from the late (greater than 1 year) postoperative lateral cephalometric radiographs indicated that 97% of patients maintained a positive overjet and that 89% maintained a positive overbite; 5% shifted to a neutral overbite.

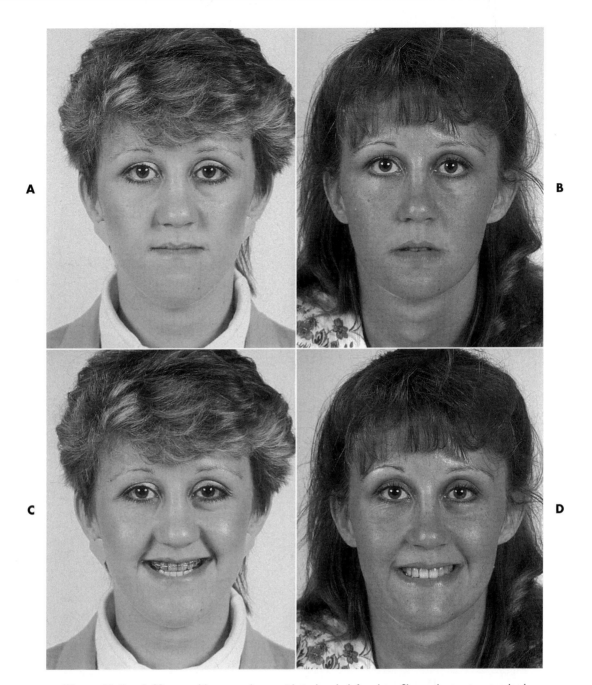

Figure 58-5. A 23-year-old woman born with isolated cleft palate. She underwent a standard maxillary Le Fort I osteotomy with horizontal advancement and a vertical reduction in horizontal advancement genioplasty. **A,** Preoperative frontal view in repose. **B,** Frontal view in repose 1 year later. **C,** Preoperative frontal view with smile. **D,** Postoperative frontal view with a smile. (From Posnick JC, Ewing MP: The role of plate and screw fixation in the treatment of cleft lip and palate jaw deformities. In Gruss JC, Manson PM, Yaremchuk MJ, editors: *Rigid fixation of the craniomaxillofacial skeleton,* Stoneham, Mass, 1992, Butterworth.) *Continued*

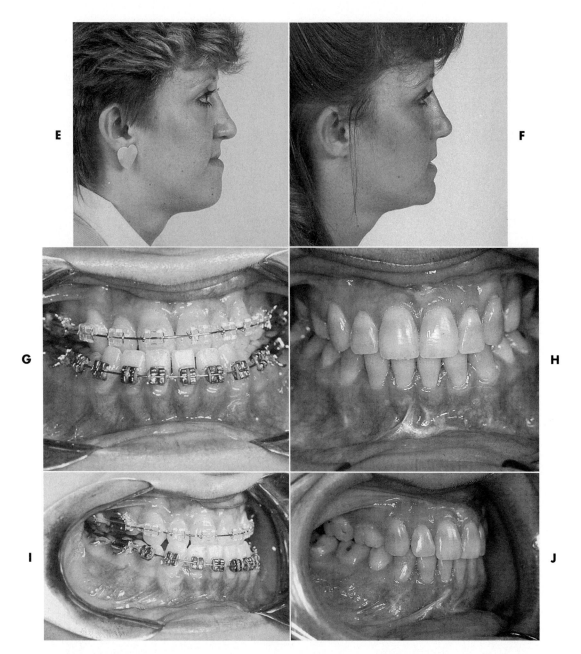

Figure 58-5, cont'd. E, Preoperative profile view. F, Postoperative profile view. G, Preoperative occlusal view. H, Postoperative occlusal view. I, Preoperative oblique occlusal view. J, Postoperative oblique occlusal view. (From Posnick JC, Ewing MP: The role of plate and screw fixation in the treatment of cleft lip and palate jaw deformities. In Gruss JC, Manson PM, Yaremchuk MJ, editors: *Rigid fixation of the craniomaxillofacial skeleton,* Stoneham, Mass, 1992, Butterworth.)   *Continued*

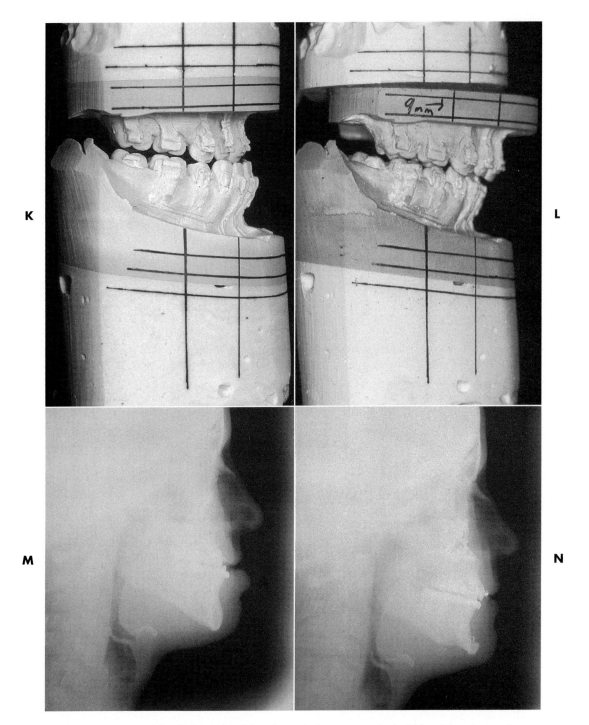

K   L   M   N

Figure 58-5, cont'd. **K,** Articulated dental casts before surgery. **L,** Articulated dental casts after surgery. **M,** Preoperative lateral cephalometric radiographs. **N,** Postoperative lateral cephalometric radiographs.

SUMMARY

The methods described to manage jaw deformities, malocclusion, residual oronasal fistulas, and bony defects in adolescents born with a cleft are safe and reliable when these methods are performed by an experienced cleft maxillofacial surgeon and team. They enhance the patient's quality of life and well-being. They also provide a stable foundation on which final soft tissue lip and nose revisions may be carried out.

REFERENCES

1. Abyholm FE, Bergland O, Semb G: Secondary bone grafting in alveolar clefts, *Scand J Plast Reconstr Surg* 15:127, 1981.

2. Bell WH: Le Fort I osteotomy for correction of maxillary deformities, *J Oral Surg* 33:412, 1975.

3. Georgiade NG: Mandibular osteotomy for the correction of facial disproportion in the cleft lip and palate patient, *Plast Reconstr Surg* 8:238-241, 1974.

4. Gillies HG, Rowe NL: L'osteotomie du maxillaire superieur envisagee essentiellement dans les cas de bec-de-lievre total, *Rev Stomat* 55:545, 1954.

5. Hall HD, Posnick JC: Early results of secondary bone grafts in 106 alveolar clefts, *J Oral Maxillofac Surg* 41:289, 1983.

6. Henderson D, Jackson IT: Combined cleft lip revision, anterior fistula closure, and maxillary osteotomy: a one-stage procedure, *Br J Oral Surg* 13:33, 1975.

7. James DR, Brook K: Maxillary hypoplasia in patients with cleft lip and palate deformity—the alterative surgical approach, *Eur J Orthod* 231, 1985.

8. Kiehn CL, Desprez JD, Brown F: Maxillary osteotomy for late correction of occlusion and appearance in cleft lip and palate patients, *Plast Reconstr Surg* 42:203, 1968.

9. Parel SM, Branemark PI, Jansson T: Osseointegration in maxillofacial prosthetics: I. Intraoral applications, *J Prosthet Dent* 55:490, 1986.

10. Poole MD, Robinson PP, Nunn ME: Maxillary advancement in cleft lip and palate patients, *J Maxillofac Surg* 14:123-127, 1986.

11. Posnick JC: Discussion: orthognathic surgery in cleft patients treated by early bone grafting, *Plast Reconstr Surg* 87:840, 1991.

12. Posnick JC: Orthognathic surgery in the cleft patient. In Russell RC, editor: *Instructional courses, Plastic Surgery Education Foundation,* vol 4, St Louis, 1991, Mosby.

13. Posnick JC, Dagys AP: Bilateral cleft deformity: an integrated surgical and orthodontic approach, *Oral Maxillofac Surg Clin North Am* 3:693, 1991.

14. Posnick JC, Dagys AP: Skeletal stability and relapse patterns after Le Fort I maxillary osteotomy fixed with miniplates: the unilateral cleft lip and palate deformity, *Plast Reconstr Surg* 94:924, 1994.

15. Posnick JC, Ewing MP: The role of plate and screw fixation in the treatment of cleft lip and palate jaw deformities. In Gruss JS, Manson PM, Yaremchuk MJ, editors: *Rigid fixation of the craniomaxillofacial skeleton,* Stoneham, Mass, 1992, Butterworth.

16. Posnick JC, Getz SB Jr: Surgical closure of end-stage palatal fistulas using anteriorly based dorsal flaps, *J Oral Maxillofac Surg* 45:907, 1987.

17. Posnick JC, Taylor M: Skeletal stability and relapse patterns after Le Fort I osteotomy using miniplate fixation in patients with isolated cleft palate, *Plast Reconstr Surg* 94:51, 1994.

18. Posnick JC, Tompson B: Cleft-orthognathic surgery: complications and long term results, *Plast Reconstr Surg* 96:255, 1995.

19. Posnick JC, Tompson B: Modification of the maxillary Le Fort I osteotomy in cleft-orthognathic surgery. The bilateral cleft lip and palate deformity, *J Oral Maxillofac Surg* 51:2, 1993.

20. Posnick JC, Tompson B: Modification of the maxillary Le Fort I osteotomy in cleft-orthognathic surgery. The unilateral cleft lip and palate deformity, *J Oral Maxillofac Surg* 50:666, 1992.

21. Posnick JC, Witzel MA, Dagys AP: Management of jaw deformities in the cleft patient. In Bardach J, Morris HL, editors: *Multidisciplinary management of the cleft lip and palate,* Philadelphia, 1990, WB Saunders.

22. Posnick JC: The staging of cleft lip and palate reconstruction: infancy through adolescence. In Posnick JC (ed): *Craniofacial and maxillofacial surgery in children and young adults,* Philadelphia, 2000, WB Saunders.

23. Posnick JC: Cleft lip and palate: bone grafting and management of residual oro-nasal fistula. In Posnick JC (ed): *Craniofacial and maxillofacial surgery in children and young adults,* Philadelphia, 2000, WB Saunders.

24. Posnick JC: Cleft-orthognathic surgery: the unilateral cleft lip and palate deformity. In Posnick JC (ed): *Craniofacial and maxillofacial surgery in children and young adults,* Philadelphia, 2000, WB Saunders.

25. Posnick JC: Cleft-orthognathic surgery: the bilateral cleft lip and palate deformity. In Posnick JC (ed): *Craniofacial and maxillofacial surgery in children and young adults,* Philadelphia, 2000, WB Saunders.

26. Posnick JC: Cleft-orthognathic surgery: the isolated cleft palate deformity. In Posnick JC (ed): *Craniofacial and maxillofacial surgery in children and young adults,* Philadelphia, 2000, WB Saunders.

27. Proffitt WR: Orthodontic treatment of clefts: yesterday, today and tomorrow. *Proceedings of the 48th Annual Meeting, American Cleft Palate-Craniofacial Association,* Hilton Head, SC, March 1991, p 32.

28. Ross RB: Treatment variables affecting facial growth in complete unilateral cleft lip and palate: 7. An overview of treatment and facial growth, *Cleft Palate J* 24:71, 1987.

29. Steinkamm W: *Die Pseudo-Progenie und ihre Behandlung,* Inaug Diss, 1938, Berlin.

30. Tessier P, Tulasne JF: Secondary repair of cleft lip deformity, *Clin Plast Surg* 11:747, 1984.

31. Tideman H, Stoelinga P, Gallia L: Le Fort I advancement with segmental palatal osteotomies in patients with cleft palates, *J Oral Surg* 38:196, 1980.

32. Ward-Booth RP, Bhatia SN, Moos KF: A cephalometric analysis of the Le Fort II osteotomy in the adult cleft patient, *J Maxillofac Surg* 12:208, 1984.

33. West A: Orthognathic surgery, *Oral Maxillofac Surg Clin North Am* 2:761, 1990.

34. Westbrook MT Jr, West RA, McNeil RW: Simultaneous maxillary advancement and closure of bilateral alveolar clefts and oronasal fistulas, *J Oral Maxillofac Surg* 41:257, 1983.

35. Willmar K: On Le Fort I osteotomy: a follow-up study of 106 operated patients with maxillofacial deformity, *Scand J Plast Reconstr Surg* (suppl 12), 1974.

36. Wunderer S: Die Prognathieoperation mittels Frontal Gestielthem Maxillafragment, *Oster Z Stomatol* 59:98, 1962.

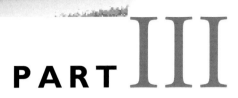

PART III

MAXILLOFACIAL SURGERY

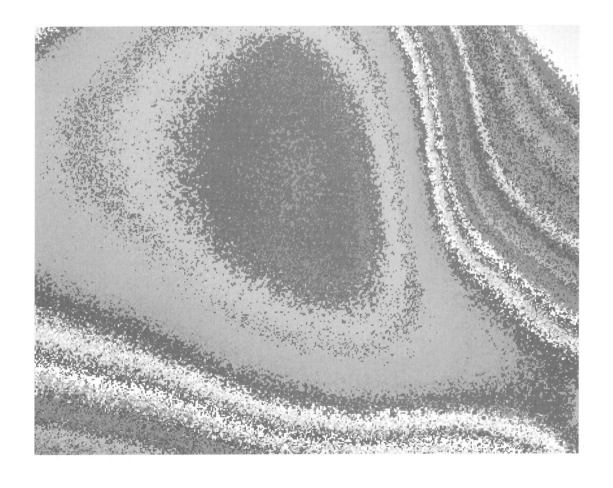

CHAPTER 59

Orthognathic Surgery

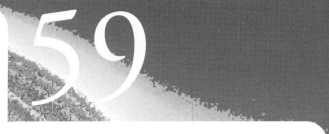

Stephen A. Schendel

Orthognathic surgery corrects malpositions of the dentofacial skeleton and incorporates both functional and aesthetic changes. The two most common conditions treated are mandibular and maxillary retrusion; maxillary vertical excess and mandibular prognathism are also common indications for surgery. This surgery requires a close working relationship between the surgeon and orthodontist. Most of these dentoskeletal deformities are developmental in nature, although some, such as maxillary retrusion, may be associated with congenital deformities, such as cleft lip and palate. Because this type of surgery involves both major functional and aesthetic changes, the optimal treatment plan includes consideration and integration of both of these factors. This chapter outlines the evaluation, diagnosis, treatment planning, and correction of the most commonly seen facial deformity types treated by orthognathic surgery.

EVALUATION

Evaluation of the orthognathic patient involves both a complete medical and dental history and physical examination. In addition to the surgeon, specialists may be called upon depending on the patient's needs. The most common dental specialists beside the orthodontist, who is a necessity in this type of treatment, are the general dentist and periodontist.

Orthognathic surgery should not be undertaken until routine dental restorative work has been completed, with the exception that permanent bridge work and crown work should await the completion of the surgical orthodontic phase. An initial psychosocial evaluation of the patient is frequently neglected, which is unfortunate because this can lead to patient dissatisfaction even in the face of acceptable surgical results. Together with the history and physical examination of the patient, records will need to be obtained. The minimum records necessary to complete an orthognathic workup include:[11,17]

1. Facial photographs in frontal, frontal smiling, profile, and three-quarter views
2. Dental study models
3. Lateral cephalometric and panographic radiographs

Additional records are frequently necessary depending on the physical examination and history and include tomographic views of the temporomandibular joints, anteroposterior cephalometric radiographs in cases of facial asymmetry, and face-bow mountings for articulation of the dental models.

The aesthetic facial evaluation is based on direct observation of the patient. Photographs are used for later reference and documentation of examination details. The aesthetic facial examination should follow a rational and systematic order. The facial type is first determined by assessing the form and shape of the face. Key features, both acceptable and unacceptable, are identified and recorded at this time. The examination includes skin and other soft tissue, muscles, and, by inference, the underlying dentoskeletal support. Vertical and anteroposterior relationships of the face are noted with attention to the face, profile, and three-quarter views. Reference aids, such as the classic canons of vertical facial thirds and width, can be used for orientation (Figure 59-1). However, the ultimate aesthetic determination may vary from classical guidelines; thus they should not be used as absolute criteria in treatment planning. The anteroposterior examination is also aided by reference to the vertical facial thirds and relative projection or retrusion of each. Individual key features should be identified and measured after establishment of the basic facial morphology. The nose is the key to the central face just as the lip-tooth relationship and chin are key features of the lower face. Although smile aesthetics and other facial movements are important and should be noted, the main treatment plan should be established from the face in repose.

The oral examination is performed only after the facial aesthetic examination is completed. This should proceed in the usual fashion, noting general oral health, state of repair of the dentition, and occlusal type based on Angle's terminology (Figure 59-2). Angle's Class I, or normal, occlusion has the mesial buccal cusp of the upper first molar occluding in the buccal groove of the mandibular first molar. The canine teeth also are related so that the mandibular canine tooth is slightly anterior to the maxillary canine tooth (see Figure 59-1). In the Class II malocclusion, the mandibular dentition lies distal to its ideal position (more posterior), and in the Class III malocclusion, the mandibular dentition lies mesial or anterior to the

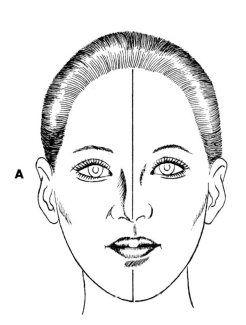

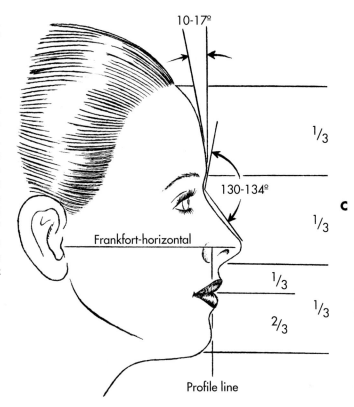

Figure 59-1. Facial canons. **A,** In the first step of the aesthetic evaluation, the face should be divided down the middle, making it possible to evaluate symmetry by comparing the right and left sides of the face. **B,** The frontal view is also divided transversely into fifths based on the width of the normal eye. Thus there should be five fifths to the normal facial width, with a one-fifth width between the eyes and a one-fifth lateral width to each eye. **C,** The vertical face is divided into thirds. The superior one third runs from the hairline to glabella, the middle one third from glabella to subnasali, and the lower one third from subnasali to the menton point of the chin. Additionally, the lower one third can be divided into thirds. The superior one third is the length of the upper lip, which runs from subnasali to stomion and is normally in the range of 19 to 22 mm. The lower two thirds runs from stomion to menton and include the lower lip and chin. The normal nasofrontal angle is 130 to 134 degrees, and the angle of the forehead from a true vertical is 10 to 17 degrees. The angle of the dorsum of the nose to true vertical also is approximately 34 to 36 degrees. A true perpendicular from the Frankfort horizontal through nasalis should cross the anterior-most projection of the chin.

ideal position. Overbite and overjet are also measured and recorded at this time, and any open bite condition, either anterior or lateral, is noted (Figure 59-3). It is important to remember that this classification system deals only with the anteroposterior relationship of the maxillary and mandibular teeth to each other; there is no reference to the occlusal position in relation to the facial skeleton or cranium with the Angle's analysis or to which jaw may actually be malposi-

tioned. In fact, a Class I occlusion will occur in many different facial types and thus this should not be the central criterion in treatment planning. Normal Class I occlusion can be found in short and long faces, as well as in protrusive and retrusive facial patterns. Thus it is only one factor that must be coordinated in the total treatment plan. Transverse occlusal relationships are also noted, and if there is a crossbite, this is referenced. Dental midlines should be evaluated in relationship with each other

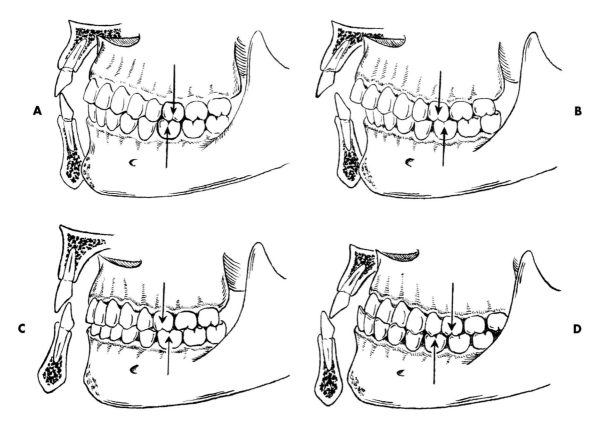

Figure 59-2. **A,** Angle's normal Class I occlusion. The mesial buccal cusp of the maxillary first molar lies in the buccal grove of the mandibular first molar. There is also a normal overjet and overbite relationship between the maxillary incisors, and the mandibular canine lies slightly anterior to the maxillary canine tooth. **B,** Class II, Division I malocclusion. There is an excessive overjet with a normal angulation to the maxillary incisor. The maxillary molar is advanced compared with the mandibular molar. Thus the maxillary mesial buccal cusp lies anterior to the buccal grove of the mandibular molar. **C,** Class II, Division 2 deep bite malocclusion has the same molar and cuspid relationship as the Class II malocclusion in **B.** However, the angulation of the maxillary incisor is more upright; thus there is a decreased amount of overjet and an increased amount of overbite. Usually there is also associated retroinclination of the mandibular incisor. **D,** Class III malocclusion demonstrates a reverse overjet with the mandibular incisor interior to the maxillary incisor. The mandibular molar also lies anterior to its normal position with the maxillary molar. Thus the mesial buccal cusp of the maxillary first molar lies behind the buccal groove of the mandibular first molar.

and with the facial midline. Lastly, any canting to the occlusal plane should be identified and its association with overall facial asymmetry noted.

A specific portion of the examination is devoted to the temporomandibular joints. The dental history is particularly important in identifying the length and severity of temporomandibular joint dysfunction. Minimal symptomatology consists of popping and clicking without pain or locking. A history of locking, either open or closed, should alert the practitioner to the potential of a displaced temporomandibular joint disk. Facial pain should also be thoroughly evaluated to determine if it is arising from the joint, masticatory muscles, or a combination of both. A significant history of temporomandibular joint dysfunction correlated with a positive physical examination should be further evaluated by specialized joint films to rule out osteoarthritic conditions or dislocation of the disk. Many patients with these symptoms will benefit from conservative temporomandibular joint therapy before initia-

tion of the orthodontic phase of treatment. Splint therapy is useful in alleviating the myofascial pain component, differentiating this from the intercapsular component, and determining the true centric relation to centric occlusion position. Further discussion of temporomandibular joint diagnosis and treatment is outside the scope of this chapter, and the reader is referred to text dealing specifically with this problem.

Cephalometry is used to classify and quantify the dentoskeletal deformity.[13,20] There are a number of different cephalometric analyses available, all with significant limitations. Cephalometric norms used in these analyses are based on statistical averages. Surgery will tend to normalize these values in most cases, yet in certain instances this will not be true and they cannot be used as absolutes. More important is the clinical experience that the surgeon has with a particular analysis and his ability to use this analysis as a means of communication with the orthodontist. The visual treatment objective as determined by the cephalometric projection tracing is more

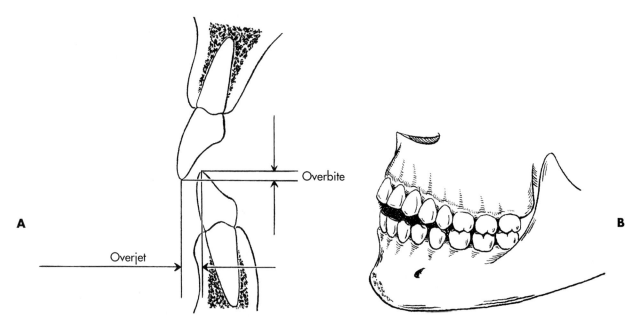

Figure 59-3. **A,** Overbite is the vertical overlap between the maxillary incisors, and overjet is the horizontal relationship between the maxillary incisors. **B,** An anterior open bite is demonstrated.

important to the surgeon than the actual cephalometric averages and norms obtained from the analysis. An understanding of the skeletal–to–soft tissue movements with surgery is crucial to a correct and predictable projection tracing. Projection analysis also allows the surgeon to try different surgical strategies and select the best one. However, all of this workup is based solely on the profile, which limits the usefulness of all analyses and their ability to predict three-dimensional soft tissue–to–skeletal movements. Computerized prediction systems have the same fault and may aggravate the situation by their oversimplification. At this time, the ultimate coordination of the profile and facial views in establishing the visual treatment objective remains up to the surgeon based on his or her ability and experience. Further compounding the situation is the inability of any of these analyses to describe beauty, which remains a subjective experience of the viewer. The visual treatment objective must be to idealize form, balance, and proportion of the face using the projection tracing and radiographs to determine the amount and direction of movement needed to obtain the desired result.[28]

Cephalometric radiographs should be taken with the teeth in centric occlusion and the lips in repose in most instances. However, when there is a significant discrepancy between centric occlusion and centric relation, or a significant skeletal open bite, an additional radiograph should be taken with the mandible in the centric relation position. Additionally, patients with true vertical shortness to the maxilla or overclosure secondary to a large prognathism should have a cephalometric radiograph taken with the mandible in rest position. This is determined most easily by having the patient close the mouth until the lips come into soft contact or having the patient pronounce "m." Anteroposterior cephalometric

radiographs are indicated when vertical discrepancies and facial asymmetries exist.

TREATMENT PLAN

Close communication between the surgeon and orthodontist is essential in establishing the treatment plan. The patient is examined by both members of the team and records are obtained. After this, a conference is held at which time the treatment plan is established. A visual treatment objective based on the projection tracing will help in determining the type of surgical procedure and the amount of movement to be obtained.[21] A knowledge of the soft tissue–to–bone ratios with skeletal movement is critical in preparing the projection tracing. In a similar manner, an orthodontic model setup is used to determine the type of orthodontic treatment and movements to be obtained before the surgical correction. The objective of all presurgical orthodontics should be to place the dentition on the respective basal bone and coordinate both arches to obtain a Class I occlusion after jaw repositioning by surgery. Treatment direction is undertaken by the orthodontist during this interval until the desired occlusion has been reached in preparation for surgery. At this time, study records are repeated and the surgeon and orthodontist meet to establish the final treatment plan and schedule surgery. After this conference, a heavy arch wire (0.45) and hooks are placed by the orthodontist in preparation for surgery. During the presurgical orthodontic treatment interval, cephalometric radiographs are valuable in determining progress. Cephalometric radiographs should also be taken in the immediate postsurgical period to determine correct positioning of the dentofacial skeleton and during the 3 to 6 months after surgery to rule out untoward changes. Immediately after surgery and for approximately the next 8 weeks, care of the patient is under the control of the surgeon. After this time period, care is gradually shifted back to the orthodontist for the final orthodontic finishing. In establishing the initial treatment plan, additional factors, such as dental prosthetic reconstruction and adjunctive surgical procedures, should be determined. This is also the ideal time for the surgeon to discuss such adjunctive procedures as rhinoplasty, liposuction, and facial bone recontouring.

In the postsurgical phase, the surgeon should monitor wound healing with particular attention to oral hygiene and adequate nutritional intake. With rigid internal fixation, intermaxillary fixation (IMF) is frequently eliminated or reduced to 1 week. My preference is 1 week of heavy elastic IMF followed by training elastics. During this training elastic period, the patient is allowed to take off the elastic on each side to eat, perform jaw physiotherapy, and brush the teeth. This interval lasts from 1 to 6 weeks. The elastics are gradually reduced to nighttime use only, followed by elimination of the elastics. Jaw opening is always reduced after surgery but is usually reestablished rapidly with jaw stretching exercises during the postoperative period. Most patients can reach 3 cm of opening by 6 weeks after surgery, and by 12 weeks, a normal opening pattern is usually reached. If this is delayed, the patient is referred to physical therapy for additional help.

MAXILLARY VERTICAL EXCESS

The long face deformity was first described in 1976.[25] Patients have a vertically long face, most evident in an increase of the lower facial third (Figure 59-4). Bilabial incompetence is present and most commonly associated with an excessive upper tooth–to–lip relationship. The normal upper lip–to–tooth ratio is 2 to 3 mm in repose. The so-called gummy smile is readily apparent. Occasional patients may have a normal lip-to-tooth relationship when there is a concomitant skeletal open bite[5] (Figure 59-5). Mentalis muscle strain is noted in attempts to obtain bilabial competency. The midfacial region, especially the paranasal portion, is usually flat. Most frequently a retrusive and vertically long chin is seen in the profile view with lip incompetence.

A Class II malocclusion is most frequently associated with this facial type, although both Class I and Class III malocclusions may be present. In addition, an open bite may be present and there is a tendency for the maxilla to be transversely narrow with a lateral crossbite. The cephalometric analysis will show a vertically long maxilla. Secondary to this will be posterior-inferior rotation of the mandible, thus contributing to the long facial pattern.[23] Variations of the vertical maxillary excess pattern exist and should be familiar to the surgeon. Usually the SNA and SNB angles are both decreased and the ANB angle is increased (SNA mean 82 degrees, SNB 80 degrees, ANB 2 to 3 degrees). However, these figures are unreliable because of variations in the cranial base angle. Thus single measurement is diagnostic.

The treatment plan should include the elimination of dental compensations and crowding before surgery. The surgical goal in this deformity is to reduce the vertical height of the maxilla to within normal limits as determined by aesthetics, mainly the lip-to-tooth relationship. The Le Fort I osteotomy with maxillary impaction is the most common procedure of choice; its biologic rationale, safety, and stability have been well demonstrated.[2,3,18,26,30] Segmental maxillary procedures may be needed in cases of large open bite or excess curve of Spee. Genioplasty is a frequently associated procedure to correct the relative chin retrusion. If the projection tracing demonstrates that the maxilla will need to move both up and posterior to obtain a Class I occlusion, the treatment plan should include mandibular surgery because, in most cases, retrusion of the maxilla will cause the aesthetic result to deteriorate. Thus a concomitant mandibular advancement is indicated using the sagittal split ramus osteotomy technique. Undesirable changes to the lips and nose can be associated with maxillary impaction. These include widening of the alar base and upturning of the nasal tip with accentuation of the supratip break. The lips may flatten and shorten with resultant loss of the amount of visible vermilion. This results in down-turning of the corners of the mouth and a lateral fullness to the cheek region. To minimize these undesirable changes, reconstruction of the lip and nose by nasolabial muscle reconstruction and a V-Y vestibular closure are indicated at the time of maxillary surgery. The amount of maxillary vertical resection is determined by the projection tracing and preoperative study model surgery based on the aesthetic examination.

Surgical Technique

The procedure is performed under general anesthesia with the patient in the supine position. Nasoendotracheal intubation is used, and the tubing is secured over the forehead utilizing either an RAE tube or a 60-degree connector. Local anesthesia is injected into the maxillary vestibule to aid with hemostasis. Blood loss is also minimized by a slight reverse Trendelenburg's position to the table and relative hypotensive anesthesia to hold a systolic blood pressure of 90 to 100. A standard facial and oral preparation is used, followed by placement of a throat pack. The lips are retracted superiorly, and a vestibular incision is made with the electrocautery starting from the mesial aspect of the first molar around to the other side. Dissection is performed at the subperiosteal plane until the piriform rim is visualized anteriorly and posteriorly and until a retractor can be placed in the pterygoid plate region (Figure 59-6). The superior dissection is stopped with visualization of the infraorbital nerve. Height of the osteotomy cuts are then marked with the use of a caliper. There should be a minimum of 4 to 5 mm between the root apexes and the inferior osteotomy. Generally this is somewhere around 32 mm anteriorly in the canine area and 26 mm in the first molar region. The amount of bone to be resected is then marked with the calipers superior to the previous marking. The amount of resected bone was previously determined by the projection tracing and dental model surgery.

Text continued on p. 881.

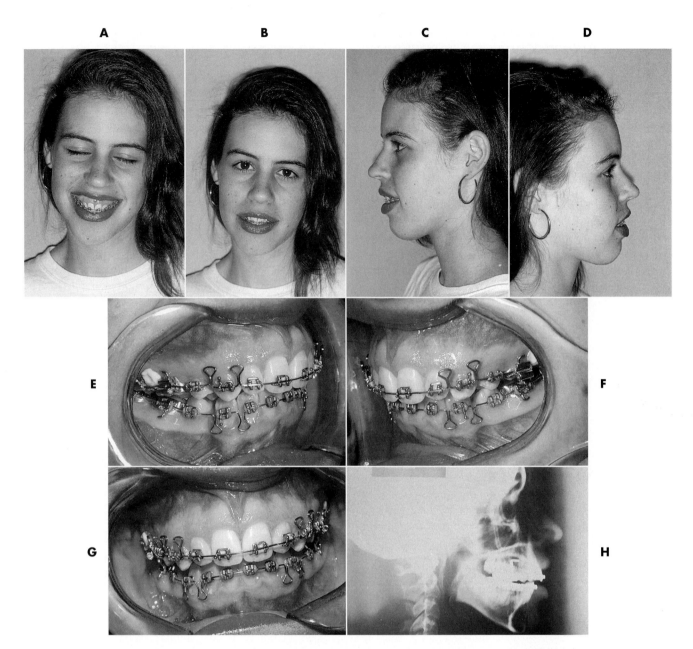

Figure 59-4. Vertical maxillary excess. **A** and **B,** Frontal views of a young woman with vertical maxillary excess demonstrating bilabial incompetence at rest and, smiling, demonstrating a large amount of gingival show. **C** and **D,** Profile views of a young woman with vertical maxillary excess demonstrating bilabial incompetence, excessive display of the incisor teeth, and a long lower vertical facial third with slight retrusion of the mandible. **E** to **G,** Occlusal views preoperatively. Presurgical orthodontics has been accomplished. A heavy arch wire has been placed and the patient's present malocclusion is now Class II. Orthodontist: G. Wadden. **H,** Preoperative lateral cephalometric radiograph demonstrating vertical maxillary excess and a large amount of bilabial incompetence. *Continued*

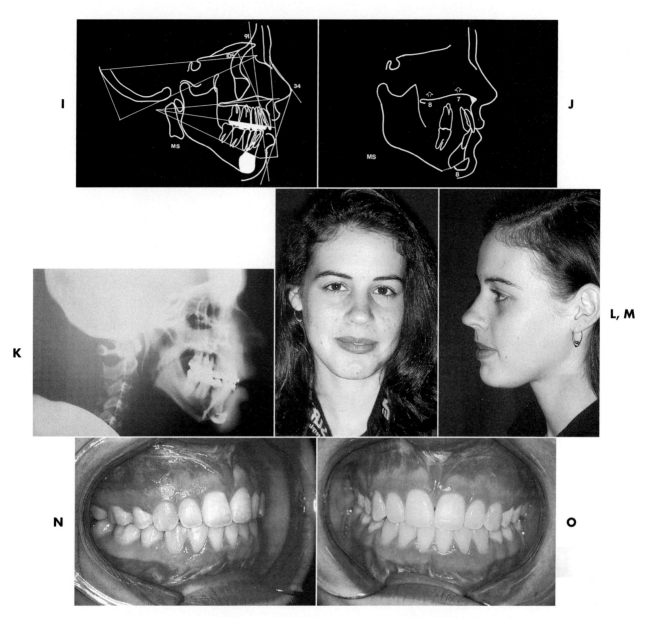

Figure 59-4, cont'd. **I,** Delaire cephalometric analysis demonstrating in the shaded portion of the maxilla the vertical excess and in the shaded portion of the mandible the excess vertical chin height. Also, there is retrusion of the chin from the desired chin point. Otherwise, cephalometric values are normal. **J,** Visual treatment objective for this patient demonstrating maxillary impaction of 7 to 8 mm associated with autorotation of the mandible and a vertical reduction advancement of the chin of 8 mm. **K,** Postoperative cephalometric radiograph. **L,** Postoperative frontal face view demonstrating equalization of the lower facial third. **M,** Lateral facial view postoperatively demonstrating normal anterior-posterior mandibular position and equalization of the facial thirds. **N** and **O,** Postoperative occlusal pictures demonstrating ideal Class I occlusion after debanding.

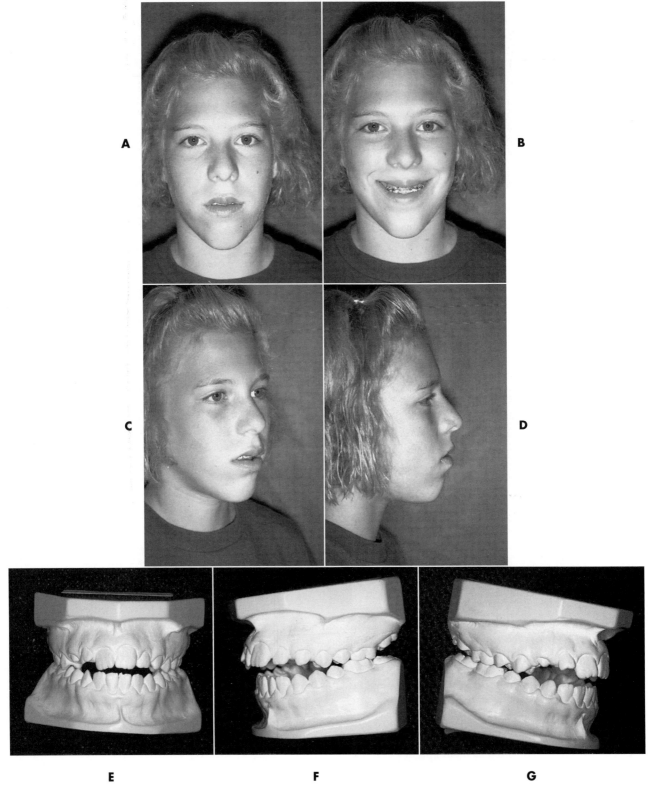

Figure 59-5. Skeletal open bite. **A** and **B**, Frontal pictures of a young woman demonstrating the normal lip-to-tooth relationship at rest and smiling. However, there is an increase in the lower facial third and an appearance of flatness to the midfacial region. **C** and **D**, Profile and oblique views demonstrating the increased lower facial third, mild bilabial incompetence, and relative retrusion of the chin. **E** to **G**, Pretreatment plaster models demonstrating large skeletal open bite and a Class II malocclusion. Contact is only on the first molar bilaterally. *Continued*

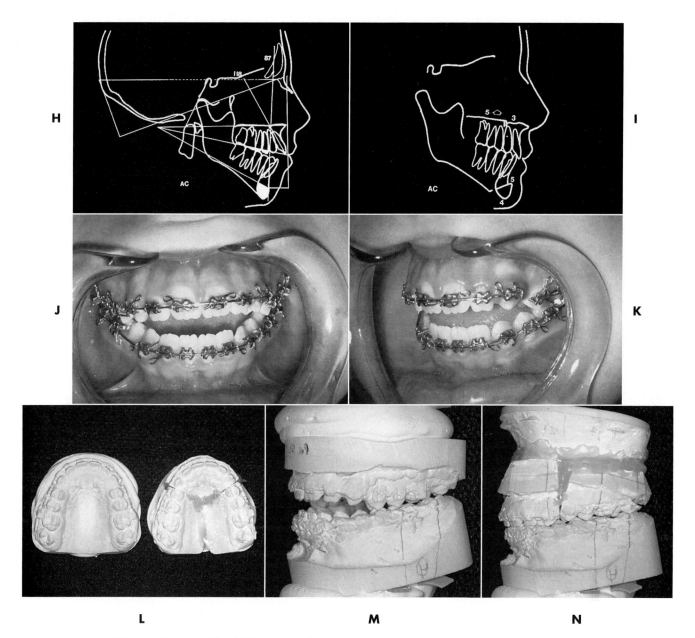

Figure 59-5, cont'd. H, Delaire cephalometric analysis demonstrating vertical excess of the posterior maxilla and normal vertical position of the incisor teeth. There is a large skeletal open bite present. There is also vertical excess to the chin that is retruded beyond its normal point. The craniofacial axis of the maxilla is 87 degrees and relatively normal otherwise. **I,** Visual treatment objective for this patient would include segmental maxillary osteotomy with impaction of 5 mm in the posterior. The anterior segments from canine to canine would be impacted only 3 mm. Associated autorotation of the mandible with the reduction genioplasty of 4 mm and advancement of 5 mm. **J** and **K,** Presurgical intraoral views demonstrating the segmental orthodontic arch wire on the maxilla with coordination of both arches without correction of the open bite before surgical treatment. Orthodontist: L. Samuels. **L** to **N,** Immediate presurgical study models and surgery models. Skeletal open bite is apparent on the uncut model. The cut model demonstrates the segmental cut between cuspid and bicuspid with correction of the skeletal open bite by impaction of the posterior maxilla. Occlusal views demonstrate the change in arch form after the impaction. Note on the uncut occlusal view that there are spaces created between the cuspid and bicuspid orthodontically to allow the surgeon to cut in this area without damaging tooth roots. *Continued*

Figure 59-5, cont'd. **O** and **P,** Postsurgical facial views demonstrating equalization of the lower facial third with the upper two facial thirds, symmetric smile line, and bilabial competence. The lip retains fullness and the nose has not widened secondary to the muscular V-to-Y closure and nasal cinch as described by Schendel. **Q** and **R,** Profile views of the same patient postoperatively. **S** to **U,** Occlusal views 1 year after surgery demonstrating maintenance of overbite and overjet relationship in a Class I occlusion.

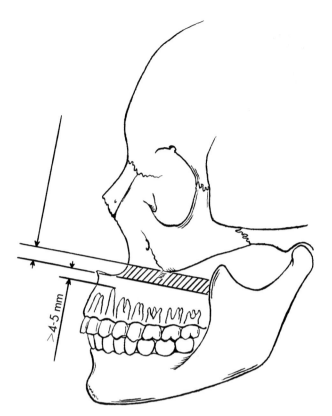

Figure 59-6. Maxillary vertical excess consists of elongation of the midface, specifically the maxillary bony structures, and results in increased maxillary tooth show and lip incompetence. Correction of this involves a vertical resection of the maxilla. The lower osteotomy cut must lie at least 4 to 5 mm superior to the apexes of the maxillary teeth. The required amount of resected bone, determined by the cephalometric radiographs, projection tracing, and model surgery, is then recorded as shown here, and the superior osteotomy is accomplished. The intervening bone is removed.

Before the osteotomies, the nasal mucosa must be dissected free from the lateral nasal wall and nasal floor and a small malleable retractor placed to protect this region. A reciprocating saw is then used to perform the osteotomies and remove the resected bone (Figure 59-7). The osteotomies frequently need to be completed using a small, straight osteotome. The osteotome is stopped on the medial cut at the perpendicular plate of the palatine bone and on the lateral cut at the pterygoid plates. A curved osteotome is then used to release the pterygoid plates from the maxilla inferior to the osteotomy only. This procedure is completed for both sides of the maxilla, and then the nasal septum is separated from the nasal crest of the maxilla using a special osteotome (Figure 59-8). A portion of the anterior nasal spine may be resected at this time to minimize the amount of nasal tip rise. The maxilla is then down-fractured by pushing inferiorly in the anterior region. The down-fracture is then completed by up-fracturing the front of the maxilla while pressure is maintained in the tuberosity region in the inferior direction. In most cases, this fully mobilizes the maxilla using finger pressure only. The vascular pedicles to the maxilla are then examined to make sure

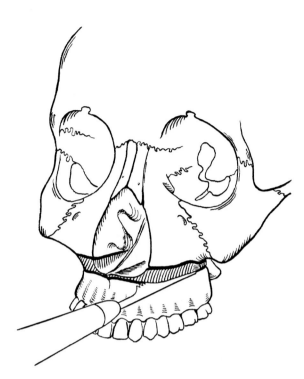

Figure 59-7. The ostectomy of the maxillary bone is done with a reciprocating saw after dissection and exposure of the maxillary wall is accomplished.

that they have not been severed. If they have been severed, they should be either liga clipped or cauterized to prevent postoperative hemorrhage. Bony interferences in the tuberosity region are frequent with maxillary impaction, and the intervening bone should be judiciously removed with a rongeur or a Kerrison forceps. The nasal crest of the maxilla is also removed to prevent buckling of the nasal septum after impaction (Figure 59-9).

If the maxilla is to be segmentalized, interdental cuts are made with a 1-mm fissure burr through the cortical bone only in the selected area. These cuts are made before down-fracturing and mobilizing the maxilla. A small spatula osteotome is then driven through these cuts until it is palpated on the palatal side without lacerating the palatal mucosa. After the down-fracture, the interdental cuts are continued across the palate with the maxilla in the down position (Figure 59-10). They are then joined and the segments mobilized. Maxillary width discrepancies can be corrected at this time by widening the maxilla in the molar region. Anywhere from several millimeters to a maximum of 10 mm can be gained by this technique. Expansion in the canine region generally is limited to 3 mm. If maxillary expansion is anticipated, parallel paramedian cuts should be made to allow transverse expansion to occur on both sides of the palate without tearing the central palatal mucosa. If no mandibular surgery is planned, the maxilla is then placed into the proper occlusion using an interocclusal acrylic wafer. The entire maxillomandibular

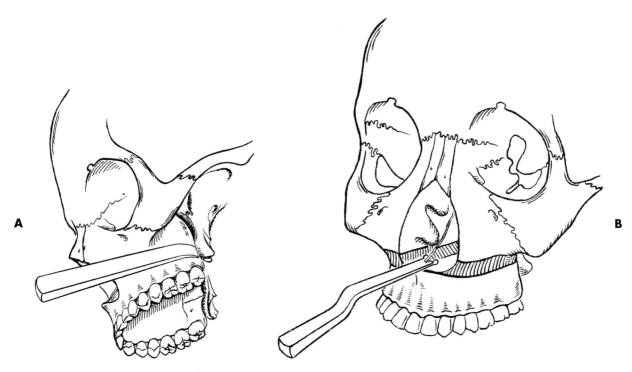

Figure 59-8. A, After the pterygoid plates have been fractured with a curved osteotome, it remains to remove the nasal septum and vomer from the maxilla before down-fracture. **B,** The septum and vomer are separated using a curved osteotome in this manner.

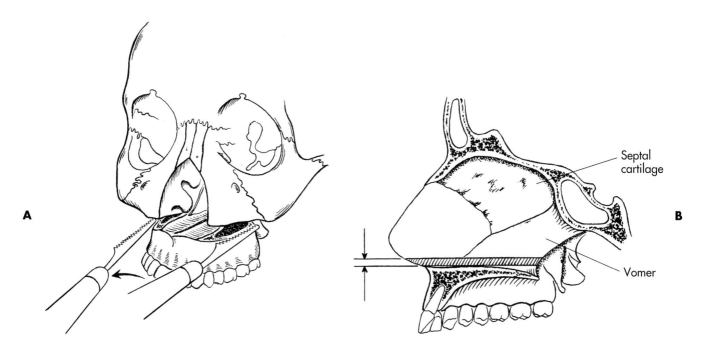

Figure 59-9. A, Le Fort I osteotomy is performed transversely above the maxillary dentition, crossing consecutively the maxillary sinus, the lateral nasal walls, the nasal cavity, and finally the septum or vomer as indicated. **B,** Maxillary impaction is necessary to remove a portion of the septal cartilage and vomer to prevent buckling of the nasal septum after vertical impaction of the maxilla.

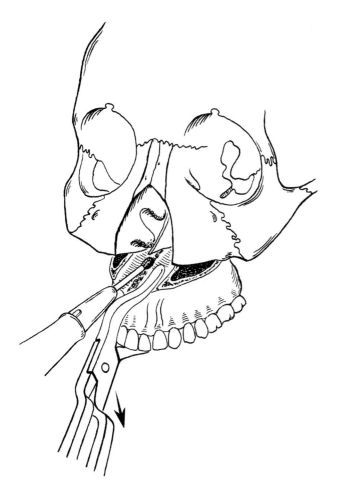

Figure 59-10. In the down-fractured position the maxilla can be segmentalized. In this drawing, a groove is being performed in the midsagittal plane to accept the nasal septum. This groove can also be deepened and the maxilla split down the midline to increase its width. Whenever segmental maxillary surgery is used, an occlusal split is obligatory.

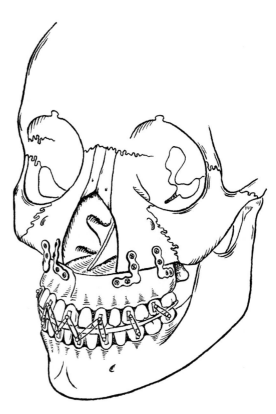

Figure 59-11. After the maxilla is superiorly autorotated, it is stabilized using miniplates as indicated.

complex is then rotated superiorly until the desired lip-to-tooth ratio has been obtained. The lateral maxillary osteotomy cuts should now be approximated. Interferences found during this maneuver are removed. Many techniques have evolved to evaluate the correct superior position of the maxilla, including internal reference lines in the bone and external measuring devices of various types. Generally these are inaccurate, and I have found the best technique is to examine the lip-to-tooth relationship while at the same time relieving any tension on the nasal complex caused by the endotracheal tube. The maxillary dental midline should also be examined at this time in relationship to the facial midline. Once the correct position of the maxilla has been determined, it is then fixed by miniplates placed in the piriform rim area on either side (Figure 59-11). Additional fixation can be obtained in the maxillary buttress region using either plates or wires. If concomitant mandibular surgery is performed, plates are recommended in the buttress region for additional stability. Any associated bone sculpting is then done, followed by closure of the incisions (Figure 59-12). The periosteum under the alar base of the nose is identified

through the vestibular incision, and a suture is placed from one side to the other and tied. This reapproximates the nasolabial muscles to their prior position in the anterior nasal spine region. A V-Y vestibular closure of the maxillary incision is then accomplished. The sutures should capture the mucosa, muscle, and periosteum but be close enough to the incisional edge so as not to shorten the vestibular depth. The leg of the Y extends upward into the upper lip and is usually approximately 1 cm in length. If this is not performed, there will be flaring of the nasal base, thinning of the upper lip with loss of vermilion show, and downturning of the corner of the mouth.[22,24]

Just before the vestibular closure, the IMF is released and the occlusion is checked. If the mandible does not articulate smoothly into the maxillary splint, the maxillary repositioning procedure should be repeated at this time. If everything is correct, the vestibular incision is closed and intermaxillary elastics are placed after removing the throat pack and placing a nasogastric (NG) tube.

If a genioplasty is planned, it is performed after rigidly fixing the maxilla and before release of the wire IMF and wound closure. A vestibular incision is used, and dissection is carried to the mental foramen bilaterally. To prevent soft tissue ptosis of the chin, dissection should not go inferior to the anterior mandibular border. The desired genioplasty is then accomplished. The posterior osteotomy should pass a minimum of 5 mm inferior to the mental foramen to avoid injury to the inferior alveolar nerve. The chin segment is mobilized and then repositioned and fixed in the desired fashion by wires or plates.[19]

Gingival anesthesia is associated with the Le Fort I procedure, especially in the anterior maxillary region. In most cases, this is resolved at the 1-year interval, but resolution can take longer. Dentoskeletal relapse has not been a significant problem with maxillary impaction. Occasional cases of late bleeding have been described, usually associated with the descending palatine vessel, but these cases are rare. Devitalization of maxillary segments is also extremely rare with this technique, as is fistula formation. Teeth may be damaged during interdental cuts, necessitating root canal treatment, but this is also uncommon.

VERTICAL MAXILLARY DEFICIENCY

The short face deformity is the converse of the long face deformity and is marked by vertical shortening of the lower third of the face.[16] The maxillary dentition is not usually visible during lip repose, and on smiling, very little of the clinical crowns are visible. The chin may appear overrotated superiorly with excessive anterior projection. The vertical shortness of the face causes a certain redundancy to the lips, and both the upper lip and lower lip tend to curl outwards excessively. This excessive soft tissue envelope may be visualized as jowling, especially in older individuals. As with long face deformity, any type of Angle's malocclusion may be associated with this deformity, although Class II appears to be the most frequent. Before rigid internal fixation with plates, relapse in the down-grafted maxilla was high. The procedure is now fairly stable.[4,9,30]

The cephalometric analysis demonstrates a shortened lower facial height frequently with increased SNA and SNB angles. There is a zero to negative tooth-to-lip ratio secondary to vertical shortness of the maxilla. The projection tracing done in this deformity is vertical lengthening of the maxilla until a normal lip-to-tooth ratio is obtained (2 to 3 mm). The occlusion should also be placed into a normal Class I. In most cases this is accomplished by only the maxillary surgery, but in some instances, a mandibular osteotomy will have to be planned concomitantly, usually to correct a Class II malocclusion. In the workup of this deformity, it is important to have a cephalometric radiograph taken with the mandible in resting position and the lips just barely touching, which will show the normal facial height. These individuals have an increased freeway space, which allows the maxilla to be down-grafted into this area and will be demonstrated by the cephalometric radiograph. Presurgical and postsurgical orthodontic treatment is similar to that associated with long face deformity except that an increased curve of Spee is corrected postsurgically by orthodontics.

Surgical Technique

Preparation of the patient is the same as that for patients with long face deformity and for other orthognathic procedures. A vestibular incision is made and osteotomy markings are accomplished in the same order. Only one osteotomy cut is needed with short face deformity; this is placed at the

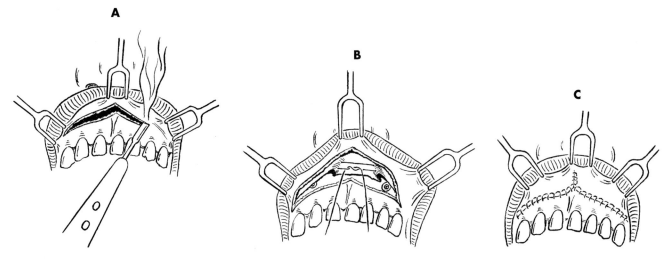

Figure 59-12. Lip and nasal reconstruction with Le Fort I osteotomy. **A,** The maxillary incision is made in the depth of the vestibule using an electrocautery on cutting. This incision goes down through the periosteum, which is then elevated at this level. After fixation of the maxilla in the appropriate position, the nose is reconstructed by suturing the periosteum and muscles underlying the nasal alae through the intraoral incision. **B,** Once this periosteum and muscle have been identified, a nonresorbable suture is passed through this area. **C,** The opposite muscle is then found and verified, a suture is passed, and these are sewn together. This inhibits morphologic changes of the alar base of the nose after Le Fort I surgery. The maxillary incision is then closed with a V-to-Y technique. The sutures must encompass both the mucosa and the periosteum.

recommended level of 4 to 5 mm above the apexes of the maxillary dentition. After down-fracture of the maxilla and mobilization, IMF is again obtained with an interocclusal acrylic wafer and 26-gauge stainless steel wire. The maxilla is then down-rotated until the proper lip-to-tooth relationship has been obtained and the osteotomy gap has opened to the predicted amount based on the visual treatment objective and dental model surgery (Figure 59-13). Intraosseous fixation is obtained with plates in both the piriform rim and maxillary buttress regions. After this, a bone graft is placed into the osteotomy gap, with my preference being cranial bone strips. Before the use of rigid internal fixation, maxillary down-grafting was associated with a high relapse tendency and overcorrection was recommended. Rigid internal fixation has demonstrated stability with this procedure and thus overcorrection is unnecessary. Very little interference will be found in the maxillary buttress region because the maxilla is being lengthened and bone will not need to be removed from the tuberosity region or the nasal crest of the maxilla. Soft tissue reconstruction is accomplished after verification of the occlusion as previously described. Postoperative care and concerns are essentially the same as with the maxillary procedure in long face deformity.

MAXILLARY RETRUSION

Maxillary retrusion is frequently idiopathic in nature but can be associated with congenital deformities, such as cleft lip and palate. The usual appearance is one of a flattened or dished-in midfacial region (Figure 59-14). Hypoplasia is most noted in the perialar and malar eminence regions.[15] Frequently the nose has a down-turned nasal tip and depressed alar bases. The upper lip may appear clinically short secondary to overclosure of the mandible. The profile view demonstrates graphically the

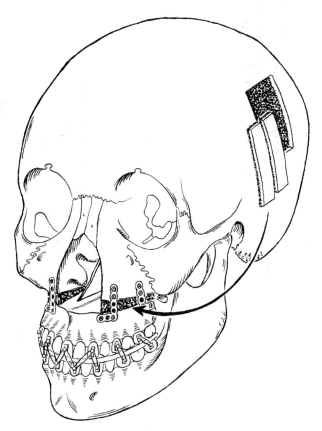

Figure 59-13. Short face surgical correction. After the Le Fort I osteotomy is performed, the maxilla is elongated, in this case by autorotation inferiorly of the mandible because no mandibular surgery is concomitantly performed. The desired amount of vertical elongation is determined presurgically by the cephalometric radiographs and aesthetic facial examination. An intervening bone graft is then placed at the appropriate width in this area, and the maxilla is stabilized using rigid fixation with many plates. This demonstrates the final result after fixation of the maxilla.

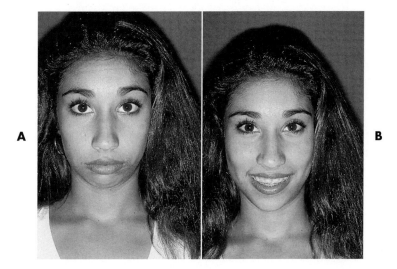

Figure 59-14. Bimaxillary retrusion. **A** and **B,** Frontal facial views of a young woman with evident decreased lower facial third vertical height and appearance of a small chin and mild flattening to the midfacial region. The smile line, however, is in the correct vertical position in relationship to the teeth and gums.

Continued

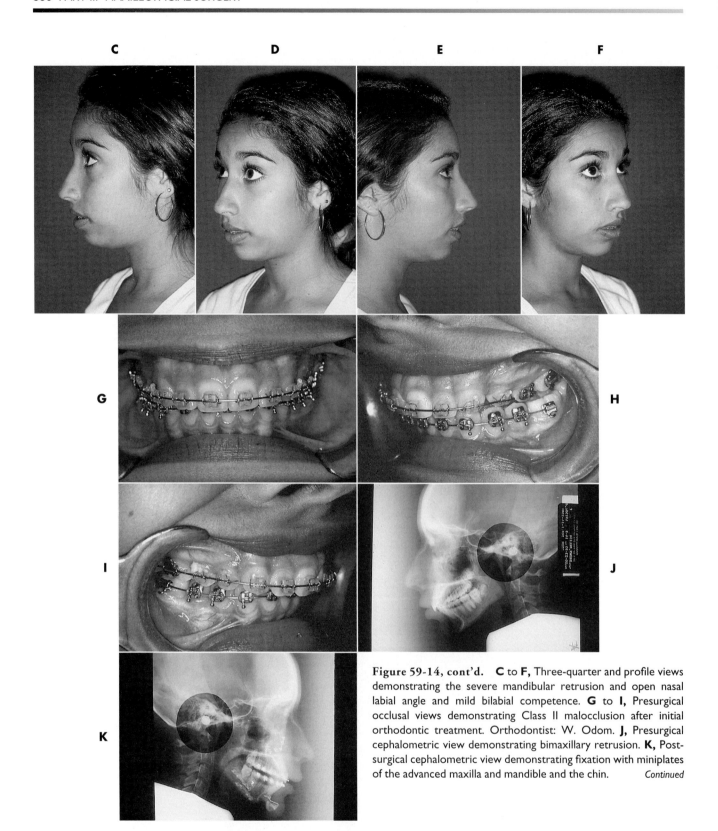

Figure 59-14, cont'd. **C** to **F**, Three-quarter and profile views demonstrating the severe mandibular retrusion and open nasal labial angle and mild bilabial competence. **G** to **I**, Presurgical occlusal views demonstrating Class II malocclusion after initial orthodontic treatment. Orthodontist: W. Odom. **J**, Presurgical cephalometric view demonstrating bimaxillary retrusion. **K**, Postsurgical cephalometric view demonstrating fixation with miniplates of the advanced maxilla and mandible and the chin. *Continued*

retrusion of the central face with either a normal chin position or anterior overrotated chin position. There may be associated shortness to the lower vertical facial height. Usually little of the maxillary dentition is visible, and in many cases of retrusion, there is an associated vertical shortness to the maxilla. Class III malocclusion is associated with this deformity with or without an open bite. There may be transverse maxillary deficiency and a crossbite associated in many cases.

The cephalometric analysis demonstrates a decreased SNA angle and a normal to larger SNB angle. There is always a negative ANB angle. The projection analysis usually indicates a need for maxillary advancement until a Class I occlusion is

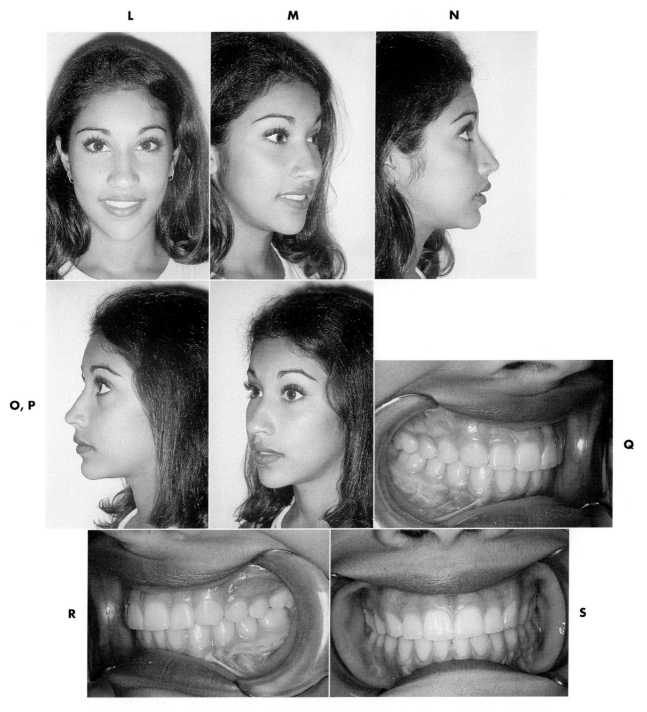

Figure 59-14, cont'd. **L,** Postoperative facial view demonstrating normalization of the face views. **M** to **P,** Profile and three-quarter views demonstrating the correct vertical and anterior-posterior positions of the facial thirds. **Q** to **S,** Postoperative occlusal views demonstrating a stable Class I occlusion.

obtained. This may include some vertical lengthening of the maxilla depending on the individual. The soft tissue of the upper lip will not follow the dentofacial skeletal advancement on a one-to-one ratio. The approximation is closest to .9 if the soft tissue lip reconstruction is performed as outlined previously. Otherwise, the ratio may fall to as much as .5 in cleft patients and .75 in other individuals. This ratio should be factored into creation of the visual treatment objective with

maxillary advancement. Projected maxillary advancements of over 5 mm generally require associated bone grafting not only for stability but also to augment the hypoplastic bone in the central face and increase the rate of bone healing.[1,7,8,15,30]

Presurgical orthodontics are done to eliminate dental crowding and any compensations present. The angulation of the maxillary incisors is particularly important for this procedure. The normal maxillary incisor–to–palatal angle is approximately 115 degrees, and the normal mandibular incisor–to–mandible plane angle is approximately 90 degrees. Excessive labial inclination of the maxillary incisors and retrusion of the mandibular incisors should be avoided in the presurgical orthodontic treatment because any postsurgical dental relapse will result in an immediate Class III malocclusion. In fact, it is frequently recommended to perform the reverse presurgical orthodontic maneuvers to retrude the maxillary incisors somewhat to allow maximum surgical advancement of the maxilla. Postsurgical finishing orthodontic treatment is similar to the other maxillary procedures.

Surgical Technique

Preparation of the patient is similar to the other maxillary Le Fort I procedures described. The Le Fort I is the same as previously described until the down-fracture has been accomplished. At this time it is necessary to stretch the soft tissues sufficiently to allow passive repositioning of the maxilla into its new anterior position. This is accomplished by use of the Rowe disimpaction forceps and gentle sustained anterior traction on the maxilla until the soft tissue relaxation has been obtained. IMF with wires is obtained in the usual manner, and the maxilla is rotated to the correct vertical position. Rigid internal fixation of the maxilla is then obtained using plates in both the piriform rim and maxillary buttress regions. Bone grafts are then placed if needed, usually wedged into the osteotomy gap that has been created. After this, the IMF is released and the occlusion is checked. Wound closure is then obtained in the manner previously described, and the patient is placed into elastic IMF after passing an NG tube and removal of the throat pack. Postoperative care is as previously described. Usually, the fixation is released at 1 to 2 weeks postoperatively followed by intermittent training elastics. In this case, training elastics should have a Class III vector to them. Routine postoperative wound care and physiotherapy are followed.

Complications associated with this procedure are as previously described for the Le Fort I osteotomy with one major exception. Relapse of the maxilla is higher in maxillary advancement cases. For this reason, some surgeons recommend an overadvancement of 1 to 2 mm in large advancements. Maxillary position should be followed closely by serial cephalometric radiographs in the postoperative period.[31]

MANDIBULAR RETRUSION

The patient with mandibular retrusion has a retruded lower facial third that is most evident in the profile view. The frontal face view usually demonstrates a normal vertical height to the lower face but occasionally may also show a reduced lower third facial height. The aesthetic soft tissue analysis of the upper and middle facial thirds is normal. In mild cases of mandibular retrusion, the appearance may be uniquely that of a small retruded chin. There may be associated excessive eversion of the lower lip with more severe mandibular

retrusions and a lack of the normal neck to mandibular soft tissue angles (cervicomental). Thus soft tissue redundancy in the submental region is frequent (Figure 59-15).

The intraoral view demonstrates a Class II malocclusion, which may further be divided into an Angle's Division 1 or 2. In Angle's Class II, Division 1, the maxillary incisor angulation is fairly normal and there is a large overjet relationship seen. In Angle's Class II, Division 2, the maxillary incisors are retroinclined, thus lessening the overjet relationship and giving the appearance of a smaller Class II malocclusion. In the Division 2 malocclusion, there is usually an associated deep bite or increased overbite relationship. The curve of Spee is thus overaccentuated, resulting in a shortened lower facial height.

The cephalometric analysis demonstrates normal parameters in the upper face with a decreased SNB angle and an increased ANB angle. In Angle's Class II, Division 1, the lower facial height is normal as previously stated, whereas in the Division 2, the lower facial height is decreased. The projection analysis is created by advancing the mandible until a normative Class I molar occlusion is achieved. In Division 2 malocclusions, this cannot be accomplished until the proper angulation of the maxillary incisors is obtained. Also in the Division 2 malocclusion, lower facial height increase is obtained by advancing the mandible before correction of the curve of Spee, creating a lateral open bite. If these open bites are closed postsurgically by orthodontic treatment, there is a resultant increase in the lower facial height that is an aesthetic benefit. If the curve of Spee is leveled orthodontically before surgery, this is usually accomplished by intruding the mandibular incisors and will result in a postsurgical short lower facial height. Genioplasty advancement is indicated in many cases of mandibular retrusion after the mandible has been advanced into a Class I condition; this should be planned accordingly. Lower facial height may also be increased by a lengthening genioplasty with an interpositional graft if needed.

The presurgical orthodontic treatment is accomplished to eliminate dental compensations and crowding. Asymmetric Class II malocclusions and very crowded lower mandibular dentitions are more difficult, and a presurgical orthodontic setup is needed to evaluate these conditions completely. It is important with mandibular retrusion to avoid any flaring of the mandibular dentition because this limits the amount of surgical advancement of the mandible. In fact, retrusion of the mandibular dentition is desirable, and in many cases this necessitates lower bicuspid extraction when substantial crowding is present. By performing these presurgical orthodontic steps, maximal mandibular advancement can be obtained. Postsurgical orthodontic finishing is done as previously described, with the exception of the Class II, Division 2 malocclusion where increase in lower facial height is desired. In this case the lateral open bites created by advancement are closed orthodontically. The surgical procedure of choice for mandibular surgery in the vast majority of cases is the sagittal split ramus osteotomy first described by Obwegeser[15] and later modified by others.[29] The biology of this technique was

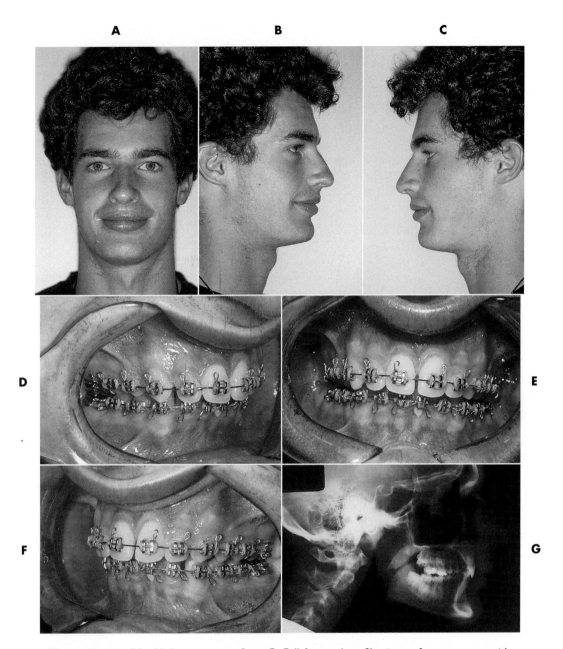

Figure 59-15. Mandibular retrusion. **A** to **C,** Full face and profile views of a young man with mandibular retrusion. Note that the facial thirds are vertically oriented in the correct manner and that the retrusion of the chin is only apparent on the lateral view. **D** to **F,** Occlusal views after preliminary orthodontic treatment demonstrating Class II malocclusion secondary to mandibular retrusion. **G,** Presurgical cephalometric radiograph demonstrating a Class II, Division 2 malocclusion before orthodontic correction of the dental compensations. Note that there is very little overjet but excessive overbite with this type of malocclusion. Presurgical orthodontics will correctly angulate the maxillary incisors with their axial inclination, creating a larger overjet that allows the mandible to thus be advanced. Orthodontist: L. Morrill. *Continued*

demonstrated by Bell and Schendel.[6] Surgical advancement of the mandible is prone to relapse, although rigid fixation has eliminated most early relapse (fixation to 3 months).[6,27,30] Late relapse secondary to condylar resorption remains a problem that is not completely understood, although there is a clear association between this relapse and preexisting temporomandibular joint symptoms. The surgical technique for the modified sagittal ramus osteotomy with plate fixation is presented.

Surgical Technique

The patient is prepared and positioned on the operating table as previously described. Local anesthetic is injected into the retromolar and ascending mandibular ramus area for hemo-

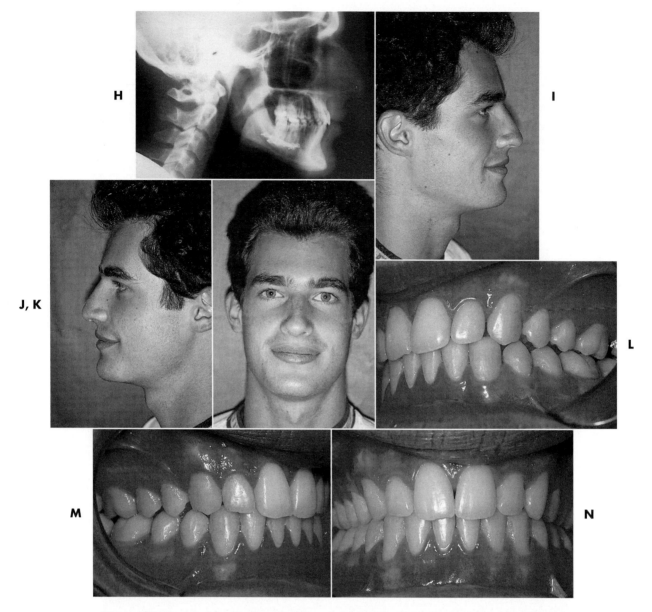

Figure 59-15, cont'd. H, Postsurgical cephalometric radiograph demonstrating advanced mandible with bilateral plate fixation of the osteotomy fragments. **I** to **K,** Postoperative photographs after mandibular advancement. Note the idealized anterior-posterior facial relationship. **L** to **N,** Postoperative occlusal result after debanding. Stable Class I occlusion is apparent.

static reasons (Figure 59-16). A small bite block is placed on the contralateral side, and cheek and tongue retraction is obtained. An incision is made starting at the mid-ascending ramus following the external oblique ridge laterally to the first mandibular molar. This incision transects the buccinator muscle along the external oblique ridge (Figure 59-17). Sufficient gingival tissue must be left buccal to the molars so that adequate closure of the incision can be obtained later. Subperiosteal dissection is undertaken to the antegonial notch and posteriorly and superiorly along the ascending ramus. A notched ramus retractor is then placed and elevated superiorly, exposing the ascending ramus. The temporalis muscle is stripped from this region until the tip of the coronoid process is reached, at which time a ramus clamp is placed. Dissection is

then taken medially along the ramus to expose the lingula. This subperiosteal dissection is best accomplished starting low, where the periosteum is easily identified, and then going superiorly. A retractor is then placed into this region, carefully guarding the inferior alveolar nerve by retracting it medially. A burr or reciprocating saw may be used to accomplish a horizontal osteotomy that goes through the cortical bone to midramal depth. This osteotomy is accomplished midway between the lingula and sigmoid notch and goes as far posteriorly as several millimeters behind the lingula. This cut should also be parallel to the mandibular occlusal plane. Anteriorly the cut is carried along the anterior border of the ascending ramus following the external oblique ridge (Figure 59-18). The osteotomy is then turned downward vertically

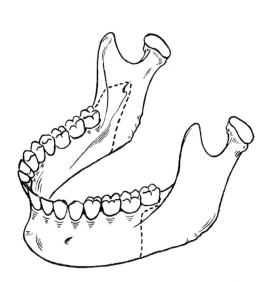

Figure 59-16. Mandibular retrusion. Correction of the mandibular retrusion by a sagittal split ramus osteotomy is indicated here. The lateral corticotomy cut is indicated in the dashed line. The mandible will then be advanced into the proper Class I occlusion.

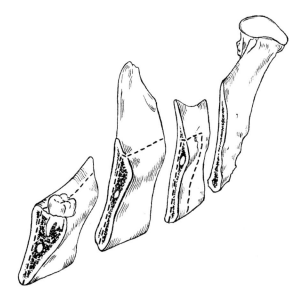

Figure 59-18. The typical appearance of the sagittal split ramus osteotomy after advancement. A coronal section demonstrating the passage of the osteotomy cut lateral to the molar tooth and nerve just under the buccal cortical bone of the lateral mandible.

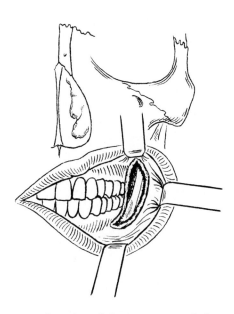

Figure 59-17. Buccal vestibular incision is made from midramal height to the distal of the first molar down through periosteum, and the flap is then reflected at this level.

Figure 59-19. The mandible is advanced to its desired occlusion, creating a gap laterally where the sagittal split has occurred. At this time it is important to see the condyle of the mandible superior and anterior of the fossa. The mandible is placed into intermaxillary fixation, and then rigid fixation is used to synthesize the proximal and distal segments after the sagittal split either with a miniplate as indicated here or with screws.

lateral to the first or second molar, depending on the amount of advancement needed. The vertical cut is carried inferiorly to the antegonial notch and around the inferior border. Completeness of the split is ascertained by a small osteotome. The split is then accomplished either with osteotomes or Smith splitters. During the split, careful attention must be paid to the position of the inferior alveolar nerve. Frequently the nerve will lie partially in a proximal segment after the split and thus will need to be gently elevated out so that the nerve damage does not occur.

After completion of the split, the segments are mobilized by stripping the residual medial pterygoid muscle from the distal segment through the split. Bony protuberances on the inside of the split segments are removed so that they will not impinge later on the alveolar nerve. At the completion of one side, the bite block is changed and the procedure is duplicated on the other side of the mandible. After both splits, the mandible is advanced and placed into the prepared acrylic wafer and IMF is obtained with wires (Figure 59-19). Fixation of the proximal and distal fragments is next performed by either screw or a plate fixation. My preference is for single-plate fixation with monocortical screws on either side. To perform this technique, a bone clamp is placed on the proximal segment, which is then rotated superiorly. A mandibular plate is then applied to this segment at a middle to inferior height position on the buccal. This plate is fixed with unicortical screws only. The proximal segment is then rotated posteriorly and superiorly with gentle pressure seating the condyle superiorly in the glenoid fossa, and the plate is fixed to the distal segment. Fixation of the mandibular proximal and distal fragments is then accomplished on the other side in a similar fashion. This technique allows the intraoral placement of plates without any cutaneous incisions. Plates are passively adapted to maintain the position of the proximal and distal fragments and thus torquing of the mandibular condyle or nerve compression is avoided. Because screws are unicortical in nature, nerve damage is eliminated yet

fixation is rigid enough to maintain stability of the segments. After placement of the plates, the IMF is released and the occlusion is checked. After ascertainment of the proper mandibular position, the wounds are closed with a resorbable suture in a running fashion. Drains may be placed in this area depending on the surgeon's preference. If an associated mandibular genioplasty is to be performed, this is accomplished after obtaining fixation of the mandibular segments and before IMF release and wound closure. Postoperative care is as previously described. Training elastics are placed in the Class II position postoperatively.

The most common problem associated with the sagittal split ramus osteotomy is mental nerve dysfunction. This is very common in the early postoperative period but resolves in the vast majority of cases over the intervening weeks to months. Very few cases have any perceptible residual mental nerve dysfunction after 6 months. The tendency for limited opening

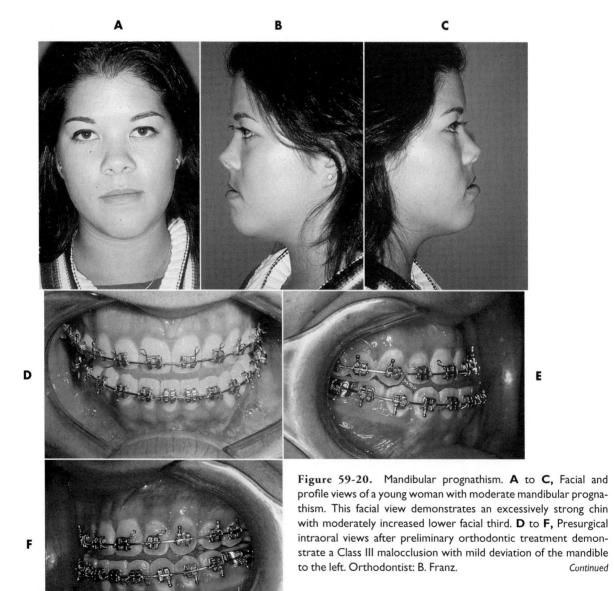

A **B** **C**

D **E**

F

Figure 59-20. Mandibular prognathism. **A** to **C,** Facial and profile views of a young woman with moderate mandibular prognathism. This facial view demonstrates an excessively strong chin with moderately increased lower facial third. **D** to **F,** Presurgical intraoral views after preliminary orthodontic treatment demonstrate a Class III malocclusion with mild deviation of the mandible to the left. Orthodontist: B. Franz. *Continued*

of the mandible postoperatively is also greater with this technique than maxillary techniques, and special attention should be taken to rehabilitate the mandibular movements in the postoperative period. Progressive condylar resorption is associated with mandibular advancement, causing occlusal relapse, and is unpredictable. It occurs in young women who have a history of temporomandibular joint dysfunction and is infrequent, occurring less than 4% of the time. Treatment should be of a conservative nature until the occlusion restabilizes. The occlusion is then corrected either orthodontically, surgically, or both.

MANDIBULAR PROGNATHISM

The aesthetic facial examination shows obvious protrusion of the mandible and lower face, especially in the profile view (Figure 59-20). Facial evaluation of the patient with mandibular prognathism also frequently demonstrates associated mild midfacial flattening. There may also be associated overclosure of the mandible, further aggravating the prognathic appearance and decreasing the lower facial third vertical height. Intraoral examination demonstrates a Class III malocclusion with or without open bite.[14] Frequently there

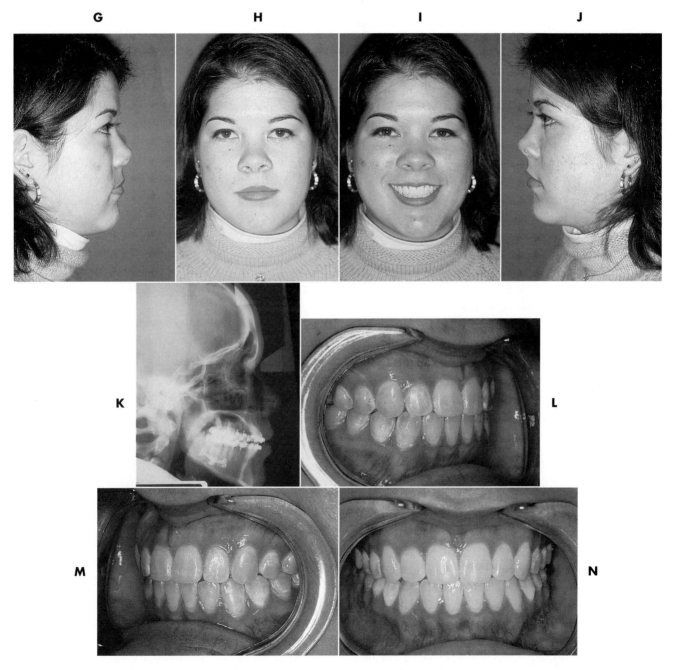

Figure 59-20, cont'd. **G** to **J,** Postsurgical facial views demonstrating the idealized facial profile after set-back of the mandible. **K,** Postoperative cephalometric radiograph demonstrating the mandible in a Class I position with miniplate fixation of the fragments. **L** to **N,** Postoperative occlusal result demonstrating a stable Class I occlusion after debanding.

is an associated bilateral transverse crossbite. If this does not correct on surgical repositioning of the jaws, maxillary expansion should be done either orthodontically or surgically depending on the situation.

The cephalometric analysis will demonstrate an increased SNB angle and negative ANB angle. The SNA angle may be normal or slightly retruded. There is always an increased overjet of a negative value, whereas overbite is variable. As with mandibular retrusion, particular attention should be paid to asymmetric Class III malocclusions and the position of the dental midlines to each other and the facial midline. The projection analysis is accomplished by setting the mandible back until a normal Class I occlusion is obtained. However, from an aesthetic standpoint, many mild Class III malocclusions secondary to mandibular prognathism are better corrected by maxillary advancement, thus filling the soft tissue envelope. Large Class III malocclusions are best corrected by combined mandibular set-back and maxillary advancement. From an aesthetic basis, very few isolated mandibular set-backs should be accomplished. The presurgical orthodontic treatment is accomplished as previously described, but retraction of the mandibular incisors and protraction of the maxillary incisors should not be done preoperatively. Moderate transverse discrepancies can be corrected by orthodontic expansion of the maxilla. However, major discrepancies will mandate an associated maxillary surgical procedure. Large mandibular set-backs are also associated with a higher relapse tendency because the intraoral space is decreased and the tongue can be compromised.[12]

Surgical Technique

In most cases the modified sagittal split ramus osteotomy is best suited for mandibular set-backs of 1 cm or less. Larger set-backs or those set-backs with extreme asymmetry or canted occlusal planes should be accomplished by intraoral vertical oblique osteotomies or inverted L osteotomies. The sagittal split technique is described here because the vast majority of set-backs are less than 1 cm.

The patient is prepared, and the procedure commences as noted for mandibular advancement sagittal split osteotomy techniques. After the splitting of the mandible, the distal segment is placed into the desired occlusal position using the interocclusal acrylic wafer and wire IMF. At this time, correct positioning of the proximal segment will demonstrate a bony overlap laterally, which should be resected (Figure 59-21). Passive positioning of the proximal segment is then accomplished, and fixation is obtained with either screws or plates. Fixation using the unicortical screws follows the same progression as described for mandibular advancement. IMF is then released and the occlusion is checked. It is my preference in correcting mandibular prognathisms to overcorrect by approximately 2 mm because there is some postsurgical rebound as the condyle repositions in the glenoid fossa. If an associated genioplasty is indicated, this is performed after rigid fixation of the mandibular segments but before IMF release. Frequently a reduction genioplasty is indicated if the chin is still strong after mandibular set-back in the projection analysis.

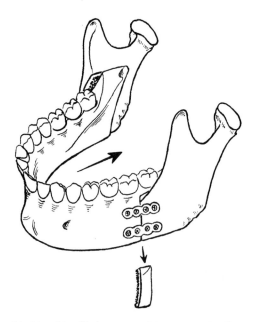

Figure 59-21. Mandibular prognathism correction by a sagittal split ramus osteotomy. After the ramus has been split and the mandible repositioned into the prepared occlusal wafer and a Class I occlusion, there is an excess of bone on the proximal mandibular segment in the lateral cortical area. This is resected and the segment is repositioned passively and fixed with rigid fixation, in this case a miniplate.

Reduction genioplasties are limited to 5 to 6 mm. If a larger chin reduction needs to be accomplished, this should be performed by shortening the posterior facial height by the ramus osteotomies and derotating the chin. Shortening the posterior facial height involves concomitant maxillary and mandibular procedures. When maxillary and mandibular procedures are done concomitantly, my preference is to perform the mandibular osteotomies first but not to complete the splits. The maxillary osteotomy is then completed and the maxilla positioned as desired. In these cases, as with any combined maxillomandibular osteotomies, an intermediary occlusal splint is frequently indicated to help position the maxilla at this stage. After rigid fixation of the maxilla, the mandibular sagittal splits are completed. The mandible is then placed into the proper occlusion as described with the maxilla using the final occlusal wafer, and rigid interfragmentary fixation of the mandible is obtained. IMF is then released and the occlusion is checked. Wound closure is then done as previously described.

Postoperative care is similar to that described for mandibular advancement surgery except that training elastics should be placed in a Class III position. Risks and complications are essentially the same as for the sagittal split in mandibular advancement.

This chapter has reviewed surgical-orthodontic correction of the most common dentofacial deformities. Only the basic surgical techniques have been covered because they account for over 90% of the procedures. Uncommon developmental and congenital deformities of the jaw are not covered, nor are all variations of maxillomandibular surgical techniques, because these are out the scope of this chapter.

REFERENCES

1. Araujo A, Schendel SA, Wolford LM, et al: Total maxillary advancement with and without bone grafting, *J Oral Surg* 36:849, 1978.

2. Bell WH: Biologic basis for maxillary osteotomies, *Am J Phys Anthropol* 38:279, 1973.

3. Bell WH: Le Fort I osteotomy for correction of maxillary deformities, *J Oral Surg* 33:412-426, 1975.

4. Bell WH: Correction of the short-face syndrome—vertical maxillary deficiency: a preliminary report, *J Oral Surg* 35:110-120, 1977.

5. Bell WH, Proffit WP: Maxillary excess. In Bell WH, Proffit JL, White D (eds): *Surgical correction of dentofacial deformities,* Philadelphia, 1980, WB Saunders.

6. Bell WH, Schendel SA: Biologic basis for modification of the sagittal split ramus osteotomy, *J Oral Surg* 35:362, 1977.

7. Carlotti AE, Schendel SA: An analysis of factors influencing stability of surgical advancement of the maxilla by Le Fort I osteotomy, *J Oral Maxillofac Surg* 45:924-928, 1987.

8. Egbert M, Hepworth B, Myall R, et al: Stability of Le Fort I osteotomy with maxillary advancement: a comparison of combined wire fixation and rigid fixation, *J Oral Maxillofac Surg* 53:243-248, 1995.

9. Ellis E, Carlson DS, Frydenlund S: Stability of midface augmentation: an experimental study of musculoskeletal interaction and fixation methods, *J Oral Maxillofac Surg* 47:1062-1068, 1989.

10. Epker BN: Modifications in the sagittal osteotomy of the mandible, *J Oral Surg* 35:157-159, 1977.

11. Epker BN, Fish LC: *Evaluation and treatment planning in dentofacial deformities: integrated orthodontic and surgical correction,* vol I, Philadelphia, 1986, WB Saunders.

12. Epker BN, Wessberg GA: Mechanisms of early skeletal relapse following surgical advancement of the mandible, *Br J Oral Surg* 20:172-176, 1982.

13. Ferraro JW: Cephalometry and cephalometric analysis. In *Fundamentals of maxillofacial surgery,* New York, 1997, Springer.

14. Hall HD: Mandibular prognathism. In Bell WH (ed): *Modern practice in orthognathic and reconstructive surgery,* vol 3, Philadelphia, 1992, WB Saunders.

15. Obwegeser HL: Surgical correction of small or retrodisplaced maxilla. The "dish face deformity," *Plast Reconstr Surg* 43:351, 1969.

16. Opdebeeck HL, Bell WH, Eisenfeld J, et al: Comparative study between the SFS and LFS rotation as a possible morphogenic mechanism, *Am J Orthod* 70:509, 1978.

17. Proffit WR, Epker BN, Ackerman JL: Systematic description of dentofacial deformities. In Bell WH, Proffit JL, White D (eds): *The data base in surgical corrections of dentofacial deformities,* vol 1, Philadelphia, 1980, WB Saunders.

18. Proffit WR, Phillips C, Turvey TA: Stability following superior repositioning of the maxilla by Le Fort I osteotomy, *Am J Orthod Dentofacial Orthop* 92:151-161, 1987.

19. Schendel SA: Genioplasty, a physiologic approach, *Ann Plast Surg* 14:506-514, 1985.

20. Schendel SA: Cephalometrics in orthognathic surgery. In Bell WH (ed): *Modern practice in orthognathic and reconstructive surgery,* Philadelphia, 1992, WB Saunders.

21. Schendel SA: Prediction tracing. In Ferraro JW (ed): *Fundamentals of maxillofacial surgery,* New York, 1997, Springer-Verlag.

22. Schendel SA, Carlotti AE: Nasal considerations in orthognathic surgery, *Am J Orthod Dentofacial Orthop* 100:197-208, 1991.

23. Schendel SA, Carlotti AE: Variations of vertical maxillary excess, *J Oral Maxillofac Surg* 43:590-596, 1985.

24. Schendel SA, Delaire J: Facial muscles: form, function and reconstruction. In Bell WH (ed): *Dentofacial deformities, new concepts,* vol 3, Philadelphia, 1985, WB Saunders.

25. Schendel SA, Eisenfeld JH, Bell WH, et al: The long face syndrome—vertical maxillary excess, *Am J Orthod* 70:398-408, 1976.

26. Schendel SA, Eisenfeld JH, Bell WH, et al: Superior repositioning of the maxilla: stability and soft tissue osseous relations, *Am J Orthod* 70:663-674, 1976.

27. Schendel SA, Epker BN: Results after mandibular advancement surgery: an analysis of 87 cases, *J Oral Surg* 38:265-282, 1980.

28. Schendel SA, Mason ME: Adverse outcomes in orthognathic surgery and management of residual problems in secondary management of craniofacial disorders, *Clin Plast Surg* 24:3, 1997.

29. Trauner R, Obwegeser H: The surgical correction of mandibular prognathism and retrognathia with consideration of genioplasty, *J Oral Surg Med Pathol* 10:677-689, 1957.

30. Van Sickels JE, Richardson DA: Stability of orthognathic surgery: a review of rigid fixation, *Br J Oral Maxillofac Surg* 34:279-285, 1996.

31. Van Sickels JE, Tucker MR: Management of delayed union and nonunion of maxillary osteotomies, *J Oral Maxillofac Surg* 48:1039-1044, 1990.

CHAPTER

TMJ Dysfunction

Russell W. Bessette

INTRODUCTION

The management of patients with facial pain is a difficult challenge. There are many causes for facial pain; some are serious, others more benign. By far one of the more common conditions is pain related to temporomandibular joint (TMJ) syndrome. This condition, often first seen by physicians, can be caused by a medical or dental problem. The medical and dental literature is replete with articles questioning the most basic concepts of TMJ anatomy, pathology, diagnostic investigations, and therapeutic management of TMJ disorders. This conclusion suggests that caution is required in managing patients with these symptoms. Given this, the practicing plastic surgeon is often confused as to a treatment pathway.

This chapter concentrates on establishing a practical diagnostic and treatment concept for patients with suspected TMJ syndrome. It is recognized that some of the treatment modalities for TMJ dysfunction are outside the usual scope or interest of the average plastic surgeon; however, the differential diagnosis of facial pain is crucial to general practice. Additionally because TMJ syndrome is commonly associated with facial trauma, it behooves the plastic surgeon to consider it in evaluating these patients.

INDICATIONS

To understand the indications for treatment of TMJ syndrome, it is necessary to look at a brief history of how we arrived at our present thinking. Early researchers often had very unclear concepts of TMJ anatomy and a lack of understanding of prime jaw function. As diagnostic techniques improved, our understanding of jaw function increased. This in turn led to significant changes in treatment methods. Most importantly, it led to more proper selection of specific treatment for specific TMJ problems.

HISTORY

In 1934, Costen[8] proposed a dental cause for TMJ dysfunction and suggested that loss of teeth produced mandibular overclosure. He reported that posterior displacement of the mandibular condyle created pressure on the auriculotemporal nerve and produced pain. Very importantly, he identified the cardinal symptoms of this condition: facial pain, TMJ click, and limited jaw opening. Although today it is believed that the cause of TMJ syndrome is more complex than jaw overclosure, these three symptoms are still diagnostic. In 1955, Schwartz[49] suggested that masticatory muscle spasm and psychologic overlay were major contributory factors. Based on his research, dental splint therapy became a prime treatment modality. His rationale was that a flat-plane dental splint could interrupt bruxism. Once the noxious influence of the occlusion was removed, the dentist could correct the bite through occlusal adjustment. The end result of this therapy was to permit relaxation in overworked masticatory muscles. He was one of the first dental researchers to advocate electromyography as a clinical tool in evaluating clinical outcome.

Despite the success of dental splint therapy in most TMJ syndrome patients, there remained a specific group of individuals who did not respond to this therapy. This finding suggested that perhaps the dental occlusion was not completely responsible for all cases. In 1978, Wilkes,[59] perfecting techniques in TMJ arthrography, coined the term *internal derangement* (ID). He described TMJ disk displacement as a primary cause in these patients. Subsequently, he went on to describe a disease classification and surgical treatment modality.

Since then, advances in diagnostic modalities have shed the most light on this disease. Notably, TMJ arthrotomography and magnetic resonance imaging (MRI)[27] improve the preoperative evaluation and reduce the number of invasive procedures. Indeed, these imaging techniques permit the clinician to separate those patients with organic surgical disease from those with functional or stress-related disorders. See Box 60-1 for staging criteria.

Box 60-1.
Staging Criteria for Internal Derangements of TMJ with Respect to Clinical, Radiologic, and Surgical Findings*

EARLY STAGE

Clinical: No significant mechanical symptoms, other than reciprocal clicking (early in opening movement, late in closing movement, and soft in intensity); no pain or limitation of motion

Radiologic: Slight forward displacement, good anatomic contour of disk, and normal tomograms

Surgical: Normal anatomic form, slight anterior placement, and passive incoordination (clicking) demonstrable

EARLY/INTERMEDIATE STAGE

Clinical: First few episodes of pain, occasional joint tenderness and related temporal headaches, beginning major mechanical problems, increase in intensity of clicking sounds, joint sounds later in opening movement, and beginning transient subluxations or joint catching and locking

Radiologic: Slight forward displacement, slight thickening of posterior edge or beginning anatomic deformity of disk, and normal tomograms

Surgical: Anterior displacement, early anatomic deformity (slight to mild thickening of posterior edge), and well-defined central articulating area

INTERMEDIATE STAGE

Clinical: Multiple episodes of pain, joint tenderness, temporal headaches, major mechanical symptoms—transient catching, locking and sustained locking (closed locks), restriction of motion, and difficulty (pain) with function

Radiologic: Anterior displacement with significant anatomic deformity/prolapse of disk (moderate to marked thickening of posterior edge) and normal tomograms

Surgical: Marked anatomic deformity with displacement, variable adhesions (anterior, lateral, and posterior recesses), and no hard tissue changes

INTERMEDIATE/LATE STAGE

Clinical: Characterized by chronicity with variable and episodic pain, headaches, variable restriction of motion, and undulating course

Radiologic: Increase in severity over intermediate stage, abnormal tomograms, and early to moderate degenerative remodeling hard tissue changes

Surgical: Increase in severity over intermediate stage, hard tissue degenerative remodeling changes of both bearing surfaces, osteophytic projections, multiple adhesions (lateral, anterior, and posterior recesses), and *no perforation* of disk or attachment

LATE STAGE

Clinical: Characterized by crepitus on examination, scraping, grating, grinding symptoms, variable and episodic pain, chronic restriction of motion, and difficulty with function

Radiologic: Anterior displacement, *perforation* with simultaneous filling of upper and lower compartments, filling defects, gross anatomic deformity of disk and hard tissues, abnormal tomograms as described, and essentially degenerative arthritic changes

Surgical: Gross degenerative changes of disk and hard tissues, perforation of posterior attachments, erosions of bearing surfaces, and multiple adhesions equivalent to degenerative arthritis (sclerosis, flattening, anvil-shaped condyle, osteophytic projections, and subcortical cystic formation)

*TMJ, Temporomandibular joint. Radiologic findings refer to arthrographic, magnetic resonance, and tomographic imaging where applicable.

OCCURRENCE

Estimates reveal that 30% of the Western population experiences symptoms suggestive of TMJ dysfunction.[6,26,52] Young women are primarily affected, with a male-to-female ratio of 1:3.[18,50] Lieberman[34] reported that 22% of children seen in an orthodontic clinic had symptoms of TMJ syndrome, but only 5% had demonstrable changes on their MRI. Similar percentages have been reported in other studies and reinforce the premise that most TMJ patients do not have organic joint pathology and therefore do not require surgical correction.

EMBRYOLOGY

The development of the TMJ begins in the human embryo at 6 weeks with the appearance of the mandibular ossification center.[37] At 8 weeks, mesenchymal condensations appear in the region of the future TMJ, which forms into the condylar and temporal blastemas. These undergo ossification at about 9 weeks at the same time that condylar cartilage appears. The articular disk forms from mesenchymal condensation between these two blastemas, with the anterior portion being derived from the condyle, the posterior portion from the temporal region, and the medial portion from the lateral pterygoid tendon. The joint spaces are developed by the process of apoptosis, which leads to the cavitation of the lower compartment by 12 weeks and the upper compartment at 14 weeks. Muscular activity is required to maintain these joint spaces once they have formed.

ANATOMY

The gross anatomy of the TMJ[7,9,16,19] is unique but typical of most diarthrodial synovial joints. The joint surfaces consist of

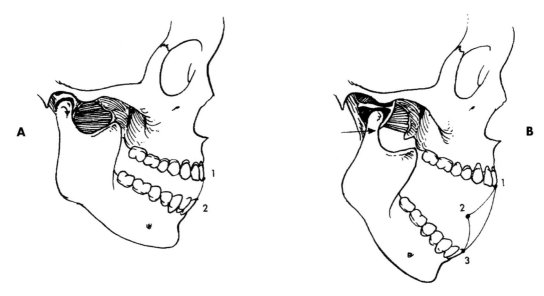

Figure 60-1. **A,** Lateral skull view during initial jaw opening. Incisor teeth distance point 1 to 2 occurs with pure hinge rotation in condyle. **B,** Maximal jaw opening. Incisor distance point 2 to 3 reflects condylar translation.

the mandibular condyles and the temporal articular surfaces. The condyles are elliptic structures measuring 15 to 20 mm medial to lateral and 8 to 10 mm anteroposteriorly. They are oriented perpendicular to the plane of the mandible, which gives them a slight medial rotation when viewed on a direct sagittal view of the skull. This anatomic fact is significant when viewing a lateral skull x-ray projection and accounts for the distortion sometimes seen in the TMJ condyles. Of major importance is that both joints function as a single unit[24] (Figure 60-1). Together they have a fixed end point, the occlusion of the teeth. This end point can change with alteration in the teeth and occlusion. For this reason, many clinicians suspect that alteration of the occlusion can lead to changes within the joint. The articular surfaces are lined by fibrocartilage, which makes the TMJ different from other synovial joints that have as their articular surface hyaline cartilage. Finally, a disk composed of dense fibrous connective tissue separates the joint into two spaces, each with a different function. Pure hinge movement is accomplished in the inferior space (ginglymus), and a sliding or translatory movement occurs in the superior space (arthrodial).

Surrounding these structures is the fibrous joint capsule, which is anchored to the zygomatic arch superiorly and the neck of the condyle inferiorly. It is reinforced anterolaterally by the temporomandibular ligament.

From a perspective of disease symptoms, the TMJ disk deserves special attention. The disk is a biconcave structure composed of dense fibrous connective tissue. It is anchored anteriorly to the superior head of the lateral pterygoid muscle and the eminentia articularis. The inferior portion attaches to the medial and lateral aspect of the mandibular condyle. The posterior part of the disk attaches in two zones to the posterior slope of the glenoid fossae. The superior attachment is composed of elastic fibers attached to the postglenoid tubercle of the squamotympanic fissure, and the inferior attachment has inelastic collagen fibers attached to the posterior aspect of

the condylar neck. Between these two posterior zones exists an area of highly vascularized and innervated loose connective tissue termed the *retrodiskal pad,* which has been implicated in the genesis of pain from TMJ disorders. It is believed that the main function of the disk is to distribute load evenly along the joint surfaces and aid in their lubrication and protection during translatory movements. This function, if lost, may have serious implications on the morphology of the affected joint. Varying changes in disk position serves as the bases for classifying TMJ ID.

HISTOLOGY

Certain histologic features of the TMJ may be important in the management of its dysfunction.[24] The articular cartilage is made up of chondrocytes in a matrix of collagen fibers and osmotically active proteoglycans, which form arcades parallel to the joint surface. The application of compressive forces to this layer leads to the expulsion of water from the hydrophilic proteoglycans and causes the cartilage to occupy a smaller volume at this point of compression. It is known that chondrocytes are incapable of regenerating new cartilage should areas be lost. These facts cast serious doubt on the validity of any procedure that involves the removal of large amounts of articular cartilage. They may also be important in the prevention of recurrent disease because it is believed that abnormal loading of the joint surface is likely to be a factor in the pathogenesis of TMJ dysfunction.

The synovium of the TMJ is known to produce synovial fluid that is essential to joint lubrication and chondrocyte nutrition. It also provides for phagocytosis of unwanted particulate material and aids in the rapid diffusion of substances in and out of the joint. For these reasons, the preservation of all but the most severely damaged, inflamed, or redundant synovium should be a high priority in any operative approach to the TMJ. Synovial fluid circulation is directly related to joint motion and as such may be crucial to the prevention of adhesions and intrinsic healing of the joint.

CHEWING AND JOINT FUNCTION

The prime function of the mandible is chewing and speech. Understanding joint mechanics is of major importance in the diagnosis and treatment of patients with TMJ syndrome.[37] During a maximal jaw opening, the TMJ undergoes two separate motions permitted by the two distinct joint spaces. The lower ginglymoid compartment is capable of simple hinge motion only, and it is here that the first 20 to 25 mm of interincisor jaw opening are achieved. The upper gliding compartment is capable of translatory motion anteriorly along the eminence and allows the last 15 to 20 mm of interincisor jaw opening to occur. It is only after translation past the height of the eminence that the additional 20 mm of rotation is possible.

At rest the mandibular condyle lies inferior to the TMJ disk. Upon jaw opening, the condyle rotates to engage the intermediate zone of the disk, causing it to move anteriorly and come in contact with the eminence. At this point, further opening is achieved by translating with the condyle along the slope of the eminence. In the final stage of opening, the condyle rotates beneath the disk. Whereas the disk and condyle lie anteriorly, the retrodiskal tissue lies free and tends to engorge with blood. This anatomic fact is easily demonstrated by moving the mandible during an open TMJ surgery.

As jaw closure commences, the condyle moves posteriorly to again lie in the glenoid fossae, causing compression and shrinkage of the retrodiskal tissue. During this phase, the superior head of the lateral pterygoid muscle contracts to control the rate at which the disk returns to its resting position. The elastic fibers in the superior zone of the posterior disk attachment allow the disk to move anteriorly and also provide the recoil necessary to return the disk to its resting position during closure.

Chewing occurs by the actions of the masticatory and suprahyoid muscles, all of which are innervated by the mandibular division of the trigeminal nerve. Sensory input from the periodontal ligament receptors of the teeth and the TMJ capsule provides final guidance for positioning of the mandible as the teeth penetrate the food bolus. Therefore malocclusion may lead to a deviated closure pattern and cause the muscle spasm. This is of major significance and reinforces the concept that myospasm is a common finding of TMJ syndrome. The spasm may occur alone or in association with ID.

EVALUATING THE PATIENT WITH FACIAL PAIN

The evaluation of the TMJ syndrome patient begins with a complete history and physical examination. Based on these findings, appropriate ancillary investigations are undertaken. In this manner, the patient is spared the cost and morbidity of tests that may not prove helpful to the diagnosis. It is important to consider and exclude the possibility of diseases that mimic TMJ dysfunction and are more serious or malignant. A partial list includes diseases of the teeth, sinuses, and ears, as well as neoplastic processes of the oral cavity and central nervous system (CNS).

Patient History

Traditionally patients with TMJ dysfunction have the classic triad of pain in the preauricular area, joint noise, and limited mandibular movement.[15,25,37]

Pain may be reported as in the joint or be more diffuse and radiate from the teeth, ear, or muscles of the face and neck. When the pain occurs may suggest its origin. Pain in the early morning may result from nocturnal bruxism causing muscular spasm, whereas joint pain later in the day after jaw function may suggest intracapsular pathology. Likewise, joint pain is commonly aggravated by chewing and tends to be constant, whereas muscle pain may be influenced by stress and may be intermittent.

The patterns of joint sounds may help the examiner identify the cause. Solitary clicks are known to occur in up to 40% of the normal population and are reversible and innocent. Pathologic clicks are usually caused by the anterior subluxation of the disk such that with jaw opening, the anteriorly displaced disk is recaptured by the condyle, causing a click. The disk subluxes as the condyle returns to the glenoid fossa with a less audible noise, leading to the so-called reciprocal clicking (Figure 60-2). It is also thought that the more stretched the posterior attachment becomes, the more likely it is that surgical intervention will be necessary to reposition the disk. Crepitus from the joint suggests the grinding of surfaces that are no longer smooth because of disruption or calcification of the disk or joint surfaces. This may be a physical sign of degenerative change in the joint.

Limited jaw motion may result from several factors, including a nonreducing anterior disk displacement, which restricts translation of the condyle and results in decreased opening (closed lock). Limited motion may also occur because of muscular restriction or adhesions within the joint, such as ankylosis, or impingement of the cornoid process and zygomatic arch.

Ear symptoms, such as tinnitus, are very commonly reported in the history. It may result from muscle spasm in the tensor tympani muscle within the ear. This muscle is innervated by a small branch of the mandibular nerve and may be a precursor of early TMJ syndrome. Experience has taught us that relief of this symptom is quite variable. If tinnitus is the only chief complaint, invasive therapy of the TMJ should only be undertaken with extreme caution.

Determining a time course for TMJ syndrome symptoms is very useful. The clinician should ask when the symptoms began, if the symptoms have changed, if there was trauma to the head, and if there is a history of bruxism. This information organized along a time continuum can strongly suggest a diagnosis. A patient may relate a fall as a child that resulted in lacerating the chin. Subsequently, there is recollection of a jaw click without pain for many years. Gradually the click became

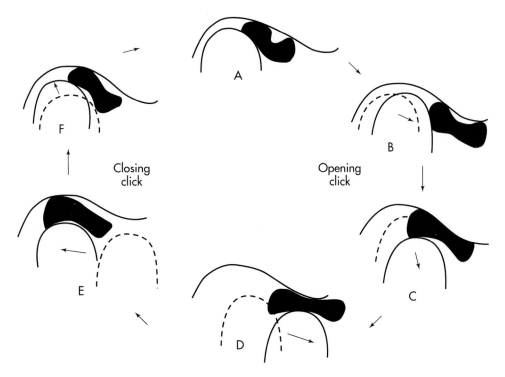

Figure 60-2. TMJ reciprocal clicking occurs with recapture and displacement of disk. **A,** Displaced disk at jaw close position. **B,** The opening click occurs as the condyle snaps under the disk and recaptures it (**C** to **E**). **F,** The closing click occurs as the disk slips off the condyle.

more noticeable and slightly painful. Perhaps there was a history of orthodontia as a teenager that suddenly was associated with decreased jaw opening. At this point in time the jaw became noticeably painful. Perhaps the locking of the jaw was intermittent followed by periods of clicking with no pain. During these times there may be recollections of mild earache or tinnitus. Eventually there may have come a time when the jaw locked and was associated with difficult chewing. Often the joint sounds may change and become crepitant. It may be described as if sand were in the joint. Although this typical history may change slightly, when it is reported, the clinician should be very suspicious of TMJ ID.

In contrast, a history that is of much shorter duration and reports brief episodes of jaw ache perhaps associated with stressful events should suggest masticatory muscle spasm secondary to bruxism. Jaw clicking may be present but does not follow a regular occurrence or pattern of advancement as described previously. In 1970, Laskin[33] believed that this picture warranted calling this condition a separate name—myofascial pain dysfunction (MPD).

Physical Examination

The examination of the patient with TMJ syndrome symptoms takes into account the entire person but obviously centers on the head, neck, and TMJ. The initial inspection begins by observing the patient as a whole, noting any evidence of stress or psychologic disorders that could confuse the accurate evaluation of a patient with chronic pain. Attention is paid to the face, observing for signs of facial asymmetry that could denote skeletal deformity. Finally, the occlusion and dentition

are inspected, looking for either malocclusion or specific pulpal problems causing pain.

When conducting the oral examination, the clinician should undertake a complete check for oral cancer. Such neoplastic tumors can often radiate pain to the ear or neck and can easily be missed unless a specific effort is made to detect them. Inspection of the ear canals and tympanic membranes are vital to the complete examination and exclude the possibility of primary otologic or sinus disease. Examination of cranial nerves II through XII can be conducted while these other structures are being assessed and help in eliminating disorders of the CNS.

Palpation of the masticatory muscles is performed to detect areas of local tenderness that suggest muscle spasm. The lateral portion of the TMJ can be palpated, denoting a click or crepitus. Sometimes these vibrations can be loud enough to transmit through the air and be heard by the examiner. The loudness of the sound does not relate directly to the pathology and sometimes can be enhanced if the patient "pops the joint." Of greater importance is differentiating the vibration as a click or crepitus (grinding). A single click should be related to the millimeters of jaw opening. A single click occurring at the maximum range of opening may signal a benign articular eminence interference. This condition occurring at 40 to 50 mm of jaw opening simply indicates a possible strike of the condyle against the articular tubercle. Crepitus, or a feeling of sandpaper in the joint, may be very suspicious for degenerative changes in the condyle or disk.

Joint motion should be assessed in all directions, beginning with the measurement of the maximal opening of the jaws. This so-called interincisor opening distance should be about

40 mm. There should be about 10 mm of lateral jaw excursion to each side, measured at the incisor midlines. All movement should be smooth and without restriction. If a condyle palpates, as if it is fixed and rotating only, this may suggest ID.

JOINT IMAGING

The recent development of many new diagnostic tools and the refinement of older techniques have led to a new era in imaging the TMJ. These studies should only be ordered if a suspicion or history suggests underlying disease. Physicians specializing in TMJ diagnosis may have instruments that more accurately predict who will benefit from MRI. These instruments include jaw tracking that can detect subtle changes in jaw movement during chewing and joint vibration analysis that will more reliably display joint sound than physical examination alone.[23]

Conventional radiography remains the investigative starting point for most patients. Transcranial views are often performed, but their interpretation in all but the most advanced disease is unreliable.[12,44,45,57] Tomograms in the mouth open and closed positions provide good data on the integrity of the osseous structure but cannot detect soft tissue disk disease. The tomogram permits elimination of tumors of bone and can describe the range of condylar motion. However, restriction of motion in the condyle can be caused by disk displacement or muscle spasm. It must be recalled that plain films may be normal in up to 85% of patients with TMJ syndrome.[53]

Arthrography using contrast material introduced into the joint spaces aids in the visualization of the ID.[4,6,43,48] Reliability of TMJ arthrography has been exceedingly high and has been reported at 100%, particularly in detecting perforations of the disk[56] (Figure 60-3). Unfortunately, the technique is painful and requires considerable experience by the radiologist. With the decreasing cost of MRI, the use of arthrography is diminishing.

Computed tomography (CT) scanning has been available for years, and its use is significant in bone ankylosis or cornoid zygomatic arch problems but is of little use in disk disorders. In a patient with acute head trauma, its use is more justifiable than in a patient with chronic jaw pain.

One of the most significant advances in imaging of the TMJ has been the MRI scan.[40,46,47] It uses nucleus alignment in a strong magnetic field to generate radio frequencies that can be detected, digitized, and analyzed by computer to produce a reconstructed image.[25] Its major advantages are that it visualizes soft tissue directly, is noninvasive, and does not use ionizing radiation. Many authors consider MRI the investigation of choice when looking for ID of the disk (Figures 60-4 and 60-5). No patient should be taken to surgery for disk repair until an MRI or arthrogram confirms disk displacement. A study by Rao et al[40] demonstrated that

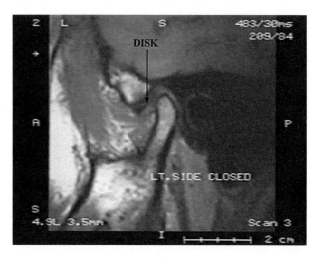

Figure 60-4. A normal left TMJ MRI taken with the jaw closed. The condyle's marrow is visualized as the bright white signal beneath the labeled TMJ disk.

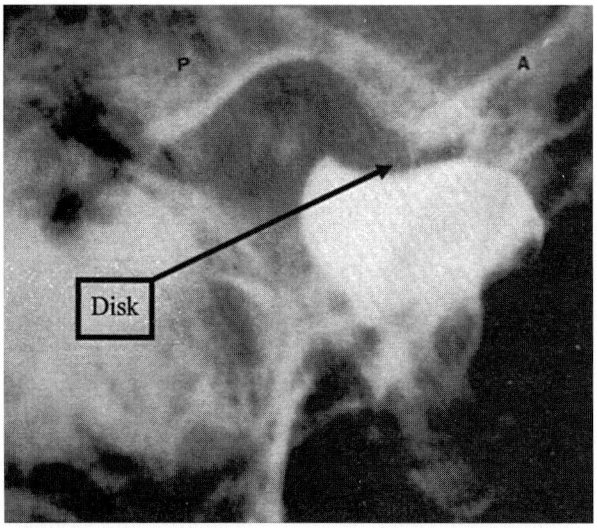

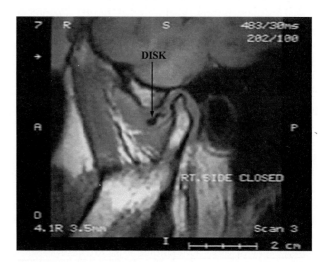

Figure 60-3. A normal right TMJ arthrogram with contrast media in the lower joint space during jaw opening (*A* = anterior, *P* = posterior). The location of the disk is visualized at the arrow.

Figure 60-5. A right TMJ MRI demonstrating a labeled disk displacement. The condyle is irregular, and the disk suggests deformity.

in 212 patients clinically suspected of ID, 94 showed normal joints.

TYPES OF TMJ DISORDERS

Myofascial Pain Dysfunction Syndrome

MPD syndrome was first described by Laskin.[33] MPD syndrome represents a constellation of symptoms, including preauricular pain, occasional joint clicking, restriction of jaw opening, tenderness localized to the masticatory muscles, and a normal radiograph. There are usually no discernible anatomic abnormalities within the TMJs.[37] The cause of MPD syndrome is multifactorial and includes occlusal prematurity, overclosure, bruxism, and anxiety. These lead to spasm of the jaw muscles and cause pain around the TMJ.[13] Some researchers believe that stress-induced bruxism is the core cause. Others believe that malocclusion causes the bruxism. In both cases, muscle spasm is the result. How the spasm is treated depends on the perceived cause.

In the absence of other features suggesting ID, further investigation, particularly with invasive testing, is not warranted. The aim of management in MPD is to break the spasm cycle that leads to an escalation of pain and anxiety. The usual starting point is the dental occlusion because this is a focal point in both stress and malocclusion. By introducing a splint between the teeth, the mandible is guided along a path that relaxes the neuromuscular system. The relaxation is believed to be a result of removal of afferent signals from dental premature contacts. Often the dentist may need to perform an occlusal adjustment after the muscles are relaxed. At this point the patient may only require the splint at night to prevent bruxism. Some investigators believe that dental splints limit the jaws to a pure hinge motion and thereby reduce the activity in the lateral pterygoids.[10,12] If the pain is exacerbated by splint therapy, ID should be suspected and disk position ascertained by MRI because a nonreducing disk may be compressed by the condyle as it seats in the fossae.

Ancillary measures may be used to assist splint therapy. This is particularly true in those patients with stress-induced bruxism. These measures include medications, such as nonsteroidal antiinflammatory agents, muscle relaxants, and other psychotropic drugs, as well as physical therapy modalities with heat, diathermy, ultrasound, and biofeedback. Dietary reduction to reduce joint stress is helpful. This may be accomplished with a simple soft diet.[37]

Despite these measures, the success rate reported in the literature for MPD is variable. After an adequate diagnostic workup and several months of compliant conservative therapy, it may be necessary to assure the patient that the diagnosis was truly MPD. If the position of the disk is in doubt, an MRI may be required. Diagnostic studies that measure jaw function and detect disk displacement may prove to be particularly helpful in reassuring both patient and physician.

Internal Derangement

ID refers to an abnormal relationship between the disk and condyle. The most common cause of ID is acute trauma. This is usually of the macro type and commonly includes automobile accidents or any blow to the head or whiplash injury. Some investigators report chronic trauma, malocclusion associated with prognathism, and open bite deformity.[37]

The pathogenesis begins with the anterior displacement of the disk relative to the superior aspect of the condyle. This in turn allows the innervated retrodiskal tissue to become trapped between the condyle and fossae. This abnormal arrangement of tissues is thought to be the source of pain. With time the altered load-bearing properties of the joint causes premature wear of articular surfaces manifested by the initial stretching and then perforation of the posterior attachment of the disk and the characteristic progressive changes of degenerative arthritis.

The current staging of ID accepted by the American Society of Maxillofacial Surgeons (ASMS) and the American Society of Plastic and Reconstructive Surgeons (ASPRS) is based on the scheme proposed by Wilkes[59] in 1989 and shown in Box 60-1. It attempts to correlate the progression of clinical findings with those expected on imaging and at operation.

The usual clinical manifestation of ID depends on the stage when first seen and includes some elements of pain, otalgia, headache, and neck ache in all but stage 1 and becomes more constant and severe as the stage progresses. Joint noises occur in most stages of ID and range from painless clicking to painful clicking with crepitus associated with degenerative arthritic changes. Motion of the joint becomes progressively more restricted as the stage advances. Movements are totally free in stage 1 and become visibly limited and distorted in advanced stages. Joint tenderness signifies intracapsular pathology and suggests ID but is more difficult to correlate with clinical stages.

The investigation of the patient with suspected ID should aim to confirm an intraarticular abnormality and exclude other unrelated causes of symptoms. If TMJ symptoms are related to other body joints, simple laboratory studies, such as erythrocyte sedimentation rate, presence of autoimmune antibodies, and uric acid levels, may uncover inflammatory causes of the arthropathy. The choice of imaging techniques may depend on the local availability of expertise, but in general, techniques that provide noninvasive information on joint integrity and that are less costly than MRI or arthrography are preferred. Once the index of suspicion is high for ID, an arthrogram or MRI is warranted.[34,40,53,56]

The management of ID is stage dependent, so it is essential that a preoperative stage be assigned as accurately as possible. Nonoperative management may be indicated in those patients with early-stage (1 or 2) disease. The intent is to reestablish the normal disk-condylar relationship. Many treatments may be similar to those described for management of MPD. Success should be seen within 2 to 6 months.[15,25,37]

OPERATIONS

Sometimes patients cannot tolerate splints, so other treatments must be considered. For those patients and those with later-stage disease, a more aggressive approach can be used because progressive stretching of the retrodiskal area makes spontaneous permanent disk reduction unlikely.[12] Currently, numerous surgical operations in the management of ID exist, and the procedure chosen will depend on the pathology and the expertise of the surgeon. The following is an attempt to outline the most common operations and to give an overview of their advantages and limitations.

TMJ LAVAGE

Recent advances demonstrate that irrigation of the TMJ with two small needles in the superior joint space may lead to marked symptom reduction. Some investigators report that such treatment removes inflammatory products responsible for pain. In early-stage disease, these attempts appear to show the most success. Other clinicians have advocated the insertion of antiinflammatory agents within the joint. Presently the long-term effect of this modality is not fully understood. In advanced-stage disease the results may not be as predictable.

TMJ ARTHROSCOPY

Arthroscopic surgery has become commonly used because of improvements in scope design and instrumentation. Simple procedures, such as arthrocentesis, biopsy, and joint lavage, are easily performed through the arthroscope.[15,25,37,41] In a series of 109 patients with ID treated with arthroscopic lysis, lavage, débridement, or a combination thereof, Mosby[19] found that 93% of patients had symptoms reduced to manageable levels with an improvement in jaw function. Less than 10% had residual dietary restrictions. Sixteen patients required reoperation, and 14 required an open arthrotomy. The long-term benefit of arthroscopic surgery is yet to be determined. Recent studies by our group demonstrate very little improvement in joint sounds after arthroscopic surgery.[30] The improvement in chewing is also uncertain because the disk position is not corrected by the procedure.

When more complex procedures are undertaken via the arthroscope, results become even more variable.[41] It is currently possible to perform anterior release of the disk with posterior cauterization or suture plication. McCain et al[36] reported on 4831 TMJs and found that 90% of patients reported excellent results. However, only 29.5% of patients were followed more than 2 years.

Recent use of lasers focused through the arthroscope has raised some controversy.[20,41] It will be necessary to follow these outcomes closely before they can be endorsed completely. It is also important to recognize the limitations of arthroscopy in advanced joint disease. In such cases the surgeon may lose the anatomic orientation, and serious complications may ensue. For example, in McCain's report,[35] hearing loss occurred in 24 patients (complete in 1), infection occurred in 14 patients, hemorrhage in 1, and neurologic damage occurred in 149 patients. Also of concern were 30 cases of facial nerve

damage, which recovered spontaneously. The conclusion is that arthroscopic surgery of the TMJ should be performed by surgeons well versed in open joint procedures with a good understanding of the joint anatomy.

TMJ ARTHROTOMY

Arthrotomy allows open inspection of the joint and permits more extensive reconstruction. The usual approach to the joint is by way of a preauricular incision, raising an anteriorly based capsular flap and then incising along the inferior border of the disk to expose the lower joint space.[2,15,25,37] Once exposed, the pathology of the joint dictates the reconstructive procedure.

Disk displacement alone requires repositioning and anchoring to prevent recurrence. This is achieved by resecting a wedge of the posterior band of the disk and retromeniscus. The cut edges are then sutured after any osteophytes on the condyle are shaved. Most studies have shown that patients treated by these procedures show a 90% improvement in pain symptoms and are pleased with the procedure. Recent studies[31] have shown that postoperative measurements of jaw function show an improvement over the preoperative tracings. These results appear to be very dependent on early postoperative physical therapy that encourages early jaw movement with condylar translation. It would appear that joint space adhesions are the single worse enemy of TMJ surgery and therefore early mobilization is to be encouraged (Figure 60-6).

Disk displacement with significant degenerative changes in the disk will prevent the surgeon from repairing the disk or ligament with suture. Often the disk is atrophic and will not cover the condyle in a normal fashion. Such tissue will not hold suture material and will fragment. The procedure of choice becomes a total meniscectomy removing all of the degenerative disk tissue. If the condyle has osteophytes, these are treated with a condylar shave using rotary drills or rasps. An emphasis is made that the arthroplasty procedure only removes obvious spurs and irregularities of bone and does not alter unaffected

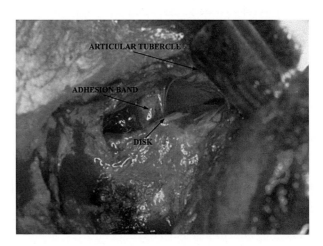

Figure 60-6. A surgical photograph of a right TMJ demonstrating a dense superior joint space adhesion band. The tubercle location and disk posterior band are labeled.

bone. In removing the posterior portion of the disk, the surgeon should exercise care in the amount of posterior ligament excised. Because of its rich vascularity, a considerable amount of bleeding can be stimulated. Some surgeons will use a carbon dioxide laser to perform the disk excision to minimize bleeding during the postoperative period.

As in the previous type of disk repair, early postoperative physical therapy is to be encouraged. Immobilization of the mandible in this group of patients appears to produce serious joint adhesions that lead to ankylosis. On the other hand, when the condyle is mobilized, early postoperative jaw function studies demonstrate that these patients can achieve near-normal ranges of motion and chewing.[32]

TMJ IMPLANTS

Perhaps no single event has set back TMJ surgery more than the overzealous use of implants within the joint. This was particularly true for the use of the Teflon-Proplast TMJ implant. Its use in young patients, often demonstrating nothing other than a disk displacement, produced consequences that will remain with these patients for years to come.[17] Smith et al[51] reported implant erosion into the middle cranial fossa. The histology on these implants demonstrates that there is an exuberant giant cell inflammation that erodes bone.

The U.S. Food and Drug Administration (FDA) and most surgical societies' recommendations indicate that patients with these implants should be imaged and followed every 6 months. The possibility of implant removal is high. Also, no attempt should be made to fill the joint space with another implant or foreign substance. Erosions into the middle cranial fossa can be treated with an inset of temporalis fascia over the glenoid fossa.[35]

Total joint replacement is still being reported in the literature; however, it should be emphasized that these implants and procedures are only indicated in severe ankylosis and degenerative disease. The surgeon should carefully evaluate his or her level of experience before attempting these operations.

ANKYLOSIS RELEASE

The incidence of ankylosis appears to be decreasing, and the techniques for its correction has improved because of the principles learned from orthognathic surgery.[3,38] It may be classified as true (intraarticular) or false (extraarticular) and also as bony or fibrous, depending on the type of fusion between the articulating elements.[28,29]

There are many causes of true ankylosis of the TMJ, but the more common include trauma, infection, and juvenile rheumatoid arthritis.[5,14,25] These conditions lead to destruction of the disk and bony elements such that a fibrous union narrows the joint space and then produces a bony fusion. The most common cause of a false ankylosis is a fracture of the zygomatic

arch with impingement on the coronoid process. This leads to a fibrous union outside the joint and immobilizes it.

These patients can display problems in nutrition and often will have serious oral hygiene problems, leading to dental decay and abscess. If the ankylosis occurred early in life, mandibular growth and facial development will be retarded and produce deformities that will subsequently require considerable orthognathic surgery to correct.

Investigation of the ankylosed TMJ is essential for treatment planning. Tomography and CT scanning provide the best views and will separate the types of ankylosis and indicate the degree of involvement. The treatment options include condylectomy and gap and interpositional arthroplasty. Condylectomy is usually performed only for cases of fibrous or early ankylosis because of the difficulty of delineating the glenoid fossa in more severe cases. Gap arthroplasty has been criticized because of a high recurrence and the tendency to produce an open bite deformity.[1,11,21,22,54,55]

In severe cases, autogenous replacement of the resected condyle with costochondral graft harvested from the contralateral fifth or sixth rib and split longitudinally except at the costochondral junction should be performed.[39,60] Preparation of the recipient site usually includes ipsilateral joint and coronoid process resection, as well as stripping of the surrounding temporalis, masseter, and medial pterygoid muscle and scar tissue. Temporalis fascia is used as an interpositional material between the graft and glenoid fossa. The graft is rigidly fixed to the lateral ramus remnant, and the patient is placed in intermaxillary fixation for 10 days. After this time, the patient must undergo intensive physical therapy to maintain motion of the newly created joint space.

Considering the importance of physical therapy and muscle strengthening, it is wise to determine muscle atrophy preoperatively. Electromyography will often detect severe hypoactivity in the temporalis and even masseter muscles. In contrast, the anterior digastric muscles may be hyperactive. Electromyography of the most important muscle, the lateral pterygoid, is nearly impossible to obtain. However, if the positioning muscles show signs of disuse atrophy, a surgical joint release may produce a relapse resulting from subsequent ankylosis.

TMJ DISLOCATIONS

Acute dislocations of the TMJ occur as the condyle extends anteriorly beyond the eminence as a result of hypermobility secondary to trauma or exaggerated mouth opening, as in yawning.[15] Spontaneous reduction usually follows, but in some cases the dislocation persists and requires manual reduction. This is accomplished by placing the surgeon's thumbs along the lower buccal sulci and the fingers along the inferior border of the mandible and exerting firm downward force to overcome the spasmed muscles, accompanied by posterior motion to replace the condyle into the fossa. Occasionally the spasm is so great as to prevent reduction, and some form of muscle relaxant or anesthesia is required.

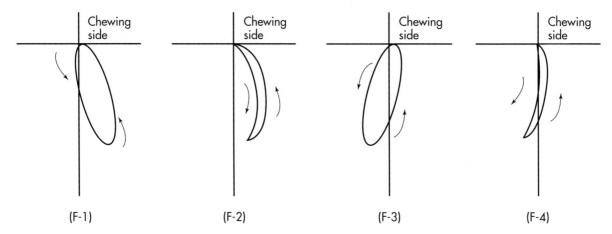

Figure 60-7. The frontal chewing patterns characterizing advancing disk pathology in the nonworking TMJ. The *F-1* pattern represents normal left side chewing. The *F-2* to *F-4* patterns demonstrate increasing deviation of the turning point towards the opposite right involved TMJ.

INFECTIOUS ARTHRITIS

The TMJ may become infected by local spread or hematogenous seeding from a distant septic focus, which is rare. Because of the availability of antibiotics, infectious arthritis is relatively infrequent, but once it is established, it may lead to osteomyelitis and ankylosis of the TMJ. Therefore, once recognized, it requires aggressive therapy with open drainage, intravenous antibiotics, and sequestrectomy if indicated.

AVASCULAR NECROSIS

Although rare, avascular necrosis of the condyle is possible after trauma or devascularization at the time of TMJ surgery. The patient will present with the typical symptoms of TMJ syndrome, including pain and limited jaw motion. Diagnostic imaging is particularly important, including MRI to detect devascularization of a portion of the condyle. The management of avascular necrosis involves the débridement of the necrotic condyle and possible condylar replacement.[42]

OUTCOMES

With the advent of managed care and increased patient information, it now behooves the surgeon to fully demonstrate the results of surgical intervention. Years ago, the main purpose of TMJ surgery was pain relief. Often this was obtained but at a significant loss of jaw function. As imaging techniques improved and methods became available to measure function, a more complete preoperative and postoperative assessment can be demonstrated.

Formerly, we believed that measuring the maximal ability of a patient to open the mouth was sufficient to evaluate treatment success. As methods using electromyography and jaw tracking improved, it became evident that there were subtle movements that took place during chewing. To see these movements, it is necessary to utilize computer technology that can display these movements in real time.

The TMJ is capable of protrusion and retrusion, as well as lateral excursion, with unilateral or bilateral movement in the upper joint spaces only. These movements are critical in mastication because they allow the cusps of the teeth to penetrate the food bolus in a shearing type of motion rather than a pure hinge motion. The large degree of side-to-side jaw motion during chewing seen in a herbivore (e.g., cow or horse) is an example of near pure translation. The vertical chewing seen in a carnivore (e.g., cat) is an example of pure hinge motion. Humans display an envelope of jaw motion composed of both hinge and translation. The chewing envelope seen from the frontal view is a tear drop shape. Techniques that measure and display these envelopes of jaw motion are called *jaw tracking*. The frontal envelopes of normal and abnormal jaw motion are depicted in Figure 60-7 (*F-1* to *F-4*).[44]

The pattern labeled *F-1* illustrates a normal TMJ's envelope of motion while chewing food on the left molar teeth. *F-2* to *F-4* demonstrate abnormal envelopes of motion seen with increasing severity of TMJ ID. As the degree of joint pathology increases in the nonchewing side TMJ, translation of the mandible to the chewing side is impeded. In other words, if a displaced disk entraps the nonchewing side condyle, the condyle cannot translate and the mandible cannot move to the chewing side. This is displayed as a distortion of the tear drop envelope in *F-1*, to a distorted envelope in *F-4*. The end result is abnormal positioning of the teeth on the chewing side.

In a patient with ID, the clinician is faced with the problem of measuring the amount of pretreatment pathology and measuring the amount of posttreatment improvement. Func-

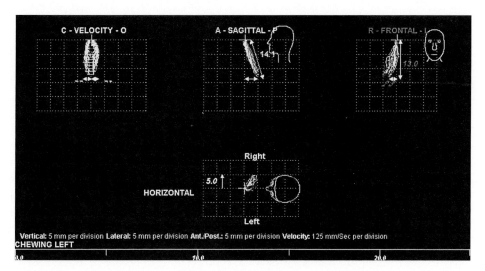

Figure 60-8. A computer screen display of gum chewing on the left dental side. The right display (frontal) displays an F-4 chewing pattern and suggests right TMJ disk displacement. The center tracing (upper) depicts the sagittal view of chewing. The left tracing reflects jaw velocity and shows a decreased speed compared with normal.

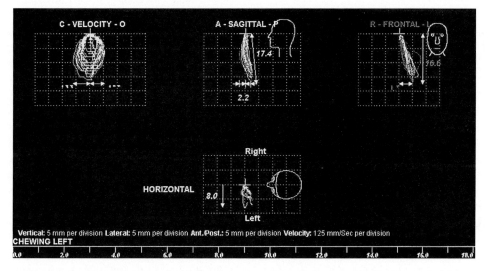

Figure 60-9. A computer screen display of normal left side chewing. The frontal pattern is F-1, and the velocity pattern reflects a smoother, symmetric envelope.

tional studies measuring chewing may provide a scale that permits quantification of pathology and success. In Figure 60-8, obtained from a preoperative patient with right disk displacement and nonreduction, a typical F-4 pattern is seen. After surgical repair of the disk, the postoperative chewing pattern displaying an F-1 chewing pattern is shown in Figure 60-9.

The advantage of this data is that it provides functional assessment of the patient that can be correlated to the clinical improvement in pain symptoms. In addition, it serves as an end point measurement in different therapeutic modalities.

As in all matters of medical management of disease, the future surgeon can be expected to document and measure the degree of pathology and the expected measurable improvement to be expected from treatment. Because of the complexity of

mandibular function, testing modalities such as these discussed should become more standardized in future years.

REFERENCES

1. Abbe R: An operation for the relief of ankylosis of the temporomandibular joint, by excision of the neck of the condyle of the lower jaw, with remarks, *NY J Med* 1880.

2. Annandale T: Displacement of the interarticular cartilage of the lower jaw, and its treatment by operation, *Lancet* 1:411, 1887.

3. Baverman J: Reconstruction of the temporomandibular joint for acquired deformity and congenital malformation, *Br J Oral Maxillofac Surg* 25:149, 1987.

4. Bell KA, Walters PJ: Videofluoroscopy during arthroscopy of the temporomandibular joint, *Radiology* 147:879, 1983.

5. Bellinger DH: Temporomandibular ankylosis and its surgical correction, *J Am Dent Assoc* 27:1563, 1940.

6. Bush FM: Prevalence of mandibular dysfunction: subjective signs and symptoms, *Plast Reconstr Surg* 55:355, 1975.

7. Chonkas NC, Sicher H: Structure of temporomandibular joint, *Oral Surg Oral Med Oral Pathol* 13:1203, 1960.

8. Costen JB: A syndrome of ear and sinus symptoms dependent upon disturbed function of the temporomandibular joint, *Ann Otorhinolaryngol* 43:1, 1934.

9. Dixon AD: Structure and functional significance of the intra-articular disc of the human temporomandibular joint, *J Oral Surg* 15:48, 1962.

10. Dolwick MF, Katzberg RW, Helms CA, et al: Arthrotomographic evaluation of the temporomandibular joint, *J Oral Surg* 37:793, 1979.

11. Esmarch F: Traitment du ressevrement cicatricel des machoires par la formation d'une fausse articulation dans la continuite de l'os maxillaire inferieur, *Arch Gen Med V Ser* 44, 1860.

12. Farrar WB, McCarty WL: The TMJ dilemma, *J Ala Dent Assoc* 63:19, 1979.

13. Foreman P: Temporomandibular joint and myofascial pain dysfunction—some current concepts. I. Diagnosis, *NZ Dent J* 81:47, 1985.

14. Freedus M, Zitoc W, Doyle P: Principles of treatment for temporomandibular ankylosis, *J Oral Surg* 33:757, 1975.

15. Greenberg SA, Jacobs JS, Bessette RW: Temporomandibular joint dysfunction: evaluation and treatment, *Clin Plast Surg* 16:707, 1989.

16. Griffin CJ, Sharpe CJ: The structure of the adult human temporomandibular meniscus, *Aust Dent J* 5:190, 1960.

17. Gundaker WE: FDA safety alert, serious problems with proplast coated TMJ implant, *US Department of Health and Human Services Bulletin,* December 1990.

18. Guralnick W, Kaban LB, Merril RG: Temporomandibular joint afflictions, *N Engl J Med* 229:123, 1978.

19. Harris HL: Anatomy of the temporomandibular articulation and adjacent structures, *J Am Dent* 19:584, 1932.

20. Hendler BH, Gateno J, Mooar P: Holmium:YAG laser arthroscopy of the temporomandibular joint, *J Oral Maxillofac Surg* 50:931, 1992.

21. Hinds CE, Pleasant JE: Reconstruction of the temporomandibular joint, *Am J Surg* 90:931, 1955.

22. Humphrey GM: Excision of the condyle of the lower jaw, *Can Med Assoc J* 160:61, 1956.

23. Ishigaki, S, Bessette RW, Maruyama T: Vibration of the temporomandibular joints with normal radiographic imagings: comparison between asymptomatic volunteers and symptomatic patients, *Journal of Craniomandibular Practice* 11:88-94, 1993.

24. Israel HA: Current concepts in the surgical management of temporomandibular joint disorders, *J Oral Maxillofac Surg* 52:289, 1994.

25. Jacobs JS, Bessette RW: Temporomandibular joint deformities. In Smith JW, Aston SJ (eds): *Grabb and Smith's plastic surgery,* Boston, 1991, Little, Brown.

26. Katzberg RW: Arthrotomography of the temporomandibular joint, *AJR Am J Roentgenol* 134:995, 1980.

27. Katzberg RW, Bessette RW, Tallents RH, et al: Normal and abnormal temporomandibular joint: MR imaging with surface coil, *Radiology* 158:183, 1986.

28. Kazanjiian VH: Ankylosis of the temporomandibular joint, *Am J Orthod Oral Surg* 24:1181, 1938.

29. Kazanjiian VH: Ankylosis of the TMJ, *Surg Gynecol Obstet* 67:333, 1938.

30. Kuwahara T, Bessette RW, Maruyama T: Chewing pattern analysis in TMD patients with and without internal derangement: Part I, *Journal of Craniomandibular Practice* 13:8-14, 1995.

31. Kuwahara T, Bessette RW, Maruyama T: Chewing pattern analysis in TMD patients with and without internal derangement: Part II, *Journal of Craniomandibular Practice* 13:93-98, 1995.

32. Kuwahara T, Bessette RW, Maruyama T: Effect of continuous passive motion on the results of TMJ meniscectomy, Part I: comparison of chewing movement, *Journal of Craniomandibular Practice* 14:190-199, 1996.

33. Laskin DM: Etiology of the pain-dysfunction syndrome, *J Am Dent Assoc* 79:147, 1969.

34. Lieberman JM, Hans MG, Rozencweig G, et al: MR imaging of the juvenile temporomandibular joint: preliminary report, *Radiology* 182:531, 1992.

35. McCain JP, Goldberg HM, De La Rue H: Preoperative and postoperative audiologic measurements in patients undergoing arthroscopy of the TMJ, *J Oral Maxillofac Surg* 47:1026-1027, 1989.

36. McCain JP, Sanders B, Koslin MG, et al: Temporomandibular joint arthroscopy, *J Oral Maxillofac Surg* 50:926, 1992.

37. McCarty WL, Farrar WB: Surgery for internal derangements of the temporomandibular joint, *J Prosthet Dent* 42:191, 1979.

38. Munro I: Simultaneous total correction of temporomandibular joint ankylosis and facial asymmetry, *Plast Reconstr Surg* 77:347, 1986.

39. Posnick JC, Goldstein JA: Surgical management of temporomandibular joint ankylosis in the pediatric population, *Plast Reconstr Surg* 91:791, 1993.

40. Rao VM, Liem MD, Farole A, et al: Elusive "stuck" disk in temporomandibular joint: diagnosis with MR imaging, *Radiology* 189:823, 1993.

41. Sanders B: Discussion of "Efficacy of temporomandibular joint arthroscopy," *J Oral Surg* 51:29, 1993.

42. Sanders B, McKelvey B, Adams D: Aseptic osteomyelitis and necrosis of the mandibular condylar head after intracapsular fracture, *Oral Surg* 43:5, 1977.

43. Schellhas KP: Medical imaging in the evaluation of facial pain, *Semin Neurol* 8:265, 1988.

44. Schellhas KP, Wilkes CH, El Deeb M, et al: Permanent proplast temporomandibular joint implants: MR imaging of destructive complications, *AJR Am J Roentgenol* 151:731, 1988.

45. Schellhas KP, Wilkes CH, Omlie MR: The diagnosis of temporomandibular joint disease: two compartment arthrogram and MR, *Am J Neuroradiol* 9:379, 1988.

46. Schellhas KP, Wilkes CH, Fritts HM, et al: MR of osteochondritis dissecans and avascular necrosis of the mandibular condyle, *Am J Neuroradiol* 103:3, 1989.

47. Schellhas KP, Wilkes CH, Fritts HM, et al: Temporomandibular joint: MR imaging internal derangements and postoperative changes, *Am J Neuroradiol* 8:1093, 1987.

48. Schellhas KP, Wilkes CH, Omlie MR, et al: Temporomandibular joint imaging. *Otolaryngol Head Neck Surg* 113:744, 1987.

49. Schwartz L: Pain associated with the temporomandibular joint, *Am Dent Assoc* 51:394, 1955.

50. Silver CM, Simon SD, Savestino AA: Meniscus injuries of the temporomandibular joint, *J Bone Surg (Am)* 38A:541, 1956.

51. Smith RM, Goldwasser MS, Sabol SR: Erosion of teflon proplast implant into the middle cranial fossa, *J Oral Maxillofac Surg* 51:1268, 1993.

52. Solberg WK, Woo MW, Houston JB: Prevalence of mandibular dysfunction in young adults, *J Am Dent Assoc* 98:25, 1979.

53. Stanson AW, Baker HL: Routine tomography of the temporomandibular joint, *Radiol Clin North Am* 14:105, 1976.

54. Topazian RG: Comparison of gap and interposition arthroplasty in the treatment of temporomandibular ankylosis, *J Oral Surg* 24:405, 1966.

55. Verneuil AS: De la creation d'une fausse articulation par section ou resection particelle de l'os maxillaire inferieur, *Arch Gen Med V Ser* 15:284, 1872.

56. Watt-Smith S, Sadler A, Baddeley H, et al: Comparison of arthrotomagraphic and magnetic resonance images of 50 temporomandibular joints with operative findings, *Br J Oral Maxillofac Surg* 31:139, 1993.

57. Weinberg LA: Role of condylar position TMJ dysfunction syndrome, *J Prosthet Dent* 41:636, 1979.

58. Wilkes C: Arthrography of the temporomandibular joint in patients with the TMJ pain dysfunction syndrome, *Minn Med* 61:465, 1978.

59. Wilkes CH: Internal derangements of the temporomandibular joint. Pathological variations, *Arch Otolaryngol Head Neck Surg* 115:469, 1989.

60. Zins JE, Smith JD, James DR: Surgical correction of temporomandibular joint ankylosis, *Clin Plast Surg* 16:725, 1989.

CHAPTER

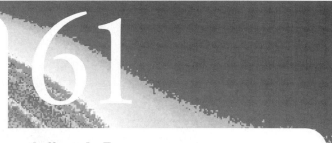

Hemifacial Microsomia

Jeffrey A. Fearon

INDICATIONS

Hemifacial microsomia is a relatively recent term, appearing in the surgical literature only in the past 50 years.[8] Hemifacial microsomia was previously referred to as *first and second branchial arch syndrome,* and the earliest case report of hemifacial microsomia has been ascribed to Kirmisson.[88] The occurrence of epibulbar dermoid, especially in conjunction with vertebral anomalies, has been designated Goldenhar's syndrome (also known as Goldenhar-Gorlin syndrome or facioauriculovertebral spectrum). These anomalies may present either unilaterally or bilaterally, with a variable expression, and with a number of associated anomalies. It is likely that all of these various entities may represent variations in severity of a similar error in morphogenesis, and the term *oculoauriculovertebral spectrum* is often applied. The frequency of occurrence is estimated to be 1:3000 to 1:5000 live births.[36] The term *craniofacial microsomia* may be used to describe individuals with hemifacial microsomia who also have unilateral orbital and cranial vault findings.

Most cases of cases with hemifacial microsomia are believed to be sporadic. Familial involvement with both autosomal dominant and recessive inheritance has been reported.[10,81,86,90] Hemifacial microsomia has occurred in monozygotic twins with concordance, although most cases in twins are discordant.[7,10,44] A mirror image has been reported in one set of monozygotic twins, lending further evidence to the speculation that an environmental factor may induce this anomaly.[83] Observations on the genetic transmission of a hemifacial microsomia-like trait in mice colonies further suggests that the same gene could produce both a unilateral and bilateral phenotype.[37,67]

Although there is evidence to support either a single gene locus mutation with reduced penetrance or environmental agents as the cause for hemifacial microsomia, at the current time a multifactorial threshold model may offer the most likely cause for this condition. Early theories suggested that hemifacial microsomia might be caused by intrauterine facial necrosis resulting from an ischemic crisis occurring in tissue supplied by the primitive stapedial artery (this is one of three successive vessels on which the first and second branchial arches are dependent from the third to fifth weeks of development). Poswillo[79] noted that focal hemorrhage in the region of the stapedial artery did lead to the phenotypic expression of hemifacial microsomia in the animal model. Studies concerning the effects of retinoic acid on animals have significantly implicated neural crest cells as playing a major role in the expression of hemifacial microsomia.[34,35] It has also been suggested that an interference in chondrogenesis may hold primary responsibility for hemifacial microsomia.[17]

DIAGNOSIS

Hemifacial microsomia encompasses a wide spectrum of deformities, which have all been well described.* The keystone to the diagnosis is hypoplasia of the hemimandible and maxillae in conjunction with an ipsilateral auricular deformity (Figure 61-1). Macrostomia, or a lateral facial cleft, is also frequently noted but is not necessary to make the diagnosis. Auricular deformities range from ear tags (which are seen anywhere on the cheek, from the lateral oral commissure to the ear) to microtia or complete anotia. Facial palsy and sensory neural hearing loss can also be associated with this syndrome and have been reported to correlate with the degree of deformity.[6] The hemimandible phenotypically may range from a mild reduction in size to marked hypoplasia with absence of a glenoid fossa and condyle and complete aplasia of the ascending ramus. Hemifacial microsomia has been reported in conjunction with an edentulous mandible; however, a review of 89 patients with hemifacial microsomia suggested that the associated mandibular deformity did not typically have an effect on dental maturation when compared with the unaffected side.[18,50] The severity of the auricular deformity appears to frequently parallel the severity of the mandibular deformity, and there may be a correlation between the development of the middle ear and the severity of the external deformity.[11] Trigeminal neuropathy has also been reported, and an autopsy on a child with hemifacial microsomia revealed not only hypoplasia of the facial nerve but also a smaller right

---

*References 13, 22, 27, 41, 80, 88.

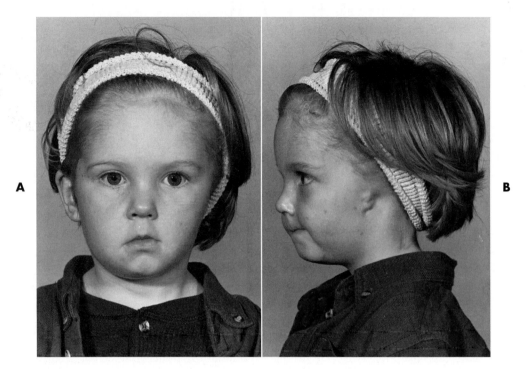

Figure 61-1. A and **B,** Hemifacial microsomia characteristically involves hypoplasia of the hemimandible and hemimaxilla in conjunction with an ipsilateral auricular deformity.

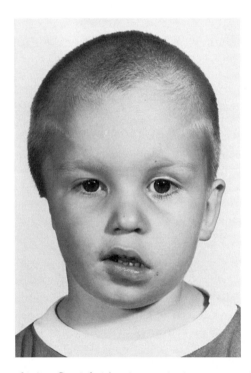

Figure 61-2. Craniofacial microsomia is an extension of hemifacial microsomia, with involvement of the orbit and frontal bones. Various degrees of frontal retrusion and orbital dystopia may be encountered.

facial nucleus in the brainstem.[1,2] Multiple ocular and adnexal findings have been reported in patients with hemifacial microsomia, and the epibulbar dermoid is one of the markers for Goldenhar's syndrome (the findings bearing the eponym of Goldenhar's syndrome consist of epibulbar dermoids, auricular appendixes, and vertebral anomalies).[25,26,29] Unilateral arrhinencephaly and multiple spinal anomalies have also been associated with Goldenhar's syndrome.[3,5] Involvement of the ipsilateral frontal bone and orbit (craniofacial microsomia) usually involves recession and a decrease in vertical height (Figure 61-2). This frontal recession does not appear to be the result of a unilateral coronal synostosis.[73] Right-sided expression of hemifacial microsomia has been reported to occur more commonly than left-sided by a 2:1 ratio, and up to 24% are reported to be bilateral.[6]

The wide spectrum of deformities seen with hemifacial microsomia has apparently inspired nosologists, the result of which is that numerous classification systems have been proposed. The very existence of such a large number of proposed classifications underscores the difficulty in accurately describing such a wide phenotypic spectrum. In 1969, Pruzansky[80] introduced a grading system from I to III that was based on the degree of mandibular hypoplasia. This system was further subdivided by Mulliken and Kaban[60] in an effort to clarify the degree of mandibular deformity in relation to surgical treatment (Box 61-1). This system has been criticized for its focus on the mandible and its failure to grade the associated anomalies of the orbit, ear, and nerve; soft tissue deficiencies; and extracraniofacial anomalies.[16,82] An anatomic/surgical classification has been proposed by Lauritzen, Munro, and Ross.[46] This skeletally based system is linked to surgical correction (Box 61-2) but has not been fully adopted, perhaps because of a lack of consensus on treatment. A TNM-style multisystem classification has been proposed using the acronym SAT to describe skeletal, auricular, and soft tissue involvement, and the OMENS-plus system is an expanded system that includes evaluation of facial nerve weakness and

Box 61-1.
Grading System based on Degree of Mandibular Hypoplasia

Type I: The mandible and glenoid fossa are small with a short ramus; this is a "mini-mandible."

Type II: The mandibular ramus is short and abnormally shaped. This type is subdivided depending on the relative position of the condyle and TMJ. Type IIA: The glenoid fossa is in acceptable functional position in reference to the opposite TMJ. Type IIB: The TMJ is abnormally placed, inferiorly, medially, and anteriorly.

Type III: There is complete absence of the ramus, glenoid fossa, and TMJ.

Box 61-2.
Skeletally Based Grading System

Type I: The facial skeleton is complete. The TMJ is intact and functional. The mandible is asymmetric, creating a lack of fullness on one side of the face. Type I may be subdivided into IA (mild) and IB (severe), depending on the degree of asymmetry.

Type II: The condylar head of the mandible is missing, that is, there is no functional TMJ. The ascending ramus of the mandible is usually vestigial and lies more medially than is normal. The zygomatic arch is present. Although there may not be a true glenoid fossa, there is adequate support for a reconstructed condyle and fossa construction is not necessary.

Type III: The mandibular condyle is missing, and the zygomatic arch is hypoplastic or absent. The glenoid fossa is absent or rudimentary and must be constructed.

Type IV: In addition to Type III defects, the lateral and inferior orbital rims are grossly recessed posteriorly.

Type V: In addition to the Type IV defects, the orbit is dystopic and frequently hypoplastic. The neurocranium is asymmetric with a flat temporal fossa.

Box 61-3.
SAT Classification

SKELETAL

S_1: Small mandible with normal shape

S_2: Condyle, ramus, and sigmoid notch identifiable but grossly distorted; mandible strikingly different in size and shape from normal

S_3: Mandible severely malformed, ranging from poorly identifiable ramal components to complete agenesis of ramus

S_4: An S_3 mandible plus orbital involvement with gross posterior recession of lateral and inferior orbital rims

S_5: The S_4 defects plus orbital dystopia and frequently hypoplasia and asymmetric neurocranium with a flat temporal fossa

AURICULAR

A_0: Normal

A_1: Small, malformed auricle retaining characteristic features

A_2: Rudimentary auricle with hook at cranial end corresponding to the helix

A_3: Malformed lobule with rest of pinna absent

SOFT TISSUE

T_1: Minimal contour defect with no cranial nerve involvement

T_2: Moderate defect

T_3: Major defect with obvious facial scoliosis, possibly severe hypoplasia of cranial nerves, parotid gland, and muscles of mastication; eye involvement; clefts of face or lips

extracraniofacial anomalies[19,30,93] (Boxes 61-3 and 61-4). Although these systems are quite descriptive, many patients seem to fall in between categories, making standardization somewhat difficult. In spite of the aforementioned shortcomings of the modified Pruzansky system, its simplicity has resulted in a widespread acceptance.

The physical examination of the child with hemifacial microsomia should begin with the forehead and the orbit, and these areas are compared for symmetry with the opposite side (if the opposite side is grossly unaffected). The extent of the auricular deformity is noted, and facial nerve function is evaluated. The globe is carefully examined for epibulbar

dermoids, and extraocular motion is assessed. The amount of chin deviation is noted. Occasionally the presence, or absence, of a temporomandibular joint (TMJ) can be palpated. If the child is old enough, he or she is asked to bite on a tongue blade to demonstrate the degree of occlusal tilt. These children usually have a Class I relationship in spite of both the marked unilateral hypoplasia of the maxilla and mandible and the associated compensatory changes on the contralateral side. Early radiologic evaluations are unnecessary, and x-ray analysis can generally be delayed until operative treatment is planned. The average child with microtia has a 50-to 55-decibel hearing loss on the affected side.[56] Therefore the importance of monitoring the opposite ear for infections and, when they do occur, treating all infections aggressively is emphasized. Frequent hearing evaluations are recommended. Up to one third of children may have velopharyngeal incompetence; therefore palatal motion is observed and speech evaluations are recommended.[52]

The surgical goals for patients with hemifacial microsomia include normalizing the occlusal tilt and, if absent, reconstructing the TMJ. Symmetry of the occlusal plane is necessary to prevent problems with the opposite TMJ, which may occur with unbalanced loading. Auricular reconstruction is also planned to restore appearance and to provide support for wearing glasses. Perhaps the most important focus of treatment is to provide facial symmetry. The normalization of appearance can bring enormous psychosocial benefits to affected individuals.

OPERATIONS

EVOLUTION OF SURGICAL SOLUTIONS

The surgical treatment for hemifacial microsomia has undergone a significant evolution over the past 40 years and is still in a state of flux. The plastic surgical approach to treating children with hemifacial microsomia has its early roots in the work of Kazanjian[43]; Gilles[24]; and Pickerill[76]; and later from Converse and Shapiro,[14,15] who described the use of free bone grafts and rib grafts placed via an intraoral incision route, as well as osteotomies of the mandible and maxilla. Longacre[51] subsequently described a more complete surgical management of hemifacial microsomia, including treatment of oral clefts, otoplasties, and bone grafts. The need to regraft the growing mandible to maintain occlusion was emphasized.

The basis for the single-stage skeletal correction of hemifacial microsomia has had its roots in the work of Obwegeser,[68,69] who described the simultaneous Le Fort I osteotomy, sagittal split osteotomy of the mandible, and reconstruction of the hypoplastic zygoma and TMJ with rib grafts. Munro[61-64] popularized the single-stage skeletal treatment of children with hemifacial microsomia, advocated treating children before growth was completed (enabling them to begin their school years with improved facial symmetry), and utilized rigid fixation to begin early range of motion (to reduce the ankylosis of reconstructed joints). Based on bone distraction techniques developed by Ilizarov,[31] Snyder et al[87] experimented with mandibular lengthening by distraction. These techniques were adapted to hemifacial microsomia by McCarthy et al[53,55] and Molina and Ortiz-Monasterio.[57] These techniques replaced the single-stage skeletal correction with a gradual distraction lengthening of the hemimandible.

AVAILABLE TECHNIQUES

Function Therapy

The use of nonsurgical, functional therapy in hemifacial microsomia has been reported.[72,85] This treatment utilizes an orthodontic activator in an attempt to induce greater-than-expected skeletal growth. Unfortunately, there is no data at the current time to support their use. A functional appliance would seem to have the greatest benefit in those patients who are most mildly affected and would not be candidates for surgical treatment.

Osteodistraction

With the introduction and continuing refinements of osteodistraction, surgeons now have a choice in the skeletal correction for hemifacial microsomia. At the time of writing, osteodistraction is currently the most commonly used technique for the treatment of hemifacial microsomia. Multiple distraction systems are available with many more in the development stages, including internal devices that will eliminate external scarring. The critical issue in surgical planning is to determine the appropriate vector of distraction. This planning is made easier by the use of devices that allow for differential distraction in various planes.

Numerous factors enter into the timing for initial surgical intervention. In favor of earlier treatment is the theory that distraction of the mandible at a young age may allow for

greater compensation of the maxilla with subsequent growth of the child. However, longitudinal studies testing this hypothesis have yet to be published. It is clear that earlier surgical intervention aimed at normalizing appearance will be of great psychosocial benefit to a child before he or she enters the school years. Arguing for later intervention is the fact that pin placement is difficult in small children secondary to the small amount of supporting bone. Pin placement is more challenging before mixed dentition because the permanent tooth buds occupy the majority of the body of the mandible.

Preoperatively, cephalometric radiographs and a Panorex are taken. These are used in planning the vector of distraction and are used to identify unerupted tooth buds. At surgery, via an intraoral incision, a corticotomy is performed in the region of the gonial angle. The inner cortex may be left intact (Figure 61-3). Pins are placed percutaneously in a location appropriate for the desired vector for elongation (Figure 61-4). Elongation is begun between the fifth and seventh postoperative days and is usually distracted at a rate of 1 mm per day. Distraction can be performed by advancing 1 mm at a single turn or by advancing 0.5 mm twice a day. If growth has not been completed, advancement is continued until the chin position is overcorrected. Once distraction is complete, the expansion device is then left on for an additional 6 to 8 weeks to allow for healing. Orthodontics may be used in conjunction with distraction and are necessary after distraction to help bring the maxillary dentition back into occlusion with the distracted mandible.

Use of the distraction lengthening device for treatment of hemifacial microsomia has many advantages. A smaller surgical procedure is required to place and remove the device than would be necessary with a full skeletal correction. In addition, distraction lengthening is technically easier and can be performed by surgeons without extensive orthognathic train-

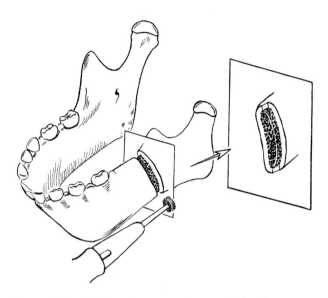

Figure 61-3. Before placement of a mandibular distractor, a corticotomy is made between the posterior molar and the mandibular angle.

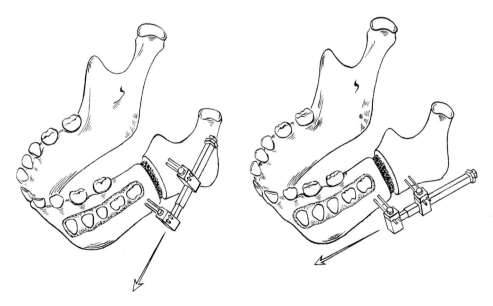

Figure 61-4. Placement of the pins for distraction determines the vector for elongation. Placement of the anterior pin may be limited by dental roots; therefore variability in placement of the posterior pin tract often determines the vector for elongation.

ing (although experienced orthodontic support is needed). Perhaps the greatest advantage to this technique is the associated elongation of the soft tissue structures, in particular the inferior alveolar nerve.

There are also multiple disadvantages with this technique. All external systems leave permanent facial scars. Hopefully, this will be eliminated in the future with subcutaneous distraction devices. Placement of external devices is also associated with mechanical problems, the most common of which is dislodgement of the pin-bone interface. As experience is accumulated using these distraction lengthening devices, complications can be greatly reduced. Surgeons familiar with these devices report that they are well tolerated by children during the 3-month treatment period. The greatest drawbacks of the distraction lengthening correction for hemifacial microsomia are that an absent TMJ is not restored and an absent zygoma is not addressed. With hypoplasia of both the hemimandible and the maxilla occurring in three planes, distraction devices are unable to bring about full three-dimensional correction. As the severity of the deformity progresses, there is a corresponding medial displacement of the ascending ramus (Figure 61-5) that is not corrected with distraction techniques. Finally, children with hemifacial microsomia usually have a Class I occlusion that is complicated by a tilt in the occlusal plane. The use of a mandibular distraction device elongates these children into a malocclusion with both an open bite and lateral crossbites. At the current time, advocates of this technique rely on orthodontics to compensate for this surgically created malocclusion; and some are utilizing orthodontia in conjunction with a hemi-Le Fort I osteotomy.[71] It would seem that mandibular distraction may be best reserved for mild cases in which the TMJ is anatomically present and there is good projection of the malar/zygomatic region. For these cases the surgeon together with the patient must decide whether the use of a distraction device followed by orthodontics is preferable to a single-stage, two-jaw procedure. For those children who are more severely affected (demonstrating malar and zygomatic hypoplasia, absent TMJs, and marked medial displacement of the vestige of the ramus), a single-stage skeletal procedure (discussed below) should be considered. The use of a distraction technique, which does not adequately correct the skeletal asymmetry, may require greater soft tissue augmentation, such as a free tissue transfer.

Skeletal Surgery

My preferred method for treating hemifacial microsomia involves a single-stage skeletal procedure. The particular procedure used will vary with the degree of deformity. Panorex and cephalometric radiographs are first obtained. CT scans with three-dimensional reconstructions are helpful in visualizing surgical planning. An occlusal splint is necessary, and dental models are made if adjustments in occlusion are planned. Those patients who have mild involvement, with an intact TMJ, may be treated with a standard two-jaw procedure. This involves a centering Le Fort I and a bilateral sagittal mandibular osteotomy. In moderate to severe cases, TMJ reconstruction along with malar and zygomatic augmentation/reconstruction is necessary.

The surgical timing depends on numerous factors. Initially, Obwegeser[69] recommended that skeletal correction be delayed until growth was completed. Following Munro's report[64] of a series in which children as young as 6 years of age were treated, Ortiz-Monasterio[70] and Kaban[38] advocated treating children as early as 3½ years of age. I prefer to delay surgery until about the age of 7 and until the child reaches approximately 20 kg. Initiating auricular reconstruction at age 6 to 7 before skeletal surgery may offer a child the often-needed psychologic "boost" as he or she enters grade school. I believe that subsequent growth of the reconstructed hemimandible with rib grafts may be less erratic when performed at an older age. Surgical planning begins with cephalometric analysis. The anterior-posterior (AP) cephalogram is used to plan the leveling of the occlusal plane (Figure 61-6). A vertical midline is established from the upper facial skeleton from a perpendicular drawn through the orbital roofs. The degree of tilt in the occlusal plane is determined by establishing a line parallel with the nasal floor and comparing this line with the horizontal line along the superior orbital rims. The vertical difference between these two horizontal lines is measured at the molars and is used to determine the amount of lengthening necessary on the affected side. Usually, in addition to lengthening the affected side, some reduction is necessary on the opposite side of the maxilla to obtain the ideal upper incisal-lip relationship. An overcorrection of 2 to 3 mm is planned in the leveling of the occlusal plane. The amount of forward rotation of the maxilla on the

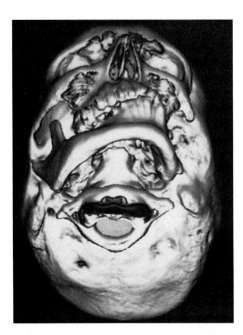

Figure 61-5. This three-dimensional reconstruction of a child with hemifacial microsomia demonstrates the marked medial dislocation of the ascending ramus and condyle. Distraction lengthening does not move this complex laterally but instead distracts the mandible from an abnormal location. Also note the incomplete formation of the zygomatic arch.

affected side is estimated on physical examination based on the measurement of the distance between the dental and facial midlines. An occlusal splint is then prepared.

Surgical exposure is achieved through a preauricular incision and both upper and lower buccal incisions. Two pen marks are placed on each upper eyelid corresponding to the central incisors and first molars, respectively. The distances between the teeth and their pen marks are measured, establishing the preoperative midfacial heights (Figure 61-7). The amount of bone to be excised from the unaffected side of the maxilla is marked. A high Le Fort I osteotomy is performed, taking care to avoid injury to unerupted tooth buds, and the maxilla is down-fractured. After down-fracturing, the maxilla is rotated forward on the affected side, bringing the dental midline into the facial midline. Lengthening of the maxilla is overcorrected by 2 to 3 mm and is confirmed by remeasuring the midfacial heights. The maxilla is then plated into position, and measurements are again taken to confirm the new maxillary position. This three-dimensional positioning of the maxilla is the most critical part of this procedure. Care must be taken not to shift the maxillary molars on the unaffected side too far laterally because this will shift the unaffected mandibular angle laterally, resulting in a undesirable appearance.

A sagittal split osteotomy is then performed on the unaffected side and, using the occlusal splint, the patient is placed into temporary interdental fixation. A rib graft with a cartilage cap is harvested from the contralateral chest, taking

advantage of the appropriate curvature. The distal 1 cm of the cartilaginous cap is cut free for creation of the glenoid fossa. A second rib graft is secured to the anterior maxillary wall medially and to the temporal bone posteriorly to create a zygomatic arch of appropriate projection. The inferior surface of the arch is burred out to accept the cut cartilaginous cap, which is then secured with a 28-gauge wire or heavy suture (Figure 61-8). The rib-cartilage graft is then inserted into a

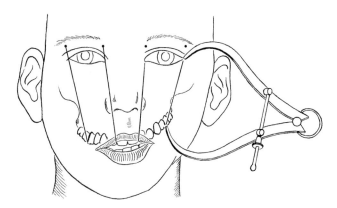

Figure 61-7. Preoperative markings are made on the upper eyelids with a pen. The distances between the lateral mark and the molar and the medial mark and the incisor are established on both the affected and unaffected sides. After the Le Fort I osteotomy, these distances are rechecked to ensure that the planned amount of vertical movement of the maxilla has been achieved.

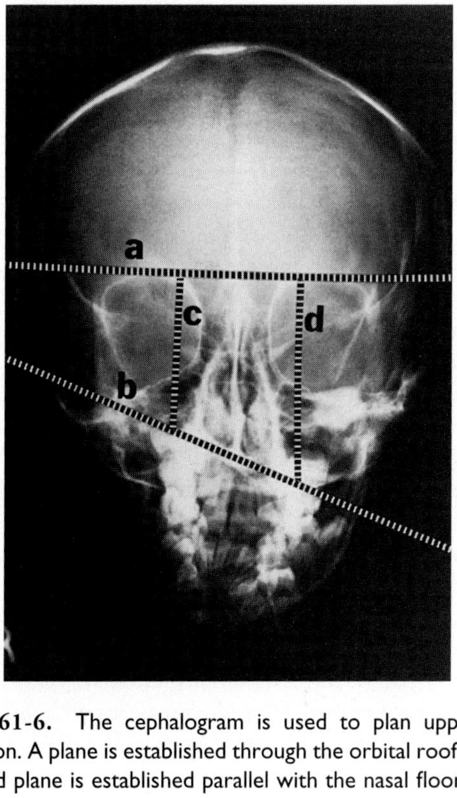

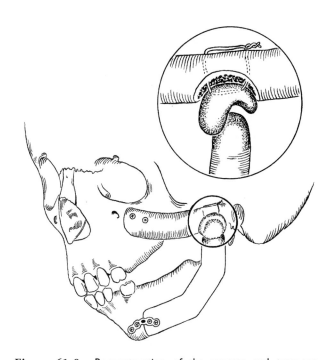

Figure 61-8. Reconstruction of the zygoma and temporomandibular joint is accomplished using rib grafts. The zygomatic arch is first reconstructed, and, using a burr, the glenoid fossa is created. This is lined with a cartilage cap that is cut with an outer lip to prevent lateral displacement of the reconstructed condyle.

Figure 61-6. The cephalogram is used to plan upper facial correction. A plane is established through the orbital roofs *(line A)*. A second plane is established parallel with the nasal floor *(line B)*. Vertical distances are established at the molars *(lines C and D)*, and the vertical differences are measured to determine the amount of lengthening on the affected side of the maxilla.

tunnel created from the body of the mandible to the preauricular incision. The cartilaginous end of the rib graft is seated firmly into the new glenoid fossa, and the distal rib is secured to the inferior border of the mandible with lag screws or a metal plate, taking care to avoid injury to unerupted tooth buds. Interdental fixation is then removed, and the occlusion is rechecked. All wounds are irrigated with antibiotic solution and closed in a layered fashion. I have recently begun to use a turnover posterior temporalis muscle flap to cover the TMJ reconstruction and am using a single drain placed through a counterincision in the temporal scalp, which runs along the mandibular rib interface. This drain is left in place for 5 days and irrigated with antibiotic solution to help prevent infection.

There are multiple advantages of the single-stage surgical treatment of the facial skeleton in hemifacial microsomia. Most importantly, this procedure is capable of restoring the congenitally absent TMJ, which when reconstructed is then able to equally share the masticatory load with the opposite side. This technique is also advantageous in that occlusion is either maintained or improved, it is performed in a single stage, and it results in a three-dimensional correction of the facial skeleton. When accurate three-dimensional skeletal correction is achieved, there is a correspondingly decreased requirement for soft tissue augmentation. The single-stage procedure is not without its disadvantages. The operation is a much larger procedure than placement of an external fixation device and usually requires a 4-to 5-day hospitalization. There is a significant infection rate, which has been reported at 6% and may be as high as 15%.[70] In an attempt to reduce this significant rate of infection, I have recently instituted antibiotic irrigation via a drainage catheter for all cases of TMJ reconstruction and bringing in a vascularized muscle flap. Although early results with this technical modification are very encouraging, conclusions cannot yet be drawn.

Autogenous reconstruction of TMJs with rib grafts has been shown to result in subsequent normal growth, but rib grafts may either undergrow or overgrow and in some circumstances may require a second orthognathic procedure to restore symmetry.

SOFT TISSUE CORRECTION

Pichler has been credited with the adage, "First the bone, then the soft tissue."[69] Augmentation of the deficient soft tissues in hemifacial microsomia was primarily limited to dermal fat grafts until 1977 when Edgerton and Marsh[21,94] suggested the use of a free tissue transfer. Since that time, many authors have reported on the successful use of microvascular free tissue transfers for the treatment of children with hemifacial microsomia.* Mordick[58] compared patients treated with both dermal fat grafts and vascularized tissue transfers and found that both were able to provide long-lasting augmentation. He concluded that dermal fat grafts were satisfactory for mild to

moderate defects and that vascularized transfers should be saved for more severe defects.

Once stable skeletal correction has been obtained, the patient's soft tissue requirements are assessed and the method of augmentation is selected. Results of augmentation are dependent on matching soft tissue contours to the opposite side. Surgical access is achieved through a preauricular face-lift incision, and careful dissection is performed to avoid injury to the facial nerve, which is often superficially displaced. In general, patients prefer undercorrection to overcorrection. Malar augmentation with alloplasts is well established in adults, and augmentation with coral blocks has been reported for the treatment of congenital hypoplasia.[33,74] I prefer to not place alloplasts in the growing facial skeleton, having observed cases in which alloplasts have eroded into the maxillary sinus in children.

AURICULAR RECONSTRUCTION

Auricular reconstruction is usually performed between the ages of 6 and 7. I prefer to have auricular reconstruction precede jaw surgery, except for cases exhibiting marked skeletal hypoplasia. For these patients it is sometimes helpful to reconstruct the facial skeleton before determining the best location for auricular reconstruction. I prefer to utilize techniques for auricular reconstruction based on Brent's elegant refinements of methods first proposed by Tanzer.[9,89]

FACIAL CLEFTS

Treatment of congenital macrostomia associated with hemifacial microsomia is usually performed early in life. The surgical goals of reconstruction include reconstituting the muscular oral sphincter (which may aid the infant with feeding) and reconstructing a natural-looking oral commissure. The techniques for closure fall into two basic categories, straight line repairs and modifications of a Z-plasty repair.[12,54] Chen and Noordholff[12] reviewed their series of macrostomia repairs and concluded the use of a vermilion flap with either an upward or downward Z-plasty produced the best aesthetic results.

CRANIOFACIAL MICROSOMIA

For those children who have both orbital dystopia and forehead involvement as a component of hemifacial microsomia, treatment is usually begun between the ages of 4 and 5. Earlier treatment is considered for severe cases of orbital dystopia to allow for central integration of the visual axis change, hopefully preventing diplopia. Surgical correction is achieved with standard craniofacial techniques, including orbital floor grafts for mild cases of dystopia and four-wall orbital osteotomies for severe cases. The forehead is advanced to achieve symmetry with the opposite side (Figure 61-9). These repairs are carried out before the orthognathic correc-

---

*References 20, 23, 40, 45, 84, 91.

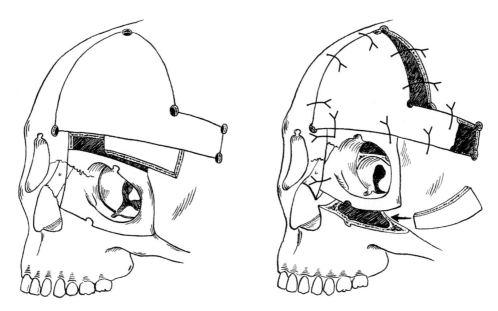

Figure 61-9. Treatment for craniofacial microsomia involves a standard unilateral frontal advancement, which may be performed in conjunction with correction of any orbital dystopia, using standard box cuts.

tion and are helpful in subsequently establishing normal facial vertical and horizontal planes.

FACIAL NERVE PARALYSIS

Most surgeons in the United States have not been treating the congenital facial paralysis associated with hemifacial microsomia. This trend toward conservatism is based on the observation that the facial paralysis associated with hemifacial microsomia is often incomplete with some residual function remaining. Iñigo et al[32] have reported their treatment of eight cases of hemifacial microsomia with cross-facial nerve grafts in children under 1 year of age. They found that the treatment of children at such a young age required a greater length of sural nerve than was available from just one leg and therefore needed to harvest sural nerve from both legs. The decision to proceed with such an operation obviously rests with the degree of paralysis and potential for functional gain posttreatment.

OUTCOMES

Hemifacial microsomia has long been thought to be a progressive skeletal and soft tissue deformity.[66] However, one recent study using long-term cephalometric analysis has suggested that the skeletal asymmetry in hemifacial microsomia may not be progressive in nature and that growth in the affected side parallels the unaffected side.[77] Further studies are needed to clearly establish whether or not the deformity progresses. If the deformity does not progress with growth,

surgical procedures should not be planned early in life for the sole purpose of unlocking growth inhibition. Other factors, such as dental maturity and the ability to achieve lasting symmetry, must be weighed in any decision concerning the timing for surgery. The most important factor to consider is the psychosocial development of the child. If early intervention will result in an affected child feeling significantly better about himself or herself, surgery should be undertaken sooner in lieu of waiting for complete skeletal maturity.

Vargervik et al[92] found that functional appliance treatment could not be shown to produce any statistically significant length increases in the affected side during treatment when compared with the nonaffected side. They also found that performing early skeletal surgery (without costochondral graft reconstruction) demonstrated a measurable increase in the length of the reconstructed ramus; however, this was on average less than the unaffected side. Kaban et al[39] demonstrated that a surgically corrected open bite during mixed dentition will level the occlusal plane without surgically treating the maxilla; however, the degree of open bite that is amenable to spontaneous closure is not discussed.

Experience with skeletal distraction of human mandibles is still relatively limited, and significant outcome studies for this mode of treatment may not be expected for another 10 years. Many questions remain to be answered for distraction techniques. If distraction does not unlock a growth potential and the affected hemimandible does not grow commensurate with the opposite side, those children treated before skeletal maturity may require a repeat distraction to maintain the mentum in the midline. The successful three-dimensional correction of the maxillary deficiency with distraction has yet to be reported. Even if distraction-created open bites can be closed with orthodontically guided maxillary dental eruption, the sagittal and transverse planes of maxillary deficiencies remain unaddressed by all currently available techniques, and a separate skeletal procedure will be necessary to correct these asymmetries.

Numerous authors report growth of a reconstructed costochondral TMJ in children with hemifacial microsomia.[59,65,75] Costochondral grafts appear to have unpredictable growth and may not grow sufficiently, may grow commensurate with the unaffected side, or may overgrow. Overgrowth of the costochondral joint may occur to varying degrees and has a reported incidence ranging from 4% to 50%.[28,61,65] These studies follow patients for an average of 4 to 6 years and do not specify how many of these patients required corrective treatment. The infection rate has been reported to be 6% and an ankylosis rate of 8%; however, these figures may run even higher.[60] There are no studies at the current time that compare patient satisfaction with various treatment options.

The goals of treatment must be the establishment of facial symmetry with normalization of occlusion and function. These goals must be met with the least amount of patient discomfort, with the shortest hospitalization, and in a cost-efficient fashion. Many studies underscore the psychosocial benefits of normalizing appearance.[4,41,47-49,78] It is these benefits that clearly offer those affected children and adults the greatest functional gains from the treatment of hemifacial microsomia.

REFERENCES

1. Aleksic S, Budzilovich G, Reuben R, et al: Congenital facial neuropathy in oculoauriculovertebral dysplasia—hemifacial microsomia (Goldenhar-Gorlin syndrome), *Bull Los Angeles Neurol Soc* 41:68, 1976.

2. Aleksic S, Budzilovich G, Reuben R, et al: Congenital trigeminal neuropathy in oculoauriculovertebral dysplasia—hemifacial microsomia (Goldenhar-Gorlin syndrome), *J Neurol Neurosurg Psychiatry* 38:1033, 1975.

3. Aleksic S, Budzilovich G, Reuben R, et al: Unilateral arhinencephaly in Goldenhar-Gorlin syndrome, *Dev Med Child Neurol* 17:498, 1975.

4. Arndt EM, Travis F, LeFebvre A, et al: Psychosocial adjustment of 20 patients with Treacher Collins syndrome before and after reconstructive surgery, *Br J Plast Surg* 40:605, 1987.

5. Avon SW, Shively JL: Orthopaedic manifestations of Goldenhar syndrome, *J Pediatr Orthop* 8:683, 1988.

6. Bassila MK, Goldberg R: The association of facial palsy and/or sensorineural hearing loss in patients with hemifacial microsomia, *Cleft Palate J* 26:287, 1989.

7. Boles DJ, Bodurtha J, Nance WE: Goldenhar complex in discordant monozygotic twins: a case report and review of the literature, *Am J Med Genet* 28:103, 1987.

8. Braithwaite F, Watson J: A report on three unusual cleft lips, *Br J Plast Surg* II:38, 1949.

9. Brent B: Auricular repair with autogenous rib cartilage grafts: two decades of experiences with 600 cases, *Plast Reconstr Surg* 90:355, 1992.

10. Burck U: Genetic aspects of hemifacial microsomia, *Hum Genet* 64:291, 1983.

11. Caldarelli DD, Hutchinson JG Jr, Pruzansky S, et al: A comparison of microtia and temporal bone anomalies in hemifacial microsomia and mandibulofacial dysostosis, *Cleft Palate J* 17:103, 1980.

12. Chen KT, Noordholff SM: Congenital macrostomia—transverse facial cleft, *Chang Keng I Hsueh* 17:239, 1994.

13. Cohen MM Jr, Rollnick BR, Kaye CI: Oculoauriculovertebral spectrum: an updated critique, *Cleft Palate J* 26:276, 1989.

14. Converse JM: Restoration of facial contour by bone grafts introduced through oral cavity, *Plast Reconstr Surg* 6:295, 1950.

15. Converse JM, Shapiro HH: Treatment of developmental malformations of the jaws, *Plast Reconstr Surg* 10:473, 1952.

16. Cousley RR: A comparison of two classification systems for hemifacial microsomia, *Br J Oral Maxillofac Surg* 31:78, 1993.

17. Cousley RR, Wilson DJ: Hemifacial microsomia: developmental consequence of perturbation of the auriculofacial cartilage model? *Am J Med Genet* 42:461, 1992.

18. Cranin AN, Gallo L: Hemifacial microsomia with an edentulous mandible: forme fruste or a new syndrome? *Oral Surg Oral Med Oral Pathol* 70:29, 1990.

19. David DJ, Mahatumarat D, Cooter RD: Hemifacial microsomia: a multisystem classification, *Plast Reconstr Surg* 80:525, 1987.

20. David DJ, Tan E: A de-epithelialized free groin flap for facial contour restoration, *J Maxillofac Surg* 6:249, 1978.

21. Edgerton MT, Marsh JL: Surgical treatment of hemifacial microsomia (first and second branchial arch syndrome), *Plast Reconstr Surg* 59:653, 1977.

22. Figueroa AA, Friede H: Craniovertebral malformations in hemifacial microsomia, *J Craniofac Genet Dev Biol Suppl* 1:167, 1985.

23. Fujino T, Tanino R, Sugimoto C: Microvascular transfer of free deltopectoral dermal-fat flap, *Plast Reconstr Surg* 55:428, 1975.

24. Gillies HD: Bone grafting to the mandible. In *Plastic surgery of the face*, London, 1920, Oxford University Press.

25. Goldenhar M: Associations malformatives de l'oeil et de l'oreille, en particulier le syndrome dermoide epibulbaire—appendices auriculaires—fistula auris congenita et ses relations avec la dysostose mandibulo-faciale, *J Genet Hum* 1:243, 1952.

26. Gorlin RJ, Jue KL, Jacobsen U, et al: Oculoauriculovertebral dysplasia, *J Pediatr* 63:991, 1963.

27. Grabb WB: The first and second branchial arch syndrome, *Plast Reconstr Surg* 36:485, 1965.

28. Guyuron B, Lasa CI Jr: Unpredictable growth pattern of costochondral graft, *Plast Reconstr Surg* 90:880, discussion 887-889, 1992.

29. Hertle RW, Quinn GE, Katowitz JA: Ocular and adnexal findings in patients with facial microsomias, *Ophthalmology* 99:114, 1992.

30. Horgan JE, Padwa BL, LaBrie RA, et al: OMENS-plus: analysis of craniofacial and extracraniofacial anomalies in hemifacial microsomia, *Cleft Palate Craniofac J* 32:405, 1995.

31. Ilizarov GA, Devyatov AA, Kamerin VK: Plastic reconstruction of longitudinal bone defects by means of compression and subsequent distraction, *Acta Chir Plast* 22:32, 1980.

32. Iñigo F, Ysunza A, Ortiz-Monasterio F, et al: Early postnatal treatment of congenital facial palsy in patients with hemifacial microsomia, *Int J Pediatr Otorhinolaryngol* 26:57, 1993.

33. Ivy EJ, Lorenc ZP, Aston SJ: Malar augmentation with silicone implants, *Plast Reconstr Surg* 96:63, 1995.

34. Johnston MC, Bronsky PT: Prenatal craniofacial development: new insights on normal and abnormal mechanisms, *Crit Rev Oral Biol Med* 6:25, 1995.

35. Johnston MC, Bronsky PT: Animal models for human craniofacial malformations, *J Craniofac Genet Dev Biol* 11:277, 1991.

36. Jones KL: *Smith's recognizable patterns of human malformation,* ed 5, Philadelphia, 1997, WB Saunders.

37. Juriloff DM, Harris MJ, Froster-Iskenius U: Hemifacial deficiency induced by a shift in dominance of the mouse mutation far: a possible genetic model for hemifacial microsomia, *J Craniofac Genet Dev Biol* 7:27, 1987.

38. Kaban LB, Moses MH, Mulliken JB: Surgical correction of hemifacial microsomia in the growing child, *Plast Reconstr Surg* 82:9, 1988.

39. Kaban LB, Moses MH, Mulliken JB: Correction of hemifacial microsomia in the growing child: a follow-up study, *Cleft Palate J Suppl* 1:50, 1986.

40. Kamiji T, Ohmori K, Takada H: Clinical experiences with patients with facial bone deformities associated with hemifacial microsomia, *J Craniofac Surg* 2:181, 1992.

41. Kapp-Simon KA, McGuire DE: Observed social interaction patterns in adolescents with and without craniofacial conditions, *Cleft Palate Craniofac J* 34:380, 1997.

42. Kaye CI, Rollnick BR, Hauck WW, et al: Microtia and associated anomalies: statistical analysis, *Am J Med Genet* 34:574, 1989.

43. Kazanjian VH: Congenital absence of the ramus of the mandible, *J Bone Joint Surg* 21:701, 1939.

44. Keusch CF, Mulliken JB, Kaplan LC: Craniofacial anomalies in twins, *Plast Reconstr Surg* 87:16, 1991.

45. LaRossa D, Whitaker L, Dabb R, et al: The use of microvascular free flaps for soft tissue augmentation of the face in children with hemifacial microsomia, *Cleft Palate J* 17:138, 1980.

46. Lauritzen C, Munro IR, Ross RB: Classification and treatment of hemifacial microsomia, *Scand J Plast Reconstr Surg* 19:33, 1985.

47. LeFebvre AM, Arndt EM: Working with facially disfigured children: a challenge in prevention, *Can J Psychiatr* 33:453, 1988.

48. Lefebvre AM, Arndt EM: Psychosocial impact of craniofacial deformities before and after reconstructive surgery, *Can J Psychiatr* 27:579, 1982.

49. LeFebvre AM, Munro IR: Psychosocial adjustment of patients with craniofacial deformities before and after surgery. In Herman P, Zann MP, Higgins TE (eds): *Physical appearance, stigma and social behavior: the Ontario symposium,* Hillsdale, NJ, 1986, Lawrence Erlbaum Associates.

50. Loevy HT, Shore SW: Dental maturation in hemifacial microsomia, *J Craniofac Genet Dev Biol Suppl* 1:267, 1985.

51. Longacre JJ, deStefano GA, Holmstrand KE: The surgical management of first and second branchial arch syndromes, *Plast Reconstr Surg* 31:507, 1963.

52. Luce EA, McGibbon B, Hoopes JE: Velopharyngeal insufficiency in hemifacial microsomia, *Plast Reconstr Surg* 60:602, 1977.

53. McCarthy JG: The role of distraction osteogenesis in the reconstruction of the mandible in unilateral craniofacial microsomia, *Clin Plast Surg* 21:625, 1994.

54. McCarthy JG, Fuleihan N: Development defects of the buccal and parotid area. In Stark RB (ed): *Plastic surgery of the head and neck,* New York, 1986, Churchill Livingstone.

55. McCarthy JG, Schreiber J, Karp N, et al: Lengthening the human mandible by gradual distraction, *Plast Reconstr Surg* 89:1, 1992.

56. Meurmann Y: Congenital microtia and meatal atresia, *Arch Otolaryngol* 66:443, 1957.

57. Molina F, Ortiz-Monasterio F: Mandibular elongation and remodeling by distraction: a farewell to major osteotomies, *Plast Reconstr Surg* 96:825, 1995.

58. Mordick TG II, LaRossa D, Whitaker L: Soft-tissue reconstruction of the face: a comparison of dermal-fat grafting and vascularized tissue transfer, *Ann Plast Surg* 29:390, 1992.

59. Mulliken JB, Ferraro NF, Vento AR: A retrospective analysis of growth of the constructed condyle-ramus in children with hemifacial microsomia, *Cleft Palate J* 26:312, 1989.

60. Mulliken JB, Kaban LB: Analysis and treatment of hemifacial microsomia in childhood, *Clin Plast Surg* 14:91, 1987.

61. Munro IR: Hemifacial microsomia: the skeletal correction, *Oper Tech Plast Reconstr Surg* 1:77, 1994.

62. Munro IR: Rigid fixation and facial asymmetry, *Clin Plast Surg* 16:187, 1989.

63. Munro IR: Treatment of craniofacial microsomia, *Clin Plast Surg* 14:177, 1987.

64. Munro IR: One-stage reconstruction of the temporomandibular joint in hemifacial microsomia, *Plast Reconstr Surg* 66:699, 1980.

65. Munro IR, Phillips JH, Griffin G: Growth after construction of the temporomandibular joint in children with hemifacial microsomia, *Cleft Palate J* 26:303, 1989.

66. Murray JE, Kaban LB, Mulliken JB: Analysis and treatment of hemifacial microsomia, *Plast Reconstr Surg* 74:186, 1984.

67. Naora H, Kimura M, Otani H, et al: Transgenic mouse model of hemifacial microsomia: cloning and characterization of insertional mutation region on chromosome 10, *Genomics* 23:515, 1994.

68. Obwegeser H: Zur Korrektur der Dysostosis Otomandibularis, *Schweiz Monatsschr Zahnheilkd* 80:331, 1970.

69. Obwegeser HL: Correction of the skeletal anomalies of oto-mandibular dysostosis, *J Maxillofac Surg* 2:73, 1974.

70. Ortiz-Monasterio F: Early mandibular and maxillary osteotomies for the correction of hemifacial microsomia. A preliminary report, *Clin Plast Surg* 9:509, 1982.

71. Ortiz-Monasterio F, Molina F, Andrade L, et al: Simultaneous mandibular and maxillary distraction in hemifacial microsomia in adults: avoiding occlusal disasters, *Plast Reconstr Surg* 100:852, 1997.

72. Ousterhout DK, Vargervik K: Surgical treatment of the jaw deformities in hemifacial microsomia, *Aust NZ J Surg* 57:77, 1987.

73. Padwa BL, Bruneteau RJ, Mulliken JB: Association between "plagiocephaly" and hemifacial microsomia, *Am J Med Genet* 47:1202, 1993.

74. Papacharalambous SK, Anastasoff KI: Natural coral skeleton used as onlay graft for contour augmentation of the face. A preliminary report, *Int J Oral Maxillofac Surg* 22:260, 1993.

75. Perrott DH, Umeda H, Kaban LB: Costochondral graft construction/reconstruction of the ramus/condyle unit: long-term follow-up, *Int J Oral Maxillofac Surg* 23:321, 1994.

76. Pickerill HP: Ankylosis of the jaw: cartilage graft restoration of the joint: a new operation, *Aust NZ J Surg* 11:197, 1942.

77. Polley JW, Figueroa AA, Jein-Wein Liou E, et al: Longitudinal analysis of mandibular asymmetry in hemifacial microsomia, *Plast Reconstr Surg* 99:328, 1997.

78. Pope AW, Ward J: Self-perceived facial appearance and psychosocial adjustment in preadolescents with craniofacial anomalies, *Cleft Palate Craniofac J* 34:396, 1997.

79. Poswillo D: Hemorrhage in development of the face, *Birth Defects* 11:61, 1975.

80. Pruzansky S: Not all dwarfed mandibles are alike, *Birth Defects* 5:120, 1969.

81. Robinow M, Reynolds JF, FitzGerald J, et al: Hemifacial microsomia, ipsilateral facial palsy, and malformed auricle in two families: an autosomal dominant malformation, *Am J Med Genet Suppl* 2:129, 1986.

82. Rodgers SF, Eppley BL, Nelson CL, et al: Hemifacial microsomia: assessment of classification systems, *J Craniofac Surg* 2:114, 1991.

83. Satoh K, Shibata Y, Tokushige H, et al: A mirror image of the first and second branchial arch syndrome associated with cleft lip and palate in monozygotic twins, *Br J Plast Surg* 48:601, 1995.

84. Siebert JW, Anson G, Longaker MT: Microsurgical correction of facial asymmetry in 60 consecutive cases, *Plast Reconstr Surg* 97:354, 1996.

85. Silvestri A, Natali G, Iannetti G: Functional therapy in hemifacial microsomia: therapeutic protocol for growing children, *J Oral Maxillofac Surg* 54:271, 1996.

86. Singer SL, Haan E, Slee J, et al: Familial hemifacial microsomia due to autosomal dominant inheritance. Case reports, *Aust Dent J* 39:287, 1994.

87. Snyder CC, Levine GA, Swanson HM, et al: Mandibular lengthening by gradual distraction: preliminary report, *Plast Reconstr Surg* 51:506, 1973.

88. Stark RB, Saunders DE: The first branchial syndrome: the oral-mandibular-auricular syndrome, *Plast Reconstr Surg* 29:229, 1962.

89. Tanzer RC: Total reconstruction of the external ear, *Plast Reconstr Surg* 23:1, 1959.

90. Taysi K, Marsh JL, Wise DM: Familial hemifacial microsomia, *Cleft Palate J* 20:47, 1983.

91. Upton J, Albin RE, Mulliken JB, et al: The use of scapular and parascapular flaps for cheek reconstruction, *Plast Reconstr Surg* 90:959, 1992.

92. Vargervik K, Ousterhout DK, Farias M: Factors affecting long-term results in hemifacial microsomia, *Cleft Palate J Suppl* 1:53, 1986.

93. Vento AR, LaBrie RA, Mulliken JB: The O.M.E.N.S. classification of hemifacial microsomia, *Cleft Palate Craniofac J* 28:68, discussion 77, 1991.

94. Wells JH, Edgerton MT: Correction of severe hemifacial atrophy with a free dermis-fat flap from the lower abdomen, *Plast Reconstr Surg* 59:223, 1977.

CHAPTER

Facial Trauma

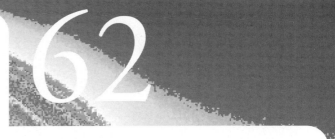

Salvatore Lettieri

INDICATIONS

The care and management of facial trauma and its deformities can be one of the most difficult yet rewarding aspects of plastic and reconstructive surgery. Injuries may be as minimal as a small laceration or as complex as true panfacial fractures. In each of these patients, thorough evaluation and management options based on sound principles should be considered and executed. Historically, craniofacial trauma has made rapid advancements in treatment principles during this past century, largely as a result of the major military conflicts. David and Simpson[8] have written an excellent review of this perspective on craniomaxillofacial trauma. With each war, more advancements have been made, particularly in the early part of this century, when Edward Angle studied posttraumatic malocclusions and also formulated his well-known classification scheme. At about the same time, Rene Le Fort in France performed his studies on 35 cadavers and reported his Le Fort I, II, and III maxillary fracture classification system in 1901.[25] Thus growing interest was borne into the literature for management of facial fractures. World War I prompted development of new levels of management in facial trauma. Sir Harold Gilles brought to the forefront the concept of a team approach, including neurosurgeons, dental surgeons, and facial trauma surgeons. World War II brought its own array of injuries. World War II was different from World War I in the increased magnitude of injury and improved ability to transport the injured soldier. The Korean War laid a foundation for rapid transfer to field hospitals, which allowed immediate management close to military fire with subsequent evacuation. During the Vietnam War, this concept of care for severely traumatized patients and better evacuation measures brought to the facial trauma surgeon many injuries in a new degree of survivors who previously would have not undergone any mode of treatment. Coincident with war advancements was improvement in the automobile, which also brought a wider spectrum of injuries.

The standards for evaluation and management of the more common facial traumas stemming from automobile accidents, assault, or penetrating injuries are presented in this chapter. The initial evaluation should include a complete examination, which can be directed with minimal injury. Usually, patients are seen in consultation, and the treating emergency room physician is the primary caregiver. Evaluation for facial injury should always begin with the integument. The underlying neuromotor function, occlusion, ocular function, and nasal passageway should follow. Along with this, clinical evaluation of the bony structures should be included.

AIRWAY

Generally, the primary care physician has already performed the airway evaluation. However, special circumstances include massive midface injuries with significant bleeding via the ethmoid sinuses, nose, and posterior pharynx. The bilateral parasymphyseal fracture is also another significant airway emergency because it allows retrusion of the mandible symphysis and collapse of the retropharynx with potentially acute airway obstruction (Figure 62-1). Because of the unstable mandible, oral endotracheal intubation can be quite difficult and emergency cricothyroidotomy may need to be performed. Nasotracheal intubation should never be attempted with severe midface fractures because this may result in impalement of the brain and/or brainstem. Similarly, a gastric tube should be placed orally. Any loose teeth, which are usually attached by soft tissue only with these severe midface injuries, should also be removed to prevent aspiration. Heroic attempts at tooth salvage should be reserved for the more stable circumstance.

Once an airway has been established, bleeding should be assessed. Ordinarily, bleeding will stop without extensive intervention, but occasionally it can be excessive. The bleeding usually occurs from fractured bone edges with overlying soft tissue injury precluding any tamponade effect. The ethmoidal and internal maxillary arteries are common culprits. The initial treatment measures include anterior and posterior nasal packing, which can control the bleeding most of the time. Exsanguination when bleeding continues, however, can occur. Key initial maneuvers are immediate closed reduction of the midface fractures, which can be performed with disimpaction forceps, followed by anterior and posterior nasal packing, along with a complete facial wrap. Should the bleeding continue through the dressing, a decision needs to be made for either transport to radiology for angiographic embolization or immediate operative intervention. Operative intervention includes ligation of the appropriate feeding vessels, the anterior

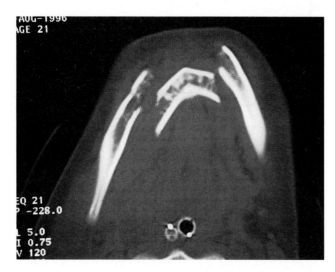

Figure 62-1. Bilateral parasymphyseal fracture with retrograde pull of the bone segment by the floor muscles attached. This can be an airway emergency because the posterior pharynx can collapse.

and posterior ethmoidal and internal maxillary arteries bilaterally. A more expedient approach is ligation of the external carotid artery distal to the lingual artery along with ligation of the superficial temporal arteries bilaterally. This controls a significant amount of the vascular inflow to the midface region, and the vessels are usually separated from the injured tissues.

EXAMINATION—INTEGUMENT

The initial inspection and examination should be directed at breaks in the integument and any ecchymoses. Lacerations can occur anywhere on the face. Usually, breaks in the skin can be from a cut or deep abrasions or so-called fracturing of the skin. This latter type of wound is more difficult to treat because there is an indeterminate zone of injury radiating from the center with necrosis of the edges. The general management for breaks in the skin is to cleanse the wound, freshen the edges, and close without undue tension on the dermis. This is generally possible. Usual lacerations that correlate to underlying fractures include the mandibular border and angle, the zygomaticofrontal region, the nasal dorsum, and the lower midforehead region overlying the frontal sinus. There are various patterns of ecchymoses that are also of particular interest. Ecchymoses in the periorbital region that occur in the lower eyelid and upper eyelid but stop at the outer edges of the eyelids have a recognizable pattern called *spectacle hematomas* indicative of underlying orbit fractures (Figure 62-2). Ecchymoses in the mastoid region can represent basilar skull fractures (Battle's sign, Figure 62-3). Intraoral ecchymosis patterns lie over fractures at the medial and lateral zygomatico-

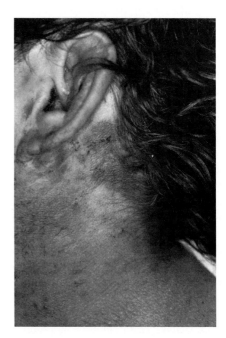

Figure 62-3. Battle's sign.

A

B

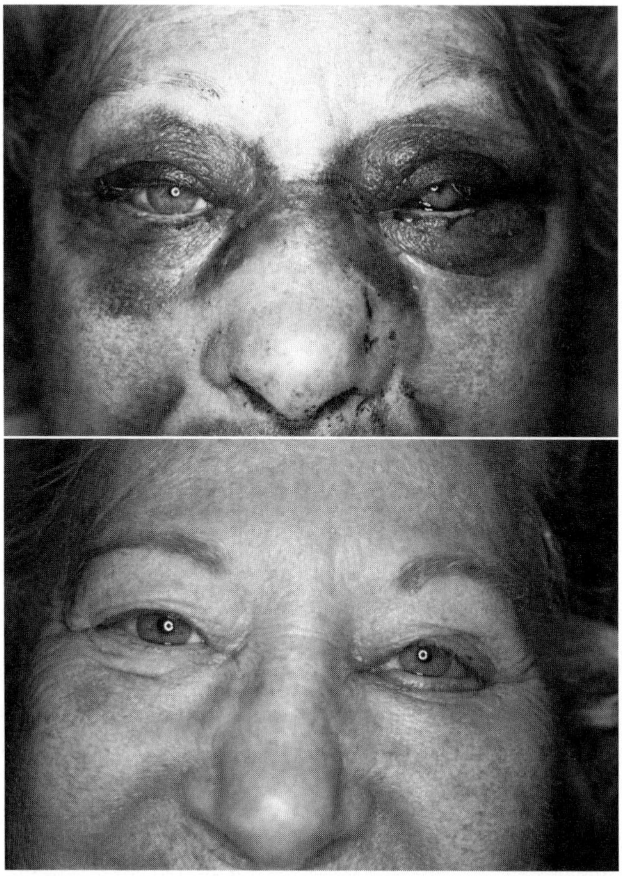

Figure 62-2. A, Bilateral spectacle hematomas. This patient had bilateral orbit floor fractures that were repaired. **B,** Postoperative photograph.

maxillary buttress if seen in the upper buccal sulci or represent mandible fractures and/or alveolar ridge fractures if in the inferior buccal sulcus.

BONE

There are common fracture patterns that occur in blunt injury, including nasal fractures with the zygomaticofrontal suture, zygomatic arch, inferior orbital rim, and the body and symphysis of the mandible, along with the angle and the upper and lower alveolar ridges. These are the usual and more common sites of fractures, which can be discerned on the physical examination. Usually, the tender areas with an associated area of ecchymosis and a suggestive history should lead to a high clinical suspicion of underlying fractures, thus prompting further diagnostic studies.

EYES

When there is severe periorbital injury, formal ophthalmologic examination is warranted. The initial examination should include inspection and evaluation of the upper and lower eyelids and the position of the medial and lateral canthi. Sometimes subtle lacerations to the medial, lower, or upper eyelid that may include the underlying canalicular structures can be missed because of severe edema and/or tenderness in the region. Visualization of the pupils and their relative reactivity, along with visualization of the conjunctiva, should be done. Usually, the lateral canthi remain attached; however, with severe fractures in the nasal orbital ethmoid region, there may be gross displacement of the medial canthi, resulting in either bilateral or unilateral telecanthus. The intercanthal and interpupillary distances should be measured. The intercanthal distance should also be broken down to the sum of its parts, that is, distance from center to the medial canthal region. For example, a patient may have an intercanthal distance of 32 mm that may be the upper limits of normal. However, when broken down to the midline, 18 mm on one side and 14 mm on the other would suggest a hemitelecanthus. A general rule of thumb is that the width of the palpebral fissure should be symmetric and also equivalent to the intercanthal distance. The anterior pupillary projection can be measured from the lateral orbital rim. Careful attention should be paid to the extraocular muscle movement, visual acuity, and accommodation.

The periorbital bony rims absorb the energy, which is distributed through the very thin orbital floor and medial and lateral walls, sparing the eye itself and the optic nerve, but there can still be injury to the eye. Visual acuity can be checked using a Snellen's card at 15 inches, and pupil diameter can also be measured. Pupil reactivity can be performed with a flashlight; in addition, a swinging flashlight test should be performed. The primary and secondary fields of gaze should be checked for diplopia. Diplopia can be absent in primary gaze but present in secondary gaze.

TEETH

Evaluation of dentition can be quite difficult. Even without injury to the upper or lower jaws or alveolar ridge, a patient can still complain that "something does not feel right" when clenching. This can be anything from an occult fracture to sensory disturbance. There can also be muscular discomfort and trismus, which can disturb the occlusion. The dental assessment should include visual inspection in addition to palpable examination. Any ecchymoses should be noted because these can be largely correlated with underlying fractures.

Most of the mandible and maxilla can be palpated bimanually for assessment of fractures. The areas that are difficult to assess are in the condylar neck and condyle region. Usually, one can be suspicious of a fracture in these regions with tenderness in the condylar region, loss of vertical height on either side, anterior open bite, or severe end incisal deviation with lateral crossbite. When the mandible is opened, the maximal incisal opening can easily approach 40 to 50 mm. Because of discomfort or fracture, this can be greatly diminished.

Inspection of dentition is also important. There are 32 teeth, and various classification schemes exist. One of the more common includes naming the right maxillary third molar as tooth number 1 extending to the left maxillary third molar as tooth number 16, numbering the intervening teeth sequentially. The left mandibular third molar is 17 and then again number these sequentially to the right mandibular third molar, 32. By convention, the portion of the tooth that is towards the midline is termed *mesial,* and the portion of the tooth that is away from the midline is *distal.* The "inner" side of the tooth is *lingual,* and the outer side is *buccal,* or *labial.* Angle's classification scheme can be divided into three categories, depending on the relationship between the maxillary and mandibular first molars (3 and 29, 14 and 19). In the Class I occlusion, the mesiobuccal cusp of the upper molar (3 and 14) occludes with the mesiobuccal groove of the lower molar (19 and 29). The lower molar is shifted mesial in the Class II occlusion and shifted distal in the Class III occlusion. One should also pay attention to the wear facets of the teeth. This can be greatly beneficial when attempting to align the teeth for placement of arch bars in mandibular and/or maxillary fractures. Loose teeth should be reseated for potential salvage. Note that the time frame of subluxation and/or frank avulsion is directly related to the tooth survival rate. Conventional thought has been to remove all teeth that have been in the line of fracture. However, many of these teeth may be salvaged.

NERVES

The two nerves most susceptible to injury are the facial and trigeminal. All of the cranial nerves, however, can be affected in varying degrees. The olfactory nerve passes through the cribriform plate, and severe frontal fractures that involve the nasal orbital ethmoid region or anterior cranial fossa along with the frontal lobes can produce injury. This is most likely a shearing type of injury to the olfactory nerves. This is very difficult to assess in the acute trauma setting. However, it should always be borne in mind to be mentioned and recorded as a potential debilitating injury because there are occupations that require olfactory sensation, such as working in a chemical laboratory.

The optic nerve passes through the optic foramen, which can be assessed by checking visual acuity or funduscopic examination in the comatose patient. The ocular, motor, trochlear, and abducent nerves all deal with extraocular muscle movement, and these exit through the superior orbital fissure. These nerves can be assessed formally by checking the extraocular muscle movement. Complete injury is termed *superior orbital fissure syndrome.* When blindness also occurs, this is an orbital apex syndrome. The trigeminal nerve has three branches. The first branch exits through the superior orbital fissure, the second branch through the foramen rotundum and then the inferior orbital fissure, and the third branch through the foramen ovale. These are most commonly injured when they exit the frontal bone, inferior orbital rim, or body of the mandible, respectively.

The facial nerve exits the stylomastoid foramen and provides motor function to the stapedius muscle; muscles of facial expression; and buccinator, posterior digastric, stylohyoid, and auricular muscles. The distal portion of the facial nerve is further broken down into five branches: temporal (or frontal), zygomatic, buccal, marginal mandibular, and cervical. As the nerve exits the stylomastoid foramen, it branches immediately into the temporal facial and cervical facial divisions and then branches out into its five distinct branches. The acoustic nerve passes through the internal meatus and can be measured by testing hearing. The costopharyngeal, vagus, and spinal accessory nerves all pass through the jugular foramen, and finally the hypoglossal nerve passes through the hypoglossal canal.

RADIOGRAPHIC IMAGING

One of the advances in medicine that has greatly facilitated facial trauma repair has been the evolution of radiographic imaging. When plain films were the only modality at hand, interpretation needed to be highly correlated with clinical examination (Figure 62-4). Imaging modalities today include the multiview facial plain films, panoramic plane view of the mandible, and computed tomography (CT). Over the past decade, CT has gone through tremendous evolution to the fast high-resolution helical scanners that are quite readily available. The standard for diagnoses of facial trauma has shifted to CT scans.[28] Many patients with severe head injuries require cranial CT scans, which can be combined with midface or mandible CT scans as the examination dictates. Multiview plain films of the face and mandible can be performed on the cooperative patient but not in patients with possible neck or intracranial inuries or those with an endotracheal tube. CT scans can be predictably performed and give a wealth of information for

determining repairs. Coronal reconstructions can also be performed, especially when these slices are 3 mm or finer; these computerized reconstructions can provide good screening of the orbital floors. Should there be any question, true coronal slices should be obtained, especially if nonoperative treatment is chosen. Should operative treatment be the choice, coronal reconstructions are adequate because exploration of the orbital floors can be performed quite readily with exposure of the infraorbital rims.

Ideally, the CT scans of the midface and mandible should be performed at the same sitting as the cranial CT scan. When there is concern over the orbits and midface, a midface true axial CT scan at 3-mm slices zero gantry with coronal reconstructions should be requested. If one also wishes evaluation of the frontal sinus, requesting a view of the frontal sinus should be done. A mandible CT can also be ordered; however, remember that most of the mandible can be assessed by physical examination and that the regions that cannot be very well assessed (i.e., the condylar neck and condyle regions) can be seen on midface axial CT. The number of negative examinations for the mandible should be quite low. The mandible slices are taken parallel to the inferior border of the mandible. There will be overlap in the condyle region along with the pterygoid regions. If there is any concern over the orbits and the patient is able to bend his or her neck after it has been cleared of any injury, coronal views to the orbit can be very helpful. One can also measure the amount of defect in the orbital floor, which can also help predict the need for repair.

FRACTURE TYPES

Mandible

The mandible is frequently involved in facial fractures, and treatment is usually needed because of the potential functional deformities.[4,6,10-12] The bone is quite strong in most areas, but there are weak areas that account for most of the fracture sites. These include the condylar neck, angle, and parasymphyseal regions. The traditional order of frequency in diminishing order is condylar neck, body, angle, parasymphyseal, and ramus. Fractures can be isolated, paired, or comminuted. All fractures need some kind of treatment, whether it is conservative, closed, or open. Clinical manifestations include a mobile mandible on examination, malocclusion, and deviation of the mandible with opening. The mandible is subject to muscular forces, which tend to add to the instability of fractures and the need for treatment. The masseter, temporalis, and medial pterygoid muscles elevate the mandible, and the geniohyoid, genioglossus, mylohyoid, and digastric muscles tend to depress the mandible. The lateral pterygoid muscle inserts into the capsule of the temporomandibular joint and tends to remain attached and pull the condyle head medial when there is a high fracture.

The primary goal in treatment is attain the premorbid occlusion and function. Treatment options include arch bar application and mandibulomaxillary fixation (MMF), open reduction and internal fixation (ORIF), open reduction and

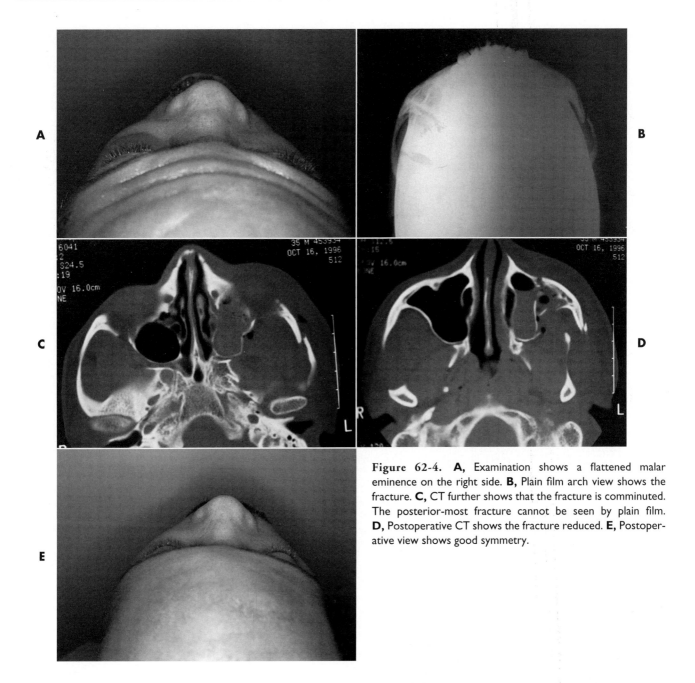

Figure 62-4. **A,** Examination shows a flattened malar eminence on the right side. **B,** Plain film arch view shows the fracture. **C,** CT further shows that the fracture is comminuted. The posterior-most fracture cannot be seen by plain film. **D,** Postoperative CT shows the fracture reduced. **E,** Postoperative view shows good symmetry.

external fixation (OREF), or a combination[10] (Figures 62-5 and 62-6). MMF can still be performed for many fractures, with the length of fixation dictated by the fracture. The problems with MMF include decreased oral intake, poor oral hygiene, gingival recession, poor communication, and chronic and varying levels of irritation and discomfort. Patients should be seen frequently and have the MMF adjusted and healing followed. Fixation will need to remain for 5 to 6 weeks before clinical and radiologic findings support removal. If a condyle fracture is present, MMF this long has a high risk of ankylosis and should not be done. By far most fractures are treated with ORIF. This type of treatment allows the patient to range the mandible sooner, to maintain oral intake, and to minimize the risk of dental or gingival morbidity. The condyle can most often be treated in a closed fashion with MMF for 10 to 14

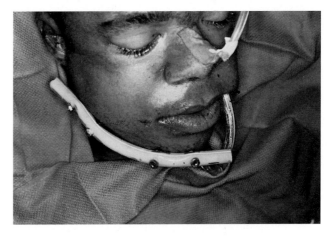

Figure 62-5. Example of application of external fixation.

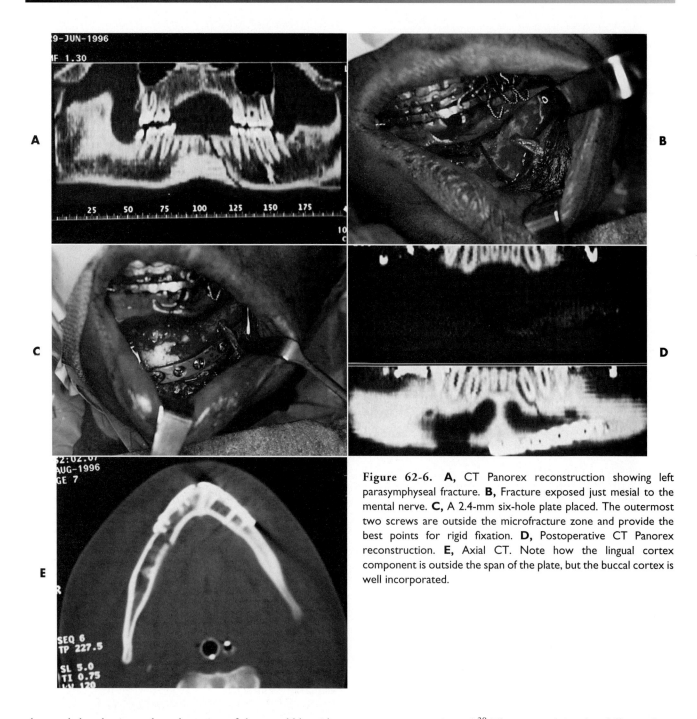

Figure 62-6. A, CT Panorex reconstruction showing left parasymphyseal fracture. **B,** Fracture exposed just mesial to the mental nerve. **C,** A 2.4-mm six-hole plate placed. The outermost two screws are outside the microfracture zone and provide the best points for rigid fixation. **D,** Postoperative CT Panorex reconstruction. **E,** Axial CT. Note how the lingual cortex component is outside the span of the plate, but the buccal cortex is well incorporated.

days and then begin graduated ranging of the mandible with elastics. Absolute indications for opening and reducing a condyle include fracture dislocation into the middle cranial fossa, intraarticular foreign body, lateral extracapsular dislocation, malocclusion or vertical shortening after conservative treatment, penetrating wound (e.g., gunshot), and complex multijaw fractures (maxilla, palate, mandible) with vertical shortening of the ramus[50] (Figure 62-7).

Palate

Fractures of the palate become more clinically significant as the surrounding structures are involved. If the maxillary alveolar ridge is involved, there is great potential for occlusal disturbance. The fractures can be sagittal, parasagittal, trans-

verse, or comminuted.[30] The approach is a bit different from that of the mandible because maintenance of occlusion while trying to open the fracture site is impossible because of the location of the fracture. The fracture can therefore be treated by fabrication of a palatal splint after obtaining dental models and performing model surgery followed by placement of the splint.[7] Another method is to open the fracture site and grossly reduce the fracture while applying semirigid fixation and then apply either the prefabricated splint or MMF.

Maxilla

The maxilla is the upper jaw, and when the fracture involves the maxillary alveolar ridge or is bilateral and freely mobile, application of MMF and rigid fixation is required. The

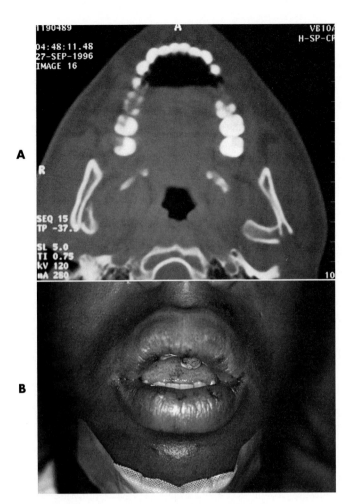

Figure 62-7. A, Bilateral condyle fractures. **B,** Open bite deformity with the bilateral condyle fractures.

decompress the infraorbital foramen where the nerve is usually pinched, and reestablish the majority of the orbit. If there is no indication for repair of the ZMC, the orbit walls and floor need to be assessed. Positive forced duction test, orbit content herniation, foreign body, and enophthalmos are indications for exploration and repair. If the orbit volume is reduced by 10%, there is an increased chance of posttraumatic enophthalmos.

Frontal Sinus

Fractures of the frontal sinus can involve the anterior or posterior tables or both. Indications for repair include an open fracture, compromised frontoethmoid drainage, depressed anterior table fracture, and a posterior table fracture that requires neurosurgical treatment.

Nasoorbital Ethmoid

Nasoorbital ethmoid (NOE) fractures are repaired when there is displacement and a widened intercanthal distance. The distance is measured from the midline to both sides and then compared, but it is difficult to assess the amount of asymmetry that will develop because of the significant amount of edema that is present in the acute trauma setting. CT is very helpful here because the segment of bone at the NOE region can be seen very clearly and, if displaced, requires treatment.

OPERATIONS

INTRAORAL APPROACHES TO THE MANDIBLE

Most of the mandible can be exposed through an intraoral approach, such as the symphyseal and parasymphyseal regions and the mid-body. The angle and the ramus can also be visualized; however, this will need the assistance of buccal cheek retractors. The advantages of intraoral approach are no visible external scar and rapid access to fractures, leaving the masseter muscle attached, which can help with fracture stabilization. The disadvantages include potential for increased operative infection rate; difficult exposure; inadequate reduction of the fractures, especially for those that are several days old and require removal of organizing hematomas; and difficult proper water-tight closure because of multiple intraoral lacerations and teeth avulsion.

The oral cavity can be cleansed with povidone-iodine (Betadine) solution and need not be scrubbed. Usually the arch bars will already have been applied. At times, application of the arch bars and seating into occlusion may be difficult with flail segments of the mandible; thus the mandible fractures should be first exposed and temporarily placed into reduction by interosseus wiring. Arch bar application with MMF is easier to perform, and then the fracture can be formally repaired. One should make the incision just on the mandible side of the deepest recess of the inferior alveolar sulcus. This may leave approximately a 5- to 8-mm cuff of mucosa and underlying muscle for secure closure. If the incision is made directly in the deepest recess, the sulcus can be obliterated on closure. Also, if

difficult scenario is when there is a freely mobile maxilla with varying degrees of comminution and bilateral condylar neck fractures. In this situation, the condylar neck fractures will need to be opened and reduced to establish the proper vertical height in addition to fixation of all the other fractures. The occlusal surface integrity will need to be maintained with MMF.[16]

Orbit and Zygomaticomaxillary Complex

The zygomaticomaxillary complex (ZMC) and orbit are addressed together because of the anatomic relationships.[17,19,37] It is impossible to have displacement of the ZMC without having a fracture of the orbit. The forces of the zygoma include the masseter muscle with a strong downward pull and the mimetic muscles. These forces, coupled with the blow to the bone, result in a tendency for the ZMC to be displaced inward and downward. The orbit volume is increased, and the eye position is back and down. There are different degrees of severity of displacement. If there is no displacement of the ZMC, there is no need for repair. If there is displacement, repair is warranted to achieve symmetry,

the incision is made too near the dental papilla, there may not be enough tissue for closure at the end of the procedure. There is a tendency for the mucosa on the mandible side of the incision to retract slightly. Once the incision is made with the knife, the muscle can then be cut with knife or cautery. The knife blade should then be turned perpendicular to the mandible and cut straight down. This will leave a cuff of muscle beneath the mucosa. The incision is made directly to the bone. Once this has been done, a periosteal elevator can then be used and swept in all directions in a strict subperiosteal plane. Note that in the parasymphyseal regions the mental nerve will be situated at the level of the first bicuspid.

The exposure needs to be modified for intraoral lacerations enough so that if there are multiple lacerations on either side of the alveolar ridge, extensive degloving could potentially devascularize the bony segments; thus an external approach should be considered. Generally, the unstable fragments of the mandible can be palpated, and the incision can be made directed over the midportion of the fracture. A trochar and buccal retractor system can be used. Usually there are two fractures to the mandible, although this is not absolute. An example would be a parasymphyseal fracture on one side and a condylar neck on the other side. A true symphyseal fracture may not have any other fractures. If the fracture is at the angle, a similar incision along the posterior buccal mucosa region made along the external oblique ridge can be done. Again using a buccal retractor and trochar system, a 2-mm plate can be placed along the external oblique ridge. The advantages are avoiding an external incision and leaving the masseter muscle attached. The disadvantages are difficulty in exposure, visualization, and proper reduction.

Once the fracture has been exposed, the site can then be cleaned of all clot and fibrinous material, the amount of which will depend on the time to repair. Various methods of fixation have been used, including interosseus wiring, stainless steel plates, Vitallium plates, and titanium plates. There are also various sizes of plating systems that can be used. Generally, for the straightforward fracture, a titanium plate designed for the mandible at 2.3 or 2.4 mm is most commonly used. For spanning multiple comminuted segments, a larger plate (2.7 mm) should be considered. The plates are usually placed along the inferior border of the mandible to avoid injury to the inferior alveolar nerves and the tooth roots. Because of this, there will be a tendency for the cephalad portion of the fracture to "open." For this reason, a tension band of some kind is required. Ordinarily, the arch bars can act as the tension band, but consideration should be given to placing a unicortical plate along the cephalad portion of the fracture.

Drill holes are placed using a low-velocity, high-torque drill. To facilitate maintaining the fracture in place, a unicortical interosseus wire can be placed, or outwardly angled drill holes can be placed and a bone tenaculum can be used. A template can be used to rapidly contour the plate. The plate should be overbent slightly. There is a tendency for the fracture to appear to be aligned, but this is only the buccal cortex; the lingual cortex can still be open. A good test for this is to distract the fracture on either side pushing inward. With this movement, if there is some time lag between the distraction of the buccal cortex or the fracture, this is suggestive of lingual cortex displacement. If there is immediate distraction of the buccal cortex of the fracture, this in turn is suggestive of lingual cortex reduction.

Once the fractures are reduced and rigidly fixed, the next step is to release the MMF and test for maintenance of occlusion. The mandible should open and close easily with seating into centric occlusion with maximal intercuspation in a repeated fashion. This should be routinely performed for any mandible fracture repair. Once this test has been performed, the patient is then re-placed into MMF. The wound should be irrigated and closed in layers. The muscle can be closed with a running 3-0 absorbable suture followed by a 4-0 absorbable suture in the mucosa. The monofilament absorbable sutures are adequate, but the knots tend to be irritating. A braided absorbable suture is less problematic. If this is the only fracture and it is a simple fracture, the patient may be released from MMF with immediate range of motion postoperatively. There is suggestive evidence, however, that there is less discomfort with resting the soft tissue by continuing MMF for 4 to 7 days with later release.

EXTERNAL APPROACHES TO THE MANDIBLE

Virtually all parts of the mandible can be approached externally. The condyle and high condylar neck regions are by far the most difficult to access. The angle and body of the mandible can be accessed through an inferior mandibular border incision approximately one to two finger breadths below the mandibular border. If the ramus and low condylar neck are the fracture sites, this incision can be placed parallel to the angle posteriorly in a similar fashion to a parotidectomy incision. A preauricular incision can be made for access to the condyle itself. The difficulties with external incisions include external scar, injury to the marginal mandibular nerve, and bleeding from the retromandibular plexus of veins. The advantages are that, once the fracture is exposed, the reduction and plating are also easier, and one can also directly visualize the lingual cortex of the mandible to assess reduction.

The condyle is one of the most difficult areas in the facial skeleton region to approach. The various branches of the facial nerve and also a multiple plexus of veins surround it. A preauricular incision is made in the skin crease. It is usually approximately 3 cm in length. The dissection is carried out along the preauricular cartilage. As long as the incision is kept within 0.5 cm of the tragus, it is relatively safe from injury to the facial nerve. The incision is carried down to the zygomatic process of the temporal bone, which is the posterior-most aspect of the arch. The condyle is just deep to this region (Figure 62-8). The periosteum overlying the posterior-most aspect of the bone is incised. The periosteum is then elevated in a posterior to anterior fashion, elevating all the soft tissue structures with this radiating outward from the bone. When done in this fashion, the nerve is safe. Usually, postoperative paresis of branches of the facial nerve is from retraction in the region. The capsule of the temporomandibular joint can then be visualized. A transverse incision is made over the capsule, leaving a cuff of approximately 2 to 3 mm for closure. The texture of the capsule will be quite tough, and the masseter muscle will be soft. Once this incision has been made, the articulating disk can usually be seen, although it may be somewhat displaced. Care should be taken to avoid tearing the disk. Usually it is still attached medially. The condyle is just inferior and usually medially displaced. Usually the superior portion of the lateral pterygoid muscle is still attached to the condyle. The condyle head can be grasped and pulled into position. It may be necessary to release the patient from MMF during the reduction of the condylar head.

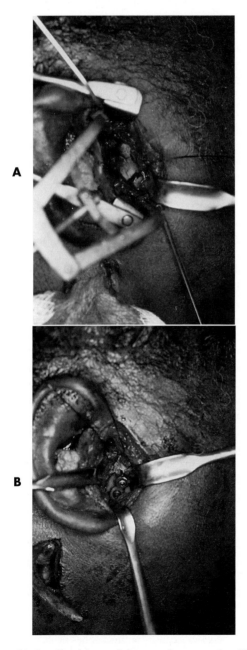

A

B

Figure 62-8. Condylar neck fracture **A,** exposed and **B,** plated.

Once the head is in position, it can be stabilized via K wire from below or held in place by clamps. It is certainly possible to strip and remove the condylar head in its entirety and then plate a portion of the head on the back table and replace it into the fossa, but this is in essence a bone graft. The medial attachments to the condyle should be left in place to allow this bone to be a vascularized piece. A four-hole or five-hole 2-mm plate can be adapted to the fracture. The angle can also be exposed to assist reduction and repair. Bicortical screws should be used. There is considerable force in this area, and the largest plate that can fit should be used. During closure, it is important to reseat the articulating disk and repair the capsule. Care should be taken to avoid large bites of tissue because the branches of the facial nerve can be grasped. The patient should be released from MMF, assessed for vertical height and centric occlusion, and then re-placed into MMF. The wound can then be irrigated and closed with deep dermal stitches and superficial stitches in a customary fashion.

PALATE STABILIZATION

Palatal fractures can be sometimes quite difficult (Figure 62-9). Treatment options include preoperative dental models with model surgery and placement on a typedont and reformation of occlusion with fabrication of an acrylic splint. For repair, usually there is a laceration overlying the fracture, which can be extended on either side of the fracture, and a small plate can be applied. Usually a 1.2- or 1.3-mm plate can be used. Sometimes mesh can be used and cut to fit the contour of the palate and also overlie the various fracture fragments for semirigid fixation. The mucosa can then be closed with interrupted absorbable suture.

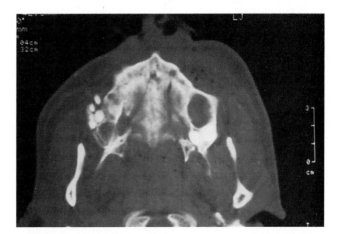

Figure 62-9. Parasagittal split palate fractures. These fractures usually have an overlying laceration through which the fractures can be approached. If repaired open, the fixation needs to be done before the MMF is applied. Usually a small plate (1.2 mm or 1.3 mm) is used to allow some movement of the bone pieces to allow a maximal intercuspation with MMF. Then the MMF will need to remain postoperatively for 7 to 10 days at minimum.

MIDFACE SURGICAL APPROACHES

Midface fractures can be difficult to approach in the trauma setting. Usually the underlying fragments in the maxillary region are comminuted and the soft tissue is attached to the periosteum. The orbital floor can be similarly fractured. There are three basic approaches to the midface fractures. The maxillary regions can be approached via upper buccal sulcus incisions. These are made on either side as needed. One should avoid direct incision at the apex of the sulcus. Similar to the mandible approach, a cuff of mucosa and muscle should be left on the maxillary side of the incision to facilitate closure. Usually the cuff of tissue is 7 to 8 mm. Retractors are placed and tension is applied followed by an incision with the knife. The mucosa is scored. One can then cut through the muscle with a knife straight down to the bone. A strict subperiosteal dissection is then carried out in the cephalad direction. Dissection usually can be made along the medial and lateral zygomaticomaxillary buttresses because the anterior maxillary wall is usually fractured with small fragments. These fragments should be saved because they may be used for bone grafting. The infraorbital nerve is also seen and usually lies in line with the medial limbus of the eye. The buttresses can be visualized by separate upper buccal sulcus incisions on either side. The frenulum in the midline should be left intact because it is quite difficult to repair if incised. There is usually also a considerable amount of blood in the maxillary sinus, which should be irrigated and removed. After fixation has been performed, the incisions are again irrigated and closed in layers as in the mandible.

SUBCILIARY INCISIONS

The subciliary incision provides access to the inferior orbital rim, the orbital floor, and potentially to the zygomaticofrontal suture. The incision that is made is usually a skin muscle flap in a stairstep fashion. A tarsal suture can be placed in the lower eyelid. Note that a forced duction test should always be performed before any procedure involving the midface and at the end of the procedure. Usually comparison from side to side is made. With careful retraction in all directions, the incision is marked approximately 2 mm below the lash line. Using a knife, the skin only is incised. The extent of the incision that is necessary is usually from just at the level of the punctum medially to the lateral canthus. It can be extended laterally as needed. Pulling cephalad on the tarsal stitch and distally with countertraction, the skin only can be incised using sharp scissors for approximately 5 mm. This maneuver will expose the underlying orbicularis ocularis muscle. The muscle can then be dissected and incised. There is an areolar plane between the orbicularis ocularis muscle and the capsulo-palpebral fascia. If the wound has been injected, there will be minimal bleeding. The dissection is carried out down to the inferior orbital rim. The rim can be quite displaced, but if one proceeds from a medial or lateral direction towards the midline, the rim can be found. The periosteum is then incised in the inferior border of the prominence of the rim. A periosteal elevator is then used; the tissue is dissected inferiorly and the periosteum is elevated off the rim. This is done to provide some tissue for resuspension of the periosteum. Usually after dissection, it is difficult to find the periosteum, and at this point, a marking stitch can be placed in the periosteum for later identification. The dissection can be carried out along the medial and lateral buttresses and on the zygomatic body laterally.

Using careful dissection with a Cottle or Freer elevator, the orbital floor can be explored. A malleable retractor and a headlight are essential. The dissection should be carried out in a strict subperiosteal plane. Again, with multiple comminuted fragments this can be difficult, but the orbital contents are gently retracted. Note that there can be an oculobradycardia from parasympathetic stimulus with retraction of the globe. The dissection should be carried out to assess any injury to the orbital floor. This can range from a small defect in the center of the floor to complete disruption extending to the medial and lateral walls. The optic canal is approximately 42 mm directly posterior to the anterior edge of the inferior orbital rim; however, the distance can vary. If the lateral wall is followed back, usually it is a safer zone to find a posterior ledge of stable bone, which is just at the anterior lip of the lateral wall of the optic canal. Reconstruction can be performed with alloplastic materials or autograft. The preferred materials used include porous polyethylene or specially designed titanium plates. These materials are fashioned to fit into the defect with the posterior-most aspect seated on the posterior shelf of stable bone. The lateral side of the orbit can often be stable and provide a suitable shelf for the implant. The implant is then rigidly fixed to the inferior rim. The porous polyethylene implant can be fixed with a position screw or have a straight plate attached, whereas the specially designed titanium plates have limbs coming off anteriorly for rigid fixation. Bone grafts include split rib grafts or split calvarial grafts. These grafts similarly can be rigidly fixed with titanium plates. All of these materials, however, must be placed under direct vision with careful retraction of the orbit soft tissue contents.

Once all the bones have been fixed and the orbit floor reconstructed as needed, then the incision can be closed. One of the crucial elements of closure is resuspension of the periosteum on the zygomatic region (Figure 62-10). Failure to repair the periosteal attachments can lead to significant soft tissue drooping after healing, which is quite difficult to repair. Usually the previously placed marking suture identifies the periosteum. Only three or four interrupted sutures are used to resuspend the periosteum along the inferior rim or to the inferior orbital rim. Another option would be to drill holes in the inferior orbital rim and place sutures through the holes. If this is done correctly, the lower eyelids can be closed tension free with multiple interrupted fast-absorbing catgut sutures (5-0 or 6-0).

The zygomaticofrontal suture can also be accessed through the subciliary incision. The lateral canthus is taken down, and a subperiosteal dissection is carried along the lateral orbital rim; with a narrow retractor pulling in a cephalad direction, the rim can be visualized. Once the rim has been rigidly fixed, it is necessary to resuspend the lateral canthus. A good point for fixation is the middle hole of the plate, which usually

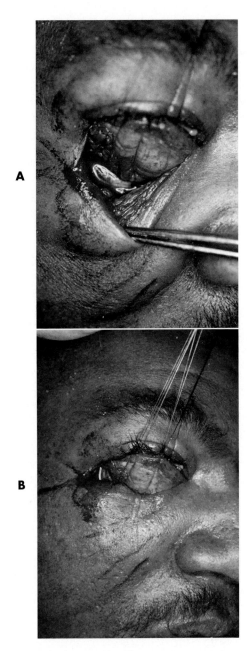

Figure 62-10. **A,** Sutures are placed into the periosteum that was degloved off the rim and **B,** pulled upward. These sutures can be tied down to the plate or to drill holes placed into the inferior rim. Although there is some portion of periosteum attached to the orbit contents that was dissected free, this edge of periosteum is usually of poor quality for good support.

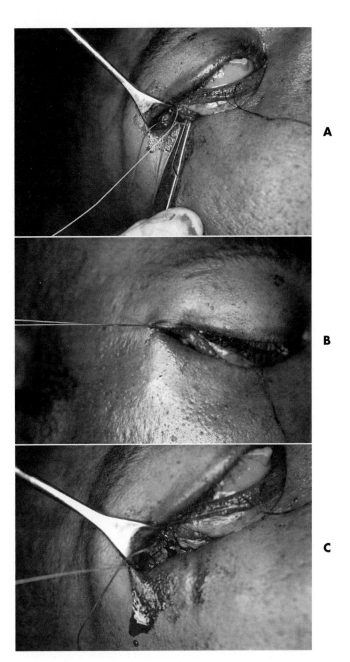

Figure 62-11. **A,** The lateral canthal tendon is grasped, and a 2-0 braided polyester suture is passed. **B,** The suture is pulled taut, and both superior and inferior tarsal plates are also tautened. **C,** The suture is then passed through the middle hole of the zygomaticofrontal plate and tied down. Because the tendon is usually grasped at just below the level of the skin, the suture in this region will bring the skin down quite close to the bone. The plate at the zygomaticofrontal suture is a good place for slight overcorrecting.

overlies the fracture site. A 2-0 braided polyester suture is placed in the lateral canthus just deep to the skin and tied down to the bone. Care must be taken so that once the suture is placed into the lateral canthus, the superior and inferior tarsus will tighten with a lateral pull. The suture can then be looped into the plate and tied down (Figure 62-11). The zygomaticofrontal suture can also be accessed through an upper blepharoplasty incision or through a direct incision overlying the fracture. If a laceration is present overlying the fracture, this opening in the skin can be extended and is usually the easiest approach.

BICORONAL INCISION

The bicoronal incision provides access to the zygomatic arch, the zygomaticofrontal suture region, and the nasoorbitalethmoid region, as well as to the frontal sinus. The bicoronal incision can be straight, have an anterior curve, or have multiple short right-angle limbs (stealth incision). Usually the limbs of the stealth incision are approximately 1.5 cm in length

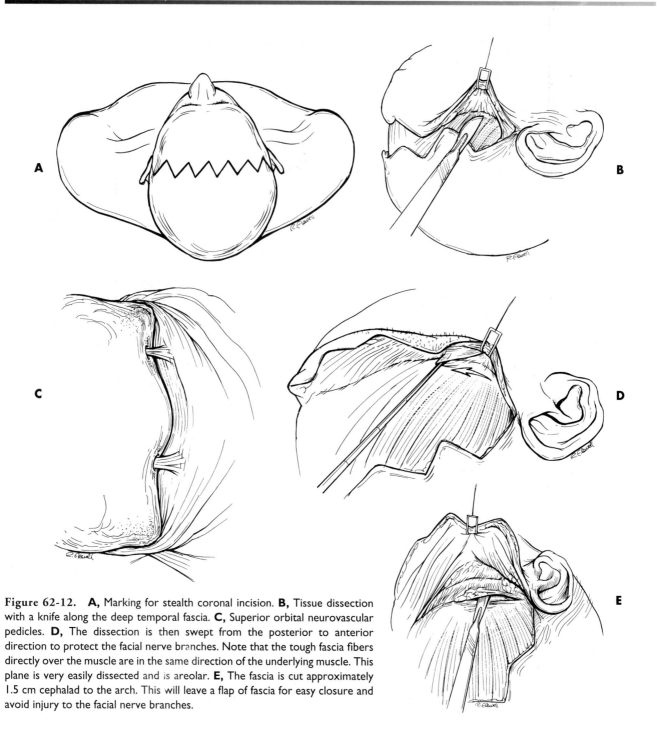

Figure 62-12. **A,** Marking for stealth coronal incision. **B,** Tissue dissection with a knife along the deep temporal fascia. **C,** Superior orbital neurovascular pedicles. **D,** The dissection is then swept from the posterior to anterior direction to protect the facial nerve branches. Note that the tough fascia fibers directly over the muscle are in the same direction of the underlying muscle. This plane is very easily dissected and is areolar. **E,** The fascia is cut approximately 1.5 cm cephalad to the arch. This will leave a flap of fascia for easy closure and avoid injury to the facial nerve branches.

and 90 degrees to each other (Figure 62-12). The hair does not need to be shaved because it can be combed to visualize the incision. The incision site is injected with epinephrine to help with hemostasis. An incision is made with a knife down to the galea, and the coronal flap is retracted anteriorly. Again, when one uses a knife, the areolar subgaleal plane can be elevated quite rapidly. When the dissection is over the temporalis muscle, care must be taken to dissect along the deep temporal fascia. This dissection can be done quite easily using a sharp knife. With retraction in the anterior direction and using a knife scoring gently through the loose superficial fascia, the

tough deep temporal fascia can be visualized. The fibers of this fascia run parallel with the muscle. The areolar plane can then be dissected with either a knife or a sharp periosteal elevator; the frontal branch of the facial nerve lies in this superficial tissue. Dissection is carried out first along the posterior aspect of the fascia down to the arch. If this dissection is carried out in a counterclockwise fashion on the right side and a clockwise fashion on the left side, the branches of the facial nerve can be protected. The superficial temporal fat can be seen through the deep temporal fascia approximately 1 to 1.5 cm cephalad to the arch itself.

Once this entire region of tissue has been elevated and the subgaleal dissection has been carried out, the bone can be exposed. Usually 2 cm from the palpable frontal orbital bandeau, the periosteum is incised and a subperiosteal dissection is performed. The supratrochlear and supraorbital neurovascular bundles are visualized. If the supraorbital neurovascular bundle is within a true foramen, it can be released by using osteotomes, allowing further retraction of the anterior flap of skin. The nasofrontal region can be visualized with strict subperiosteal dissection. Note that when there are fractures in this region, care must be taken to avoid releasing the medial canthal ligament from the bone. A majority of the time the medial canthal ligament is still attached; thus displaced bone fragments lead to telecanthus as opposed to true disruption of the tendon from the bone. Also note that the strict periosteal dissection should be carried out in a region of the trochlea because injury here is irreparable. Exposure of the arch can be performed by incising the deep temporal fascia cephalad to the arch with a knife and then cut directly down toward the arch, incising along the superior border. If the dissection is carried out superficial to the deep temporal fascia and then incised below this, a cuff of fascia is left, facilitating closure and minimizing injury to the facial nerve. The dissection is carried out along the arch from a posterior-to-anterior direction in a sweeping fashion. The approach allows excellent visualization of the upper midface and its fractures.

After adequate fixation and treatment of all the various injuries, the bicoronal flap can be closed quite rapidly. The deep temporal fascia should be resuspended. If this is not done, again there can be problematic soft tissue drooping that is quite difficult to repair. This suspension is done with a 3-0 absorbable suture in an interrupted fashion. A drain can be left. With the stealth incision, galeal sutures can be placed at the apexes only, which provide good approximation of the wound, followed by staples. An en bloc running locking suture can also be placed.

MIDFACE FRACTURES

The midface fractures include the ZMC fractures and the various Le Fort level fractures. Orbital and nasal fractures along with NOE complex fractures can be included. Frontal sinus fractures are discussed separately. Invariably, there is significant overlap with all of these fractures, and only a minority of the time are the classic Le Fort fractures seen. Usually there are multiple components of each. The classic ZMC fracture usually has a fracture at the infraorbital rim just above the inferior alveolar nerve, the zygomaticofrontal suture region, along the arch at the region of the zygomaticotemporal suture, the lateral zygomaticomaxillary buttresses, and the lateral orbit at the zygomaticosphenoid suture. The medial buttresses can be intact. The orbit floor by definition is also fractured but may not require repair because it is not comminuted or the defect is minimal. If the arch is not comminuted, reduction via subciliary and upper buccal sulcus

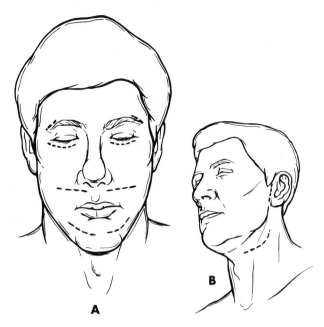

Figure 62-13. Anterior approach incisions for **A,** midface and **B,** mandible fractures.

incisions is usually all that is required (Figure 62-13). One of the keys to anatomic reduction is to visualize the zygomaticosphenoid suture during the orbital floor exploration. This is an especially important landmark when there is significant comminution to the fractures. Usually, the plates used are 1.2 or 1.3 mm along the inferior rim. A similar plate or a 1.5-mm plate at the zygomaticofrontal region and a 2-mm plate along the zygomaticomaxillary buttresses. Although the zygomaticofrontal suture allows the best rigid fixation, it is the least reliable for anatomic reduction. Once these external regions have been fixed, the orbit floor can be visualized. For smaller defects with stable ledges of bone on both sides and posteriorly, a 1.5-mm porous polyethylene implant can be used. For larger defects, split calvarial bone graft, rib graft, or an orbital floor plate can be used (Figure 62-14).

True bilateral Le Fort I fractures require application of arch bars and MMF after reduction of the maxillary segment. The maxillary segment can be reduced with disimpaction forceps. Once it has been done, there is usually good alignment of the fractures, and 2-mm plates can be placed at each of the medial and lateral buttresses. A Le Fort II level fracture is differentiated from the Le Fort I level fracture in that, with manipulation of the maxilla, the entire nasal complex moves in the Le Fort II fracture (Figure 62-15). Again, with minimal or no comminution, these can be plated across the fractures. The Le Fort III level fractures can be approached similarly to the ZMC fracture. When there are multiple segments of the various Le Fort fractures on either one side or both and there is severe comminution, all the fracture segments can be temporarily reduced with interosseus wires and then assessed at the key points of anatomic reduction, followed by rigid fixation. Should there be comminution or medial displacement with difficulty in reduction of the arch, a bicoronal incision is needed.

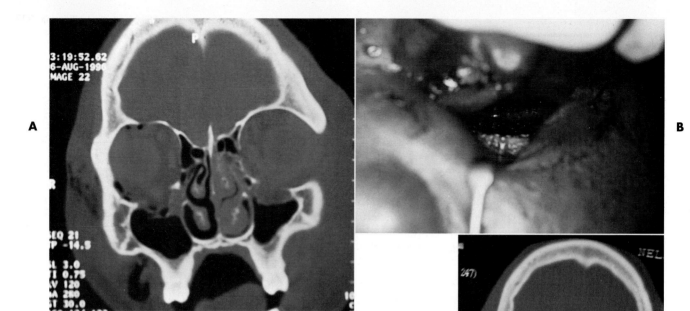

Figure 62-14. **A,** Coronal CT showing bilateral orbit floor fractures. **B,** Specialized titanium orbit floor plate placed on the floor with the posterior aspect sitting on the lateral portion of the anterior-most bone of the optic canal. The plate is placed under direct vision and then rigidly fixed to the anterior rim. **C,** Postoperative CT shows anatomic alignment of the orbital floor plates.

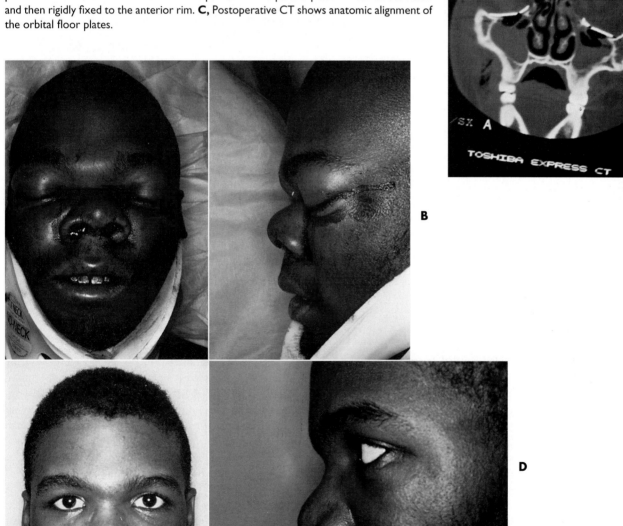

Figure 62-15. **A,** Front view of patient with classic bilateral Le Fort II fractures. The midface is impacted with the pyramidal fracture pattern across the nasofrontal region. **B,** Lateral view. **C,** Postoperative frontal and **D,** lateral views.

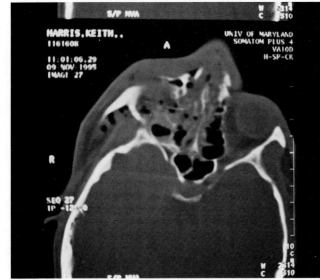

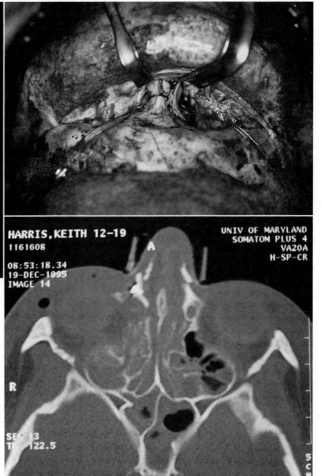

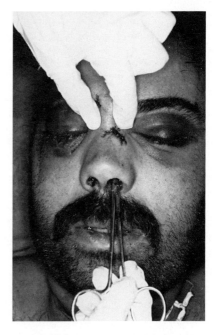

Figure 62-16. **A,** NOE fracture with displacement. **B,** Fracture fragments are shown with transnasal wires passed from side to side. One wire is passed anteriorly and the second wire is passed posteriorly. The two ends are twisted together to compress the segment. If the medial canthal ligament is detached, it can be reattached to the wires as they are twisted down. A 2-0 braided polyester suture is used. **C,** Postoperative CT scan.

Simple nasal fractures can be taken care of by closed reduction. However, complex displaced nasal fractures will require more treatment, such as immediate bone grafting using split calvarial bone graft or rib graft. This provides good projection and minimizes the need for secondary nasal reconstruction. NOE fractures can be one of the most challenging regions to repair. Usually the fragments are quite small and comminuted. If care has been taken to avoid stripping of the medial canthal ligament, one can place transnasal wires. Usually, two wires can be placed. A 26-gauge wire is placed transnasally in the NOE region posteriorly, and then a second wire can be placed 4 to 5 mm anterior to this. Once these two wires, which are parallel to each other, are placed, these can be twisted down on either side. If the medial canthal ligament is detached, it can then be sutured with a 2-0 braided polyester suture and tied to the wires. As these are twisted down, the bone segments will then close (Figures 62-16 and 62-17). It is best to seemingly overcorrect the medial canthal ligament to reattachment; as the soft tissues relax, overcorrection is rarely a problem.[33,42,43] If there are clear fractures that are not comminuted, these bony segments can be plated. Nasal bone grafting requires scissor dissection in a blunt fashion across the dorsum of the nose, staying superficial to the bone and the cartilage, creating a pocket for graft placement.

Figure 62-17. Test for stability of NOE segment. A mosquito clamp is placed into the nasal passage and the segment is tested with bimanual palpation. It is important to place the fingers (of the left hand here) posteriorly into the lacrimal crest region to achieve a true test.

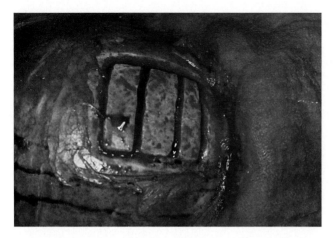

Figure 62-18. Split calvarial bone graft. Multiple strips are taken. The trough is first made with a round bur down into the diploë layer. The best place for grafts is in the parietal bone segment at least 1.5 cm away from the sagittal suture and preferably away from any of the other sutures. A pineapple bur is then used to smooth off the edges. A curved osteotome is used to get the split started, and then a straight osteotome is used. The osteotome needs to be parallel to the skull and the position changed frequently around the periphery of the graft as multiple small advances of the osteotome are made until the graft is split off. Usually 40-mm grafts can be split without breaking.

Usually this requires harvesting a 40-mm segment of split calvarial bone graft (Figure 62-18). This can be approximately 3 to 4 mm in diameter and beveled on either side for a smooth contour. A notch can be burred proximally so it will seat into the nasofrontal region. The graft is rigidly fixed in a cantilever fashion.

FRONTAL SINUS

Frontal sinus fractures are approached through bicoronal incisions. At times, open frontal sinus fractures have a large enough incision to allow a direct approach. The keys to the treatment of frontal sinus fractures are the nasofrontal ducts and the posterior table. If the nasofrontal ducts are compromised, the frontal sinus will need to be defunctionalized. This means that the mucosa needs to be removed and the nasofrontal ducts obliterated. If frontal bone flaps are removed for repair of dural tears or evacuation of a hematoma, the frontal sinus can be cranialized. This would include removal of all the posterior table of the frontal sinus and plugging of the nasofrontal ducts. This can be done with split calvarial bone graft or can be harvested from the posterior table of the frontal bone flap. If the entire ethmoid roof is destroyed, plugging will not work, and a large bone graft can be contoured to seat as a new ethmoid roof. All of these repairs can be covered with a pericranial flap. If the posterior table is intact and the nasofrontal ducts are plugged, the frontal sinus is obliterated. Various substances have been used, including fat, cancellous bone graft, methyl-

methacrylate, and hydroxyapatite. Whichever modality is used for obliteration, it is of utmost importance that all the mucosa be removed. This is done with a curette and a diamond burr to smooth all the surfaces of the sinus. There are invaginations of the mucosa into the bone, which can be problematic in the future.[41]

OUTCOMES

ORBIT

The reported incidents of blindness after facial trauma have been between 0.67% and 3%.[49] Another reported rare complication is cavernous sinus carotid fistula. The usual signs of ophthalmoplegia and auditive homolateral sensation, along with proptosis and potentially a pulsatile globe, are present.[34] The more usual problems that develop are convergence insufficiency and postoperative enophthalmos. Convergence insufficiency can be as high as 21%, of which 82% may recover by 6 months with the remaining being potentially permanent.[1] This may be due to neurologic injury versus extraocular muscle injury or a combination of both. For management outcome of orbit fractures, one must consider repair versus nonrepair.[36,38,47] One of the keys to preventing enophthalmos is proper anatomic alignment and restoring orbital volume. It is hoped that this can prevent postoperative enophthalmos. There is a higher percentage of patients with postoperative enophthalmos when the initial injury is not corrected. In the past, it has been thought that the fat atrophies leads to enophthalmos, but the main culprit is most likely incomplete restoration of orbital volume. The usual sites are posterior on the medial or lateral side. There is either nonrestoration of the medial wall or incomplete alignment of the lateral wall at the zygomatic sphenoid junction. In one study in which the orbital volume was measured, there was a mean difference of 17.9% between the normal side and the side with the enophthalmos. There was a measured increase in volume between 3.4 ml and 7.1 ml for 2.5 to 3 and 3.5 to 5 mm, respectively. There was no evidence of fat atrophy.[39]

FRONTAL SINUS FRACTURES

The usual complications of frontal sinus fractures include infection, postoperative deformity, and mucopyocele.[23] In a recent study, 71 patients were treated and bone graft was used in all. Meningitis occurred in two patients, and a mucopyocele occurred in one patient. There has been considerable debate over the years as to what is the best substance for obliteration. The complication rates should be relatively low. The key to an obliteration may be less in the substance used and more in the preparation. It is essential that the communication between the nose and the front sinus cavity be blocked and that all of the mucosa be removed. Invariably, when there is a mucopyocele or a mucocele that has developed, it is from an incomplete removal. Nonsurgical treatment of frontal sinus fractures has had complication rates of approximately 10%. When the complications occur, however, they can be quite significant and difficult with which to deal. The general consensus is to err on the side of treating frontal sinus fractures.[48]

ZYGOMATICOMAXILLARY COMPLEX FRACTURES

The functional deficit from nonrepair of the ZMC fractures exclusive of the orbit, nose, and condyle is largely related to maintaining facial width and projection. There can be persistent paresthesia or anesthesia in the infraorbital nerve distribution. As many as one third of patients can have significant degrees of injury to the nerve, with more likely resolution after repair versus nonrepair.[46] This makes a case for operative intervention and reduction of the fracture with decompression of the infraorbital foramen. The zygomatic arch and its relationship to midface fractures for the reconstitution of the proper orbitozygomatic relationships are quite important.

MANDIBLE FRACTURES

Mandible fractures can be one of most frustrating parts of craniofacial surgery. Complications include function, infection, occlusion, and neurologic complications. There can be occlusal interference as high as 38% in patients with teeth left in the line of fracture. However, when the same criteria are used in healthy volunteers, as many as 28% of those can have similar problems. These can be corrected with minor procedures. This further illustrates the difficulty of evaluating occlusal problems because many times minor occlusal interference can be treated with grinding and are not counted as complications. It has been implied that mandibular third molars increase fracture rates. When evaluated retrospectively, patients with mandibular third molars have an approximately 3.8-fold increase in angle fractures compared with those who do not. Many times it is worthwhile to remove the third molar when it is included in the line of fracture because it is not necessary for occlusion.[45] Furthermore, the infection rate of mandibular fractures with miniplate (i.e., semirigid versus rigid fixation) can be significantly different. Infection rates as high as 12.3% versus 2.3% have been reported for miniplate versus rigid fixation, respectively. The removal rate is also higher for the miniplate fixation. The potential for facial nerve injury, however, is higher for rigid plate fixation; this is largely related to the approach used. The difficult mandible fracture to care for is the atrophic edentulous mandible.[44] Various approaches have been used with success. Approximately 7% of these fractures have required acute bone grafting. Overall there is a 96.5% rate of primary healing (in all groups). Those who had nonunions were in the severely atrophic (less than 10 mm) group.[27]

PANFACIAL FRACTURES

Overall, the outcome of panfacial fractures is quite difficult to assess. Invariably, its management is the sum of its parts; if a careful steplike approach is carried out, as has been advocated,[29,32] optimal results can be obtained. The key to restoration of the facial fractures is the proper anatomic realignment and rigid fixation of the bony skeleton. The soft tissue will follow. It must be stressed, however, that the soft tissue must be repaired also.

REFERENCES

1. al-Quainy IA: Convergence insufficiency and failure of accommodation following midfacial trauma, *Br J Oral Maxillofac Surg* 33:71-75, 1995.
2. Berne JC, Butler PE, Brady FA: Cervical spine injuries in patients with facial fractures: a 1-year prospective study, *Int J Oral Maxillofac Surg* 24:26-29, 1995.
3. Birrer RB, Robinson T, Papachristos P: Orbital emphysems: how common, how significant? *Ann Emerg Med* 24:1115-1118, 1994.
4. Buchbinder D: Treatment of fractures of the edentulous mandible, 1943 to 1993: a review of the literature, *J Oral Maxillofac Surg* 51:1174-1180, 1993.
5. Campiglio GL, Gignorini M, Candiani P: Superior orbital fissure syndrome complicating zygomatic fractures. Pathogenesis and report of a case, *Scand J Plast Reconstr Surg Hand Surg* 29:69-72, 1995.
6. Chu L, Gussack GS, Muller T: A treatment protocol for mandible fractures, *J Trauma* 36:48-52, 1994.
7. Cohen SR, Leonard DK, Markowitz BL, et al: Acrylic splints for dental alignment in complex facial injuries, *Ann Plast Surg* 31:406-412, 1993.
8. David DJ, Simpson DA: *Craniomaxillofacial trauma,* New York, 1995, Churchill Livingstone.
9. Ellis E III: Complications of rigid internal fixation for mandibular fractures, *J Craniomax Trauma* 2:32-39, 1996.
10. Ellis E III: Treatment methods for fractures of the mandibular angle, *J Craniomax Trauma* 2:28-36, 1996.
11. Ellis E III, Dean J: Rigid fixation of mandibular condyle fractures, *Oral Surg* 76:6-15, 1993.
12. Ellis E III, Sinn DP: Treatment of mandibular angle fractures usng two 2.4 mm dynamic compression plates, *J Oral Maxillofac Surg* 51:969-973, 1993.
13. Evans GR, Clark N, Manson PN: Identification and management of minimally displaced nasoethmoidal orbital fractures, *Ann Plast Surg* 35:469-473, 1995.
14. Giudice M, Colella G, Marra A: The complications and outcomes of fractures of the orbital-maxillary-zygomatic complex, *Minerva Stomatol* 43:37-41, 1994.
15. Glassman RD, Manson PN, Vander Kolk CA, et al: Rigid fixation of internal orbital fractures, *Plast Reconstr Surg* 86:1103-1109, 1990.

16. Gruss JS, Mackinnon SE: Complex maxillary fractures: the role of buttress reconstruction and immediate bone grafting, *Plast Reconstr Surg* 75:17-24, 1985.

17. Gruss JS, Van Wyck L, Phillips JH, et al: The importance of the zygomatic arch in complex midfacial fracture repair and correction of posttraumatic orbitozygomatic deformities, *Plast Reconstr Surg* 85:878-890, 1990.

18. Huag RH, Schwimmer A: Fibrous union of the mandible: a review of 27 patients, *J Oral Maxillofac Surg* 52:832-839, 1994.

19. Jackson IT: Classification and treatment of orbitozygomatic and orbitoethmoid fractures. The place of bone grafting and plate fixation, *Clin Plast Surg* 16:77-91, 1989.

20. Jayamanne DG, Gillie RF: Do patients with midfacial trauma to the orbito-zygomatic region also sustain significant ocular injuries? *J R Coll Surg Edinb* 41:200-203, 1996.

21. Jimenez DF, Sundrani S, Barone CM: Posttraumatic anosmia in craniofacial trauma, *J Craniomax Trauma* 3:8-15, 1997.

22. Koury ME, Perrott DH, Kaban LB: The use of rigid internal fixation in mandibular fractures complicated by osteomyelitis, *J Oral Maxillofac Surg* 52:1114-1119, 1994.

23. Larrabee WF, Travis LW, Tabb HG: Injuries of the nasofrontal orifices in frontal sinus fractures, *Laryngoscope* 97:728-731, 1987.

24. Lauer SA: Commentary: management of traumatic optic neuropathy, *J Craniomax Trauma* 2:27, 1996.

25. Le Fort R: Etude experimental sur les fractures de la machoire superiore, Parts I,II,III, *Rev Chir (Paris)* 23:208, 1901.

26. Lin KY, Bartlett SP, Yaremchuk MJ, et al: The effect of rigid fixation on the survival of onlay bone grafts: an experimental study, *Plast Reconstr Surg* 86:449-456, 1990.

27. Luhr HG, Reidick T, Merten HA: Results of treatment of fractures of the atrophic edentulous mandible by compression plating: a retrospective evaluation of 84 cases, *J Oral Maxillofac Surg* 54:250-254, 1996.

28. Manson PN, Markowitz B, Mirvis S, et al: Toward CT-based facial fracture treatment, *Plast Reconstr Surg* 85:202-212, 1990.

29. Manson PN, Clark N, Robertson B, et al: Comprehensive management of pan-facial fractures, *J Craniomax Trauma* 1:43-56, 1995.

30. Manson PN, Glassman D, Vander Kolk C, et al: Rigid stabilization of sagittal fractures of the maxilla and palate, *Plast Reconstr Surg* 85:711-717, 1990.

31. Manson PN, Glassman D, Illiff NT, et al: Rigid fixation of orbital fractures, *Plast Reconstr Surg* 86:1103-1109, 1990.

32. Manson PN, Hoopes JE, Su CT: Structural pillars of the facial skeleton: an approach to the management of Le Fort fractures, *Plast Reconstr Surg* 66:54-61, 1980.

33. Markowitz B, Manson PN, Sargent L: Management of the medial canthal ligament in nasoethmoidal orbital fractures, *Plast Reconstr Surg* 87:843, 1991.

34. Nocini P, Lo Muzio L, Cortelazzi R, et al: Cavernous sinus-carotid fistula: a complication of maxillofacial surgery, *Int J Oral Maxillofac Surg* 24:276-278, 1995.

35. Paskert JP, Manson PN: The bimanual examination for assessing instability in naso-orbito-ethmoidal injuries, *Plast Reconstr Surg* 83:165-167, 1989.

36. Pearl RM: Surgical management of volumetric changes in the bony orbit, *Ann Plast Surg* 19:349-358, 1987.

37. Rohrich RJ, Hollier LH, Watumull D: Optimizing the management of orbitozygomatic fractures, *Clin Plast Surg* 19:149-165, 1992.

38. Roncevic R, Stajcic Z: Surgical treatment of posttraumatic enophthalmos: a study of 72 patients, *Ann Plast Surg* 32:288-294, 1994.

39. Schuknecht B, Carls F, Valavanis A, et al: CT assessment of orbital volume in late post-traumatic enophthalmos, *Neuroradiology* 38:470-475, 1996.

40. Spoor TC, McHenry JG: Management of traumatic optic neuropathy, *J Craniomax Trauma* 2:14-26, 1996.

41. Stevens M, Kline SN: Management of frontal sinus fractures, *J Craniomax Trauma* 1:29-37, 1995.

42. Stranc MF: Primary treatment of naso-ethmoid injuries with increased inter-canthal distance, *Br J Plast Surg* 28:8, 1970.

43. Stranc MF, Robertson GA: A classification of injuries of the nasal skeleton, *Ann Plast Surg* 2:468-474, 1979.

44. Thaller SR: Fractures of the edentulous mandible: a retrospective review, *J Craniofac Surg* 4:91-94, 1993.

45. Thaller SR, Mabourakh S: Teeth located in the line of mandibular fracture, *J Craniofac Surg* 5:16-19, 1994.

46. Vriens JP, Moos KF: Morbidity of the infraorbital nerve following orbitozygomatic complex fractures, *J Craniomaxillofac Surg* 23:363-368, 1995.

47. Wolfe SA: Treatment of post-traumatic orbital deformities, *Clin Plast Surg* 15:225-238, 1988.

48. Wolfe SA, Johnson P: Frontal sinus injuries: primary care and management of late complications, *Plast Reconstr Surg* 82:781-789, 1988.

49. Zachariades N, Papavassiliou D, Christopoulos P: Blindness after facial trauma, *Oral Surg Oral Med Oral Pathol Oral Radiol Endod* 81:34-37, 1996.

50. Zide MF, Kent JN: Indications for open reduction of mandibular condyle fractures, *J Oral Maxillofac Surg* 41:89-98, 1983.

CHAPTER

Pediatric Facial Trauma

Kevin J. Kelly

INTRODUCTION

The purpose of this chapter is to familiarize the reader with pediatric fracture management. Each region of the face is discussed. This includes appropriate clinical findings, indications, and operations for a particular injury. Outcomes vary, depending on many different factors. Some potential outcomes of these injuries and treatments are discussed in each section.

By definition of The American Academy of Pediatrics, pediatric medicine deals with the age-group of birth to 21 years of age. How fractures are handled in children and areas of similarities and differences between adult and pediatric treatment are addressed.

Many bones of the facial and cranial skeleton in children can be secured with plate and screw fixation as early as 3 months of age. However, the developing dentition and skeletal changes occurring in a growing child make management of pediatric facial fractures a great challenge. Many of the rigid plate and screw fixation techniques that are used in adults are not easily applied with similar fractures in children because they may cause injury or disruption of the developing dentition or bony skeleton. Therefore the management of pediatric fractures becomes a science unto itself.

Automobile accidents are the greatest cause of facial fractures in the adult population. When studying the etiology of facial fractures in children at Vanderbilt University Medical Center (a Level I Trauma Referral Center), we also found that motor vehicle accidents were responsible for most children's facial fractures, 65% (Figure 63-1). The frequency of fracture types varies between the pediatric and adult populations. In the adult population, nasal bone fractures are the most frequent facial fractures. In contrast, mandible fractures are the highest percentage of bony injuries in children, 31% (Figure 63-2). The adult nose is very prominent. If an adult is struck in the face, the nose is most often the first place that would be impacted and fractured. With children, the mandible, although relatively small, is most often fractured. There is also a tremendous amount of cartilage in a pediatric nose, enabling it to flex rather than to fracture. In evaluating pediatric trauma and following children from birth to 16 years of age, we see

that, as children get older, more fractures are seen (Figure 63-3). In the early years of life, children are in a protected environment. As they start getting older, children become active, playing sports, climbing trees, and having more contact with other children. Although there is some variability in fracture frequency studies from different centers around the country, this may reflect the nature of the referral pattern in a particular city and the socioeconomic status of the population in that region. Numbers of fractures may vary, depending on the age of the study. Studies including the 1970s and 1980s may not reflect the effect of intense public education efforts to place children in automobile restraint seats.

Facial fractures are rare in children. Of all pediatric trauma admissions, facial fractures make up less than 5%. Head injuries make up about 60%.[7,15] In children, there is a much greater incidence of skull fractures than facial fractures. This can be understood if we look at the facial-to-cranial proportions of children. There is a much greater cranial volume–to–facial volume ratio in children than in adults.[8,34] If a child sustains a frontal impact, he or she has a much greater chance of sustaining a skull fracture than a facial injury. In an adult's head, there is a significant increase in the facial bone–to–cranial bone ratio (Figure 63-4). An adult is therefore more apt to fracture facial bones than cranial bones.[15]

At birth, the cranial-to-facial proportion is about 8 to 1. An adult has a cranial-to-facial proportion of about 2 to 1.[8,30] Therefore, in addition to overall surface area increases with growth, there is a significant change in the cranial-to-facial proportions as one grows older.

When a child does sustain a facial bone fracture, it is most often a greenstick fracture. Greenstick fractures are more common in children than in adults. Children's bones seem to be more elastic. There are also rudimentary paranasal sinuses (see the more extensive discussion in the Maxillary Fractures section). Large cartilaginous growth centers contribute to more flexibility of facial bones.[7] The small facial-to-cranial ratio increases the potential that force from an impact may be directed to the cranium, therefore decreasing the direct force to the face. There is a greater cancellous–to–cortical bone ratio in children's bones, which also leads to more greenstick injuries.[32,33] There is thinner cortical bone with ill-defined margins between the medullary and cortical bones in children.

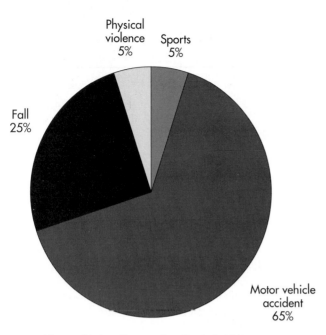

Figure 63-1. Causes of pediatric facial fractures.

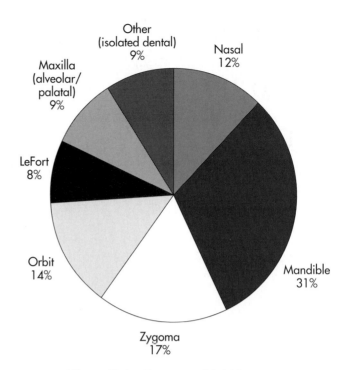

Figure 63-2. Frequency of facial fractures.

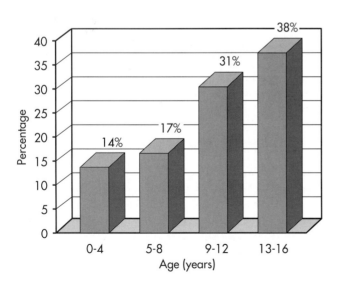

Figure 63-3. Fracture trends with age.

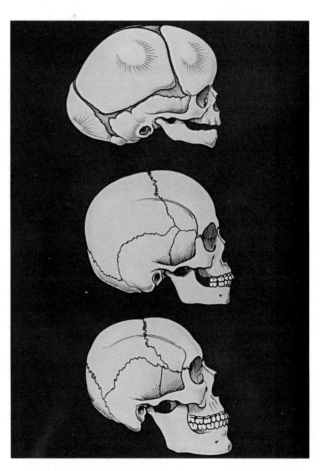

Figure 63-4. Cranial-to-facial proportions in the skull of a newborn, a 5-year-old, and an adult. The cranial-to-facial ratio at birth is 8:1. At 5 years of age, the ratio is 4:1, and by adulthood, the ratio becomes 2:1. Note that the frontal bone is more prominent the younger a child is.

A child's skeleton has very active growth occurring, so all of the soft cellular matrix involved with growth has a tendency to be more flexible than the dense, more brittle bones of the adult skeleton.[28] Although it has often been cited in the literature that there is more subcutaneous fat in children's faces than in those of adults, resulting in more greenstick injuries, it is unlikely this small difference provides enough of a cushion to change the course of a facial impact. A factor that does play a role is the high tooth-to-bone ratio in children (Figure 63-5). Developing tooth buds fill a tremendous amount of the mandible and midface of children. Even though part of a tooth bud is hard tissue, what generates the tooth as it develops is a rich soft tissue matrix. This adds a tremendous amount of flexibility to these areas of the mandible and maxilla, therefore making fractures less common in these regions of the face than in adults and more likely to be greenstick if the bone does fracture.

During clinical examination to diagnose fractures, we use the same parameters for children that we do for adults (i.e., palpation and x-rays). With children, it is much more difficult to obtain a good clinical examination. The physician should deal with children in such a way as to develop their trust so they will allow an examination. A normal child coming into the office at 3 years of age for an elective examination can sometimes be a challenge. A child who has experienced a tremendous amount of trauma and is suddenly sitting in a frightening emergency room is under a great deal of stress. The same is true when obtaining x-rays. It is very difficult to get a good series of films. Despite the difficulty, the physician should make certain not to accept studies that are less than optimal. It may be necessary to sedate a child, even to the point of placing him or her under general anesthesia, to get a thorough physical examination and adequate x-rays. One should never formulate a treatment plan with less-than-optimal films or a less-than-optimal physical examination.

OPERATIONS AND INDICATIONS

DENTAL AND ALVEOLAR BONE INJURIES

The discussion of dental anatomy, dental injuries, and replantation of teeth in children is a vast topic beyond the scope of this chapter[1,2,20]; however, some facts must be emphasized because they pertain to children's facial fractures. When dealing with dental injuries, it is important to remember that children's deciduous teeth (the primary teeth) are space maintainers. Each pediatric tooth maintains a place for the eruption of an adult tooth (Figure 63-6). If a child has lost a molar, it can have a significant effect on disrupting the normal development of the entire adult dental arch. Too often, I have

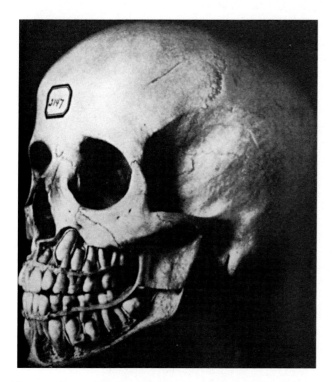

Figure 63-5. The cross-section of the maxilla and the mandible in a 3½- to 4-year-old. Note the high tooth-to-bone ratio. (From Dufresne CR, Manson PN: Pediatric facial trauma In McCarthy JG [ed]: *Plastic surgery,* ed 2, Philadelphia, 1990, WB Saunders.)

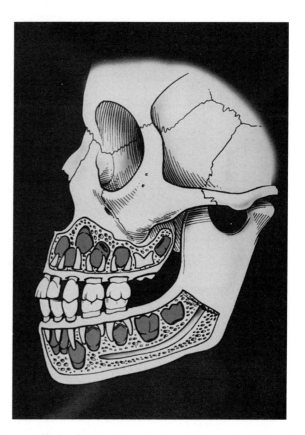

Figure 63-6. Relationship of the deciduous teeth to the developing adult tooth buds. Each deciduous tooth maintains a place for eruption of an adult tooth. The loss of one of these deciduous teeth will result in drift of the adult dentition as it erupts, potentially disrupting the normal configuration of the dental arch of the maxilla and mandible.

heard a surgeon say if confronted with a loose or avulsed deciduous tooth, "It's only a baby tooth; just discard it, it's not important." Although there is not an indication to replant a deciduous tooth, it is imperative to consider maintaining the space it once occupied. When confronted with a lost deciduous tooth as a result of trauma, the physician must refer that child to a pediatric dentist. The dentist can make a cantilevered apparatus that will maintain that space. Therefore, when the adult dentition erupts, it can develop in a normal position. This also holds true for the loss of adult teeth in the mixed dentition stage. It is imperative to maintain space to avoid shifting of the dentition. Some surgeons may also rationalize that it is not important if the occlusion is off a little and that children can always get orthodontics later to align or correct a bite. A full-mouth orthodontic reconstruction may cost $4000 to $5000 and require more than a year of orthodontic braces. Most children are self-conscious about braces, and in light of the expense, it is a shame to commit a child to that course because he or she was not sent to a dentist to have a $150 space maintainer made.

Intact, evulsed permanent teeth in children should be replanted in an attempt to save them if they meet the criteria for replantation.[1,2] They are secured to an arch bar or acrylic splint.

There will be times when the surgeon is unable to salvage intact teeth. If there is an alveolar injury where the supporting bone is lost (Figure 63-7, A and B), it is not possible to place the root back into soft tissue alone and expect it to survive. The tooth needs to be removed and the wound closed to obtain as water-tight a seal as possible. Injury to the primary dentition may transmit force superiorly to the developing, underlying adult tooth buds (Figure 63-7, C). Parents must be warned that an injury such as this may result in abnormal eruption or no eruption of the developing adult teeth in this region of the mouth.

Isolated alveolar fractures bearing secure teeth are managed by stabilizing the involved dentition to adjacent teeth in stable bone. This is accomplished by using an arch bar or acrylic splint.

MANDIBULAR INJURIES

Mandibular Body, Symphysis, and Ramus

Children with mandibular fractures may present with the same clinical findings seen in adults with similar injuries. Pain, edema, malocclusion, intraoral lacerations, hematoma, facial lacerations, paresthesias, and tenderness can all be clues to the

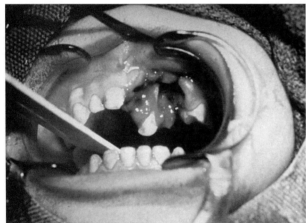
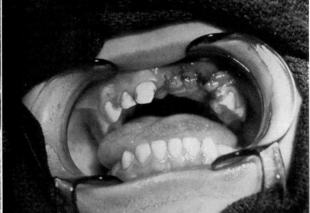
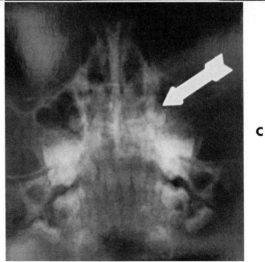

Figure 63-7.   **A,** A traumatic injury to the alveolus of a child, resulting in the evulsion of bone. Note exposed tooth root superiorly. **B,** Soft tissue closure after extraction of the tooth. **C,** Developing adult tooth bud in the maxilla along the piriform rim deep to the traumatized region. Transmission of force to this tooth bud can disrupt its development.

nature of a fracture. Most pediatric mandibular fractures will be nondisplaced greenstick injuries. These should be managed with a conservative approach when possible, which consists of a soft diet and careful observation. Careful observation does not mean seeing the child in the emergency room, putting him or her on a soft diet, and seeing him or her again in 6 weeks. It means watching the child on a weekly basis. If there is any change in the occlusion when following the child and the occlusion does not look perfect, the surgeon must do another x-ray examination of the child and make certain that he or she has not had some distraction of the fracture, which would require a more aggressive treatment.

Infants are in a protected environment, making fractures rare, although with child abuse on the rise, more infant injuries are being seen. Infants are already on liquid or soft diets. A greenstick fracture is easily managed conservatively by continuing the normal diet and observation. With unstable fractures

of the infant mandible (or maxilla), the surgeon must rely on splint fixation because there is no dentition erupted to use for maxillomandibular fixation. There is almost no indication to open an infant's fracture because the abundance of developing teeth in the bone makes fixation almost impossible without damaging these structures. The outcome with a conservative approach is very good. The fractures heal rapidly and the children function well.

The first deciduous teeth, the incisors, erupt in children at about 6 months of age (Figure 63-8). As the incisors continue to develop, the molars begin to erupt, followed by the cuspids. An important thing to understand is the root developed in the primary dentition. At about 3 years of age, and until about the age of 6, there is enough tooth root to be able to secure a primary tooth to an arch bar without avulsing it and obtain support for the arch bars for maxillomandibular fixation. After the age of 12, maxillomandibular fixation with arch bars can be established in the same way that it is in adults because the adult

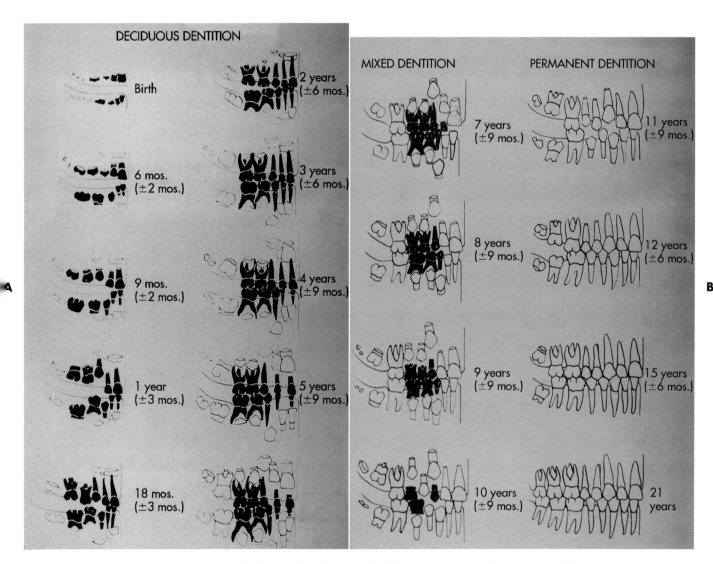

Figure 63-8. **A** and **B,** Stages of deciduous and adult dentition from birth to 21 years of age. (From Graber TM: Growth and development. In Graber TM [ed]: *Orthodontics principles and practice,* Philadelphia, 1972, WB Saunders.)

dentition has erupted and root formation has matured enough to provide necessary support.

Between 6 and 12 years of age is a stage of mixed dentition (adult and primary teeth together in the oral cavity) when obtaining support for an arch bar to place a patient in maxillomandibular fixation using the teeth becomes very difficult. In this age-group, children are starting to resorb the roots of the primary dentition and are starting to have various stages of eruption of the adult dentition. Thus the roots of the primary teeth are disappearing, but the roots of the adult teeth are not yet well formed. Therefore, if the physician places a wire around a tooth that does not have adequate root support, as the wire is tightened firmly, it may evulse that tooth. It is frustrating to be trying to place an arch bar and then suddenly find that as the surgeon tightens the dental wires, he or she is left holding a collection of free teeth and has no support for the arch bar (Figure 63-9). Although from age 6 to age 12, the surgeon may be able to gently apply an arch bar without avulsing the teeth and place the patient in maxillomandibular fixation, if that child tries to open his or her mouth, those teeth may wind up ligated to the arch bar and out of the gingiva, leaving a loose arch bar.

The very early stages of resorption of the primary dentition roots are at about 5 years of age. The first adult tooth (first molar), which starts to appear at about 6 years of age, does not have well-formed roots. In addition, the crown is not very prominent through the gingiva; therefore it is difficult to get a wire below the height of tooth contour to stabilize an arch bar. As a child progresses in age, he or she loses more of the roots of the primary dentition while the adult dentition slowly starts to develop more root structure. From 6 to 12 years of age, there is a tremendous amount of flux in the development and stability of teeth caused by the various stages of root development; this may vary from child to child. A surgeon must have a thorough understanding of the developing dentition to manage maxillomandibular fixation and fractures in children.

It is difficult to recall the exact configuration of each tooth root at each age even when working with the dentition daily. Therefore it will be helpful to use an x-ray to evaluate the dentition. A Panorex can be extremely helpful (Figure 63-10). Evaluate each of the teeth. Assess which teeth have stable roots and which teeth are starting to lose their root support. The occlusal fixation has to be planned based on where the child is in terms of dental development. (If the surgeon intends to open a fracture, this Panorex can also help assess where developing tooth buds are to avoid injuring them.) Some older techniques, such as splints and circumferential bone wires, which were once used for adult fractures, are still used to secure maxillomandibular fixation in children when teeth will not provide stability for an arch bar. An acrylic splint is fabricated and the patient placed into fixation, stabilizing the splint by securing it to the bone using circumferential wires (circummandibular wires, orbital rim wires, cranial suspension wires, circumzygomatic wires, piriform aperture wires, or nasal spine wires) (Figure 63-11). All of these circumferential wires provide a means to stabilize the splint to the teeth, then stabilize the splint to the next most stable section of the facial skeleton. Therefore the surgeon can establish maxillomandibular fixation (normal occlusion), which is a critical step in fracture treatment while taking stress off the dentition. This technique may also afford an opportunity to stabilize a fracture without doing an open reduction (Figure 63-12).

It is often helpful to place a maxillary and mandibular arch bar and secure it to stable bone using a circumferential bone wiring technique (this provides direct bone support for the arch bar and does not rely on the dentition for support). Then a splint can be placed into position and maxillomandibular fixation can be applied by wiring from the upper to the lower

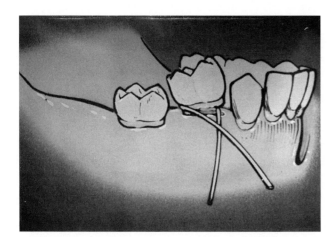

Figure 63-9. Attempting ligation of deciduous teeth with significant root resorption can result in avulsion of those teeth. Understanding the stages of dental development of each child is critical for managing fractures.

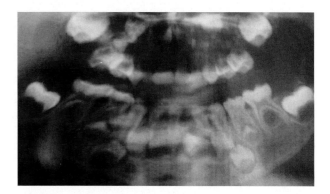

Figure 63-10. A Panorex can be extremely helpful for evaluating the deciduous and adult dentition at the various stages of development. Note that this is useful not only for planning maxillomandibular fixation but also to help identify the position of the tooth buds to avoid injury should open reduction and internal fixation be necessary.

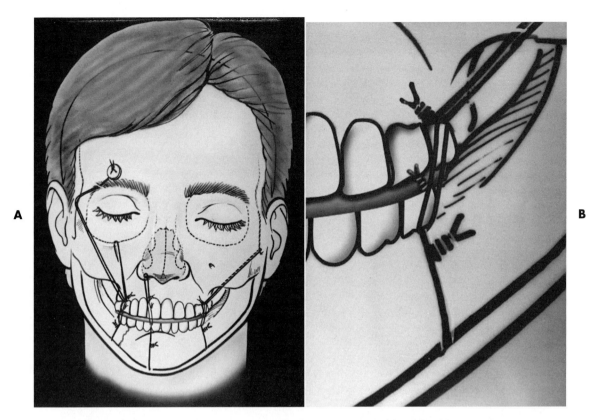

Figure 63-11. A, Options for circumferential bone wire techniques: circummandibular, infraorbital rim, piriform rim, cranial suspension wire, and circumzygomatic technique to stabilize splint fixation for maxillomandibular immobilization. Ideally, three points of fixation should be used on each side of the splint to stabilize it (three wires around the mandible, and three wires from the midface). **B,** Note use of interpositional wire securing the upper circumferential bone wire to the lower mandibular wires.

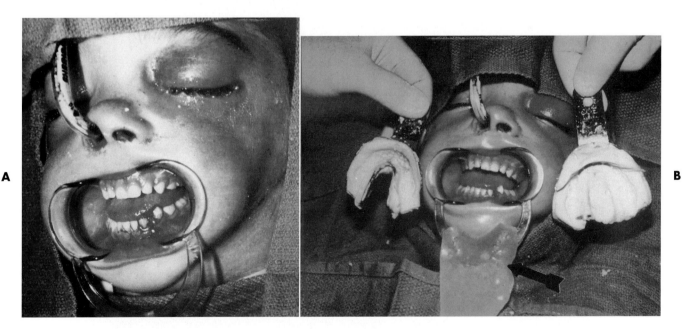

Figure 63-12. A, A child with a displaced left mandibular parasymphyseal fracture. **B,** Upper and lower geltrate impressions. The arrow depicts a wax bite registration to determine the relationship of the upper to the lower dentition on the nonfractured side. (The vast majority of children will require anesthetic to facilitate taking these impressions. They will not tolerate having this done under local anesthetic.)

Continued

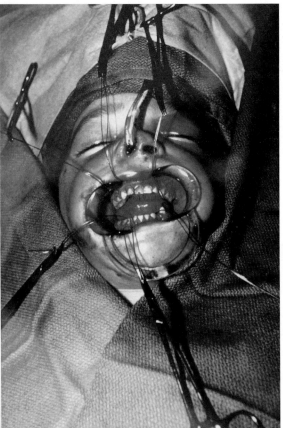

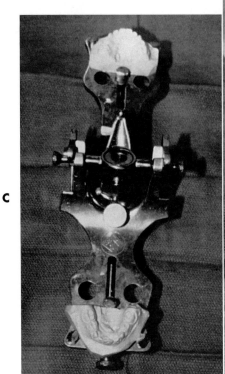

C

D

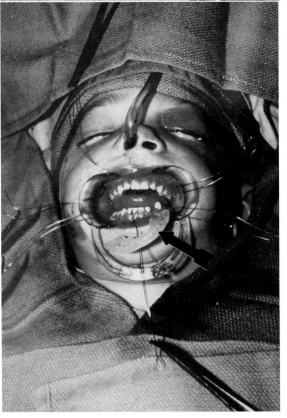

E

Figure 63-12, cont'd. **C,** Mounted dental models. The impressions are used to create a stone model. The stone models are mounted on an articulator. The stone is cut with a saw to reproduce the fracture line. The occlusion is realigned into the desirable postoperative occlusion. An acrylic splint is then produced from these models. **D,** Three circummandibular wires are placed, a percutaneous right circumzygomatic and percutaneous left circumzygomatic wire, along with a right piriform aperture wire. **E,** The splint *(arrow)* has been fabricated from the model. The teeth are set into the splint. The bone suspension wires are then secured, stabilizing the dentition to the splint, establishing maxillomandibular fixation. This can be accomplished from impressions to fixation during one operative procedure.

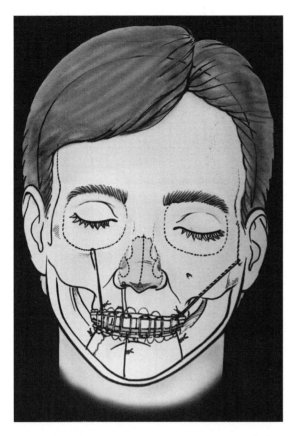

Figure 63-13. Circumferential bone wires secured directly to arch bars with application of splint and arch bar to arch bar wiring, securing maxillomandibular fixation.

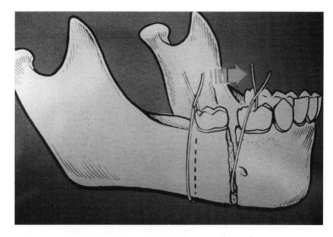

Figure 63-14. When placing circumferential bone wires, caution must be used to avoid drawing the wire through the fracture site and transecting through the mandible.

arch bar. Therefore, if the surgeon needs to take the child out of maxillomandibular fixation temporarily for any reason (e.g., nausea), this can easily be done by cutting only the upper-to-lower arch bar wires. The patient can be placed back into fixation without a second trip to the operating room to replace cut circumferential bone wires (Figure 63-13), which would be necessary if the upper circumferential bone wires were fastened directly to the lower bone wires. A similar goal can be accomplished by eliminating the arch bar having an interconnecting wire between the upper and lower circumferential bone wires, but these may be more difficult to replace if it is necessary to cut these wires (see Figure 63-11, *B*).

One must be careful with any fracture when placing circummandibular wires. The surgeon is standing anterior to the patient when placing these wires. The tendency is to pull those wires forward as they are being tightened. The wire may start to migrate forward. If the surgeon is not careful about placing the circummandibular wires, they may slip into the fracture site (Figure 63-14). As the surgeon continues tightening a wire in the fracture site, it may act like a Gigli's saw and cut through the mandible. Therefore it is important when using these circumferential bone wires to know how the fracture lines are inclined and plan how to fixate the splint to be certain there is stable bone in the region where each wire will be placed.

A conservative approach is the best approach to consider first for a mandible fracture. However, with unstable fractures that cannot be secured with closed reduction techniques, an open reduction and internal fixation becomes necessary (Figure 63-15, *A*). These injuries are approached by taking an impression and fabricating a splint. The fracture is manipulated and the patient is put into maxillomandibular fixation using the technique appropriate for the child's dental development. If the surgeon is still not satisfied with the reduction, the fracture is opened and internal fixation is applied (Figure 63-15, *B*). After finishing the internal fixation, it is critical to make sure the condylar heads are not dislocated. Take the patient out of maxillomandibular fixation and make certain it is possible to range the mandible passively and obtain normal intercuspation. After this has been checked, the child may be placed back into maxillomandibular fixation using the splint.

Some surgeons are intimidated by children's fractures and will accept a less-than-ideal result to avoid opening the fracture site. The surgeon does want to be conservative, but with displaced or unstable segments after closed reduction, he or she must use more aggressive techniques to reestablish normal preinjury anatomic relationships. With open reduction and internal fixation, whether the surgeon is an advocate of using a rigid plate or wire fixation, keep in mind where tooth buds are located in the bone at all times. In a child's mandible, particularly in the body, there is very little room for bone fixation devices (see Figure 63-5). To place a plate or a wire on the mandibular body, the surgeon must hug the inferior border. If he or she drifts superiorly at all, the developing tooth buds will be damaged. There is slightly more room at the mandibular angle and symphyseal regions for fixation. As seen in Figure 63-5, the mandibular canal passes through the bone of the mandible. This must also be carefully considered when placing hardware. The placement of rigid fixation can be difficult with maxillary fractures, as well. The tooth buds are located very close to the piriform buttress, providing very little room for fixation. There is almost a horizontal plane between

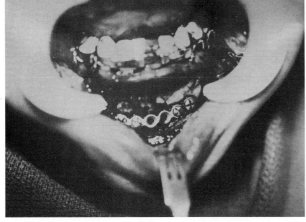

Figure 63-15. **A,** A displaced mandibular symphysis fracture. **B,** Open reduction and internal fixation. After reduction, the patient is taken out of maxillomandibular fixation, the splint is removed, and the mandible is ranged to check the occlusion to be certain the condylar heads are seated properly in the glenoid fossas. Occlusion is checked before removing the child from the operating room. The maxillomandibular fixation may then be reapplied.

the zygoma and maxilla in children, leaving little room for fixation at the zygomaticomaxillary buttress. Therefore it is critical for a surgeon to develop a thorough understanding of conservative splint fixation with circumferential wiring techniques to avoid opening a fracture if possible. However, if a fracture must be opened, it is important to pay attention to the location of developing tooth buds and tooth roots for the age of the child and utilize well what little room is available for fixation.

Many of the basic techniques and principles used for adults apply to children. The boy in Figure 63-16, *A,* was shot by his 4-year-old brother playing with a handgun and lost part of his mandible (Figure 63-16, *B*). With this injury, an external fixation device is helpful. The wound is débrided multiple times to be sure that the surgeon is dealing only with viable tissue. Once confident that there is only healthy tissue, a reconstruction can then be performed. (In this child's case, a fibular osteocutaneous microvascular transfer was utilized.)

Care must be taken when placing an external fixation device to be aware of the location of tooth buds (Figure 63-16, *C*). The surgeon not only has to place the pins in an area on the mandible away from the zone of the injury but also must stay away from the developing teeth. In children, the posterior molars may be very high in the ramus. This is easily seen in the Panorex of this child. The left posterior mandibular molar bud is a large tooth bud, located in the ascending ramus (Figure 63-16, *D*). The concern with this child's arch is that this is the only tooth that is going to erupt and function in the left proximal mandibular segment. This tooth will provide a posterior stop and bridge abutment for reconstruction of a dental prosthesis. It can play an important role in stabilization of dental implants. Better function will be obtained in the years to come if that tooth bud is saved. It would be an injustice to this child to inadvertently place an external fixation pin in that tooth bud and destroy it.

Condylar Head Injuries

Upper mandibular injuries (condylar head and neck injuries) present with the same clinical findings seen in the adult population: deviation of the fracture toward the side of the fracture because of the pull of the lateral pterygoid muscle on the nonfractured side (Figure 63-17). Pain on opening, open bite, and ecchymosis may all be present.

Condylar head injuries become important because of the mandibular growth occurring in these regions. A large portion of the growth of the mandible is centered at the condyles and the posterior aspect of the ramus. Development is by bony deposition posteriorly and superiorly, involving a major remodeling of these regions as growth progresses. The condyle and ramus of the mandible play an adaptive role, responding to the growth of the cranial base, midface, and surrounding soft tissue influences.[9,21-23] When teeth start to erupt as a child gets older, the alveolar bone develops more fully. Although this is a simplistic summary of mandibular growth, which is a very complex process of deposition and remodeling, clinically one will perceive a downward and forward growth of the mandible (Figure 63-18). The mandibular condyle in children is a major region of growth, able to change in any direction to accommodate surrounding anatomic stimuli. The best way to think of the condyle head is as a large, vascular, trabecular sponge. It is not firm or rigid as in adults. The head of the condyle is soft up until approximately 3 years of age; then this "sponge" starts to ossify and form a more rigid structure.[4,33] When a child strikes his or her chin, the force of impact is transmitted back to the condylar head, and that sponge may get crushed. A crush injury is more likely than a routine fracture in a child less than 3 years of age. Anything that disrupts the condyle circulation, causing bleeding or scarring in this area, will create a risk of temporomandibular joint ankylosis. In addition, anything that disrupts the condylar head can also disrupt the growth of the mandible.[4,20] Therefore the age at which a child sustains a condylar injury becomes significant. Before 3 years of age, one might see a severe growth deformity resulting from a trauma to this region.[7,14,27] After about 12 years of age, the same type of trauma may have fewer problems regarding development. The

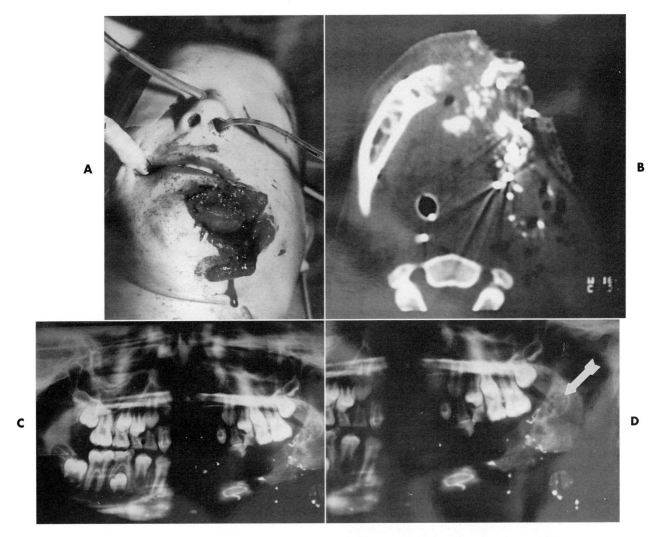

Figure 63-16. **A,** Child with an extensive loss of soft tissue and bone secondary to a gunshot wound to the left side of his face. **B,** Axial CT scan showing the extensive bone loss. **C,** A Panorex showing the abundance of developing teeth in the mandibular and maxillary bone. **D,** A Panorex taken after osteocutaneous microvascular transfer of soft tissue and bone to reconstruct the mandible. Note the developing mandibular tooth bud in the left ramus *(arrow)*. Very meticulous care must be taken to avoid injury to that tooth bud either when doing the bony reconstruction or at the time of placement of an external fixation device.

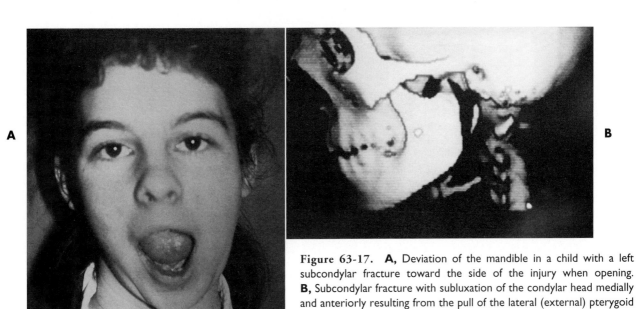

Figure 63-17. **A,** Deviation of the mandible in a child with a left subcondylar fracture toward the side of the injury when opening. **B,** Subcondylar fracture with subluxation of the condylar head medially and anteriorly resulting from the pull of the lateral (external) pterygoid muscle. Note the decrease in the vertical height of the ramus and subsequent open bite.

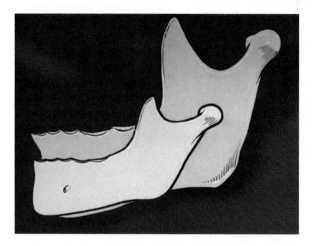

Figure 63-18. Condylar growth is a very complex remodeling process of the infant mandible. The diagram depicts the development of the mandible from infancy *(smaller maxilla in front)* to adulthood *(larger maxilla in back)*. Note that most deposition occurs at the posterior and superior regions of the mandible, with additional bony deposition occurring at the alveolus with the development of the dentition. (From Rally DM: Development of growth by anatomic divisions. In Rally DM [ed]: *A synopsis of craniofacial growth,* Stamford, Conn, 1980, Appleton & Lange.)

fracture location can also have a significant effect on a child's growth. A condylar fracture has a greater potential to result in a developmental deformity than if the fracture were to involve the body of the mandible. After the age of 3, the body contributes less to the development of the mandible than the condyle does. Therefore the location of the injury and the age of the child are significant factors to consider when evaluating a mandibular fracture. A condyle injury can have a significant effect on growth. The young man with a mandibular asymmetry (Figure 63-19, *A*) presented at the office and indicated that his mother was told by doctors that he injured his "jawbone in front of his ear" when he was 2 years of age. Ever since then, his mother reported his "jaw has grown off to the side." He sustained a left condylar injury. He had normal growth on one side, but on the fractured side, growth was inhibited. This caused the mandible to rotate around the midfacial axis toward the affected side (Figure 63-19, *B*).

The location of the condylar injury affects the management of the patient. An intracapsular injury, by definition, involves the condylar head within the confines of the capsule. This injury should be managed with immediate mobilization. A child with this type of injury can be given chewing gum to stimulate mobility and allowed to eat a regular diet. There should not be a decrease in the vertical height of the ramus,

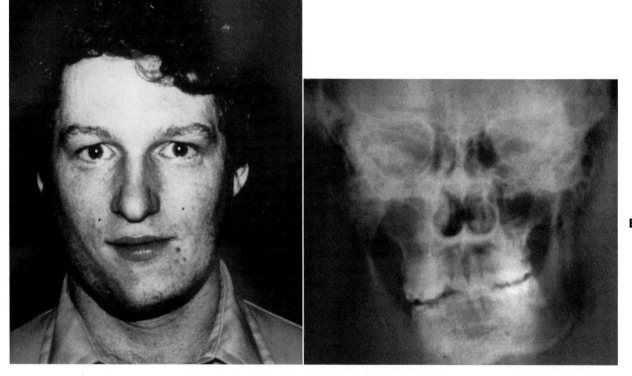

Figure 63-19. **A,** Mandibular asymmetry resulting from a condylar injury in early childhood. **B,** Posteroanterior radiograph showing the degree of mandibular asymmetry.

which would cause an open bite, with an intracapsular injury. There is a significant risk of ankylosis of the joint if these injuries are immobilized. Evaluate the child in the office weekly and encourage continued movement. Discuss with the parents ways to stimulate the child to range the joint. Chewing gum is good because it promotes movement, but the physician has to find ways for parents to get a child to fully range his or her joint (a large sandwich can be a good stimulus for a child to open the mouth widely).

With condylar injuries, a conservative approach is by far the best approach. There are almost no indications to open a child's temporomandibular joint,[27] with the exception of a foreign body in the joint space or absolute inability to reestablish occlusion. A condyle that has been pushed into the middle cranial fossa would be another indication but is extremely rare. By opening the joint capsule and exploring the condylar head for a high capsular injury, the circulation may be disrupted in this very important region of growth. Because this region is basically a large vascular sponge in a child who is less than 3 years of age, there is little chance of fixating bony fragments because there is little bone that is dense enough to secure a pin, plate, or screw. All that this will accomplish is to generate a great deal of bleeding and scarring, worsening the injury iatrogenically and increasing the risk of ankylosis. Even if the condylar head has been subluxed, there is such active growth and adaptation in young children in this area that the condyle has been reported to remodel and reestablish a normal anatomic relationship with the glenoid fossa. This is more apt to occur, and with better function than one can obtain by attempting a reduction of the condylar head surgically. A conservative approach with careful observation and immediate mobilization is the best approach for these intracapsular injuries. This is also true in older children. There are many textbook discussions about intermaxillary fixation for 2 or more weeks, but this is not the ideal approach for these injuries.

Subcondylar Fractures

Subcondylar fractures are more common than high articular fractures in children older than 5 years of age.[7] Most are greenstick fractures. After the age of 5, the condylar head starts to become more calcified, and the neck of the condyle becomes more refined and the weakest area of the mandibular ramus. These injuries have few problems with long-term sequelae unless they are bilateral. A bilateral injury represents more force; consequently, there is more potential for disruption of growth.[33] Greenstick injuries can be managed with a soft diet and careful observation of occlusion. Subcondylar injuries with loss of ramus height are treated by closed reduction techniques. A child is placed into maxillomandibular fixation. Children heal rapidly, and fixation is rarely necessary longer than 2 to 3 weeks.

In young children, the approach would be to make a splint and establish occlusion, placing circummandibular wires and maxillary suspension wires to secure the splint. The surgeon should be equally concerned about mobilizing a subcondylar injury as about mobilizing an intracapsular injury. A child should not remain in fixation for extended periods because ankylosis can occur even if the joint is not directly injured. It is important to remove the mandibular fixation after 2 to 3 weeks and mobilize the joints. You can get the child ranging by using the same methods discussed previously.

The fixation becomes even more significant with bilateral subcondylar injuries because of a greater potential of developing an open bite than a unilateral subcondylar fracture. With a bilateral injury, fixation should be left slightly longer, 3 full weeks, to enable the bone to become more rigid and maintain the ramus height. A standard rule of thumb would be 2 to 3 weeks of fixation is all that is required for a unilateral subcondylar neck fracture in children. With a bilateral fracture, a full 3-week period of fixation is required.

LE FORT FRACTURES

Midfacial fractures in children show many of the symptoms seen in adults, such as a mobile or impacted maxilla, malocclusion, periorbital ecchymosis, lacerations around the midface, hematoma, edema, paresthesia, and bony step-offs. Midfacial fractures are rare in children. In the population of less than 12 years of age, they make up only 0.5% of all fractures.[7,26] When they do occur, they are most often greenstick in nature.

Le Fort I fractures are rare in children because of the elasticity of the maxilla and absence of a well-developed maxillary sinus with thin cortical bone walls. Looking at the LeFort I region of the maxilla in a 4-year-old (see Figure 63-5), the majority of the maxilla is supported with developing tooth buds that have a high concentration of soft tissue, making the maxilla more flexible and more resistant to fracturing. This concept is better understood when looking at maxillary sinus development. There is not a well-pneumonized sinus with thin cortical walls in children as is seen in adults. In a newborn, there is a small, rudimentary maxillary sinus (Figure 63-20). It is hardly pneumonized at all. It is very small and localized along the piriform buttresses, medial to the infraorbital nerve.

At about 5 years of age, the sinus is starting to pneumonize more significantly. The sinus is centered almost entirely behind the infraorbital nerve. The sinus has expanded significantly, but the maxilla is still filled with developing tooth buds. By the time a person reaches adulthood, the maxillary sinus is well defined and the walls are made up of thin cortical bone. The teeth have erupted, and there is less soft tissue present in the maxilla, making it less forgiving when traumatized. If children do sustain Le Fort injuries, Le Fort II fractures are more common because the nasal ethmoidal area is delicate in children, and there is not the soft tissue of the developing tooth buds in that region to support it.

To manage maxillary fractures, a conservative approach is by far the best approach. Greenstick injuries most often can be managed with a soft diet and careful observation of occlusion. With more complete fractures, it is necessary to reduce the fracture and stabilize it with closed techniques using splints,

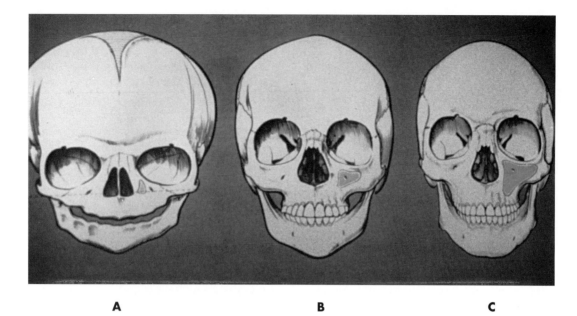

A   **B**   **C**

Figure 63-20. The skull at birth **(A)**, 5 years of age **(B)**, and adulthood **(C).** There is a significant increase in the size of the maxillary sinus from birth to adulthood. The sinus is very small and rudimentary in the early years of life and increases greatly as a person ages. (From Kazanjian VH, Converse JM: *Surgical treatment of facial injuries*, Baltimore, 1974, Williams & Wilkins.)

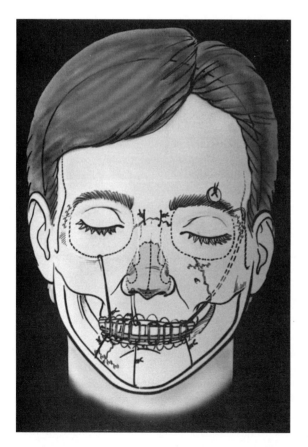

Figure 63-21. A combination of open reduction and internal fixation with midfacial suspension wires and circummandibular wires in a child with mixed dentition. The circummandibular and midfacial circumferential wires are relegated to the role of stabilizing the maxillomandibular fixation (splint).

maxillomandibular fixation, and circumferential bone wires. Fixation is left in place for 3 to 4 weeks. One must keep in mind with circumferential bone wires to go to the next highest stable portion of the facial skeleton to obtain support. With a Le Fort III fracture, for instance, circumzygomatic wires cannot be used to stabilize the splint because that region of the midface is fractured. The next highest portion of stable bone must be used, which would necessitate using cranial suspension wires. If the reduction using splints and suspension wires is not satisfactory, or if there is still displacement or instability, an open reduction and internal fixation would be necessary. The proper facial width, height, and projection will only be reestablished in these cases with interfragmentary bone stabilization, particularly with more complex injuries involving the middle and upper facial skeleton. The circumferential suspension wires therefore are relegated to the role of supporting a splint for maxillomandibular fixation during the ages when dental structures alone will not support arch bars (Figure 63-21).

Tooth buds can be very superficial in the maxillary walls and must be respected if opening a maxillary fracture in a child. In the areas of the maxilla between the buttresses, the developing tooth buds in young children may be separated from the mucosa only by a thin layer of periosteum and may not have a well-developed bony cortex. Therefore, when opening these regions, the surgeon must be careful not to plunge into the underlying tooth buds.

Although maxillary growth is in a forward and downward direction and is a very complex process, there is a generalized remodeling that occurs (Figure 63-22). Cleft lip and palate surgery has taught that there are some localized, very active

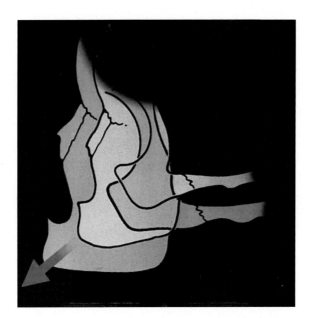

Figure 63-22. Maxillary growth is a generalized remodeling, resulting in an overall downward and forward growth of the facial skeleton. The child's maxilla *(smaller)* as it grows into an adult maxilla *(larger maxilla)*. (From Graber TM: Growth and development. In Graber TM [ed]: *Orthodontics principles and practice,* Philadelphia, 1972, WB Saunders.)

regions of growth in the maxilla, such as the region of the septum. However, because of the more generalized remodeling in the maxilla, "growth centers" seem to play a less critical role in the development of the maxilla than the condyle does with the mandible. Therefore maxillary trauma has less potential to have a negative effect on growth.[6,7,19]

Maxillary fractures heal extremely rapidly in a period of about 2 to 4 weeks. Therefore early treatment is imperative. Because of this rapid healing, these fractures need to be addressed within the first 3 to 4 days of the occurrence of the injury. It is a much more difficult problem once the maxilla has healed in a child in an abnormal position to perform an elective osteotomy because of the potential injury to tooth buds. It is therefore critical that a Le Fort fracture in a child be recognized and addressed early. The best chance of a perfect reconstruction is at the time of the primary injury and early in the course of that injury.

ORBITAL FRACTURES

The etiology of orbital injuries in children is very similar to that in adults. The clinical findings are also identical to those in adults. It is important to consider children's orbital development. At approximately the age of 2, the orbits have almost reached their adult size. The orbits will have reached their full adult size by the time the child reaches about 7 years of age. The small maxillary sinuses and flexible bone results in fewer blowout fractures in children. The orbital floor is supported by developing tooth buds in very young children, particularly in the inferior medial region of the floor. Because there is little

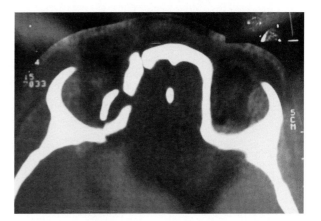

Figure 63-23. Medial orbital fracture with significant displacement of bone segments.

development of the maxillary sinus, there is often not a large void for the orbital floor to be extruded into, but displacement can occur. With orbital injuries, just as with all children's injuries, a conservative approach is best. Nondisplaced fractures need only be carefully followed. There are some circumstances in which conservatism is not possible (Figure 63-23). Indications for open reduction and internal fixation of orbital fractures include diplopia (with positive force duction test), enophthalmos, vertical malposition of the globe, displacement of the zygoma or orbital walls, and infraorbital nerve paresthesia or anesthesia. Infraorbital nerve paresthesia or anesthesia would certainly not be an indication to explore as an isolated finding, but in conjunction with any one of the above, it would certainly reinforce the need to be aggressive. When exploring, the goal is to align bony fragments and to release entrapped orbital soft tissue. Early exploration in orbital injuries in children is indicated if a conservative approach is not possible. Delayed repair is a much more difficult problem in children because of their tendency to rapidly heal. The surgeon has to be careful of the tooth buds and their proximity to the orbital floor. When exploring an orbital floor, the tooth bud of the cuspid tooth may be found very close to the medial anterior portion of the orbital floor. The surgeon must be careful when trying to reelevate bony fragments not to drift into this developing tooth bud (Figure 63-24). Obviously, the surgeon must exercise extreme caution regarding the optic nerve and globe itself, being aware that the depth of the orbit will vary significantly with age. Many of the same techniques used to reconstruct adult orbits apply to the repair of children's fractures. Many materials can be used to reconstruct a child's orbit. Although various synthetic materials have been used by many surgeons, bone grafting in a growing child is still the best approach. Numerous bone sources are available, including ilium, rib, and split cranial bone. Rib is abundant and easily

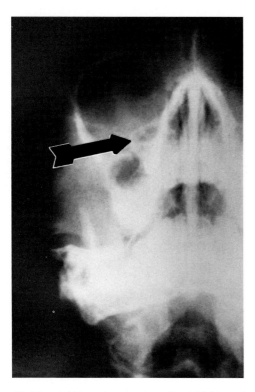

Figure 63-24. A Waters' x-ray view of a child. Note the close proximity of the developing cuspid tooth bud *(arrow)* to the medial anterior orbital floor.

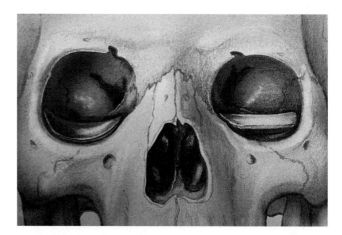

Figure 63-25. The right orbit depicting the desirable position and contour of a bone graft for reconstruction of an orbital injury. The left orbit showing bridging of a poorly contoured graft, decreasing orbital volume.

contoured. The cranial bone is an excellent bone source but more difficult to contour. In addition, the surgeon must be cautious about harvesting split cranial bone in children. Depending on the child's age, there may not be a well-formed diploë. (This is discussed more completely in the Cranial Reconstruction with Bone Loss section in this chapter.) The inner table of the ilium is a good donor source. The surgeon has to avoid the iliac crest in very young children and make certain to confine the harvest to the inner table of the pelvis. The iliac crest is a growth center for the pelvis, and disruption of that area at a young age may result in asymmetry of the ilium. No matter which bone source is used for orbital reconstruction, it is imperative that close attention be paid to contouring the bone to the orbit to reestablish normal orbital volume. Orbital soft tissue contents are elevated from the maxilla into the orbit and the floor grafted. The graft must be contoured and supported well to prevent it from dropping, which would increase orbital volume. The surgeon must also be careful not to bridge over the circumference of the orbit so as to create a decrease in the orbital volume (Figure 63-25). This may result in an iatrogenic problem, proptosis, and continued diplopia. It is vital to reestablish normal orbit volume.

It is imperative that the surgeon obtain a thorough ophthalmologic examination on a child who has sustained an orbital injury. *An undiagnosed preoperative condition becomes a postoperative complication.* It is extremely difficult to evaluate the site of an adult who has an orbital injury. In children, it becomes a much greater challenge. They are injured, frightened, and very reluctant to allow the physician to examine them. Therefore a thorough ophthalmologist's examination to evaluate the globe would be a critical requirement in managing orbital injuries in children. If visual deficiencies are not documented in the chart before a child is taken to surgery, any visual difficulties noted postoperatively will certainly be attributed to the surgery and not to the mechanism of injury.

ZYGOMA FRACTURES

Zygoma fractures in children are rare. The maxillary sinus is not well developed; therefore there is good support for the zygomaticomaxillary buttress. Tooth buds in this buttress region contribute to the ability to absorb energy. Because the zygoma is a dense, stable bone, displacement is usually caused by a significant force. Although considering potential cerebral spine injuries in all facial fractures is important, this becomes more significant when seeing a zygoma fracture in a child.

In the pediatric population, the surgeon will see all the same clinical findings seen in adults with zygoma injuries. Indications for surgical exploration of the zygoma are asymmetry, a palpable infraorbital rim step-off, global malposition, persistent diplopia with a positive force duction test, and radiographic evidence of bony displacement.[15] Zygoma fractures need to be repaired in the first 4 to 5 days after the occurrence of the injury.[7] Earlier than that would be even more ideal. Children have a tremendous potential to heal very rapidly and consequently will form a strong fibrous union in a very short time. Secondary reconstruction and osteotomies are extremely difficult because they may jeopardize developing tooth buds. Therefore early intervention and accurate treatment are critical. The orbital floor is routinely explored after a zygoma fracture has been opened and reduced. It is imperative, after reducing the fracture, that the surgeon check the orbital floor for stability, even if he or she did not suspect instability of the

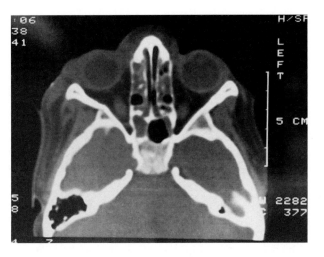

Figure 63-26. **A,** The posterior displacement of a fractured zygoma, supporting fractured segments of orbital floor. **B,** The loss of stability of the orbital floor after reducing the zygoma fracture, resulting in an increase in orbital volume. It is therefore imperative to explore the orbital floor after reducing a zygoma fracture to be certain that stability has not been lost.

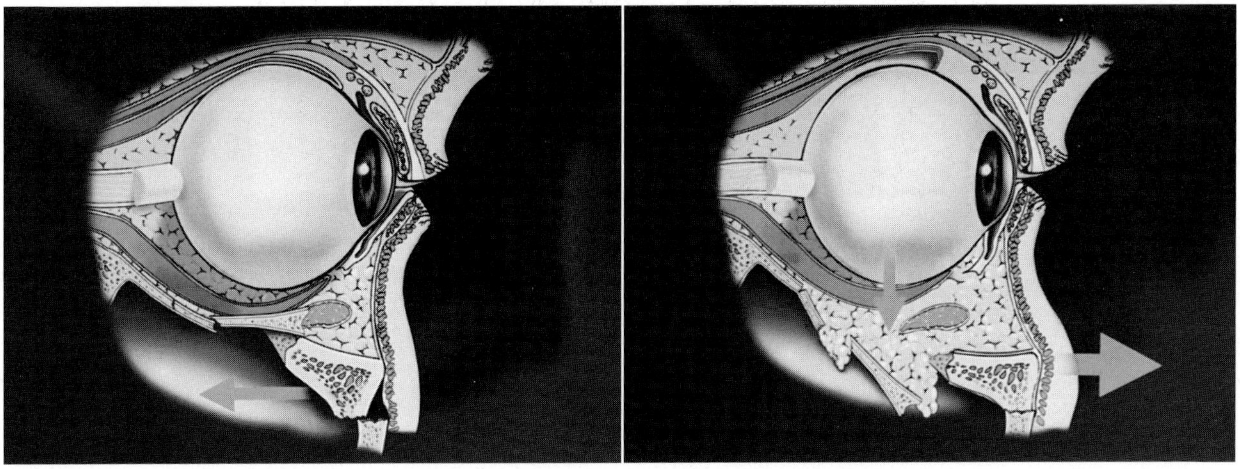

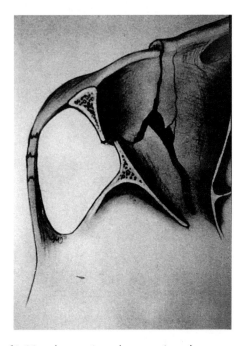

Figure 63-27. Axial CT scan of a right zygoma fracture. Note the malalignment of the zygoma with the sphenoid wing, disrupting the lateral orbital wall, resulting in an increased orbital volume. Note the straight line that the left sphenoid wing makes with the zygoma on the nonfractured left side. Anatomically, they create a lateral orbital wall that is a flat plane. Alignment of the sphenoid wing, creating a flat plane in the region of the lateral orbital wall, is a critical guide to reestablishing the normal three-dimensional position of the zygoma in space during reduction.

Figure 63-28. A comminuted zygomatic arch may appear well reduced but in fact still allow displacement of the zygoma and increased orbital volume. (Courtesy Paul Manson, MD.)

floor preoperatively. Because most zygoma fractures result in a posterior displacement of the zygoma, it may be pushed underneath fractured fragments of the orbital floor and support them. Upon reduction, as the zygoma is brought forward, the support for the orbital floor may be lost. It is extremely frustrating to reduce the zygoma, stabilize it, and then postoperatively find that there is a change in orbital volume that was not appreciated preoperatively (Figure 63-26).

The sphenoid wing is the critical guide to reestablishing the normal three-dimensional position of the zygoma in space (Figure 63-27). The plane between the sphenoid wing and

zygoma in the region of the lateral orbit is a flat plane. This plane can act as a guide to reduce the zygoma properly. Many surgeons have advocated the use of the zygomatic arch as a guide to reestablish the proper three-dimensional position of the zygoma. Although that can be an excellent technique, with a comminuted zygomatic arch there may be a potential to make the arch too rounded and not realize it, consequently allowing the zygoma to remain posterior and lateral in position (Figure 63-28). This increases the orbital volume. The zygomatic arch is not an arch in the architectural sense. A significant portion of it is actually a flat plane (Figure 63-29).

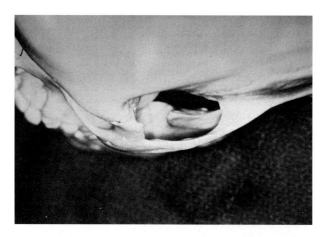

Figure 63-29. Coronal view of zygomatic arch. Note that a significant portion of the zygomatic arch is a flat plane.

Realignment of the lateral wall of the orbit (sphenoid wing and the zygoma) into a straight plane will enable the surgeon to reestablish normal orbital volume with less potential for error. Once the zygoma is secured with rigid fixation, it is possible to go back and reconstruct the zygomatic arch, confident that the zygoma is in its proper position three-dimensionally and the orbital volume has been restored.

The child in Figure 63-30 was struck in the face with a brick that was thrown from a moving convertible as she was walking down the street with her mother. She sustained a right zygoma fracture with an orbital floor blowout. Clinical signs revealed periorbital ecchymosis, subconjunctival ecchymosis, diplopia, and edema. An increase in the orbital volume is depicted by the malalignment of the sphenoid wing and lateral orbit (zygoma) on the right side in comparison with the nonfractured left side (Figure 63-30, C). Reduction is performed through an upper

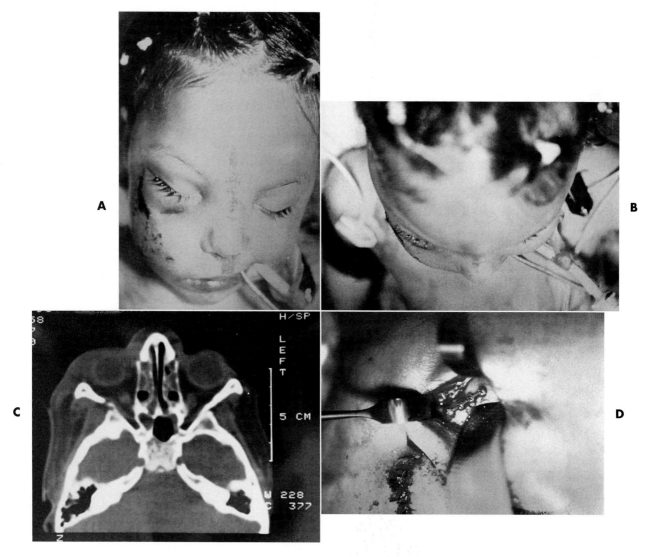

Figure 63-30. A 5-year-old was struck with a brick from a moving car, resulting in a right zygoma fracture and right orbital blow-out fracture: **A,** Front view. **B,** Coronal view. **C,** Axial CT scan showing the malalignment of lateral wall of the orbit and increased orbital volume. Note the straight alignment of the zygoma and the sphenoid wing on the nonfractured left side. **D,** Microplate fixation of the frontal zygomatic suture area through an upper blepharoplasty incision. *Continued*

blepharoplasty incision and a subciliary incision. Some surgeons have used a lateral brow incision. Brows on children are very thin, which can lead to a more noticeable scar than an upper blepharoplasty incision to gain access to the frontal zygomatic suture area. A major consideration in all pediatric fractures is to obtain access to a fracture with the least amount of periosteal stripping to avoid potential disruption of growth. Microplate fixation was used to stabilize the fracture, and the orbital floor was bone grafted (Figure 63-30, *D* to *F*). Postsurgically, we have reestablished her normal orbital

volume and normal orbital function, along with a satisfactory aesthetic result (Figure 63-30, *G*).

NASAL FRACTURES

Nasal fractures will present with the same clinical findings seen in adults (bruising, swelling, deviation, bleeding, retrusion of the nose, and septal deviation). Nasal fractures are more common than zygoma fractures or maxillary fractures in the pediatric population. The nose is very cartilaginous at an early age, which makes it flexible. Fractures of the nose are very difficult to diagnosis because of the tremendous amount of cartilage.[7] Clinical evaluation is very important. Hematoma may cause cartilage necrosis of the septum, making it imperative to evaluate the septum completely.[33,36] The surgeon also must be very careful to evaluate the lateral cartilaginous structures (examining the intranasal lining, along with the skin) to look for hematomas, which may put pressure on the upper and lower lateral cartilages and disrupt their development. The surgeon needs to be aggressive about draining nasal pyramid and septal hematomas in children.

Treatment of nasal fractures in children is very similar to treatment in adults, with elevation of displaced segments, alignment of the septum, osteotomy if it is an old injury, placing intranasal packing, splint fixation to stabilize the nasal pyramid and septum, and bone grafting as needed for significant crush injuries.

There are two nasal growth spurts. One is from birth to 5 years of age, and the other is from 10 to 15 years of age.[7] Injuries during these times have a much greater potential for disruption of growth. The physician needs to make parents aware that children must be followed on a long-term basis to be certain that injuries will not result in deformity.

NASOORBITAL ETHMOIDAL FRACTURES

Nasoorbital ethmoidal (NOE) injuries may result in a child presenting with telecanthus, a saddle nose deformity, periorbital ecchymosis (Figure 63-31), a blunting of the medial palpebral fissure, or nasal bleeding. It is important to consider the potential for intracranial injury in children with NOE fractures. Pneumocephalus on computed tomography (CT) and cerebrospinal fluid (CSF) rhinorrhea can alert the physician to the potential disruption of the dural seal. In children, the frontal sinus is often not well pneumonized until approximately the early teens. On rare occasions, one may see a well-developed frontal sinus in a child who is 1 to 6 years of age, but usually the sinus is very rudimentary. Because the frontal sinuses are often not well developed in young children, a frontal impact does not have the "crush zone" that is seen in adult foreheads. Therefore, in children, the structure immediately deep to the frontal bone often is not frontal sinus but the brain. Consequently, the surgeon must be acutely aware of an NOE injury or frontal bone fracture in children having potential intracranial sequelae. Treatment of mobile (positive

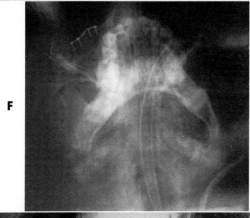
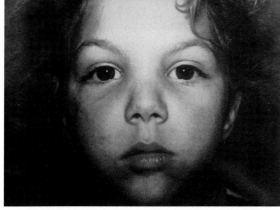

Figure 63-30, cont'd. E, Microplate fixation of the infraorbital rim through subciliary incision. **F,** Postoperative x-ray showing microplate fixation. **G,** Postoperative view with reestablishment of orbital volume and zygomatic contour.

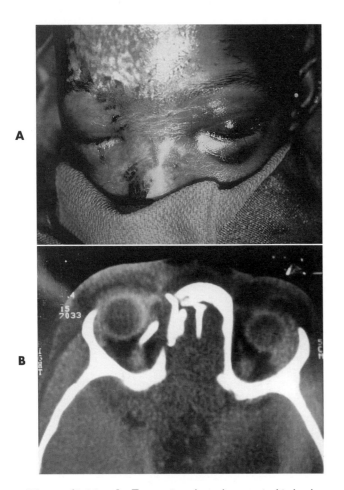

Figure 63-31. **A,** Traumatic telecanthus, periorbital edema, and ecchymosis with depression of the nasal dorsum secondary to nasal orbit ethmoidal fracture. **B,** Axial CT scan of nasal orbit ethmoidal injury.

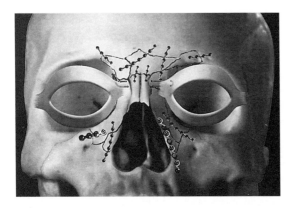

Figure 63-32. Transnasal medial orbital fixation of the medial canthal tendons with reconstruction of midfacial fractures (NOE fracture).

intranasal clump test)[16] or displaced NOE fractures in children is very similar to that in adults, with open reduction, transnasal medial orbital fixation, and interfragmentary wiring or rigid fixation (Figure 63-32). The surgeon must be very careful to avoid detachment of the medial canthal tendon from bone fragments when proceeding with the dissection of the medial

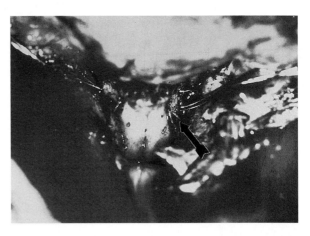

Figure 63-33. Transnasal medial orbital reduction wires placed through a bone graft *(arrow)*. The medial canthal tendon is then sutured to the transnasal wire with 2-0 braided nylon suture. As the wire is tightened, the bone graft is drawn medially, and the canthal tendon follows.

orbit because that would complicate the reconstruction. Of all pediatric fractures, NOE injuries need to be treated the most aggressively to reestablish the normal intercanthal distance. A conservative approach without stabilizing the medial orbital segment will often result in telecanthus, even if this is not evident at the time of injury. If bone has been lost in the area of the fracture, a bone graft, using the transnasal wire to stabilize the bone graft and attaching the canthal tendon to that wire, will reestablish the normal canthal configuration (Figure 63-33). It is imperative to reestablish the normal three-dimensional configuration of the medial orbit (height, projection, and width). Transnasal medial orbital wiring will enable the surgeon to reestablish the nasal width by reestablishing the intercanthal distance. To determine if the canthus is positioned properly vertically, the various bone fragments around the medial orbit must be reconstructed carefully from superior to inferior, so as to reestablish the normal continuity (circumference) of the medial orbit. This will automatically reestablish the facial (orbital rim) projection in this region.

FRONTAL BONE AND FRONTAL SINUS FRACTURES

Children have a smaller face-to-head ratio than adults, as discussed previously. Therefore, when sustaining frontal blows to the head and neck, children are more apt to sustain cranial fractures than facial fractures. As mentioned previously, the frontal sinus in children is not developed to any great extent until the teen years (it may first be seen in its rudimentary stages from the ages of 1 year to 6 years). With frontal bone and frontal sinus fractures, the surgeon obviously wants to be as conservative as possible, but the management of sinus injuries will be similar to that of an adult. Frontal sinus fracture

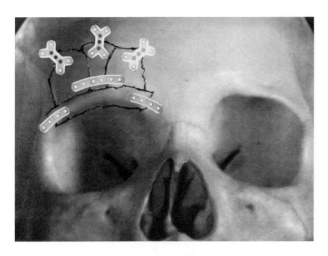

Figure 63-34. Reconstruction of frontal bone and superior orbit, reestablishing the normal superior orbital arch contour. Note resorbable plate and screw fixation.

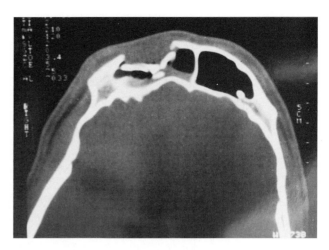

Figure 63-35. Axial CT scan of asymmetric frontal bone fracture with involvement of the frontal sinus.

management is an area of great controversy in the literature. There are numerous management options available, depending on the nature of the injury[16]:

1. Fractures of the anterior sinus wall can be managed by obliterating or reconstructing the sinus.
2. Fractures of the posterior wall are managed by reconstructing, obliterating, or cranializing the sinus.

Involvement of the frontal nasal duct becomes a major consideration regarding the ability to reconstruct the frontal sinus and establish drainage. If the frontal duct has been involved in the injury, drainage from the frontal sinus may be obstructed. If the surgeon opts to reconstruct a sinus, reestablishing the patency of the frontal duct is imperative. Persistent air fluid levels in a frontal sinus that has been reconstructed will require a more aggressive approach (removal of all frontal sinus mucosa with cranialization or obliteration).

Displaced cranial bone segments will require open reduction and fixation. Close cooperation with the neurosurgery team to deal with intracranial injuries is imperative. When reconstructing the frontal bone or the superior orbit, it is important to maintain the normal configuration of the superior orbital circumference, similar to the importance of maintaining the normal circumference of the inferior orbital rim and floor (Figure 63-34). In a situation in which the frontal bone has been comminuted with hemorrhage of surrounding soft tissue, this can lead to alteration of bony circulation and disruption of symmetric growth to the forehead (Figure 63-35). Despite careful alignment and fixation of cranial bone fractures, asymmetry and irregularities may still develop as a child continues to grow. Resorption of bone fragments and "pseudogrowth" of fractures are rare, but parents must be made aware that children with skull fractures need to be followed in the future for potentially irregular cranial growth.

CRANIAL RECONSTRUCTION WITH BONE LOSS

Often, we are consulted to reconstruct children who have sustained cranial injuries with loss of bone. There are many autogenous sources of bone available for reconstruction (rib, ilium, and split cranial bone). Synthetic materials, methylmethacrylate, and titanium prosthetic plates have been very popular in neurosurgery for many years but should be avoided in children. Bone graft would certainly be the first choice for reconstructing any cranium, particularly a growing child's cranium. Split cranial bone is an excellent source of bone (Figure 63-36). When planning to harvest split cranial bone for grafting, the age of the child and the development of the diploë must be carefully evaluated. Although some sections of the skull have a diploë at 3 to 6 months of age, this is not well developed and it is difficult to obtain very much bone. At 3 years of age, the diploë starts to become better defined and is more reliable for harvesting a split cranial bone graft. However, the diploë at this age is thin and there may still be sections where the inner and outer tables of the skull are still not well separated in some children. It is not until about 9 years of age that there is usually a wide, well-established diploë. Therefore, from 3 to 9 years of age, when opting to harvest a split cranial bone graft, it is best to take a full-thickness cranial graft and split that on the operating room table utilizing the various sections, one for the reconstruction as desired and the other to repair the donor defect. This is the safest method to avoid intracranial injury. After 9 years of age, the diploë is much better defined, and harvesting an in situ split cranial bone graft becomes safe.[13] (However, it is still prudent to obtain a CT scan to confirm that the diploë is well formed.) An in situ graft harvest is very useful for harvesting moderate amounts of bone to reconstruct a nose or orbital floors. If a large section of bone is needed as a single unit, it is much simpler to harvest a large, full-thickness portion of the skull. This is true even in older

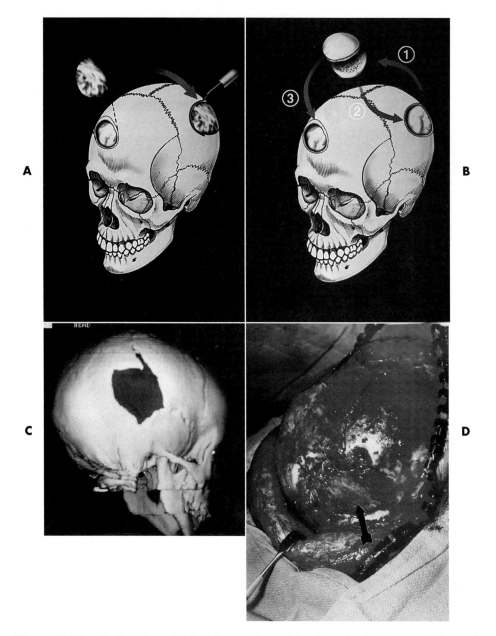

Figure 63-36. **A,** Technique of full-thickness split cranial grafting. Sterile aluminum foil is used to outline the skull defect for reconstruction. This is transferred to a portion of the skull with a desirable contour (suture lines are avoided), and the bone is marked. **B,** A full-thickness portion of cranium is then harvested and split. The outer table of the diploë is used to reconstruct the traumatic defect, and the inner table is replaced. (note: an in situ split cranial harvest may be possible if the child's age is appropriate. See text for details.). **C,** Posterior traumatic cranial defect. **D,** Posterior skull defect exposed through a coronal incision (*arrow marking the dura*). *Continued*

children and can be helpful in adults, as well. Because of the rounded contour of the skull, it is not easy to split the skull without the potential to penetrate the inner table. Therefore it is safer to split the skull on a back operating room table and then utilize the various segments for the reconstruction as needed. This can add an increased margin of safety when harvesting extremely large bone grafts, avoiding penetration of the inner table of the skull and potential intracranial injury. It is best to avoid in situ split cranial grafts in children who have

had intracranial hemorrhage or multiple skull fractures to avoid introducing a new source of trauma.

Rib provides another good source of bone for skull reconstruction. The young man in Figure 63-37 sustained frontal and parietal bone loss (see Figure 63-37, *A*). Harvesting multiple split ribs was used for reconstructing this defect. Using bone-contouring forceps, each rib is contoured, positioned, and fixated. Each rib is positioned like a bricklayer builds a brick wall, layer after layer until the defect is

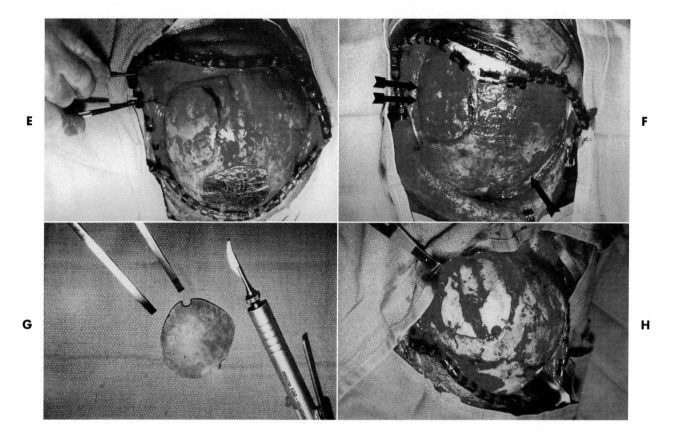

Figure 63-36, cont'd. **E,** Sterile aluminum foil is used to create a template of the defect. It is then brought to a portion of the skull where the contour is most in keeping with the desirable contour for the reconstruction. Suture regions of the skull are avoided. **F,** A full-thickness graft has been taken *(double arrows)* from the opposite side of the skull from the traumatic defect *(single arrow).* **G,** The full-thickness cranial graft is split. **H,** The inner cortex is replaced where the graft is harvested, and the outer cortex is used for the defect, shown here secured to the peripheral bone.

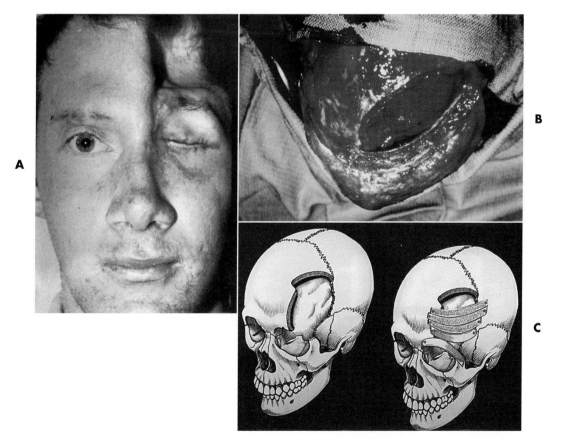

Figure 63-37. **A,** Young man with evulsion of frontal bone and parietal bone. **B,** Operative view of split ribs being contoured and layered to repair the defect. **C,** Diagrammatic representation of the skull defect and split rib reconstruction.

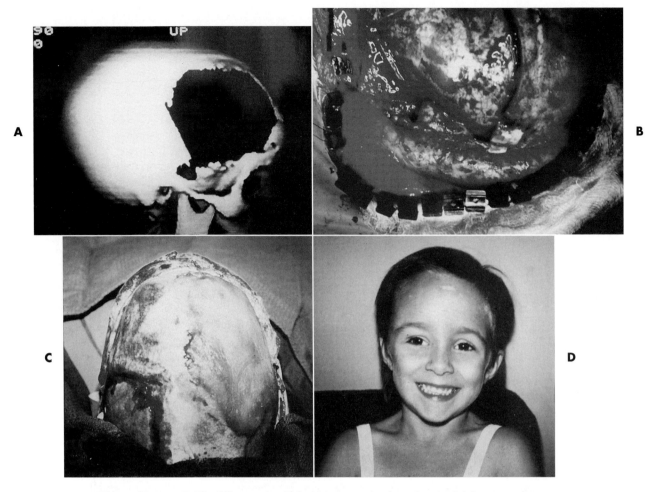

Figure 63-38. **A,** The CT scan of a child with an extensive frontal parietal defect secondary to a motor vehicle accident. **B,** Bony skull defect with the dura exposed. **C,** Skull (coronal view). Note right frontal parietal reconstruction. **D,** Postoperative view depicting the reconstructed skull showing forehead appearance.

reconstructed (see Figure 63-37, *B* and *C*). This may have a tendency to leave an irregular surface in the region of the reconstruction. Therefore this technique is often best used beneath hair-bearing areas of the scalp.

Under rare circumstances, synthetic materials may be used if the skull growth has been completed or other sources of bone have been exhausted. The CT in Figure 63-38, *A,* depicts a child who has had a large section of bone evulsed from her skull. She was ejected from a car. After a prolonged stay in the intensive care unit, she completely recovered neurologically from her injury, leaving a skull defect requiring reconstruction (Figure 63-38, *B*). Although our first choice was to use bone graft, other factors prevented us from doing so. Therefore we reconstructed her defect with methylmethacrylate (Figure 63-38, *C*). The majority of her skull growth had been completed at the time of her presentation. Although bone graft should always be considered a first choice, this may not always be possible and other modalities may need to be considered. This reconstruction left her with a pleasing cranial contour and protection for her brain (Figure 63-38, *D*). The use of methylmethacrylate is still controversial, even in adult skull

surgery.[17,18,24,38] As with any synthetic material, one should avoid using it in a growing skull, in a region of infection, in the region of a sinus, or where soft tissue coverage is less than ideal.

Another option for skull reconstruction is a prefabricated prosthesis. The 16-year-old boy depicted in Figure 63-39 is an individual who sustained an extensive cranial injury from an explosion, resulting in the loss of his superior orbit, left eye, and a portion of his frontal and parietal bones, resulting in the defect seen here (see Figure 63-39, *B* and *C*). A three-dimensional CT scan is obtained and is sent out to one of several companies, which will create a three-dimensional model of the skull defect. Lorenz Surgical (Jacksonville, Fla.) is one of the companies performing this service. Their prosthesis is made of glass beads coated with hydroxyapatite. The skull model is sent back to the surgeon, who checks it to make certain that it accurately reflects the cranial defect. After the model has been thoroughly examined and it is determined to be accurate, then a prosthesis can be fabricated (see Figure 63-39, *D*). The prosthesis is placed into position and lag screwed for stability (see Figure 63-39, *E*). The temporalis muscle is suspended. Figure 63-39, *F,* shows this young man

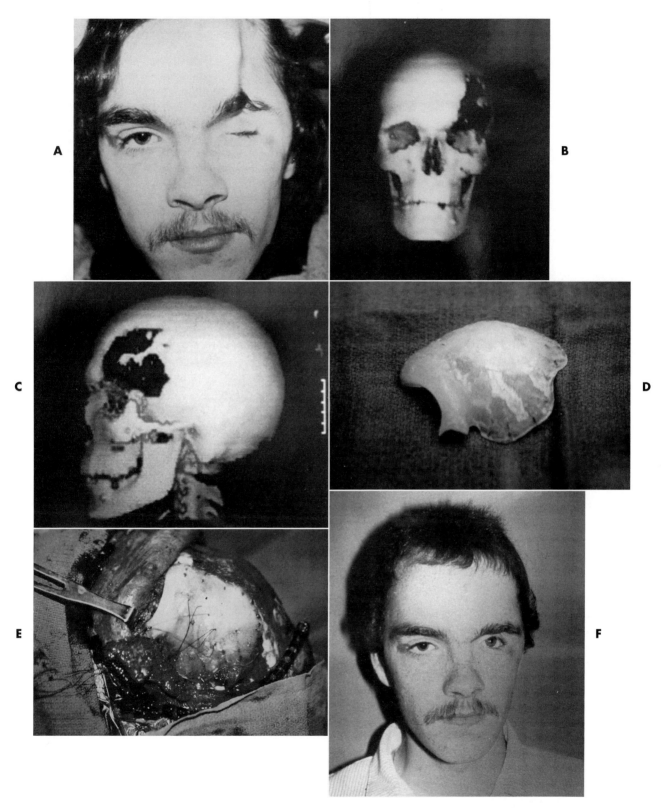

Figure 63-39. **A,** A 16-year-old boy who sustained a blast injury to the cranium, resulting in loss of his left eye and evulsion of the left frontal and parietal region of the skull. **B,** Frontal CT view showing the defect. **C,** Lateral CT view of defect. **D,** Skull prosthesis constructed from a three-dimensional model fabricated from the three-dimensional CT scan. **E,** Prosthesis in position, lag screwed for stability. Note that the horizontal mattress sutures pass through the prosthesis to elevate the temporalis muscle. **F,** Postoperative view.

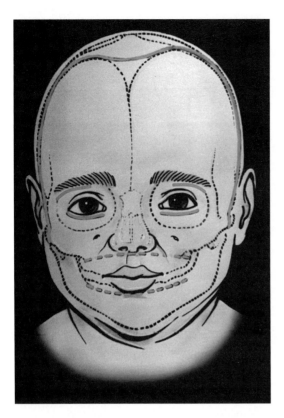

Figure 63-40. Incisions for access to the facial skeleton: coronal, lateral brow, subciliary, transconjunctival, intraoral. NOTE: Facial lacerations can also provide access to facial fractures.

many years after his surgical reconstruction. Flaps have been used around his lids to facilitate placement of an ocular prosthesis. His normal cranial contour has been reestablished along with protection for his brain.

Complications that can result from cranial reconstruction include:

Synthetic materials (avoid in children):
1. Infection
2. Rejection
3. A growing skull changes and can leave irregularities in the area of the reconstruction
4. Loosening of the prosthesis
Bone graft:
1. Infection of the operative site
2. Resorption of graft
3. Donor site complications:
   Scar
   Infection
   Loss of the inner table of the skull from the donor (full-thickness harvests), resulting in a newly created defect
4. Malunion (donor or recipient site)

It is important to reiterate that, in growing skulls, autogenous bone is the best choice to reconstruct defects. Therefore the age of a child and the amount of skull growth completed by the time of presentation must be considered.

FRACTURE EXPOSURE

Surgical exposure in children is very similar to that in adults. The coronal incision, the upper blepharoplasty incisions, transconjunctival incisions, and subciliary incisions provide good access to the upper facial skeleton (Figure 63-40).[16] Intraoral mucosal incisions are used to expose the anterior walls of the maxilla and the mandible from angle to angle. Lacerations may also be used. The goal is to obtain the best access to a fracture with the least amount of periosteal stripping possible.

OUTCOMES

Fortunately, the majority of pediatric fractures go on to heal uneventfully if treated properly. Complications may arise with children's injuries, such as aspiration, nonunion of fracture segments, malunion, osteomyelitis, ankylosis, hypoplastic bone development, asymmetric development of the facial skeleton, nerve paresthesia, globe dysfunction, and abnormal globe position. Additional complications include dental complications and loss of teeth.[10] With tooth buds in the line of fracture, there is a 20% incidence of malformation and developing malocclusion.[3,7,35] CSF rhinorrhea may be another complication secondary to NOE fractures or skull fractures. After open reduction of midfacial fractures, there is only a 5% chance of persistent obstruction of the lacrimal system if there are no lacerations present.[15] Therefore it is important not to introduce an iatrogenic source of lacrimal injury by cannulating the punctum unless there is a laceration present or one is placing transnasal orbital wires to reduce an NOE fracture. Facial fractures around the lacrimal apparatus are best managed by fracture reduction. If epiphora is persistent, reconstruction of the lacrimal drainage system can be undertaken on an elective basis. Laceration in the region of the medial canthus will require more aggressive exploration and immediate repair of lacrimal injuries.[12]

In children under 5 years of age, it is best to avoid a tracheostomy. Fifty percent have complications such as pneumothorax, emphysema, tracheal erosion, tracheal stenosis, and occlusion of the tracheal airway because of the small diameter of the cannula.[5,25]

PEDIATRIC FRACTURES AND GROWTH

At about 3 months of age a child has reached approximately 50% of his adult facial size, and at 2 years of age about 70% of his adult size. By the time a child reaches 5½ years of age, the facial skeleton has reached almost 80% of its adult size.[8,30] Facial growth after properly treated fractures usually proceeds well with no long-term difficulties. However, growth problems

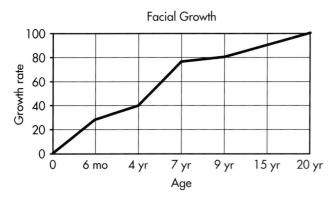

Figure 63-41. Growth curve, birth to 20 years. (Modified from Schultz RC: Facial trauma in children. In *Facial injuries,* ed 3, St Louis, 1988, Mosby.)

can be a complication of facial fractures.* No one has all the answers of what effect fractures may have on facial growth in any particular child. Pediatric facial growth needs to be considered when dealing with any fracture. It is difficult to quantitate the extent of trauma and disruption of growth. A minor injury may result in significant problems, and a major injury may not have any effect on growth whatsoever. Therefore it is very difficult to predict with certainty the potential of a child's growth after an injury. Maxillary hypoplasia does appear to be a rare entity. Posttraumatic development problems seem, more often, to affect the mandible, especially if the child is younger than 5 years of age.

Facial growth is not something that starts at birth and continues on at a steady rate until 16 to 18 years of age, then suddenly stops. There are several growth "spurts," or periods when children are very active in their growth (Figure 63-41). The most active periods are from birth to 6 months and from 4 years to 7 years of age. Fractures during rapid growth periods obviously have a more significant potential to disrupt growth.[32] It is common sense that younger children may experience more severe growth problems resulting from injuries than older children with similar injuries who have completed most of their growth. (There is obviously a much greater potential for disruption of growth in a fracture in someone who is 2 years of age than in someone who is 16 years of age).[7,21,27] Some occlusal changes occur with growth. However, if we have made the decision to do an open reduction and internal fixation, we must strive to reestablish the occlusion into its normal anatomic condition before the time of injury. Children do not necessarily "grow back into a normal occlusal pattern," and a child who has a displaced mandible cannot be expected to miraculously reestablish a normal occlusion. Some surgeons erroneously believe that the occlusion will improve with growth if they do not establish good intercuspation at the time of fracture reduction. This can set up a child for a poor result.

Although fractures themselves can have an effect on growth, it is difficult to ascertain the impact surgery with periosteal stripping and internal fixation may have on growth. Most children's fractures do continue to grow in a normal pattern, but stripping periosteum further disrupts the blood supply to bone, and if the child is predisposed to growth difficulties secondary to an injury, this may potentially worsen the outcome. Although there is always the concern that surgery may disrupt growth, it must be realized that a fracture itself has the potential to disrupt growth. It also must be recognized that a child who has a mandible that is significantly displaced, or a maxilla that is significantly displaced, certainly does have a functional problem and requires correction of that defect. If the child needs an operation to attempt to reestablish normal anatomic configuration, one certainly should not be intimidated by the fact that it is a young child. A conservative approach (observation or closed reduction) should always be considered first. If that is not feasible, the surgeon must be prepared to take the necessary steps to reconstruct a child's fracture defect, opening the fracture to reestablish preinjury anatomy. It is imperative that the surgeon talk extensively to parents, letting them know that there is a potential for disruption of bone growth and/or disruption of developing tooth buds in certain fractures. This will help parents understand the need for long-term follow-up.

The placement, translocation, and removal of hardware is a topic that is drawing a great deal of attention in craniofacial surgery at the time of this publication. Fixation plates in a growing skeleton have been a significant consideration for many years now. Placing a periorbital microplate on a 2-year-old child's orbit is of greater concern than placing it on a 14-year-old because of the amount of growth to be realized. Therefore the age of a child plays a role in how aggressive the surgeon is with fixation. Some surgeons have advocated the use of wires as being a modality that will disrupt growth to a lesser degree than rigid titanium fixation plates.[33] Rigid plate fixation has been used for many years in children but not followed long enough to precisely define its influence on growth at this time. Well-controlled studies regarding the effect of rigid fixation on growth over long periods of time are scant. Resorbable fixation plates made of polymers of lactic and glycolic acid, which will dissolve over time, have just recently been introduced. These plates are in the early stages of development and have brought a new dimension to the treatment of children's fractures. However, at the time of this publication, the U.S. Food and Drug Administration (FDA) has not approved these plates for load-bearing bone fractures (e.g., a mandibular fracture between dental-bearing segments). There are some advantages and disadvantages of resorbable plate use (e.g., expense, size, time of application). Therefore this technology must progress further before it becomes a panacea.

Long-term follow-up through the growth years of children is the only thing that is going to give outcome information. Will a resorbable plate prove to be better than a piece of wire?

---

*References 7, 11, 14, 15, 29, 31, 34, 36, 37.

As a specialty, surgeons are obligated to take a very close look in the years to come to determine what the best approach to a growing facial skeleton may be (resorbable plate, nonresorbable plate, wire fixation).

There have been no indications at the time of this publication that it is necessary to risk a second anesthetic or second surgical procedure to remove plates and screws from children who have had fractures repaired. Obviously, a resorbable plate that dissolves in a short period of time and one that still has the rigid characteristic nature necessary to stabilize a fracture until it heals is the best of all worlds. We can only hope that this is something that will be satisfactory and can be offered to children for all fractures as the technology advances in this field over the next 10 to 20 years. It is imperative that the surgeon explain to parents that the effect that hardware may have on their child's growth is not known, but unfortunately at this time, it is all that is available.

Obviously, a conservative approach, observation, using splint fixation where all hardware is removable, would be ideal, but under some circumstances, as discussed extensively in this chapter, this will not always provide a reduction that will facilitate adequate function. When opening a fracture, doing as little periosteal stripping as possible, placing the least amount of hardware possible to get the job accomplished, and using autogenous bone for reconstruction of defects when needed are all sound principles to remember when dealing with the growing skeleton of a child.

REFERENCES

1. Andreasen JO: Luxation of permanent teeth due to trauma, *Scand J Dent Res* 78:273, 1970.

2. Andreasen JO: Treatment of fractured and avulsed teeth, *J Dent Child* 28:29, 1971.

3. Andreasen JO, Sundstron B, Raven JJ: The effect of traumatic injuries to primary teeth on their permanent successors, *Scand J Dent Res* 79:284, 1971.

4. Blackwood HJ: Vascularization of the condylar cartilage of the human mandible, *J Anat* 99:550-563, 1965.

5. Bridges CP, Ryan RF, Longenecker CG, et al: Tracheostomy in children: a twenty year study at Charity Hospital in New Orleans, *Plast Reconstr Surg* 37:117, 1966.

6. Converse JM: Facial injuries in children. In Mustard JC (ed): *Plastic surgery in infancy and childhood,* Edinburgh, 1979, Churchill Livingstone.

7. Dufresne CR, Manson PN: Pediatric facial trauma. In McCarthy JG (ed): *Plastic surgery,* vol 2, Philadelphia, 1990, WB Saunders.

8. Enlow DH: *Handbook of facial growth,* ed 2, Philadelphia, 1982, WB Saunders.

9. Enlow DH: Postnatal craniofacial growth and development. In McCarthy JG (ed): *Plastic surgery,* vol 4, Philadelphia, 1990, WB Saunders.

10. Gelbier S: Injured anterior teeth in a preliminary discussion, *Br Dent J* 123:331, 1967.

11. Jazbi B: Subluxation of the nasal septum in the newborn's etiology, diagnosis and treatment, *Otolaryngol Clin North Am* 10:125-138, 1977.

12. Jelks GW, Smith BC: Reconstruction of the eyelids and associated structures In McCarthy JG (ed): *Plastic surgery,* Philadelphia, 1990, WB Saunders.

13. Koenig WJ, Donovan M, Pensler J: Cranial bone grafting in children. In: *Plastic and reconstructive surgery,* Baltimore, 1995, Williams & Wilkins.

14. Maclennan W: Consideration of 180 cases of typical fractures of the mandible & condylar process, *Br J Plast Surg* 5:122, 1952.

15. Manson PN: Skull and midfacial injuries. In Mustard JC, Jackson IT (eds): *Plastic surgery in infancy and childhood,* New York, 1988, Churchill Livingstone.

16. Manson PN: Facial injuries. In McCarthy JG (ed): *Plastic surgery,* Philadelphia, 1990, WB Saunders.

17. Manson RN, Crawley WA, Hooper JE: Frontal cranioplasty, risk factors and choice of cranial vault reconstructive material, *Plast Reconstr Surg* 77:888, 1986.

18. Marchac D: Deformities of the scalp and cranial vault. In McCarthy JG (ed): *Plastic surgery,* vol 2, Philadelphia, 1990, WB Saunders.

19. McCoy FJ: Late results in facial fractures. In Goldwyn RM (ed): *Long term results in plastic and reconstructive surgery,* vol 2, Boston, 1980, Little, Brown.

20. Moos KF, El-Attar A: Mandible and dental injuries. In Mustard JC, Jackson IT (eds): *Plastic surgery in infancy and childhood,* ed 3, New York, 1988, Churchill Livingstone.

21. Moss ML: The primacy of functional matrices in orofacial growth, *Dent Pract Dent Rec* 19:65, 1968.

22. Moss ML, Rankow R: The role of the functional matrix in mandibular growth, *Ann Orthod* 38:95, 1968.

23. Moss ML, Salentijn L: The capsular matrix, *Am J Orthod* 56:474, 1969.

24. Munro IR, Guyuron B: Split rib cranioplasty, *Ann Plast Surg* 7:341, 1981.

25. Oliver P, Richardson JR, Clubb RW, et al: Tracheostomy in children, *N Engl J Med* 267:631, 1962.

26. Rowe NL: Fractures of the facial skeleton in children, *J Oral Surg* 26:505, 1968.

27. Rowe NL: Fractures of the jaws in children, *J Oral Surg* 27:497-507, 1969.

28. Rowe NL, Winter GB: Traumatic lesions of the jaws and teeth. In Mustard JC (ed): *Plastic surgery in infancy and childhood,* Edinburgh, 1971, Churchill Livingstone.

29. Sarnat Gans BJ: Growth of bones, methods of assessing, and clinical importance, *Plast Reconstr Surg* 9:140, 1952.

30. Scott JH: Further studies on the growth of the human face, *Proc R Soc Med* 52:263, 1959.

31. Scott JH, Symonds NE: *Introduction to dental anatomy,* ed 5, Edinburgh, 1967, Churchill Livingstone.

32. Shultz RC: Facial trauma in children. In *Facial injuries,* ed 3, St Louis, 1988, Mosby.

33. Shultz RC: Facial fractures in children and adolescents. In Cohen M (ed): *Mastery of plastic and reconstructive surgery,* vol 2, Boston, 1994, Little, Brown.

34. Shultz RC, Meilman J: Complications of facial fractures. In Goldwyn RM (ed): *The unfavorable result in plastic surgery,* Boston, 1984, Little, Brown.

35. Sneider SS, Stern M: Teeth in the line of mandibular fractures, *J Oral Surg* 29:107, 1971.

36. Stucker FJ, Bryarly C, Shockley W: Management of nasal trauma in children, *Arch Otolaryngol* 110:190-192, 1984.

37. Walker DG: The mandibular condyle: fifty cases demonstrating arrest in development, *Dent Pract* 7:160, 1957.

38. Wolfe SA: Discussion of Manson et al paper, *Plast Reconstr Surg* 77:901, 1986.

39. Zide BM: The temporomandibular joint. In McCarthy JG (ed): *Plastic surgery,* vol 2, Philadelphia, 1990, WB Saunders.

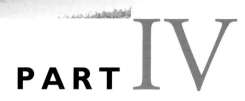

PART IV

PEDIATRIC PLASTIC SURGERY

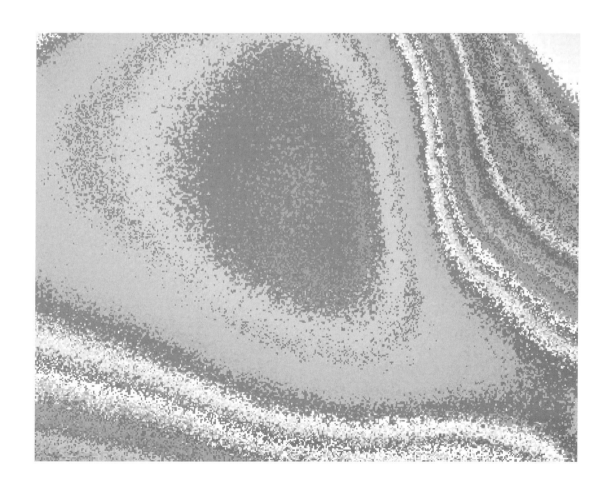

CHAPTER

The Management of Hemangiomas and Vascular Malformations of the Head and Neck

Craig R. Dufresne

INDICATIONS

The head and neck area is a region that maintains a vast, concentrated network of veins and arteries. This vasculature nourishes the facial soft and specialized tissues, as well as the central nervous system. This region comprises less than 14% of the total body surface area in the adult; however, more than one half (56%) of all vascular anomalies occur in this region.[32,40,42] Possibly as a result of this concentrated vascular network, errors in the growth and development of these structures are more frequent, thus leading to this preponderance of vascular problems.

Hemangiomas and vascular malformations are the most common congenital lesions noted in infancy, with an estimated incidence of 0.54 per 1000 live births.[32,42] Most anomalies are noted, watched, concealed, and simply fade away in time. However, a small percentage (up to 5%) of others, despite their benign histologic appearances, can result in rapid growth, facial distortion, ulceration, infection, pain, bleeding, occlusion of luminal structures, congestive heart failure, thrombocytopenia, or even lethal complications because of their location or development.* When the hemangiomas are located in the visible areas of the facial and neck regions, they can occasionally produce devastating physical deformities with associated psychologic trauma. Because of the complexity and diversity of these lesions, the choice of therapy must be determined on an individual basis. The treatment will depend on the diagnostic determination of the type of tumor, its size, anatomic location, stage of growth and development, and its clinical course.

The selection of the most appropriate treatment can be quite difficult and hinges mainly on accurately predicting the natural progression of the lesion. Often, because of the complexity of these lesions, a multidisciplinary approach is required for the best treatment.[11,12,15,20,44]

It is extremely important for patient, parents, and physician to appreciate the complexity and variability of these lesions. It is equally important to try to predict the natural history of each tumor to prepare the family for the specific treatments available and the reasonable expectations.[7,11,25,27,46] To this end, it is essential for the physician to accurately diagnose and classify the lesion in question. This is often difficult because of the cumbersome and at times confusing nomenclature that surrounds these problems. In the past, classification of these anomalies has taken many forms and added to the confusion in the literature. Any useful classification system can only be justified if it has diagnostic applicability, aids in therapeutic planning, and guides future studies of pathogenesis.[26,27,32,33] I believe that present studies performed on the endothelial features and clinical evolution of these cutaneous vascular birthmarks will permit separation or classification of these lesions into three major categories: hemangiomas, malformations, and ectasias.[15,32,33]

The term *hemangioma* is used to denote a vascular tumor with increased endothelial turnover during the proliferative phase of development that may involute by progressive cellular death or fibrosis. The term *malformation* is used to describe a vascular anomaly with a normal endothelial cell cycle. These vascular malformations are inborn errors of vascular channel morphogenesis formed by any combination of abnormal capillary, arterial, venous, or lymphatic channels with or without shunting. This type of anomaly is present at birth and tends to be neither proliferative nor potentially involute but grows commensurate with the individual. These lesions will often expand with time. Some are dormant and only start to grow after a trigger or stimulating factor occurs. The term

*References 6, 8, 16, 22, 23, 26, 32, 44.

ectasia is used to describe lesions with normal endothelial turnover having vascular dilation. These lesions are vascular anomalies and not tumors and represent lesions such as cherry angioma or spider angioma.

HEMANGIOMAS

Seventy percent of hemangiomas are evident at birth and therefore constitute the most common congenital anomaly noted in humans. Of the remaining 30%, approximately half develop within the first year of life, with their clinical course being similar to that of newborns. Most hemangiomas appearing in the adult population are probably present earlier in life but are not recognized until a growing mass or some other symptom develops resulting from the establishment of an increased blood flow and until expansion occurs. Multiple lesions are present in 10% to 15% of cases.[12,15,33,38,40]

A female predominance is clearly noted in the hemangioma patient population, with a female-to-male ratio of 2:1 to 3:1.[15,16,25,32,36] There is no clear explanation available for this preponderance, although the cells in these lesions will often have estrogen receptors and will demonstrate growth with certain hormonal changes or administration. The development or appearance of vascular lesions, such as arterial spiders, palmar erythema, and cutaneous and gingival hemangiomas, is frequently seen during pregnancy. This phenomenon has been attributed to the powerful variations in endocrine secretion in the female. It is not infrequent that these lesions will demonstrate regression in the postpartum period, suggesting that steroidal hormones may play an etiologic role in their development.[32,33,41]

Distribution along racial differences is also noted. Hemangiomas are often seen in the white population, whereas they are relatively rare in the African-American population (comprising only 0.1% of those affected).[32,40]

Capillary (Strawberry) Hemangioma

The most common "birthmark" seen in the general population is the capillary, or strawberry, hemangioma. The pathology of this congenital vascular anomaly is characterized as either capillary, cavernous, or mixed type. These terms are used to describe the relative sizes of the vascular spaces involved within the lesion. This terminology is often confusing because a single lesion may be composed of compact masses of endothelial cells, with both capillary and cavernous components. Pathologists try to apply the usage of these terms to describe the major or predominant component of the vascular lesion. Unfortunately, even the detailed histologic and ultrastructural studies do not always reveal any distinctive features that can be correlated to prognosis.[32,33,39] In proliferating hemangiomas, however, it has been noted that there are 30 to 40 times the number of mast cells as expected in normal tissue. The granules found in mast cells contain amines, prostaglandins, and leukotrienes, thus playing an integral role in vasoproliferation and neovascularization. When the hemangioma starts to involute, the number of mast cells returns to normal.[32,33]

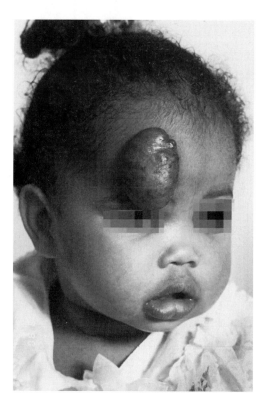

Figure 64-1. This 2-year-old child demonstrates an involuting capillary hemangioma with a significant cavernous portion. The surface is turning a gray color as its starts to change and as the overall volume starts to decrease.

Hemangiomas may exhibit various types of behavior in that they may expand, remain stable, or completely involute. Prognosis or prediction of behavior is often very difficult. The assignment of a given lesion to a specific pathologic subgroup usually does not offer any prognosis of its natural history. Similarly, the pathologic location of a hemangioma predominantly in the dermis or hypodermis has no predictive value on its ultimate growth or development. However, when hemangiomas are associated with other mesenchymal tissue anomalies, such as a lymphohemangioma or hemangiolipoma, the lesions are less likely to resolve than pure hemangiomas.[38-40]

Most hemangiomas that occur in the neonatal period will evolve from a "herald spot." This represents a pale, well-demarcated flat area on the body that is believed to represent an underperfused or nonperfused vascular sequestrum. This area will then undergo a vascularization and neovascularization process. The enhanced blood flow will then transform the herald spot, sometimes dramatically, into a rapidly expanding, irregular, pebbly, crimson hemangioma (Figure 64-1). In the congenital lesions noted at birth, these events are presumed to occur in utero.[7,12,15,20]

Once a hemangioma presents itself, it grows rapidly for the first 4 to 6 months of life. It may then maintain its size for the following 6 months and then begin a slow but variable process of involution. The involution process is heralded by the appearance of a central pallor and coalescence of blue-gray areas on the surface. The pebbly appearance and raised surface will start to

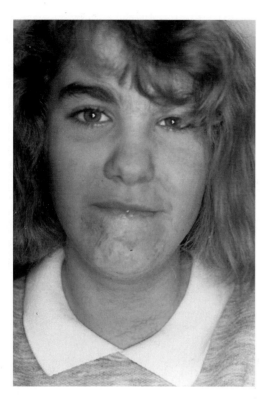

Figure 64-2. This 11-year-old child had an extensive capillary hemangioma over the left side of the face, chin, and neck. As the involution process continues, the volume decreases, but in massive cases the skin takes on a crepy, scarred appearance with residual telangiectasias.

recede. Finally, there will appear a reduction in volume. The involution process, whether partial or complete, usually is completed by age 5 to 7, although the process can continue through adolescence.* At times the residual anomaly leaves redundant skin, telangiectasias, or a thin, crepelike appearance to the tissue (Figure 64-2).

Studies of the vascularization process of capillary hemangiomas have shown that each lesion is supplied by a single afferent arterial vessel from a normal-appearing subcutaneous artery. The blood outflow leaving the lesion does so by way of multiple veins exiting into the periphery. The potential for growth or regression depends on the location and patency of those feeder vessels.[38,39]

Spontaneous regression of the lesion occurs as thrombosis of the feeder vessels occurs. Clinically this spontaneous regression can be monitored as the number of arteriovenous (A-V) fistulas (as determined by Doppler examination of the lesion) begins to diminish.[4,6] Nevertheless, it is still unknown whether regression is secondary to spontaneous cessation of the arterial blood supply or to the involution of the hemangiomas themselves.[38-40]

If all hemangiomas behaved the same and all were to spontaneously resolve, no therapy would be required. Unfortunately, this is not the case, so the clinician has to rely on experience and close observation of the lesions. Determination

of intervention, however, is only appropriate when it will improve the clinical course and final outcome, particularly in the head and neck area.

In reviewing several of the major series, it may be noted that some degree of spontaneous involution was noted in 75% to 95% of hemangiomas without the need for any intervention.[15,18,38] Several factors were examined in hopes of being able to determine the course or prognosis of the lesions. In the young patients followed, neither the size of the hemangiomas nor the gender of the patient appeared to influence the speed or the completeness of involution. The anatomic site of the lesion had a minimal effect on the final result, except that lesions of the mucous membranes of the lip were found to regress less completely than those elsewhere in the body. The presence of multiple lesions did not appear to have any prognostic influence. The patients with multiple hemangiomatous lesions did not necessarily resolve all the lesions at the same time or at the same speed. Lesions that did not grow or expand early in infancy did not necessarily have a better prognosis or involute any greater than those that exhibited explosive growth patterns. Most of the expanding hemangiomatous lesions did not appear to grow after the twelfth month of life. There also was no correlation between the date of appearance of the lesion or when it started the involution process. Ultimately, all had a satisfactory result, even those that persisted beyond the fourth year of age when they started the involution process.[5,15,18,38,41]

Other dramatic changes could be noted with the involution process, but again little correlation could be associated with some of these findings. The appearance of superficial ulcerations occurred in 10% of hemangiomatous lesions. The ulcerations were confined to the intermediate-and large-sized lesions during the expanding growth phase and nearly always healed within a few weeks. Unfortunately, however, the presence of the ulceration did not have any prognostic significance as it related to ultimate resolution of the hemangioma. It was, however, associated with leaving noticeable scars and residual telangiectasia.[5,12]

Despite the high rate of spontaneous involution and healing of the hemangiomas, there are still a considerable number of lesions and situations that require treatment or specific means of intervention. The consensus of opinion is that early and aggressive treatment is justified in specific cases when the patient's life, special sensory organs, or well-being is in jeopardy. Those conditions are as follows*:

1. Obstruction of the airway
2. Cardiovascular decompensation
3. Uncontrollable ulceration and bleeding
4. Unmanageable infections (chronic, recurrent)
5. Thrombocytopenia
6. Obstruction of luminal structures (e.g., auditory canal, nasopharynx, and alimentary tract)
7. Obstruction of the visual axis
8. Skeletal distortion or atypical skeletal and soft tissue growth patterns

---

*References 12, 14, 17, 30, 32, 33, 42.

*References 12, 15, 16, 23, 24, 26, 33.

9. Small lesions (localized in such an area that excision can be performed without any cosmetic or functional risk to the patient)

10. Pain

When the lesion involves the tracheal or bronchial regions, progressive airway obstruction can occur, thus requiring immediate intervention. In infants, who are by nature obligate nasal breathers, progressive enlargement of nasopharyngeal hemangiomas may be cause for immediate intervention. If they develop slowly, they can result in the infant transferring to the oral airway for breathing purposes. However, if compromise of the airway is occurring, emergency intervention is required to save the patient.[16,18,21,37,41]

Cardiovascular decompensation can occur as a result of A-V shunting leading to high-output congestive heart failure. This potentially lethal condition can often be seen in those individuals who are noted to have multiple cutaneous and visceral hemangiomas. Affected infants will usually develop symptoms early in life, within 2 to 8 weeks. The triad of congestive heart failure, anemia, and hepatomegaly is most often present. Jaundice, abdominal bruits, and internal hemorrhage within the abdominal cavity or within the alimentary tract can also be noted.[12,14,15,41]

Hemorrhage from the surface of the lesions can result from minor trauma or may result from platelet-trapping coagulopathy (i.e., Kasabach-Merritt syndrome). Whenever this is evident, it will require multiple modalities of intervention to stabilize the clinical condition.*

When progressive necrosis is evident along the surface of the hemangiomas, problems with recurrent infection can be evident. This is particularly true in instances in which there is involvement of the surfaces that are easily traumatized, such as the lips or mucous membranes.[12,15,33]

Early intervention is also indicated when vision is sufficiently obscured to cause amblyopia, astigmatism, or permanent damage to the visual axis. A linear relationship between the duration of complete visual obstruction and eventual loss of visual acuity has been identified and was found especially significant when obstruction was greater than 3 months. The period most vulnerable is before the first year of life but extends to 3 years of age. The degree of visual obstruction also relates to the degree of permanent damage, that is, if greater than one half of the lids are involved, the degree of visual obstruction and the permanent damage will be greater.[15,33]

Small lesions that are localized to areas that can be easily excised without cosmetic or functional risk to the patient are also ideal for early intervention. The late or delayed treatment of lesions that have not completely resolved may yield contour or color deformities and may require tissue replacement or resurfacing. These particular deformities have to be handled in a very individualized manner.[7,11,12]

Some of the more challenging problems lie with the effect on growth of the developing skeleton. It is not simply a matter of enhanced blood flow but actually other factors that may influence asymmetric development of the underlying tissue (Figure 64-3). Sometimes, by removing the primary lesion,

*References 12, 14, 21, 33, 34, 35, 37, 44.

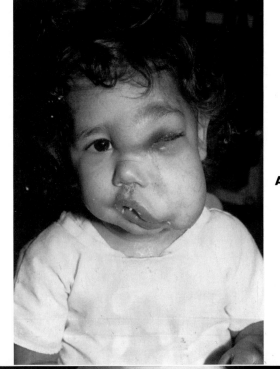

A

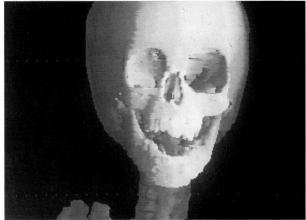

B

Figure 64-3. A, This young child had an underlying lymphovenous hemangioma that has resulted in amblyopia of the left eye because of delayed treatment. **B,** The facial skeleton has also developed bony hypertrophy on the involved side of the face.

you can arrest the effect on the underlying skeleton and reconstruct the disturbing soft tissue deformities.[33,42,44,45]

Pain is not a frequent finding in patients with hemangiomas; however, it can be seen in patients who experience repeated trauma to the lesions that further evolves into recurrent bouts of phlebitis. Often multiple phleboliths will be noted in the most tender and painful areas. Once removed with resection of the surrounding vascular anomaly, the patient will often experience relief of these symptoms[33] (Figure 64-4).

MALFORMATIONS

Vascular malformations are structural abnormalities resulting from faulty morphogenesis of the embryonic vascular plexuses.

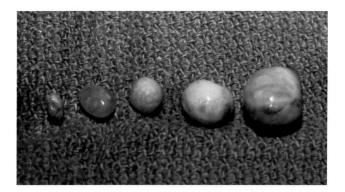

Figure 64-4. Phleboliths can be found in hemangiomas in which there has been trauma, inflammation, or sclerotherapy delivered to the lesion. Often the patient will complain of pain or tenderness in the area of the phleboliths. These phleboliths were taken from a female patient who had repeated trauma to the area. The region was a single, large network of cavernous veins that had started to swell and become painful.

By definition, a vascular malformation is always present at birth, although the anomaly may not become obvious until the early neonatal period. These lesions grow commensurate with the child. There is no evidence that they proliferate by cellular hyperplasia or invade adjacent tissue. The hemodynamic and lymphodynamic characteristics will determine the natural history of these lesions. Usually one type of abnormal vascular channel may predominate in a vascular malformation, frequently combined with capillary, arterial, venous, and lymphatic components, as well as some complex combined anomalies often referred to as specific syndromes (e.g., Klippel-Trénaunay-Weber syndrome, Maffucci's syndrome, Proteus syndrome).[15,37,41,44]

These malformations can be either isolated or one localization of a systemic disease, such as neurofibromatosis, Osler-Weber-Rendu disease, or Sturge-Weber syndrome. Most of these lesions are "low-flow" types.[33,44]

Port-Wine Stain (Nevus Flammeus)

The port-wine stain is an intradermal vascular malformation that is present at birth and persists throughout life, showing no spontaneous regression. It occurs in 0.3% to 0.5% of newborns. Its early light red color may become a deep purple with age. The lesion may also develop a nodular hyperkeratotic appearance in adult years. Port-wine stains may be associated with an underlying cavernous element capable of assuming arteriovenous connections[38,40] (Figures 64-5 and 64-6).

The characteristics of Sturge-Weber syndrome include facial nevus flammeus, seizures secondary to hemangiomatous meningeal involvement, and glaucoma. It should be suspected in patients with port-wine stains involving either the ophthalmic or the maxillary division of the fifth cranial nerve. There are often ipsilateral vascular malformations of the choroid and leptomeninges either with or without calcifications, usually overlying the posterior parietal and occipital lobes. There is also a high risk of developing glaucoma as the patient ages. Ophthalmologic and neurologic consultations are indicated in the management of these patients[15,25-27] (Figure 64-7).

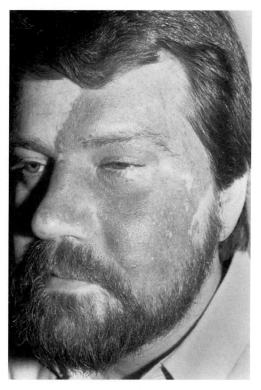

Figure 64-5. This 32-year-old patient demonstrates an extensive port-wine stain malformation with only the earliest signs of surface changes. Clinical examination of the lesion demonstrates that the vascular malformation extends over each component of the left fifth cranial nerve distribution, and a clinical history reveals long-standing glaucoma in the left eye. Together these symptoms confirm the diagnosis of Sturge-Weber syndrome.

Cosmetic reasons generally dictate the treatment of port-wine stains, although developing A-V connections can convert them into aggressive lesions with high attendant morbidity. However, efforts to permanently remove port-wine stains surgically have been disappointing. Excision and grafting, dermal overgrafting, and flap replacement have all been attempted but only substitute contour and scar deformities for color deformity.[8] Tattooing procedures once recommended are no longer advocated because of the difficulties with pigment matching and pigment fading.[16] Heavy makeup (e.g., Covermark, Lydia O'Leary), though not ideal, is still an acceptable form of management. Steroids, radiation, cryotherapy, and electrocoagulation have been tried for port-wine stains with little success in some of the difficult lesions. Recent developments in laser technology have now made treatment more predictable and aesthetically acceptable. In some cases, multiple modalities have to be used to achieve satisfactory results.[16,33]

Arteriovenous Malformations

The most difficult lesions to treat are the arteriovenous malformations (AVMs), which contain fistulas and demonstrate "high-flow" characteristics, such as pulsations, bruits, thrills, and increased skin temperature. These hemodynamically active lesions can expand with alterations in pressure or flow and with collateral formation secondary to trauma or attempts at operative therapy. Some malformations may enlarge by hormonal

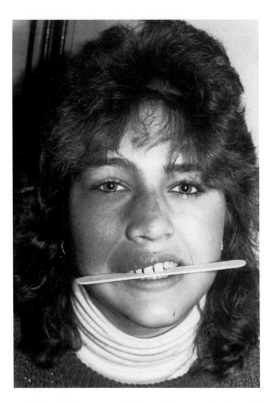

Figure 64-6. This young girl reveals a port-wine stain that extends over the maxillary distribution of the fifth cranial nerve. The bony skeleton is also hypertrophied under this malformation, as demonstrated by the occlusal cant.

modulations during puberty, pregnancy, or estrogen therapy. The low-flow lesions are often associated with skeletal hypertrophy, whereas the high-flow lesions are more likely to cause destruction of adjacent skeletal structures.*

The high-flow arterial malformations are clinically labeled unstable because of their tendency to cause acute, often emergent problems. Expansion of such a lesion may be a precipitous event, for example, after trauma to the area, infection, or an attempted operative resection. In some patients, increased cardiac output may progress to a state of high-output congestive failure. A-V anomalies of the extremities can result in ischemic necrosis of the distal limb, whereas the lesions of the facial region can present with frightening hemorrhage after minor trauma or routine dental extraction. Some of these malformations induce a grotesque appearance and are extremely difficult to treat. The therapeutic challenge will depend on the extension, the localization, and the tissues involved.[12,15]

The clinical examination will separate these malformations associated with pulsating enlarged vessels, thrill, and audible bruit from those that are soft, bluish, can be depressed but reconstitute their volume rapidly, and have no thrill and no audible bruit. Angiography will confirm in the first group that the arterial feeders are enlarged with rapid A-V shunting and rapid filling of the abnormal network of the AVM. The second group will show arteries of normal size, no A-V shunting, and

*References 10, 11, 18, 41, 44, 45, 47.

normal capillary phase of sometimes late faint pooling of contrast. This group consists of cavernous or venous types of malformations.[15,40]

OPERATIONS

The clinical management of vascular lesions carries with it several modalities of treatment, including: (1) surgical ablation, (2) embolic therapy or sclerotherapy, (3) steroid therapy, (4) chemotherapy, (5) compressive therapy, (6) radiation therapy, (7) thermal therapy and/or cryotherapy, and (8) laser therapy.[12,15,33]

Surgical ablation may be very simple and direct or combined with sclerotherapy or embolization. Hemangiomas that are persistent, repeatedly traumatized, and less than 1 to 2 cm in diameter located in nonvital, cosmetically covered areas may be elliptically excised without waiting for involution (Figure 64-8). Lesions of the nasal tip have been often excised in the past, but a more conservative treatment may also be more appropriate in this setting unless the deformity is quite disfiguring. Prophylactic excision of hemangiomas before pregnancies has been recommended, especially those lesions of the lip, because of their tremendous growth potential before parturition.

The management of massive hemangiomas, which assume large A-V plexiform communications, cause extensive deformity, and encroach on underlying deeper structures, is complex and must be individualized. There is no way of predicting those that will spontaneously regress from those that will not and will need treatment. Angiography will usually show normal arteries without significant early A-V shunting, but the capillary phase will show many irregular capillaries with pooling of contrast in the tissue of the hemangioma. Embolization is usually carried out with particles if the lesion is significant in size. This can trigger and accelerate the involution process. It can decrease the mass effect of the tongue, the compression of the airway, or the swelling of the eyelid. Vascular malformations have to be properly classified into those with enlarged arterial feeders and A-V shunts and those with normal-sized arterial feeders, slow flow, and no fast A-V shunting but sometimes late pooling of contrast. The indications and techniques of embolization, and thus the treatment course, depend on this classification.[12,30,31,34,37]

The treatment of such A-V malformations is often challenging, frustrating, and potentially as life threatening as the lesion itself. The treacherous natural course of these lesions is often only briefly interrupted by courageous attempts at resection, resulting in further tissue loss and "malignant" hemodynamic enlargement of persistent anomalous channels and collaterals. Several therapeutic principles have been learned from past misadventures and mistakes. Whenever possible, the entire lesion must be excised as if treating a "cancer." Any residual anomalous vascular tissue at the margin of excision only invites

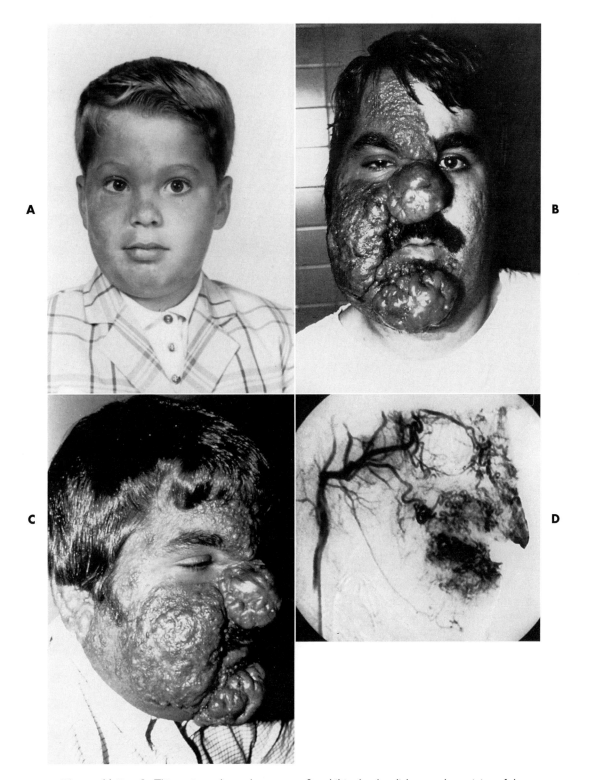

Figure 64-7. **A,** This patient, shown here at age 8, exhibited only a light vascular staining of the left side of his face along the distribution of the fifth cranial nerve. This patient did develop seizures and other signs consistent with the diagnosis of Sturge-Weber syndrome. **B** and **C,** By the time the patient was in his mid-twenties, hypertrophy of the lesion, recurrent infections in the involved areas, and significant facial disfigurement developed. The patient became a recluse and suffered significant psychologic trauma as a result. **D,** Angiography of the external carotid system demonstrates the abnormal vasculature throughout the facial region. Embolization and resection was required to treat the main portions of the vascular malformation.

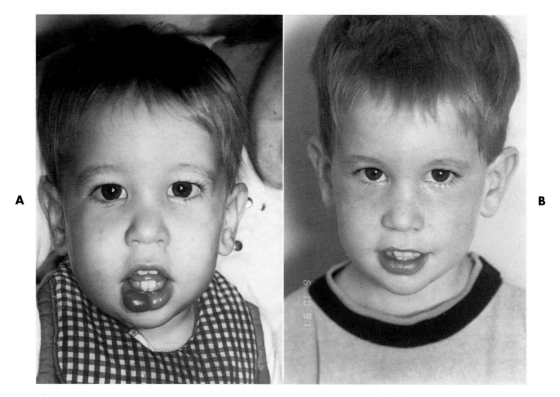

Figure 64-8. **A,** This young child was noted to have a hemangioma of the lower lip that grew progressively shortly after birth. **B,** Continued monitoring of the lesion noted only partial involution. It was decided because of its location and repeated trauma during eating that simple elliptical resection would offer the best solution.

further "recurrence" and expansion of the lesion. Numerous surgical disasters have taught surgeons never to ligate "feeding" vessels proximal to an A-V malformation. If there is an underlying coagulation defect secondary to thrombotic consumption, this must be preoperatively treated with heparin or other medical modalities.[12,15,40]

Treatment of the large and more extensive lesions with intravascular selective angiography and embolization offers the best and most consistent therapeutic approach. This is usually carried out as a preliminary-stage procedure with embolization followed by wide surgical extirpation within 24 to 48 hours. Provisions for extensive blood replacement, hypotensive anesthesia, and possible cardiopulmonary bypass with deep hypothermic circulatory arrest should be considered whenever resection is anticipated. Under these conditions, the best opportunities for complete resection and thus cure are met. After the wide resection, the defect should be reconstructed if possible with local axial flaps or microvascular free-tissue transfers. All of these factors and the postembolization films have to be analyzed carefully to ensure viable reconstruction.[3,12,33,37]

ALTERNATIVE TREATMENTS

Steroid Therapy
In 1967, Zarem and Edgerton[48] by serendipity made the observation that expanding strawberry hemangiomas responded well to steroid therapy. Their report and observations were repeated

and confirmed in numerous case reports and series.[4,9,15,18,48] It was also noted that proliferating lesions in patients younger than 10 months usually responded well to steroid therapy. Not all vascular lesions respond, however, to this mode of treatment. Cavernous hemangiomas in adults, arteriovenous fistulas, port-wine stains, and lymphangiomas have not been found to respond to steroid management. The doses vary with the series reviewed; however, the generally accepted dosage is 2 to 3 mg/kg/day of prednisone given systemically or orally over a 2- to 3-week period. Hemangiomas that are sensitive will respond within a period of 7 to 10 days. At this stage the dosage can be lowered to 0.75 mg/kg/day. Slowly responding lesions can be treated with a 4- to 6-week course followed by an interval of 3 to 4 weeks and then another course (Figure 64-9). If there is no response, there is no reason to continue the therapy. It is important to note the need to carefully monitor the child's growth milestones, metabolic status, and exposure to infections. If these show signs of disturbance, the therapy is modified or terminated.[4,9,15,16,48]

On occasion, rebound phenomena can be seen with reduced steroid levels. In these instances, the patients can be treated with 2- to 3-week cycles at reduced dosages until continued regression and involution is noted. Sometimes three cycles are needed to initiate involution.[4,9,33]

Chemotherapy
The cellular and biochemical bases of steroid effect remain to be defined, although Sasaki and Pang[36] recently demonstrated

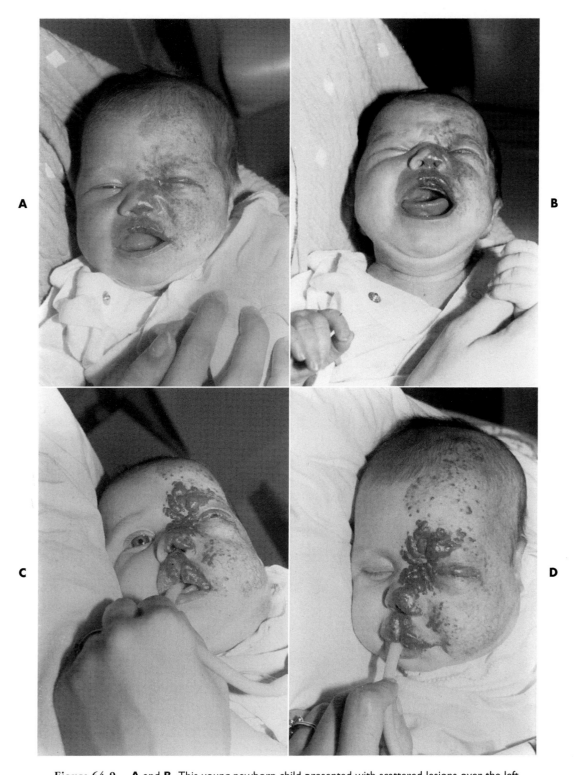

Figure 64-9. **A** and **B,** This young newborn child presented with scattered lesions over the left side of the face that were relatively flat in nature; however, there was repeated ulceration of the upper lip and persistent swelling around the left eye. **C** and **D,** Within 6 weeks the facial skin lesions had become more raised and the ulcerations of the lip deeper. The columella had become ulcerated and portions necrotic. The left eyelids became more involved with the hemangioma, resulting in visual obstruction.   *Continued*

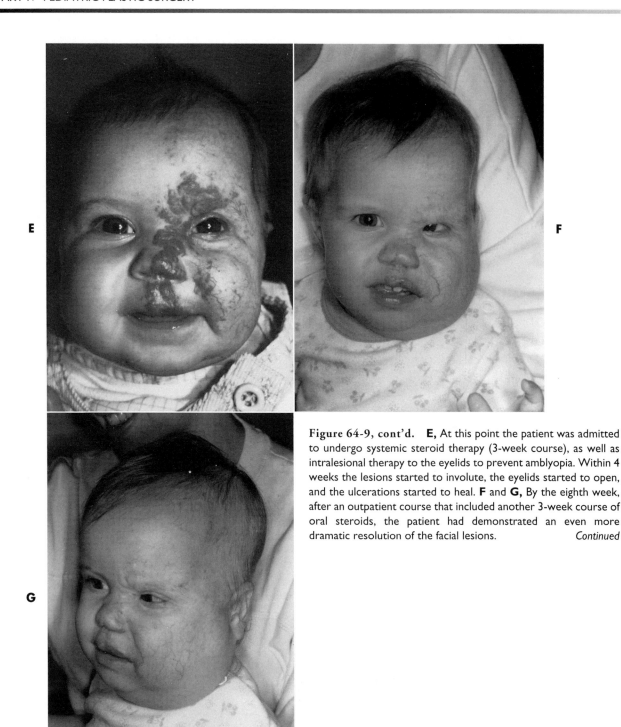

Figure 64-9, cont'd. E, At this point the patient was admitted to undergo systemic steroid therapy (3-week course), as well as intralesional therapy to the eyelids to prevent amblyopia. Within 4 weeks the lesions started to involute, the eyelids started to open, and the ulcerations started to heal. **F** and **G,** By the eighth week, after an outpatient course that included another 3-week course of oral steroids, the patient had demonstrated an even more dramatic resolution of the facial lesions. *Continued*

that virtually all juvenile strawberry hemangiomas contain estrogen receptors. No evidence for hormonal markers are found in vascular malformations. Previous studies suggest that steroids (1) augment sensitivity of the terminal vascular bed to catecholamines and (2) inhibit fibroplasia. Direct intralesional injections of methylprednisolone and triamcinolone/beta-methasone have been very successful in obtaining excellent results, especially for periorbital lesions.[4,9,14,16]

Recently, cyclophosphamide and α-interferon have been added to the armamentarium to inhibit the growth of massive hemangiomas associated with platelet trapping and congestive heart failure when such lesions are too large to allow complete resection.[16,21,22,43] Based on diurnal cortisol activity, α-interferon is given at 3 million U/m^2/day intravenously in the evening during a 4- to 9-week period.[43]

Pressure Therapy

When carefully applied, compression treatment of hemangiomas is noninvasive, safe, and effective as demonstrated by numerous case reports.[16,28] Today this method can be used in

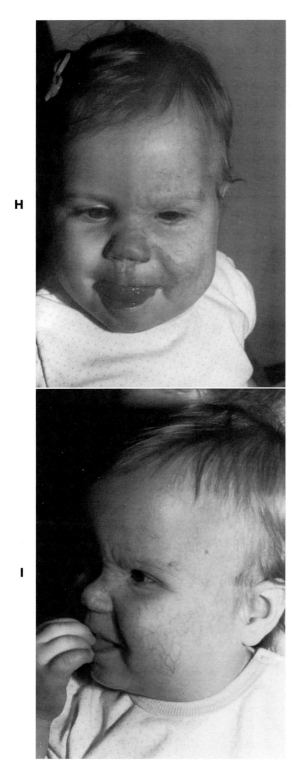

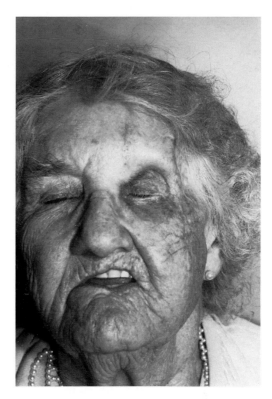

Figure 64-10. This elderly woman had undergone thermal destruction of port-wine stain malformation as a young child. This has resulted in a permanent disfigurement and chronic pain for the patient over the left facial and orbital region without successful removal of the vascular malformation.

Sometimes these attempts were partially successful; however, most often they resulted in extensive tissue damage and scarring (Figures 64-10 and 64-11).[12,15,33] Sometimes the successes reported in the early literature were actually believed to be attributed to the normal involution process of the hemangioma occurring coincidentally with treatment.

Radiation Therapy

Radiation has been used almost since its discovery for the treatment of vascular lesions. Many authors who reviewed series of patients treated with various forms of irradiation and compared those treated with observation only have concluded that the ultimate results were equally satisfactory. Despite these early encouraging reports, most authors believe that irradiation has no place in the treatment of hemangiomas. Edgerton[15] states that "gamma or beta irradiation therapy should never be used to treat any form of hemangioma," basing his opinion on the fact that irradiation has been associated with damage to epiphyses, breast, gonads, skin, ocular lens, thyroid, growing structures, and the possibility of late tumor induction.[12,15,33] Other authors observed that the complications were 10 times that in the untreated patients[16] (Figure 64-12).

Laser Therapy

Improved laser technology and better microscopic evaluation of the laser-tissue interactions has led to a better understanding of the tissue response. The efficacy of the laser is dependent on the laser-tissue interactions and thermal coagulation that

Figure 64-9, cont'd. H and **I,** Three months after the use of steroid therapy, only the patient was left with some telangiectasia and some slight skin scarring.

combination with other modalities. There is, however, no clear explanation for its mechanism of action, but ischemia and necrosis are theorized.

Thermal Therapy/Cryotherapy

Use of burning and freezing techniques have been described for hundreds of years in attempts to control these lesions.

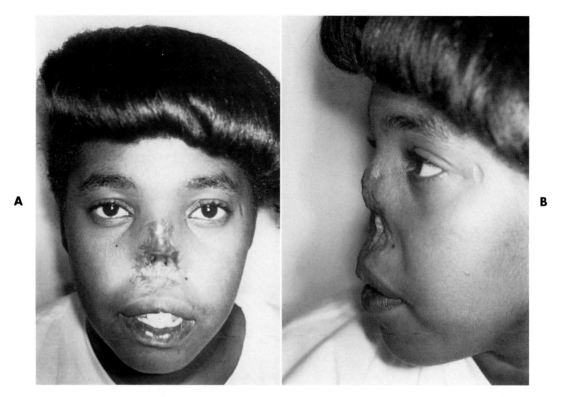

Figure 64-11. **A** and **B,** This teenage patient had a nasal capillary hemangioma treated with cauterization as a young child. The resultant scarring and contraction has left her with significant nasal stenosis and aesthetic deformity.

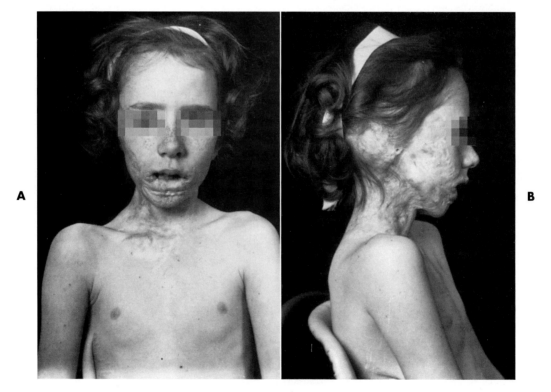

Figure 64-12. **A** and **B,** This patient had developed a capillary hemangioma shortly after birth that affected the right side of the face, ear, and neck region. Irradiation as a young child for this patient resulted in the necrosis of the right ear down to the internal auditory meatus, hypoplasia of the right facial skeleton, vocal cord fibrosis, and irradiation necrosis and scarring of the facial and skeleton.

results. This interaction results in cell necrosis, hemostasis, and gross alteration of the extracellular matrix at specific temperature-heating time combinations. Laser surgery is a controlled thermal coagulation or burn with the surgeon controlling the intensity and location of the heat injury. The relatively low-power continuous lasers, such as the CO_2 and the argon-ion, and the rapid-pulse (continuous) lasers, such as copper vapor and potassium titanyl phosphate (KTP) lasers, usually cause a well-controlled superficial partial-thickness burn. The pulsed yellow dye lasers designed for selective photothermolysis of microvascular lesions in contrast causes selective burns in the microvessels. The selective photothermolysis uses selective ab-

sorption of light pulses by pigmented targets, such as blood vessels, pigmented cells, and tattoo ink particles, to achieve selectively thermally mediated injury. The short pulses that are necessary to deposit energy in the targets before they cool off achieves extreme localized heating, thermal coagulation, and thermally mediated mechanical damage. The degree of the damage is dependent on the rate of energy deposition in the target area[1,2,10,19] (Figure 64-13).

With the use of a greater array of lasers, much greater success has been achieved over many vascular lesions with resultant improved aesthetic results. As this technology improves, greater sophistication and selectivity have allowed more

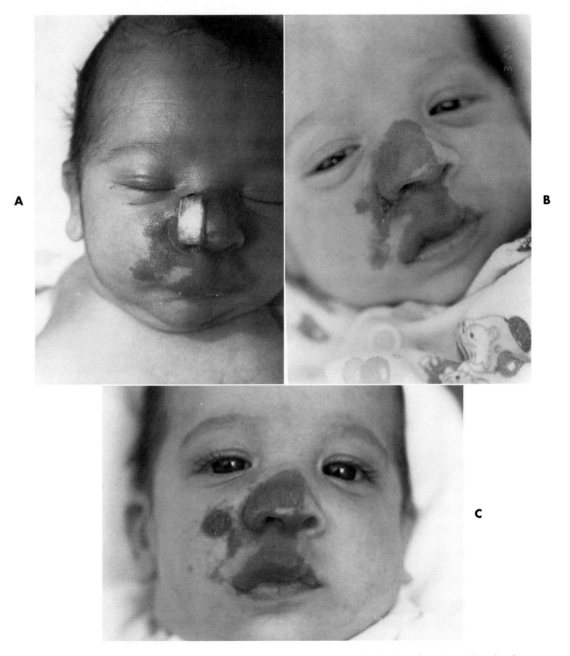

Figure 64-13. **A,** This 1-day-old infant was noted to have pulsatile bleeding from the right side of the nose shortly after birth. Chemical cauterization, Gelfoam, and pressure stopped the bleeding until the child was able to be transferred to a hospital that could carry out angiography and surgical resection. **B,** Treatment consisted of exploration of the facial artery, embolization, and resection of the malformation. **C,** The cutaneous portion of the malformation persisted. *Continued*

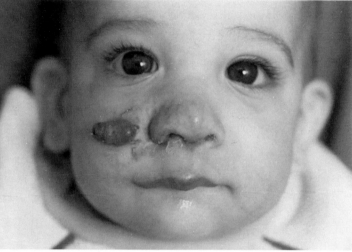

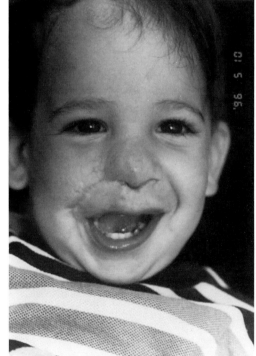

Figure 64-13, cont'd. **D** and **E,** The cutaneous portion was treated with a vascular laser with good results. **F,** A cutaneous recurrence was noted to persist in the cheek area and was resected with very satisfactory results.

The limitations in advancing into a vessel depend on the loops and hairpin turns of the vessel. After three or four sharp loops, the friction between the vessel and catheter but also between the catheter and the guide wire limit the advancement of the catheter. This limitation will sometimes dictate the type of material used for embolization. As a general principle, the more aggressive the embolic material, the more selective the catheter has to be in relation to the malformation being treated.[12,34,37]

It is now routine to advance into the branches of the division of the ascending pharyngeal artery, occipital artery, lingual or facial artery, and middle meningeal or superficial temporal artery, as well as other tributaries and collaterals of the external carotid artery.[12,29-31] This allows more selective ablation with less chance of unwarranted injury to vital structures nearby.

The materials used for embolization are divided into solid and liquid agents. Particles of polyvinyl alcohol foam (PVA) are among the most used solid materials. They come in calibrated sizes ranging from 150 Fm to 1 mm. The shape of the particles is very irregular, with many spicules that adhere to the vessel wall. They can be injected in association with 30% ethanol, which increases the occlusion and thrombosis of vessels to the malformation. However, using ethanol also increases the risk of tissue necrosis. PVA particles are not permanent occlusive material but are used preoperatively to prepare the operative area. Surgical ablation should be carried out ideally within 24 to 48 hours of embolization to achieve the best results[12,37] (Figure 64-14).

Coils can be used for permanent occlusion of a vessel. They are made of platinum, which is poorly thrombogenic. The thrombogenicity of the coils is increased by adding fibers

complete ablation of the lesions in younger patients, leaving less scarring.[1,2,19]

Embolization and Sclerotherapy

The management of complex vascular anomalies has been revolutionized by improvements in the technology of embolization. The embolization procedures consist of using artificial emboli to block the vessels going to the tumor or vascular malformation. The catheters clinically available allow superselective catheterization of vessels close to 1 mm in size. Their flexibility and maneuverability are also constantly improving.

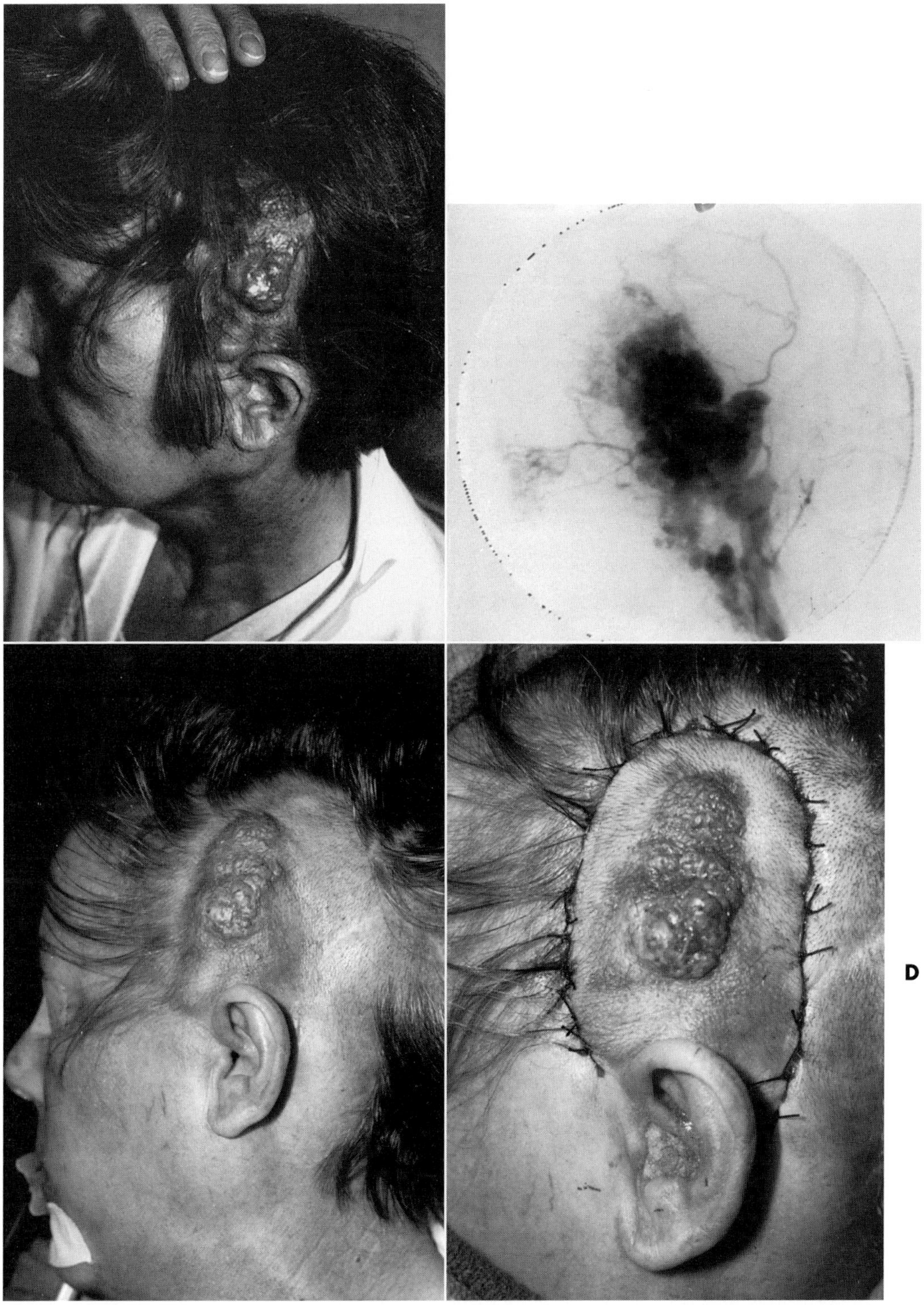

Figure 64-14. **A,** This postmenopausal woman noted this lesion after being treated with hormonal replacement therapy. **B,** This extensive AVM was embolized with PVA and prepared for resection with 24 hours. **C,** The mass had decreased in size and color lightened after embolization. **D,** Blocking sutures are placed at times to further decrease bleeding that is expected in the resection of large AVM lesions. *Continued*

attached to the coil. They come in different sizes, lengths, and shapes. They can be straight or curved with a known radius after being detached. They advance easily inside the guiding catheter and are pushed with a "pusher" guide wire.[12]

Gelfoam pieces or foam were previously very common but are now less often used. However, a large plug of Gelfoam can be used for protection of a territory that should not be embolized. Recanalization occurs more frequently and quicker after Gelfoam embolization than after PVA embolization.[3,12,33]

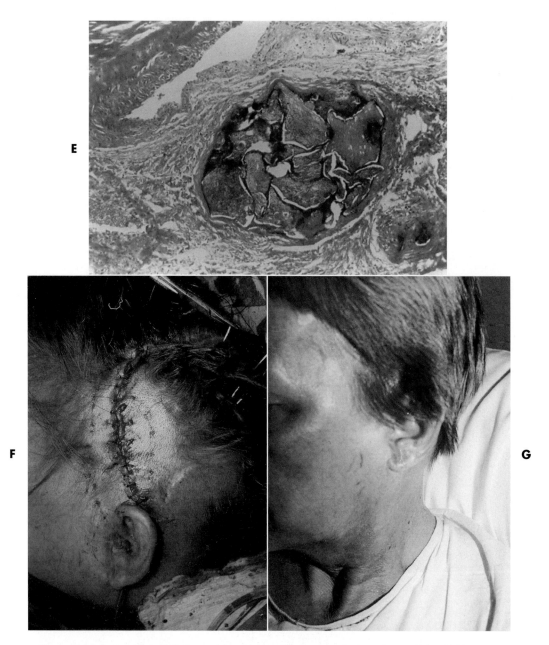

Figure 64-14, cont'd. **E,** PVA particles are noted in the resected specimen of the AVM associated with clot and thrombosis with the lumen of the vessels. **F,** After wide resection, local flaps were used for reconstruction. **G,** The postoperative appearance 4 months later was quite acceptable.

Various types of liquid agents can be used. Silicone can be made radiopaque by mixing it with tantalum powder, bismuth powder, or tungsten powder. It solidifies in several minutes to hours, depending on the components used. Some silicone has a fixed polymerizing time, depending on the amount of catalyst used. Most of these mixtures have a substantial viscosity. They should be used if one thinks that a complete cure of the vascular lesion can be obtained. The risk of tissue necrosis is increased versus solid particles. Silicone should not be used when there is a large and fast A-V shunt.[3,12,33]

Hydroxy-ethylmethacylic glue can also be made radiopaque by mixing it with tantalum or tungsten powder. Adding Pantopaque to the acrylic glue increases the polymerizing time.

Pure glue solidifies in 1 or 2 seconds when it is in contact with blood. It is an excellent agent when occluding fistulas with fast A-V shunting. However, great care must be taken when using it in tumors because the risk of tissue necrosis is substantial. In widespread lesions it assists the surgeon in many ways to reduce the blood loss and allows for a better and more complete resection (Figures 64-15 and 64-16). The use of acrylic glue is discouraged in cases of fistulas or high-flow A-V malformations.

Pure ethanol is an excellent agent for sclerotherapy to be used for direct injection into a venous or vascular malformation with slow flow. It should be used carefully because of the risk of tissue necrosis. It is indicated in venous angiomas,

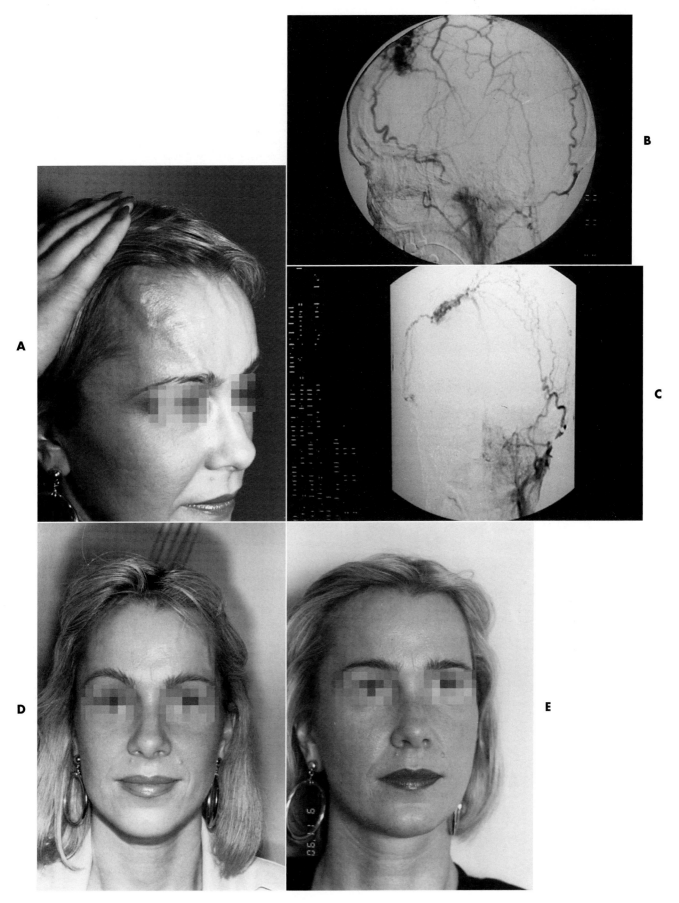

Figure 64-15. **A,** This patient had always had a red blush in the region of the right forehead. After a rhytidectomy with ligation of the right superficial temporal vessels, a pulsatile growing lesion developed with a bruit audible to the patient. **B** and **C,** Arteriography revealed recruitment from the contralateral temporal vessels and the occipital vessels. After embolization with acrylic glue, resection was complete with a satisfactory result being noted at 3 months **(D)** and 5 years **(E).**

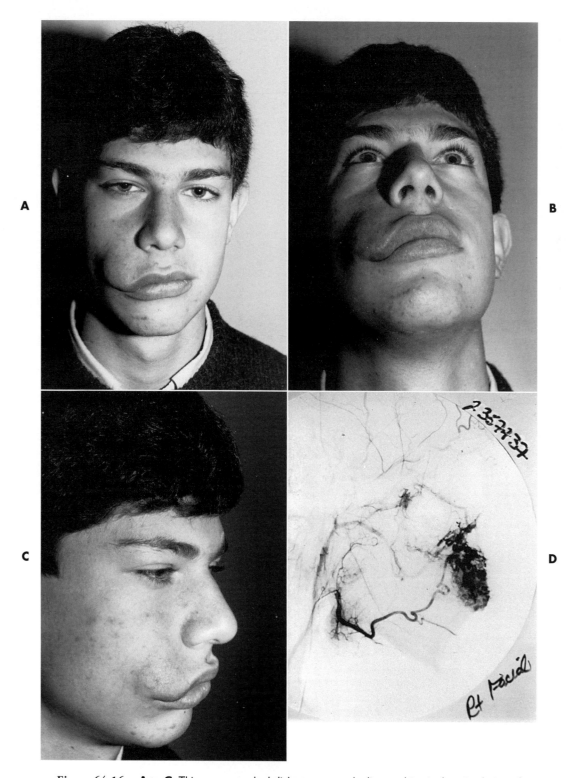

Figure 64-16. **A** to **C,** This young man had slight trauma to the lip, resulting in the stimulation of growth for this AVM. Arterial ligation of the blood supply further increased growth. Embolization and resection within a 24-hour period was proposed for treatment. **D,** Arteriography through the right internal maxillary artery and the right facial artery defined the source of inflow for embolization. *Continued*

Figure 64-16, cont'd. **E** to **G,** One-year followup reveals good symmetry and function with no evidence of recurrence.

but it should not be injected intraarterially in fast-flow A-V malformations[3,12,33] (Figures 64-17 and 64-18).

OUTCOMES

COMPLICATIONS

Most surgical procedures for vascular malformations can be done safely, with the vast majority of these vascular embolizations being achieved without complications. A good knowledge of the anatomy, careful superselective angiography of excellent quality, and large experience with the different clinical situations diminish the risk. Good communication between specialists and surgeons is needed to ensure good results ultimately for the patient.

The collaterals of the external carotid artery (ECA) are well known and are usually considered safe territory for embolization because there is very little risk of brain damage. In fact, any embolization of the ECA has to be done very carefully by interventionalists who know the anatomic variations of the ECA branches. Several areas of anastomosis are important in the head and neck area. The occipital artery and the ascending pharyngeal artery are very often if not always anastomosed with the vertebral artery. This dangerous anastomosis may or may not be seen during selective angiography of these two vessels depending on the position of the tip of the catheter and multiple hemodynamic factors (speed, strength of injection of contrast, and quantity

injected). Even when it is seen, it does not mean that embolization cannot be done but that it has to be done under visualized and flow-controlled injection. It is also possible to protect the anastomosis with a plug of Gelfoam before embolization.[3,29,34]

The second most dangerous anastomosis is between the middle meningeal artery and the ophthalmic artery. There are multiple embryonic variants of these connections, but one realizes that when they do exist, embolic material injected into the middle meningeal artery can reach the central artery to the retina and induce monocular blindness or can reach the internal carotid artery (ICA) and its distal branches. The third dangerous connection exists between the distal internal maxillary artery and the carotid siphon or the ophthalmic artery. Finally, the distal facial artery with its angular branch is connected to the ophthalmic artery.[12,34]

Besides the dangerous connections between the ECA and ICA territory, one has to consider the risk of necrosis of normal tissue whenever the tip of the catheter cannot be advanced selectively enough. This occurs when embolization of the internal maxillary artery or the facial artery is carried out. It is not always possible to deliver the embolic material only to the target area, and therefore the risks of embolization have to be weighed against the advantages. It is possible then to select an embolic agent that is not too toxic and carry out embolization that is not too aggressive.

In cases of deep extensive vascular malformations, reflux of particles or liquid agents into the cerebral vessels is exceptional but can induce a catastrophic stroke when it happens. A certain

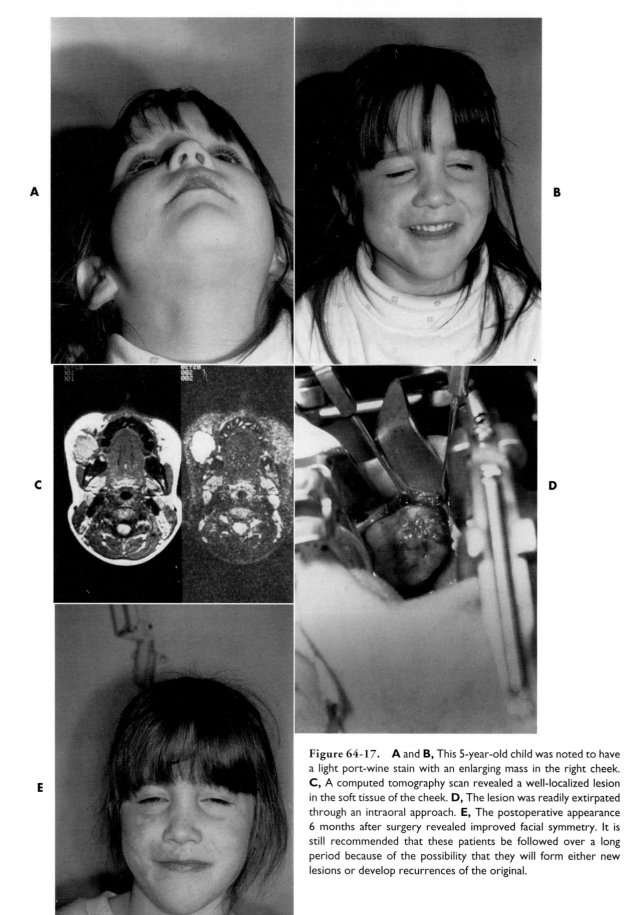

Figure 64-17. **A** and **B,** This 5-year-old child was noted to have a light port-wine stain with an enlarging mass in the right cheek. **C,** A computed tomography scan revealed a well-localized lesion in the soft tissue of the cheek. **D,** The lesion was readily extirpated through an intraoral approach. **E,** The postoperative appearance 6 months after surgery revealed improved facial symmetry. It is still recommended that these patients be followed over a long period because of the possibility that they will form either new lesions or develop recurrences of the original.

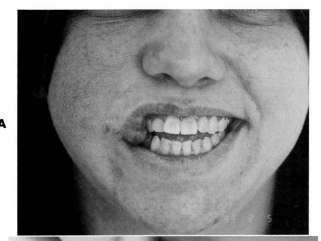

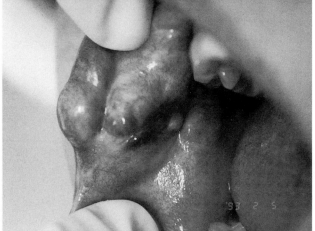

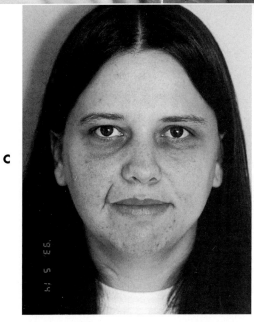

Figure 64-18. **A** and **B,** This patient had developed an enlarging venous malformation after her pregnancy and the birth of her child. The lesion did not regress after completion of the pregnancy and left her with a significant aesthetic deformity that was also easily traumatized. **C,** Sclerosing with absolute alcohol followed in 3 weeks with full-thickness cheek resection was performed. Adhering to aesthetic principles, resection of the malformation and reconstruction of the commissure were performed that enabled a satisfactory reconstruction with good function.

number of cranial nerves can be damaged by the embolization. The posterior branch of division of the ascending pharyngeal artery, which gives blood supply to the ninth, tenth, eleventh, and twelfth cranial nerves, is more safely embolized with particles than with liquid agents to avoid ischemic complications or inducement of ischemic changes within these nerves.[3,12,33]

The middle meningeal artery is a dangerous artery to embolize. The connections with the ophthalmic artery and the ICA have already been reviewed with particular attention at the important risks associated with embolization in this area. There is also a recurrent branch at the level of the foramen spinosum, which gives blood supply to the seventh nerve. This nerve can be damaged during embolization of this artery and during embolization of the ascending pharyngeal artery or of the stylomastoid artery off the occipital artery. This complication rarely occurs but is more likely to occur with aggressive material, such as liquid agents, than with calibrated solid particles. Most of the time the facial palsy will resolve but sometimes only after several months.

Tissue necrosis is more frequently seen when liquid embolic agents are used than when particles agents are used. It is rarely severe enough a complication that would necessitate complete excision and grafting of the area. Most of the time it is limited and heals spontaneously.[3,12]

AESTHETIC RESULTS

As greater superselective embolization is carried out, more selective destruction of the malformations can be achieved. Earlier intervention has also allowed better ablation and therefore better aesthetic results for some of these patients. However, adherence to traditional plastic surgical techniques and principles is essential for the surgeon to obtain the best aesthetic improvements. Rotational flaps, free grafts, and free-tissue transfers all have a role the reconstructive process, but as in any ablative reconstructive procedure, strict adherence to aesthetic units is the only way of ensuring better aesthetic results. The application of new laser technology holds great promise in reducing facial scarring, controlling the treatment of the superficial portion of the lesions, and allowing earlier intervention.

PHYSICAL FUNCTIONING

Earlier intervention and a better understanding of the gamut of vascular lesions leads to better physical well-being and function. Earlier and more precise involvement actually makes the area treated smaller and thus less destructive. Multiple modalities are often necessary to obliterate these lesions and "cure" the patient. Chronic bleeding, pain, or infections have to be dealt with to control the vascular anomaly. Functionally, it has been found that earlier intervention and complete removal of these more complex lesions will result in a better outcome.

QUALITY OF LIFE

The management of patients with vascular hemangiomas and malformations of the head and neck area has evolved into an art that requires the team effort between physicians involved in different specialties. Most often the lesions are benign in nature and self-limited in extent. However, mismanagement may result in a greater problem than the one that was initially noted. Experience coupled with proper diagnosis and evaluations will allow for more successful results in the multidisciplinary management of these problems. Caution also must be exercised when great risks are taken for cosmetic reasons. However, with the recent technologic advances, successful results can be performed with interdisciplinary experts working together. These patients should be followed for several years as in other anomalies, such as cleft lip and palate. Patients with A-V malformations are at particular risk for recurrence or with such events as pregnancy or hormonal manipulation. It is critical that the patient is educated and informed of these potential problems.

COSTS OF CARE

The cost-effectiveness of treating these lesions has to be based on the anomaly's specific diagnosis and the predicted evolution of the lesion. The overwhelming majority of these lesions are easily handled with conservative observation and patience, which will lead to a minimal cost for treatment. However, lesions that are expected to grow and develop significant clinical sequelae should be dealt with early and aggressively. In these cases, conservative treatment or minimal intervention may be a disservice resulting in bigger treatment operations, greater disfigurement, and a greater psychologic impact on the patient.

Radiologic angiography and embolizations will often require hospital admissions with subsequent surgical intervention. This will in some cases result in a several-day hospitalization, which in today's medical world may be difficult to get approval for but will ultimately result in a higher "cure" rate. Angiography rates will range from $5000 to $10,000 for the evaluation, with the cost of embolization driving up the initial cost of the treatment. However, this is often offset by the fact that subsequent additional surgeries will multiply the economic burden of treatment by several times.

PATIENT SATISFACTION

The ultimate goal of treatment for any disease process or anomaly is the control or eradication of the process or, in cases of congenital deformity, restoration of normal form, contour, aesthetics, and function. This is not always able to be achieved but must be strived for in each case. The best cure rates and reconstruction have in many of these complex cases only been achieved with a multidisciplinary team approach using multiple new modalities.

REFERENCES

1. Anderson RR: Laser-tissue interactions. In Goldman MP, Fitzpatrick RE (eds): *Cutaneous laser surgery: the art and science of selective photothermolysis,* St Louis, 1996, Mosby.

2. Apfeldberger DB, Maser MR, Lash H: Extended clinical use of the argon laser for cutaneous lesions, *Arch Dermatol* 115:719, 1979.

3. Azzolini A, Bertani A, Riberti C: Superselective embolization and immediate surgical treatment: our present approach to treatment of large vasular hemangiomas of the face, *Ann Plast Surg* 9:42, 1982.

4. Bartoshesky LE, Bull M, Feingold M: Corticosteroid treatment of cutaneous hemangiomas: how effective? A report on 24 children, *Clin Pediatr* 17:625, 1978.

5. Bingham HG: Predicting the course of a congenital hemangioma, *Plast Reconstr Surg* 63:161, 1979.

6. Bingham HG, Lichti EL: The Doppler as an aid in predicting the behavior of congenital cutaneous hemangiomas, *Plast Reconstr Surg* 47.580, 1971.

7. Bowers RE, Graham EA, Tomlinson KM: The natural history of the strawberry nevus, *Arch Dermatol* 82:59, 1960.

8. Clodius L: Excision and grafting of extensive facial hemangiomas, *Br J Plast Surg* 30:185, 1977.

9. Cohen SR, Wang CI: Steroid treatment of hemangioma of the head and neck in children, *Ann Otol* 81:584, 1972.

10. Cosman B: Experience in the argon laser therapy of port wine stains, *Plast Reconstr Surg* 65:119, 1980.

11. Crikelair GF, Cosman B: Histologically benign, clinically malignant lesions of the head and neck, *Plast Reconstr Surg* 42:343, 1968.

12. Debrun GM, Dufresne CR: Vascular malformations. In Dufresne CR, Carson BS, Zinreich SJ (eds): *Complex craniofacial problems,* New York, 1992, Churchill Livingstone.

13. Dufresne CR, Hoopes JE: Pseudomalignancies, *Clin Plast Surg* 14:367, 1987.

14. Edgerton MT: The treatment of hemangiomas: with special reference to the role of steroid therapy, *Ann Surg* 183:517, 1976.

15. Edgerton MT, Hiebert JM: Vascular and lymphatic tumors in infancy, childhood and adulthood: challenge of diagnosis and treatment, *Curr Probl Cancer* 2:1, 1978.

16. Edgerton MT, Morgan RF: Hemangiomas: congenital hamartomas. In Welch KJ, Randolph JG, Ravitch M (eds): *Pediatric surgery,* St Louis, 1986, Mosby.

17. Folkman J: Tumor angiogenesis: a possible control point in tumor growth, *Ann Intern Med* 82:96, 1975.

18. Fost NC, Esterly NB: Successful treatment of juvenile hemangiomas with prednisone, *J Pediatr* 72:351, 1968.

19. Goldman, PM, Fitzpatrick RE (ed): *Cutaneous laser surgery: the art and science of selective photothermolysis,* St Louis, 1996, Mosby.

20. Grabb WC, Dingman RO, O'Neal RM, et al: Facial hamartomas in children: neurofibroma, lymphangioma, and hemangioma, *Plast Reconstr Surg* 66:509, 1980.

21. Hanna BD, Bernstein M: Tranexamic acid in the treatment of Kasabach-Merritt syndrome in infants, *Am J Pediatr Hematol Oncol* 11:191, 1989.

22. Hurvitz CH, Alkalay AL, Sloninsky L, et al: Cyclophosphamide therapy in like-threatening vascular tumors, *J Pediatr* 109:360, 1986.

23. Lasjaunias P, Doyou D: The ascending pharyngeal artery and the blood supply of the lower cranial nerves, *J Neuroradiol* 5:267, 1978.

24. Lasjaunias P, Moret J: Normal and non-pathological variations in the angiographic aspects of the arteries of the middle ear, *Neuroradiology* 15:213, 1978.

25. Martin LW, MacCollum DW: Hemangiomas in infants and children, *Am J Surg* 101:571, 1961.

26. Margileth AM, Museles M: Current concepts in diagnosis and management of congenital cutaneous hemangiomas, *Pediatrics* 36:410, 1965.

27. Merland JJ, Riche MC, Monteil JP: Classification actuelle des malformations vasculaires, *Ann Chir Plast* 25:105, 1980.

28. Miller SH, Smith RL, Shochat SJ: Compression treatment of hemangiomas, *Plast Reconstr Surg* 58:573, 1976.

29. Moret J: Blood supply of the ear and cerebellopontine angle, *J Neuroradiol* 9:215, 1982.

30. Moret J: Abnormal vessels in the middle ear, *J Neuroradiol* 9:227, 1982.

31. Moret J: Vascular architecture of tympanojugular glomus tumors, *J Neuroradiol* 9:237, 1982.

32. Mulliken JB, Glowacki J: Hemangiomas and vascular malformations in infants and children: a classification based on endothelial characteristics, *Plast Reconstr Surg* 69:412, 1982.

33. Mulliken JB, Young AE: *Vascular birthmarks,* Philadelphia, 1988, WB Saunders.

34. Natali J, Merland JJ: Superselective arteriography and therapeutic embolism for vascular malformations (angiodysplasias), *J Cardiovasc Surg* 17:465, 1976.

35. Neidhart JA, Roach RW: Successful treatment of skeletal hemangioma and Kasabach-Merritt syndrome with aminocaproic acid, *Am J Med* 73:434, 1982.

36. Sasaki GH, Pang CY, Wittliff JL: Pathogenesis and treatment of infant skin strawberry hemangiomas: clinical and in vitro studies of hormonal effects, *Plast Reconstr Surg* 73:359, 1984.

37. Stanley P, Gomperts E, Woolley MM: Kasabach-Merrit syndrome treated by therapeutic embolization with polyvinyl alcohol, *Am J Pediatr* 109:308, 1986.

38. Wallace HJ: The conservative treatment of hemangiomatous nevi, *Br J Plast Surg* 63:161, 1979.

39. Walsh TS Jr, Tompkins VN: Some observations on the strawberry nevus of infancy, *Cancer* 9:869, 1956.

40. Watson WL, McCarthy WD: Blood and lymph vessel tumors: a report of 1056 cases, *Surg Gynecol Obstet* 71:569, 1940.

41. Weber TR, West KW, Cohen M, et al: Massive hemangioma in infants: therapeutic considerations, *J Vasc Surg* 1:423, 1984.

42. Weber TR, Connors RH, Tracy TF, et al: Complex hemangiomas of infants and children, *Arch Surg* 125:1017, 1990.

43. White CW, Sondheimer HM, Crouch EC, et al: Treatment of pulmonary hemangiomatosis with recombinant interferon alpha-2a, *N Engl J Med* 320:1197, 1989.

44. Williams HB: Vascular neoplasms, *Clin Plast Surg* 7:397, 1980.

45. Williams HB: Facial bone changes with vascular tumors in children, *Plast Reconstr Surg* 63:309, 1979.

46. Wolf JE Jr, Hubler WR: Tumor angiogenic factor and human skin tumors, *Arch Dermatol* 3:321, 1975.

47. Young AE: Congenital mixed vascular deformities of the limbs and their associated lesions, *Birth Defects* 14:289, 1978.

48. Zarem HA, Edgerton MT: Induced resolution of cavernous hemangiomas following prednisolone therapy, *Plast Reconstr Surg* 39:76, 1967.

CHAPTER

Congenital Nevus

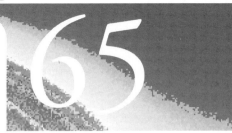

Bruce S. Bauer
Andreas N. Chimonides

INTRODUCTION

Imagine the birth of a healthy, beautiful child as an occasion of excitement, anticipation, and incredible joy for parents and family alike. Although every parent is faced with fears and anxiety about the future and how this newborn will fare in the coming years, this is a time of great wonder and beauty. Now suppose that, on first look at the child, this picture is marred by the appearance of a deeply pigmented birthmark covering a major portion of the baby's face, trunk, or extremity. This time of joy can be suddenly transformed into one of horror, concern, despair, and fear. This transformation is not often softened by the lack of readily available information about what the lesion is (if it is malignant or benign, and if there are other problems associated with it) and even less knowledge of what can be done to eliminate its presence and lessen the impact of the lesion on this child's future. Unfortunately, there is often a delay in gaining this information.

Regardless of the size of the "birthmark," early consultation with a knowledgeable physician is critical to the family's ability to bond with their newborn, and that physician, whether he or she is a dermatologist or plastic surgeon, must be armed with the information to present the family with a straightforward, easily understood discussion of the nature of the lesion, the varied approaches to treatment, and an overview of the outcomes of the varied methods of treatment. If well presented in a compassionate manner, even the prescription for multiple surgeries over a many-year period can at least offer these new parents the hope that eventually their child will be able to integrate normally into the world. It is the purpose of this chapter to lay the groundwork for such a discussion and outline an approach to treatment based on experience with more than 200 large and giant nevi, as well as many more small to medium lesions, pigmented and nonpigmented, treated over a 17-year experience on an active pediatric plastic surgical service (with close ties to a pediatric dermatology service). The treatment plan outlined has evolved over this period based on careful consideration of the effectiveness of each different treatment modality in each body region with similar-size lesions. Refinements and modifications in treatment have come about

through a desire to improve cosmetic and functional outcomes and to minimize the likelihood of late corrective surgery for problems encountered in the early treatment. We begin with an overview of the lesions treated and the indications for treatment, and then we concentrate on the pros and cons of different treatment modalities. Although we expect that these treatment "protocols" will continue to evolve over the coming years, we believe that this chapter represents a large step in the direction of dealing with these often problematic lesions.

INDICATIONS

Congenital nevus is any nevus present at birth. The word *nevus* refers to an abnormal or faulty growth in the skin that is generally synonymous with the term *hamartoma*. It is a nonspecific term that applies to a wide variety of cutaneous lesions. The term is derived from the Sanskrit root *-gha* and the Latin root *-gen,* both referring to birth. It is descriptive of a histologic clustering of cells into nests that share embryologic origin but in an ectopic location. Although most physicians and patients use the word *nevus* to describe pigmented lesions, this term applies to a variety of cutaneous malformations, (e.g., epidermal nevus, sebaceous nevus), many of them not present at birth.[23]

Most congenital nevi are made up of congenital melanocytic nevi (CMN). At birth, approximately 2.5% of children have pigmented lesions, and 1% of newborns have congenital melanocytic nevi.[2,7,39,51] CMN result from an aberration in the normal development of the neuroblast cells. Melanoblasts, which are precursors of melanocytes, migrate during the early embryologic stage from the neural crest not only to the skin but also to mucous membranes, eyes, meninges, ears, mesentery, and the chromaffin system, where they differentiate between the eight and tenth weeks of gestation into dendritic melanocytes. When the normal differentiation and migration of those cells is disturbed, the result is an ectopic population of cells seen in nevus. Nevus cells in the dermis are classified into types A (epithelioid) found in the superficial dermis, type B (lymphoid) found in the mid-dermis, and type C (fibrocytic) found in the deep dermis. They are distinguished from fibroblasts and Schwann cells by staining with immunoperoxidases, including the S-100 stain and myelin basic protein stain.[23]

CMN are characterized at birth by a thickened skin that may be smooth, rough, nodular, or verrucous with variations in shades of brown and blue throughout the lesion. Many of them are covered with hair that is coarse, larger, and more pigmented than the patient's normal hair (Figure 65-1). There are often multiple satellite pigmented papules beyond the periphery of the main lesion; some may be faint or barely visible at birth, increasing in depth of pigmentation over the first 6 to 12 months. As the infant grows, the involved areas become thicker and frequently darker, the surface is more irregular, and verrucous nodules frequently develop.[23,40] Giant nevi located in the head and neck and posterior trunk may be

associated with leptomeningeal melanocytosis and neurologic disorders, such as epilepsy.[22] Those that overlie the vertebral column may have underlying spinal defects, such as meningomyelocele or spina bifida. In some cases of giant nevus, computed tomography (CT) and magnetic resonance imaging (MRI) studies may reveal neural lesions, particularly in the temporal lobe, which may or may not be associated with a seizure disorder.[14]

CMN can be divided into three groups, depending on size (see Figure 65-1).[26] Small congenital nevi are defined as those less than 1.5 cm in diameter, most of which are easily excised in a single operative procedure and are found in 1% of newborns.[39] Medium congenital nevi are defined as those greater than 1.5 cm but less than 20 cm in diameter and are seen in 0.6% of newborns. Large and giant congenital nevi have been defined variously as those larger than 20 cm, those greater in total area than 100 cm^2, or those that cannot be completely

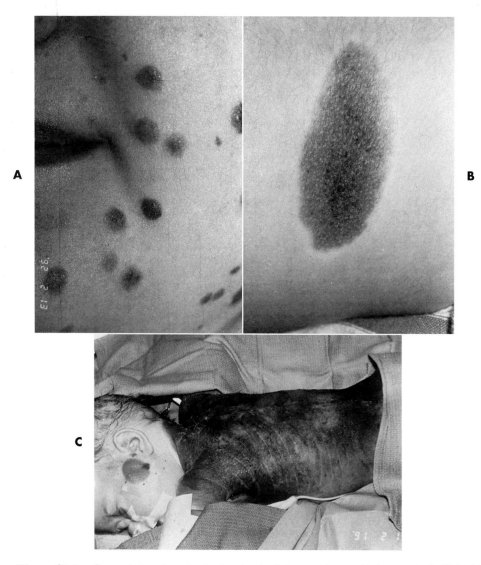

Figure 65-1. Congenital nevi, varying in size, depth of pigmentation, and hair growth. **A,** Multiple small nevi of the face in a child with giant nevus of the trunk, showing marked variation in thickness, color, and texture. **B,** Medium (7-cm) nevus of the flank with typical variegated pigment within the lesion. **C,** Giant nevus of entire back with dense pigmentation and hair growth.

excised without a significant deformity.[44] Other authors have defined large and giant nevi as those measuring greater than 2% of total body surface (TBS)[4,20,37] (the definition we have followed).[4] This rare variant occurs in less than 1 in 20,000 newborns.[4,20,37,44]

The differentiation of congenital from acquired melanocytic nevi carries an important treatment connotation. There is controversy about whether specific histologic changes can differentiate congenital from acquired melanocytic nevi.[23,40] According to Mark et al,[32] congenital melanocytic nevi differ histologically from acquired nevi. In contrast to acquired melanocytic nevi, a congenital nevus is generally a deeper lesion with melanocytes distributed far down into the dermis and sometimes even in the subcutaneous fat. The nevus cells tend to be grouped around adnexal structures, nerves, blood vessels, and lymphatics. These features, however, are not specific to congenital nevi and can occasionally be seen in acquired nevi.

One of the most important elements of the diagnosis of CMN concerns the likelihood of the development of melanoma (and for giant nevi, the possibility of degeneration into either melanoma or sarcoma).[4,52] Although the association between large and giant congenital melanocytic nevi and malignant melanoma has been established beyond reasonable doubt, the magnitude of risk of malignant transformation has varied in the literature from as little as 2% to as high as 31%.* Many of these studies were significantly skewed by the sample population examined. Quaba and Wallace,[37] in their 1986 review of the subject, attempted to put the widely different figures into perspective, and they have calculated an 8.51% incidence of melanoma developing with larger than 2% of the TBS during the first 15 years of life. The opinion that complete prophylactic excision of all giant nevi should be accomplished in infancy and early childhood is well supported in the literature.[3,25,41,48,54] Approximately 50% of malignancies that have occurred in giant nevi developed in the first 3 years of life, 60% by childhood, and 70% before puberty. The lifetime risk of melanoma in patients with giant CMN may be as high as 15%.[24] The nature and magnitude of the association between small CMN and melanoma is still controversial.[23,39] Obtaining accurate data on malignancy of small CMN is very difficult because establishing their congenital nature based on history taken by an older child or adult is often inaccurate. Careful statistical analysis estimates a 21-fold increased risk of melanoma for individuals with small CMN when nevi were ascertained by history, and a threefold to tenfold increase in risk when nevi were uncertain by histopathologic criteria (the presence of cytologically benign nevocellular nevi in the dermis immediately adjacent to invasive melanoma). Although history and histology are not infallible determinants and the strength of association is entirely dependent on methods used for ascertainment of CMN, the observed frequency of association is several orders of magnitude greater than expected based on surface area considerations and chance alone.[39] The lifetime risk of melanoma in patients with small CMN as stated by Rhodes and

Melski[39] lies between 0.8% and 2.6% by histologic method of determination and 4.9% by historic assessment. The risk of melanoma before puberty is 1:200,000 or near 0, with the risk increasing in the years following.

Aside from the potential for malignancy, the cosmetic deformity and psychologic impact of CMN on a child are profound.[4,30,37,44] In certain instances the parents will reject and even abandon a newborn infant with this condition. Modern plastic surgical techniques can often greatly ameliorate the cosmetic defects, and parents should be given a realistic appraisal of this condition. The benefits both from a risk of malignant degeneration standpoint and aesthetic concern of excising the large and giant lesions before school age cannot be overemphasized because the procedures involved are often significantly better tolerated during infancy and early childhood.[4]

There are several variants of congenital melanocytic nevi that are important because they can simulate melanoma histologically. Blue nevi, Mongolian spots, and the nevi of Ota and Ito are benign melanocytic nevi frequently present at birth that are characterized by proliferation of melanocytes that are located wholly in the dermis. They occur secondary to an arrest in embryonal migration of melanocytes bound for the dermal-epidermal junction. They most likely represent different stages of the same physiologic process.[23]

MONGOLIAN SPOTS

Mongolian spots are flat, deep brown or blue-gray, often poorly circumscribed, large macular lesions with a predilection for certain locations and racial groups.[11,29] They are often found over the lumbosacral region and buttocks. Occasionally they are seen in the upper extremities and shoulder. Infrequently they appear on the abdomen, chest, and rarely on the palms or soles. Approximately 96% of black infants, 46% of Hispanic infants, and about 10% of white infants are born with these lesions.[11] They may be single or multiple and vary in size from a few millimeters to 10 cm or more in diameter. Although they may occasionally persist into adulthood, Mongolian spots are usually self-limited and therapy is unnecessary.[29]

BLUE NEVUS

Blue nevi, although often seen in childhood, occasionally are present at birth.[23] These lesions are histologic variants of the intradermal nevus found in the mid-dermis to deep dermis. They are divided into two types: simple and cellular.[42] The common blue nevus is a small, round or oval, blue-black to slate grey, smooth-surfaced, sharply circumscribed, mildly elevated nodule that is usually less than 1 cm in diameter. Although they may occur in any part of the body, they are most commonly seen in the extremities, especially the backs of the hands and feet, the lumbosacral region, and the head. They can be single or multiple, and women are twice as frequently affected as men. Cellular blue nevi are considerably less

---

*References 4, 23, 30, 32, 37, 38, 44.

common than ordinary blue nevi and are characterized by irregular shape, lighter color, and frequently size larger than 1 cm in diameter with predilection for the lumbosacral region.[42] The individual cells in a blue nevus have an elongated dendritic appearance and may be associated with densely aggregated macrophages that have phagocytized the pigment. It is the presence of this dense pigmentation at the deeper layers of the dermis that impart the bluish coloration to these lesions.

Although the common blue nevi remain benign lesions, there is a low but distinct chance of malignant transformation in the cellular variety of this lesion.[16,35] Although relatively few cases of malignant degeneration have been reported, these lesions may exhibit aggressive behavior and metastasize.[16,35] For this reason, it is generally recommended that blue nevi be excised.

NEVUS OF OTA AND NEVUS OF ITO

The nevus of Ota and the nevus of Ito are clinical forms of blue nevus with a distribution correlated with specific dermatome patterns.[23,28] Nevus of Ota was first described in Japan in 1939.[28] Since then, multiple cases have been recorded from around the world, most commonly in Indians and blacks. Females account for 75% of all reported cases. Approximately 50% of lesions are congenital and 40% appear at puberty.[31] Nevus of Ota is a flat, irregular, gray-blue patch of the face supplied by the first and second divisions of the trigeminal nerve, particularly the periorbital region, temple, forehead, malar region, and nose.[28] More than 50% of patients will have involvement of the sclera of the ipsilateral eye and occasionally

the conjunctiva, cornea, and retina. Mucous membrane involvement, especially the lips, pharynx, hard palate, and nasal mucosa, is occasionally seen. In about 5% of cases the nevus of Ota is found bilaterally. The nevus of Ito has the same features as the nevus of Ota, except that is seen in the distribution of the posterior supraclavicular and lateral cutaneous branches to the shoulder, neck, and supraclavicular areas. Unlike Mongolian spots, nevi of Ota and Ito do not disappear spontaneously and hyperpigmentation frequently occurs after puberty. Although these lesions are benign, there have been at least 37 cases of associated melanoma reported in the English-language literature.[46] Because microscopically melanocytes are found in the upper dermis, Q-switched ruby and argon lasers have been used for ablation of these lesions with excellent results.[15]

NEURAL NEVUS

The neural nevus is distinguishable histologically as a type C form of intradermal nevus.[23] The cells of the neural nevus have a similar histologic appearance to Schwann cells and nerve organelles (pacinian and Meissner's corpuscles). They may in some cases resemble neurofibromatosis. These lesions frequently appear as smooth, lobulated, hairless nodules varying from light tan to dark black appearance. Some have a soft, flabby consistency, often hanging in folds (Figure 65-2). They are commonly found within congenital giant pigmented nevi, particularly in the midline region of the back. Some authors have suggested that there is a high association of neural nevus with malignancies in these areas,[23,52] whereas some patholo-

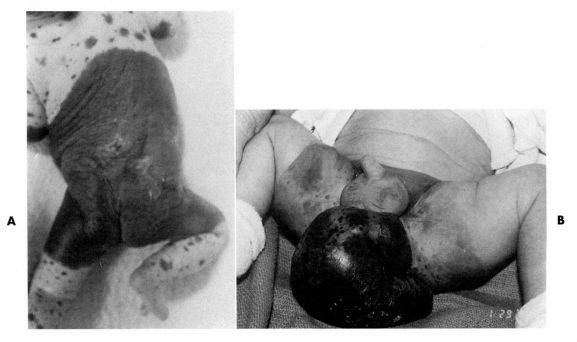

Figure 65-2. **A,** An infant with a giant nevus of the trunk showing the thickened folds of a neural nevus in the lumbosacral area. **B,** A rare bulky nevocytoma, a variant of neural nevus in the midst of a giant bathing trunk nevus.

gists believe that these lesions have been not infrequently confused with melanomas on histologic examination. Given the fact that there may be this increased association, it is recommended that these portions of a giant nevus be either excised early or at least biopsied if definitive treatment will be delayed.

NEVUS SPILUS

Nevus spilus is a sharply demarcated, flat brown patch, speckled with smaller dark brown to black-brown areas of pigmentation (Figure 65-3).[9] This is a relatively common lesion found in 1% to 3% of the adult population with equal gender prevalence; it is frequently seen on the trunk and extremities.[27] Although frequently present at birth, it may occur in infancy or childhood. Its size may vary from 1 to 20 cm in diameter, almost always solitary. Histologically, the epidermis shows increased pigment in the basal layer with an increased number of melanocytes throughout the lesion and elongation of rete ridges. The darker spots are melanocytic nevi of the junctional and compound types.[9] Although there are reports of malignant transformation developing in nevus spilus, routine clinical observation is indicated unless suspicious changes are seen or if the lesion is clearly congenital in nature.[50] Some of these lesions, particularly when large and in prominent locations, may warrant excision for aesthetic reasons alone.

EPIDERMAL NEVUS

Epidermal nevus is a benign hamartoma characterized by hyperkeratosis, acanthosis, and hypertrophy of the epidermis.[43,45,47] Onset at birth occurs in 60% of cases; 80% are evident by 1 year of age and 95% by 7 years of age. It affects both genders equally, and lesions can be unilateral or

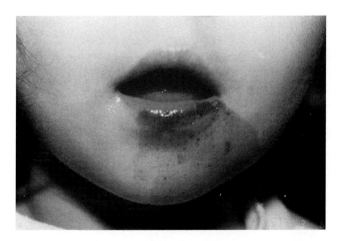

Figure 65-3. The typical features of a nevus spilus are visible in this large lesion of the lower lip and chin. The lightly speckled pigmentation is interspersed with melanocytic nevus along the vermilion and in darker spots within the lighter lesion.

symmetric, solitary, or extensive.[43] Typical lesions are hyperpigmented, linear, velvety, or papillomatous. They are often found in the extremities, although they may occur anywhere in the body, frequently in a dermatomal distribution. Four variants have been described[36,43,45]: Nevus verrucous is a localized, solitary lesion often present at birth, linear or oval in shape. Most are 2 to 3 cm in size, often noted on the trunk or extremities but may occur on the head or neck. Nevus unius lateralis are extensive, systematized forms of epidermal nevus that can often cover more than one half of the body. Ichthyosis hystrix refers to widespread epidermal lesions in irregular geometric patterns that follow Blaschko's lines. Epidermal nevi in which inflammation is present are known as inflammatory linea verrucous epidermal nevus (ILVEN). They are erythematous, pruritic, scaling linear plaques that can be misdiagnosed as psoriasis.[36,45]

The association of epidermal nevi with other congenital anomalies is termed *epidermal nevus syndrome* (Figure 65-4).[36,43,45,47] Typical anomalies include skeletal abnormalities (in approximately two thirds of patients, with kyphoscoliosis the most common), central nervous system abnormalities (in approximately one third of patients as hydrocephaly, mental retardation, or seizures), and ocular abnormalities (in approximately one fifth of patients as epibulbar dermoids and colobomata of the retina, iris, or lid). Less commonly, anomalies of the urogenital tract and cardiovascular system are seen. The risk of malignant degeneration with epidermal nevi is unknown but not believed to be common. Most tumors reported are low-grade, such as Bowen's disease, keratoacanthoma, or basal cell carcinoma.[17] In addition, affected individuals may show increase incidence of noncutaneous systemic malignancies.

Although surgery may be effective for removal of localized lesions, it may provide little relief in the treatment of extensive (see Figure 65-4) lesions because surgical intervention is rarely indicated in infancy and the extent of involvement with thick, hyperkeratotic lesions later may even render tissue expansion of little benefit. It is also the lead author's personal impression that excision of these lesions may for unknown reasons be associated with significantly greater risk of hypertrophic scarring, and at the very least this factor should be taken into consideration when deciding on the optimal treatment modality. Although cryosurgery, dermabrasion, or electrodesiccation and curettage may produce gratifying results initially, recurrences are common. At the same time, these later treatment approaches, if properly applied, may give benefit without the risk of unsightly and potentially deforming scarring. In some cases, reepithelialization after dermabrasion or dermaplaning may be followed by a flat appearance without discoloration that may remain as such for many years.[36]

SEBACEOUS NEVUS

Nevus sebaceus was described in 1895 by the German dermatologist Jadassohn.[17,33] It is a congenital hamartoma of sebaceous glands. They present as yellowish-tan, waxy or velvety plaques, most commonly located on the head and neck

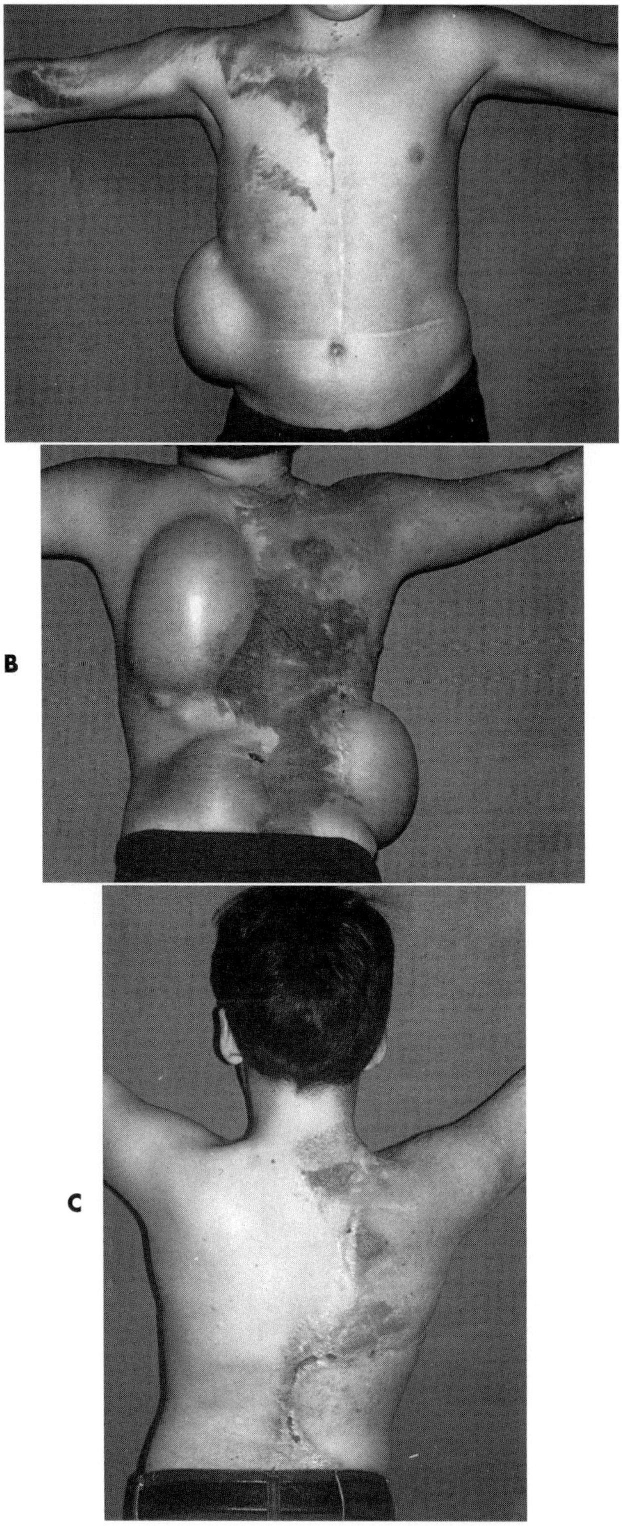

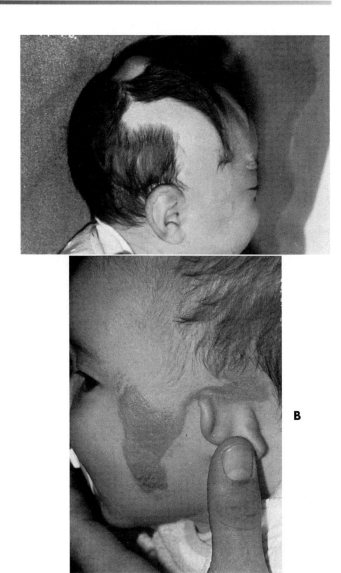

Figure 65-4. A 10-year-old child with epidermal nevus syndrome. **A,** Anterior view with typical linear epidermal nevi of the shoulder and upper arm. **B,** Giant epidermal nevus of the back with tissue expanders in the back before reduction of the nevus. **C,** After partial excision of the back nevus and advancement of the adjacent flaps.

Figure 65-5. The varied presentation of a sebaceous nevus are evident in the two infants illustrated here. **A,** A giant sebaceous nevus of the scalp is seen in a child with sebaceous nevus syndrome who had a severe seizure disorder. **B,** A typical waxy, pinkish, orange nevus of the cheek and superior auricular sulcus.

(Figure 65-5). The lesion is usually solitary, round, oval, or linear, and varies in size from a few millimeters to several centimeters in diameter.[18] Typically, lesions over the face and neck are linear where scalp lesions are oval, appearing as an area of alopecia.[53] Although congenital in origin, some may not be apparent early and appear to arise in early childhood and rarely in adulthood. They are estimated to occur in 0.3% of births. Although familial cases have been described, they are usually sporadic without gender preference.[17,53] As the child grows, hormonal changes during puberty bring on a series of changes of these lesions. By adolescence these lesions have often shown progressive thickening with the surface changing from waxy smooth to verrucous with hypoplasia of sebaceous gland associated with itching, drainage, and occasional intermittent inflammation. Large, linear sebaceous nevi in the head and neck have been associated with a seizure disorder in 10% of cases.[53] Even more extensive lesions, again particularly in the head and neck, may be associated with other manifestations and neurologic symptoms. Nevus sebaceus syndrome refers to this constellation of symptoms, seen in these patients, including sebaceous nevus, ocular dermoid, major ophthalmic abnormalities, mental retardation, skeletal abnormalities, and seizure disorders.[10,13,31]

The primary indication for excision of sebaceous nevus is the well-recognized risk of malignant degeneration, which has been reported to be between 15% and 20%.[13] The most common neoplasm arising from this disorder is basal cell carcinoma. Other tumors arising from lesions of nevus sebaceus include syringocystadenoma papilliferum; keratoacanthoma; leiomyoma; piloleiomyoma hydradenoma; apocrine cystadenoma; squamous cell carcinoma; and, rarely, aggressive apocrine carcinoma and malignant eccrine poroma. Malignant degeneration, although on occasion reported during adolescence, rarely occurs before early adult life (the third decade).[13] Although the risk of malignant transformation is low in infancy and early childhood, larger lesions may be more readily excised during this period, avoiding the more complicated reconstructive procedures at a time that the child may not tolerate them as well. This approach may also avoid the embarrassment of the change in appearance and cellular activity (with increased thickness, discharge, etc.) that occurs in these lesions as a child goes through the hormonal changes of puberty. Treatment of extensive lesions often requires tissue expansion and is approached in a similar fashion to that described below for congenital pigmented nevi. However, unlike the latter, it is recommended that tissue expander placement be carried out through an incision beyond the border of the sebaceous nevus rather than within the lesion. At the same time, excision of the smaller lesions can easily be left until the child is old enough to undergoes the procedure under local anesthesia in an office setting.

SPITZ NEVUS

Although not a congenital nevus, this lesion is worth mentioning briefly because it is commonly seen in young children and may be confused with other congenital lesions. The Spitz nevus is a distinct histologic and clinical entity.[18,23] Originally described as "juvenile melanoma" and readily confused with the latter lesion under the microscope (without the knowledge of the context in which the lesion is seen), these lesions have been reclassified as a variant of an acquired nevus. Typically appearing as a firm, pinkish, raised lesion that may even be confused with a vascular lesion, they may also be pigmented with wide variegation in color (Figure 65-6). They are quite common on the face but may even appear as large clusters of lesions in an area on the trunk or extremity. Histologically, these lesions exhibit clusters of nonpigmented spindle and epithelioid nevomelanocytes in the lower epidermis with elongated nevomelanocytes "raining down" into the upper dermis.[18,23]

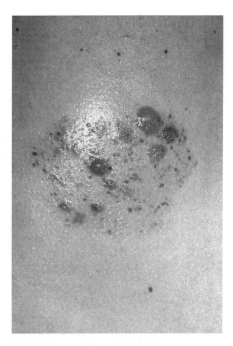

Figure 65-6. A large cluster of Spitz nevi with typical firm, pink nodules, presented on this teenager's upper thigh.

Although there is no evidence that Spitz nevus is a precursor of melanoma, these lesions may recur and enlarge rapidly if not completely excised, with the histologic appearance seeming to become more disorganized and increasing the concerns about the true nature of the lesion. This being the case, excision with a few-millimeter margin is recommended and has been effective in treating even recurrent lesions in our experience.

OPERATIONS

Although much of the following discussion of operations pertains to experience gained in the treatment of congenital pigmented nevi, the treatment of large sebaceous nevi, problematic epidermal nevi, etc., can follow the approaches described. Some variations are mentioned in the Indications section; others will be touched on here.

Over the past two decades, the approach to the management of congenital nevi has evolved. Cronin,[12] Johnson,[21] and others[34] originally advocated dermabrasion and split-thickness excision of large nevi to diminish significant cosmetic deformity (Figure 65-7). Although these techniques may improve the appearance and decrease the overall "nevus cells load," they do not address the nevus cells located in the deep dermis, around hair follicles, nerves, and lymphatics.[40]

Curettage and a Q-switched ruby laser therapy have most recently been suggested for removal of CMN. Although these therapeutic approaches may give fairly favorable cosmetic results, they do not necessarily remove all nevus cells and

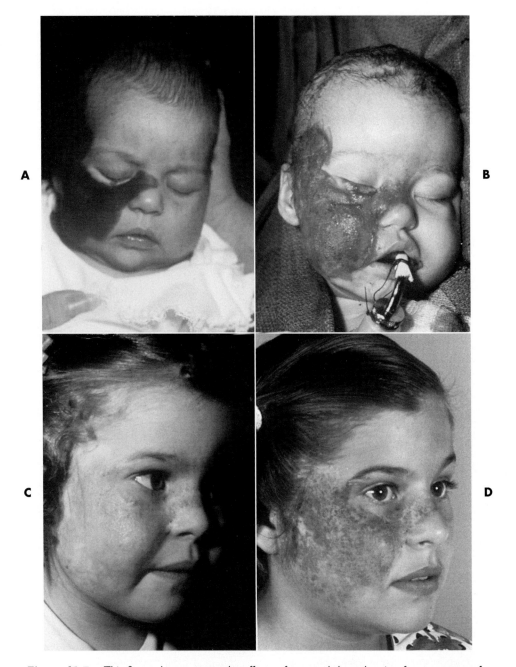

Figure 65-7. This figure demonstrates the effects of neonatal dermabrasion for treatment of a giant nevus of the face and the potential problem of late "bleed through" of the remaining deep nevus requiring subsequent excision and flap reconstruction. **A,** An infant with a giant nevus of the face. **B,** Dermabrasion of the face at 1 month of age. **C,** At age 3 years showing a reasonably good cosmetic result of the procedure. **D,** At 6 years of age the nevus is now visible with deep pigment throughout the area previously dermabraded.

thereby are not recommended. Either of these treatment modalities may be associated with late "bleed through" of the pigment from the residual deeper portions of the nevus occurring often when the child is approaching school. This presents a greater treatment dilemma than it would have had the definitive treatment been carried out earlier (see Figure 65-7).[4,6] At the same time, there may be a role for these less invasive treatment modalities for very extensive lesions or those not lending themselves well to treatment. In these cases the ability

to lighten the pigment may represent a significant advantage even if the effect of this treatment on risk of malignant change were not seemingly significantly altered.[4]

The most appropriate treatment of CMN is based primarily on considerations of lesion size, location, histology, and patient age. Because the risk of malignant change in small CMN is extremely low during the first decade of life,[37,39] our approach is to delay excision until the child is older and able to undergo the procedure under local anesthesia. Exceptions to

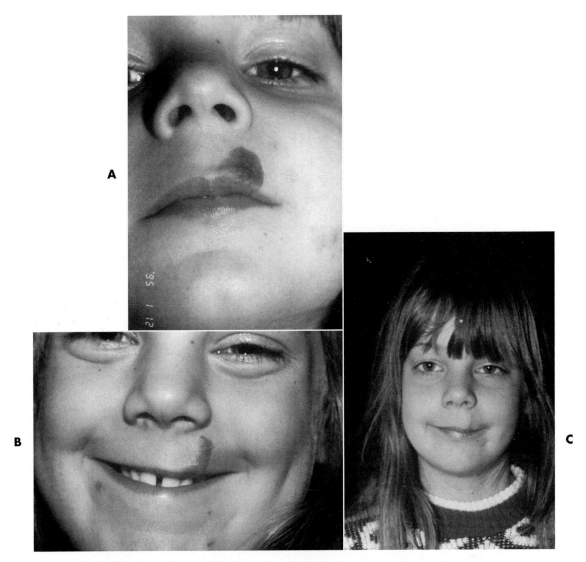

Figure 65-8. Because of their location, some small lesions may require staged excisions to both optimize the outcome and minimize the need for complex flaps or grafts. **A** to **C,** This nevus of the lip was excised in three stages, with the first involving both adjacent advancement of lip skin and a smaller wedge excision through the lip, followed by further advancement along the vermilion-cutaneous junction.

this rule would be if the lesion were located in an area where excision under local would be poorly tolerated (e.g., periorbital area) or if the lesion lies in a region that the complexity of the reconstruction would still require a general anesthetic even in an older child (e.g., lips, nasal tip or alar margin, eyelids). Most of these lesions can be excised primarily, but not infrequently those on the face may be better excised in two stages to minimize the length of the final scar and avoid the need for more complicated flap procedures (Figure 65-8). Dissection should be carried down to the underlying fascia to remove all nevus cells in most cases, except in the facial area where for smaller lesions, excision well into the underlying fat may be acceptable. Even medium-size lesions, because of the tissue requirements and the need to avoid distortion of key anatomic landmarks of the particular region, may require more complex methods of excision and reconstruction. These include serial excisions or reconstruction with skin grafts, local flaps, or flaps generated using tissue expansion (Figure 65-9). This may frequently be the case with lesions of the scalp, face, and distal extremities.

Giant CMN present a reconstructive challenge for both the novice and even many experienced plastic surgeons. Although complete early excision of giant CMN is often looked on as an insurmountable task, newer approaches to excision and reconstruction gained with further experience with tissue expansion,[4,6,19,49] including varied methods of flap design[8] to maximize the benefits of the tissue gained through expansion, along with the addition of microsurgical refinements, allow the excision to begin as early as 6 months of age and to be completed in early childhood.[4] In many cases this evolution of technique has enabled excision of larger and larger lesions without the need for skin grafting.[8] As we have gained more experience with the

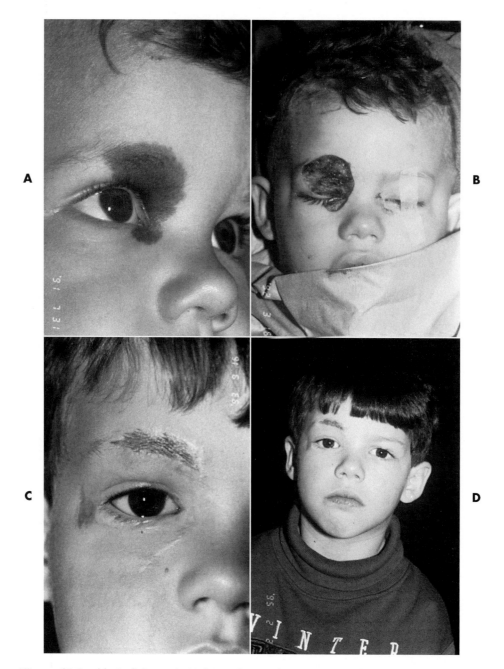

Figure 65-9. Nevi of the periorbital area frequently require a combination of graft and flap techniques for the excision and reconstruction. This nevus of lids, canthus, and medial brow was excised in a single stage using a full-thickness skin graft in combination with an island flap reconstruction of the brow. The brow flap was then thinned. **A,** The nevus before excision. **B,** The result 1 year after excision. **C** and **D,** The result 3 years postoperatively.

technical aspects of these varied reconstructions and have been able to evaluate the outcomes of the varied treatment modalities, in each given area, we have continued to add refinements that should minimize the likelihood of poor aesthetic and functional outcomes, as well as to minimize the likelihood of additional procedures in later life to address those problems. We will look at treatment of large and giant nevi by body region, looking at the techniques used and which of the spectrum of techniques have proven most effective in each different area. Within the discussion of the operative planning for excision of congenital nevi of the head and neck we include some

generalized discussion of expander type, placement, use of expanded full-thickness grafts, and postoperative management of the expander patient.

LARGE AND GIANT MELANOCYTIC NEVI OF THE SCALP

Tissue expansion is the primary treatment modality used for excision and reconstruction of large congenital nevi of the scalp, as well as a part of the treatment plan for most other lesions of the head and neck.[4] Unless dealing with nevi of greater than 50% of the scalp, when the initial options for reconstruction are limited, every effort should be made to orient hair (particularly along the anterior hairline) correctly. Although tissue expansion can begin as early as 3 months of age with no evidence of residual cranial malformation (although temporary molding may occur that will reshape in the months after expander removal), in patients in whom serial expansion will be required or in whom a large expander (500 ml or greater) will be positioned, expansion at 6 months of age is preferred. The most critical element in accomplishing early excision and avoiding complications is meticulous preoperative planning. Experience has shown that the spherical shape of the scalp and the ungiving nature of the galea necessitates the routine use of large or multiple tissue expanders. Even smaller lesions of the scalp may be treated with initial tissue expansion of the adjacent scalp to minimize problems in healing that result from undue tension. Tissue expanders are placed through incisions just within the margin of the nevus whenever possible (see Sebaceous Nevus above). The incisions are made after infiltration with 0.5% lidocaine with 1:200,000 epinephrine and are carried down into the subgaleal plane in the scalp and the subfrontalis plane in the forehead. In general, dissection can be accomplished easily using malleable retractors under the flap. When difficulty is encountered in reaching over the curve of the scalp, dissection can be continued using a urethral sound. The dissection is carried to a dimension of at least 1 cm greater than the expander base in all directions. A narrow path is dissected for the injection port, which is placed far away from the tissue expander (a miniport or low-profile injection port is both well tolerated and readily injected in the preauricular region; the area of the mastoid prominence should be avoided) to allow for safe, full expansion. If necessary, the miniport is secured to the tissues with absorbable sutures (if working in a pocket large enough to see the port) or secured with a carefully placed suture (through the skin and around the tubing) and secured with a gauze bolster on the skin to avoid migration and accidental deflation of the expander. As in all cases in which tissue expanders are being used, after placement of the expander, the injection port is tested. Every effort should be made to avoid surface folds on the expander because this will put the overlying skin flap at risk for possible necrosis. Kinks or bends of the injection port should be prevented to avoid difficulties with inflation of the expander, and care should be taken when using large expanders to ensure that the injection port is far enough from the expander to prevent difficulty in expansion when the expander is approaching maximal size. This may entail adding additional tubing between expander and port in some cases. In addition, some standard (higher-profile) injection ports may prove too high a profile beneath the scalp of an infant or young child, thereby representing a risk to the overlying skin blood supply. These should be avoided. One or more 19-gauge butterfly intravenous (IV) tube drains are routinely placed in all patients (generally one drain per expander), and the needle end of the drain is placed into Vacutainer tubes at the completion of the case. Closure of the incisions is carried in two layers, with 4-0 clear nylon on the galea and 4-0 blue nylon on the scalp. Typically the sutures are left in place throughout

the expansion process, only being removed if there is undue irritation.

Expansion is usually accomplished over a period of 10 to 12 weeks, expanding once per week in most cases but increasing to every fourth or fifth day when early expansion has been proceeding uneventfully. Expanders have varied in size from 100 to 550 ml, with most larger lesions being addressed with expanders in the 300-to 550-ml range. We have used rectangular expanders with a reinforced backing in virtually all cases. The amount injected will depend on the area expanded and size of the expander. In the scalp, expansion with 20 to 40 ml is routine once the initial weeks of expansion have demonstrated good healing and the parents are comfortable with the expansion routine (approximately two thirds of the expanders being injected by a family member in our more recent series).

The choice of flap, whether direct advancement, transposition, or rotation, will depend on the amount of tissue obtained, the location of the nevus, and recognition of differences in hair direction (Figure 65-10). Whereas early in our experience we, along with others, used a preponderance of advancement flaps, we have found an increasing benefit both in expedience of covering large areas with less need for serial expansion and improved reconstruction of hairline and hair direction using transposition flaps (see Outcomes section).

LARGE AND GIANT CONGENITAL MELANOCYTIC NEVI OF THE FACE (CHEEK, FOREHEAD, NOSE, EAR)

Although tissue expansion is routinely used for excision and reconstruction of large and giant nevi of the face, areas including the periorbital region (including eyelids), nose, and ears may be best treated with either nonexpanded or expanded full-thickness skin grafts[5] (Figures 65-11 and 65-12). Where little or no normal adjacent tissue is available for expansion, these expanded full-thickness grafts can be used to cover complete facial aesthetic units. More recently, the use of the prefabricated flaps for the central facial and nasal area have improved final aesthetic and functional outcome over full-thickness grafts where immediately adjacent normal regional tissue is unavailable. These prefabricated flaps have the obvious advantage of the added thickness of subcutaneous tissue and improved skin characteristics over full-thickness grafts. Meticulous preoperative planning is critical to avoid the risk of distortion of the eyebrow and temporal hairline in treatment of large and giant nevi of the forehead and also to avoid distortion of the lateral canthus (see Figure 65-11), ectropion, distortion of the oral commissure, and hollowing of the cheek secondary to atrophy of the subcutaneous fat of the cheek for lesions of the midface. Expanders are placed on either side of nevi of the central forehead with 100-to 200-ml expanders used in most cases and flap advancement carried out along the brow. When advancing and rotating a flap from the hemiforehead to the opposite side, great care must be taken to avoid elevation of the brow on the side opposite the nevus and repeat expansion may be needed. Transposition flaps may provide an

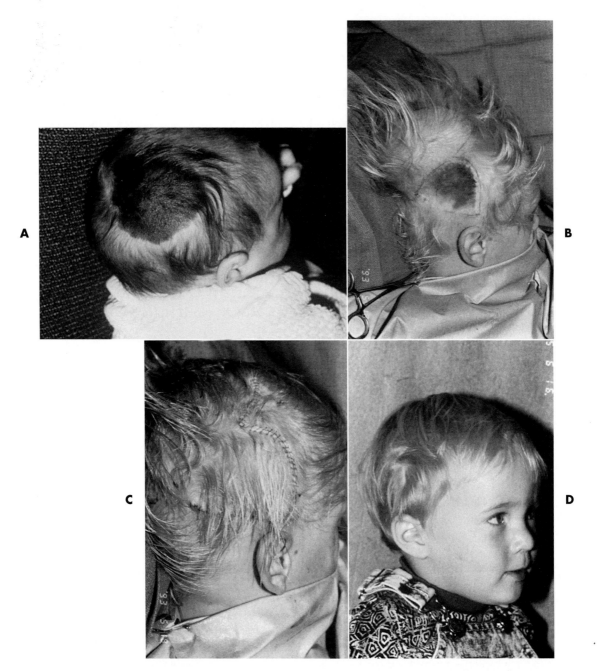

Figure 65-10. Excision and reconstruction of large and giant nevi of the scalp is facilitated by use of transposition flaps rather than straight advancement flaps in many cases because of the ease of covering large areas and better orienting the flaps for optimal hair pattern. **A,** A large nevus of the occipitoparietal area, **B** and **C,** With single expander placed posteromedially, showing the outline of the flap and transposition of the flap. **D,** The result at 6 months after excision.

additional means of avoiding brow elevation by interposing extra tissue between the hairline and brow. Expansion for excision of nevi of the cheek may be more readily accomplished, particularly when the lesion lies from the level of the lateral canthus medially, by a prior elevation and advancement of the flap with partial excision of the nevus without expansion first. This approach will allow better positioning of the expander to deal with the medial cheek, lip, and commissure area and thereby minimize the likelihood of distorting these areas.

The expansion of full-thickness donor sites for facial reconstruction after nevus excision has been accomplished using postauricular skin, clavicular skin (Figure 65-12), and submental skin (where bearded skin was desired for an upper lip graft in a single case). The donor site expansion is continued until there is enough tissue to harvest the full-thickness graft and close the donor site without tension. Preoperatively, a pattern of the aesthetic unit to be reconstructed is made using x-ray film and used to harvest the appropriate graft. Recognizing the potential difficulties of

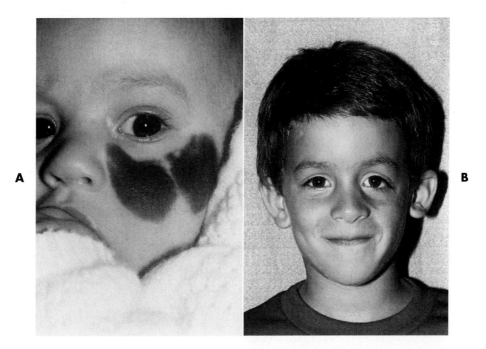

Figure 65-11. **A,** This large nevus of the medial cheek and infraorbital area was treated by both upward advancement of an expanded flap from below the lesion and advancement downward of some of the skin above the orbital rim. **B,** The result at 5 years after excision shows the persistent effects of an approach that allowed downward pull rather than lateral and upward pull of the flaps on the canthus. This distortion and relative tissue shortage can be hard to correct later.

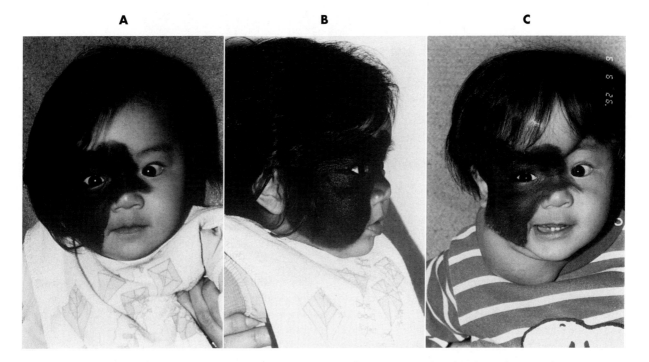

Figure 65-12. This giant nevus of the face and adjacent temporal scalp required repeated expansion and a combination of flap and expanded graft reconstruction. **A** and **B,** Anterior and lateral views of the lesion. **C,** Initial expansion of the forehead and neck/postauricular skin with subsequent flap advancement into the forehead, island flap from the dome of the expanded scalp for the eyebrow reconstruction, and transposition of the neck/postauricular flap into the cheek.   *Continued*

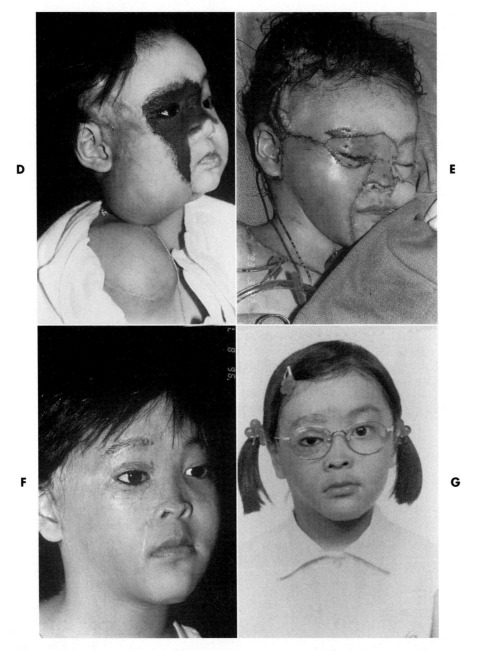

Figure 65-12, cont'd. D, The second expansion was carried out beneath the cheek flap and scalp and at the clavicular expanded skin graft donor site. **E,** After completion of the nevus excision (except ciliary margin) and flap and graft reconstruction. **F,** Result at 3 years postoperatively before revision of the eyelid. **G,** Result at 4 years after the excision.

getting a large full-thickness graft to take over the facial contours, meticulous hemostasis, central tacking sutures, and a suture dressing should be used. Xeroform gauze, cotton soaked in saline and mineral water, and adhesive Reston foam secured beyond the graft margins with skin adhesive and sutures is routinely used for extensive grafts. An alternative to an expanded full-thickness skin graft for medium-size lesions such as both lids or the entire anterior ear would be the harvest of the entire postauricular skin with closure of this donor site using a full-thickness skin graft from the groin.

The pigmentation difference in the latter graft being in the postauricular donor region is not a concern, and the benefits of a large, postauricular graft to the visible face are fully gained.

When applying full-thickness grafts on the face or extensive grafts (both full- and split-thickness on the trunk or extremity), movement between the graft and bed is further minimized by placing the child on a combination of analgesics and sedation, with diphenhydramine (Benadryl) and chloral hydrate (each of these drugs on a q8h regimen but alternated q4h). The graft is examined in most cases at 3 to 5 days for full-thickness grafts and 5 to 7 days postoperatively for large split-thickness grafts on the posterior trunk.

LARGE AND GIANT CONGENITAL PIGMENTED NEVI OF THE TRUNK

Some of the largest congenital melanocytic nevi are seen over the trunk. They may involve either the anterior or posterior trunk, with the majority being seen in the posterior trunk, with capelike and bathing trunk distributions common. The treatment varies with each location.

Anterior trunk nevi, located in a transverse direction across the abdomen, may be excised and the defect may be closed in an abdominoplasty fashion either in a single procedure or in serial procedures. Dissection is carried down to the abdominal fascia, similar to an abdominoplasty, preferably with electrocautery to minimize blood loss and transfusions. If the nevus cannot be excised and the defect closed primarily in the first procedure, the risk of excessive tension and scar spread can be minimized by using tissue expansion. Large expanders (500 to 1000 ml) are routinely used and placed above the abdominal fascia either above, below, or along either margin of the lesion. Selection of tissue expander site is very critical because dissection in the immediate area of the breast buds should be avoided to prevent distortion of the position of the nipple-areolar complex and subsequent breast growth. Expander ports are typically placed down on the anterior thigh, where they can be readily palpated, or for expanders in the upper abdomen overlying the lower ribcage or sternum, where there is firm skeletal tissue beneath the port.

With careful planning and adequate expansion (frequently overexpanding the expanders), the need for extensive release of the capsule will be minimized. Under no circumstances should the capsule be excised because this will lead to a significant increase in blood loss and may well compromise the vascular supply to the flap. Even limited capsule release should be done very carefully to avoid injuring the blood supply to the skin flaps. In the majority of cases involving the anterior trunk, excisions are accomplished with direct advancement flap closure whether the flaps are expanded or not. Lesions involving the immediate breast or nipple-areolar area present a treatment dilemma. Excision in infancy or early childhood carries a significant risk of injury or even excision of the breast bud with subsequent breast deformity or absence. Attempting to expand the tissue in the same area and move it elsewhere may have similar consequences. It is our recommendation that these lesions be left alone until after thelarche (Figure 65-13). At this time the excision and reconstruction may be carried out more safely. Large nevi may be more easily excised and reconstructed using an expanded full-thickness graft for coverage rather than adjacent expanded skin. Lesions involving the entire breast are relatively rare, and few have been

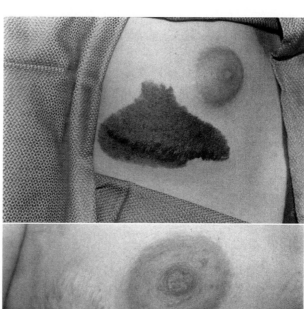

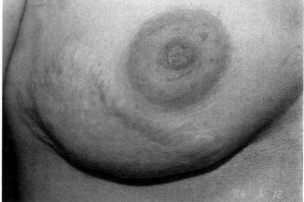

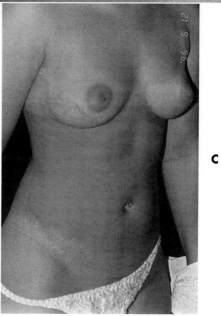

Figure 65-13. This case demonstrates the use of an expanded full-thickness skin graft in treatment of a large nevus of the breast. This approach was chosen to ensure that the breast shape was not violated and to confine the scars to the breast above the inframammary fold. **A,** Shows the nevus was treated by a relatively ineffective partial excision in early childhood, then left for the definitive excision until after thelarche. **B,** Close-up view of the expanded graft on the breast 7 years after excision and graft. **C,** Both the breast and the donor site scar in the groin along the bikini tan line.

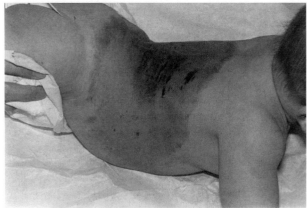

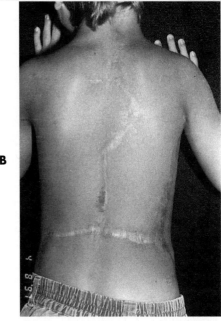

Figure 65-14. A, Giant nevi of the mid-back are generally easily treated with expanders placed above and below the nevus and the expanded flaps advanced both toward one another and some skin recruited from the flanks. **B,** The result is shown 7 years after the reconstruction.

treated. Reconstruction in these cases may need to follow principles of standard breast reconstruction for coverage to provide optimal shape, skin coverage, and limited risk of distortion of the surrounding chest and adjacent breast. Lesions of the shoulder, both anterior and posterior, are discussed below.

Our approach of posterior trunk nevi has changed dramatically over the last decade (Figures 65-14 and 65-15). Large segment excision with immediate sheet grafting was routinely practiced and published in our 1988 review of the first 76 patients in which varied treatment modalities for large and giant nevi were reviewed. We now believe that many of the extensive posterior trunk lesions, even those covering the buttock, perineal, and perianal areas, can be excised and reconstructed using tissue expansion alone. Large tissue expanders

placed over the flanks allow for construction of large transposition "angel wing" flaps, which can be frequently advanced to cover most of the back and buttocks. Expanders are placed either cephalad or caudal to the nevus, typically using 500- to 550-ml expanders in infants. These expanders can be inflated to as much as 1200 ml each and provide substantial transposition flaps with excellent blood supply and the ability to cover considerably longer distances than the typical advancement flaps used by many surgeons. Careful design of these flaps to include large paraspinal perforators increases their length and survival. The routine use of hand-held Dopplers preoperatively to map out these vessels is very beneficial. Dissection of tissue expander pockets is as described above and is usually started at 6 months of age while the infant skin is most mobile. Expansion of the buttock and upper thigh skin used in combination with repeat expansion of previously expanded and transposed flaps will allow coverage of the entire buttock area with the scars at completion in a very favorable position to avoid late contracture problems. "Intermediate-size" giant nevi in the mid-back have in some cases been excised by others (who prefer to use expanders as little as possible) without the use of tissue expansion, but we believe that even in these cases the excision is simplified by the added tissue gained through the expansion process. In these instances the excision is accomplished with gradual recruitment of surrounding skin and serial excision.

The shoulder area along with the adjacent neck and deltoid area presents additional challenges of reconstruction in an area with varied contour, skin thickness, and a propensity for wide and often hypertrophic scarring. Expansion of the upper back and anterior chest to recruit tissue into this area may potentially distort the breast and carry the scars that much further down the back. Although excision and grafting would be considered by many as the treatment of choice, the contour defect that may remain, as well as the color and texture difference expected with an extensive graft, have made use of this option less than ideal. In an effort to address these concerns, we have applied microvascular techniques to our armamentarium of procedures for treatment of giant nevi. Given the size of the defects that may need to be covered in this area, we have elected to use either a preexpanded or nonexpanded free TRAM flap, recognizing that the flap will need contouring after inset (Figures 65-16 and 65-17). The contouring is done readily with liposuction in combination with final excision of the border of the nevus, which is left in place at the time of the initial flap inset. Although novel in approach, we believe that the outcome seems to warrant this innovation.

LARGE AND GIANT CONGENITAL PIGMENTED NEVI OF EXTREMITIES

Our management of CMN of the extremities has evolved over the last few years, as well. The choice of technique is determined by the location and extent of the lesion. Although tissue

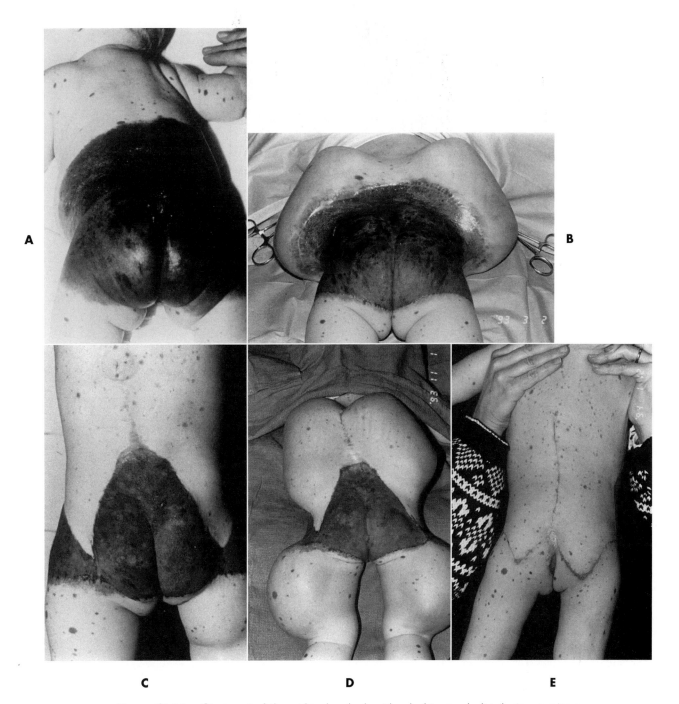

Figure 65-15. Giant nevi of the mid-to low back with a bathing trunk distribution require a different flap design. **A,** This 3-month-old presented with involvement of the entire perineal and perianal area, buttocks, and back. **B,** Two 500-ml expanders were placed cephalad to the nevus at the same time some upward advancement of buttock/thigh skin was carried out without expansion. The expanders are shown expanded to approximately 700 ml each over 12 weeks. **C,** Expanded transposition flaps shown before placement of new expanders. **D,** After expansion of both the previous back flaps and the buttock/thigh flaps. **E,** The result after excision of remaining nevus except for a thin strip of nevus along one edge of the anal verge, left for excision once other scars were stable (to minimize risk of circumferential scar or wound problem during flap transfer).

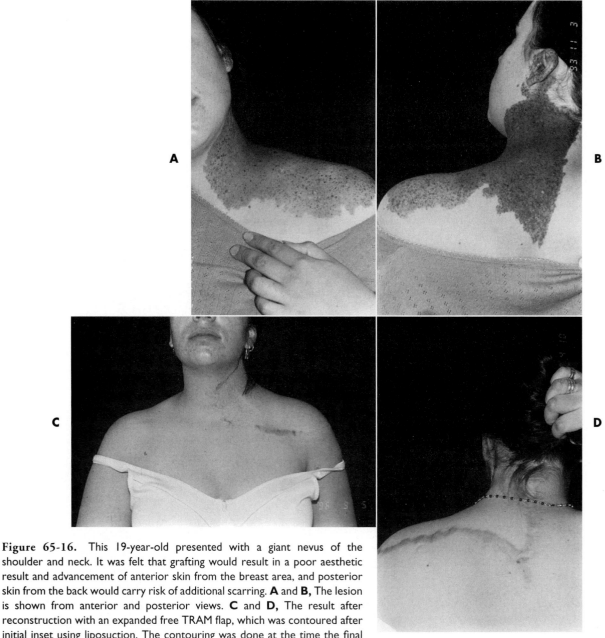

Figure 65-16. This 19-year-old presented with a giant nevus of the shoulder and neck. It was felt that grafting would result in a poor aesthetic result and advancement of anterior skin from the breast area, and posterior skin from the back would carry risk of additional scarring. **A** and **B,** The lesion is shown from anterior and posterior views. **C** and **D,** The result after reconstruction with an expanded free TRAM flap, which was contoured after initial inset using liposuction. The contouring was done at the time the final excision of a rim of nevus, left bordering the inset flap. Note excellent contour of both neck and shoulder with this approach.

expansion has been a primary modality of treatment in the head and neck and is also readily accomplished in the trunk, tissue expansion for excision of nevi of the extremities has not been as readily accomplished. This fact is more the result of the limitations imposed by the geometry of the extremities and limitations this geometry imposes on flap design and movement than the greater likelihood on expander complications in the extremities. Although the risk of expander complications can be significantly reduced with careful planning, placement through a remote incision, and at times endoscopic expander placement, the greater likelihood of scars imposing a restriction on later movement and unsightly contour defects after reconstruction

still present a significant concern. When used, expanders must be carefully selected to ensure placement without folds or edges that will compromise the overlying flap or risk breakdown of the incision used for the expander placement. Expander placement through a distant incision, possibly aided by the endoscope, may minimize the risk of expander exposure. The expanders will vary in size based on where on the extremity they are being placed, the size of the lesion to be excised, and the age of the child at the time of treatment. Expanders vary from 100 to 500 ml. This is an area in which the replacement of an expander in the same pocket with an even bigger expander and continuation of expansion before nevus excision may be of

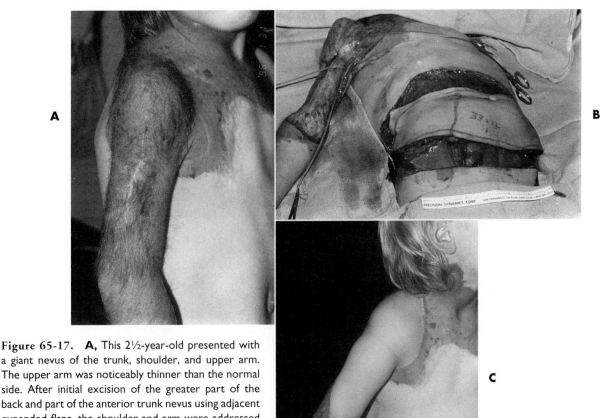

Figure 65-17. **A,** This 2½-year-old presented with a giant nevus of the trunk, shoulder, and upper arm. The upper arm was noticeably thinner than the normal side. After initial excision of the greater part of the back and part of the anterior trunk nevus using adjacent expanded flaps, the shoulder and arm were addressed with an expanded free TRAM flap as well. **B,** The expanded TRAM flap is shown with the recipient site prepared by partial excision of the nevus. The brachial vessels were used as recipient vessels. **C,** Nine months after the free flap showing excellent contour of both the shoulder and arm.

great efficacy (so-called in situ serial expansion). This approach may involve significantly less risk of complication than attempting to reexpand the previously advanced skin flap with its adjacent scar.

Lesions of the deltoid can be addressed by expanding the upper back/scapular area and transposing an epaulet type of flap into place. This will avoid potential narrowing of the proximal extremity and scarring into the axilla with limitation of movement. We have applied a similar principle to that mentioned for the shoulder and neck for the entire shoulder and upper neck using a large expanded free TRAM flap with good success. As we move further down the upper extremity, our previous choice for circumferential lesions was the use of either split-thickness or, more ideally, expanded full-thickness skin grafts. Again with this approach we are faced with the aesthetic problems of poor color, contour, and the potential functional problems of graft contracture and loss of range of motion. To that end, we have approached some of these lesions with either expanded or nonexpanded pedicle flaps from the flank/abdomen (Figure

65-18). These flaps can provide the supple skin with subcutaneous tissue necessary to avoid carrying scars up or down the arm (that might be needed to move adjacent expanded skin flaps) and leave the donor site in a relatively less visible area. Although this approach requires more staging than simple excision and skin graft, the ultimate outcome both aesthetically and functionally is superior. When it comes to large and giant nevi of the hand, skin grafts, particularly expanded full-thickness grafts, remain our treatment modality of choice. An expanded full-thickness skin graft can provide both excellent aesthetic and functional results in this area (Figure 65-19).

The lower extremity provides an even greater challenge than does the upper. Large but not giant nevi of the thigh generally lend themselves well to excision using expansion, at times carrying out a partial excision at the time of tissue expander placement. Tissue expansion is effective for medium to large lesions of the lower leg, as well, but the limitations of the area impose themselves more the farther distal the lesion. Expanded full-thickness grafts have provided a means of improving on

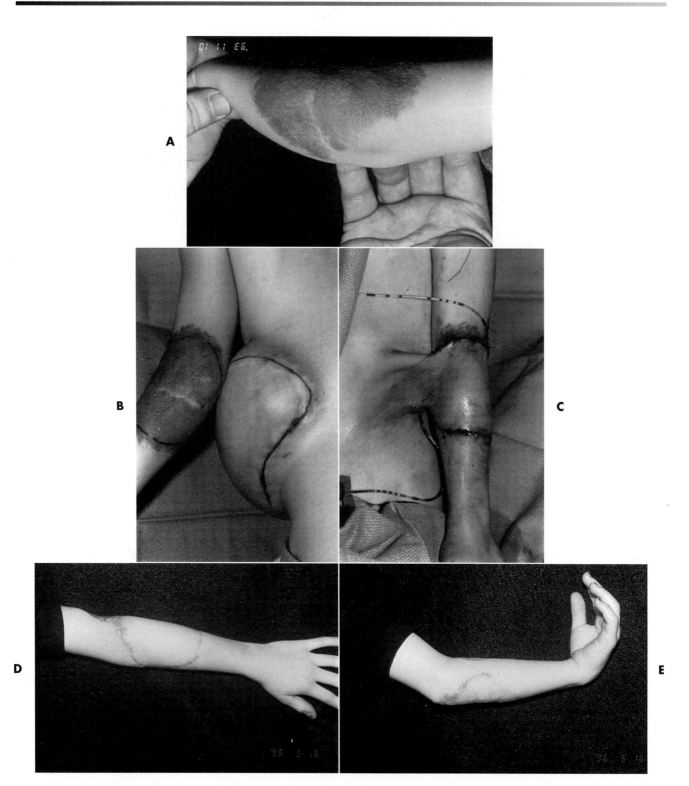

Figure 65-18.   In an effort to improve on the aesthetic result of excision of a near-circumferential nevus of the arm, where a graft frequently leaves a contour defect, and expansion of flaps above and below may even if able to cover the defect require carrying scars above and below the area of nevus, a pedicled flap is planned from the adjacent flank. **A,** Lateral view of the nevus. **B,** Posterior view of the nevus and expander in the flank with outline of the proposed flap. **C,** Anterior view of the initial flap attachment. **D** and **E,** Two views of the inset flap after complete excision and flap inset. Note maintenance of soft tissue contour and absence of any scar outside the initial area of involvement.

A   B   C   D

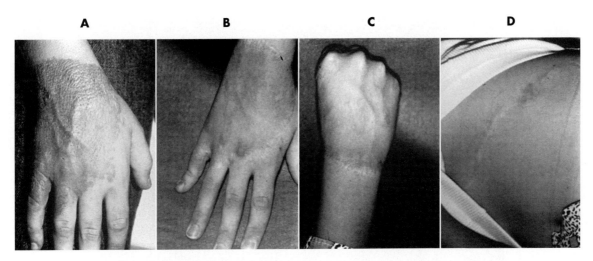

Figure 65-19.   An expanded full-thickness skin graft used for treatment of a giant nevus of the dorsum of a hand. **A** and **B,** Preoperative and postoperative views of the nevus and graft 5 years after reconstruction. **C** and **D,** Additional view of the grafted hand and the groin donor site.

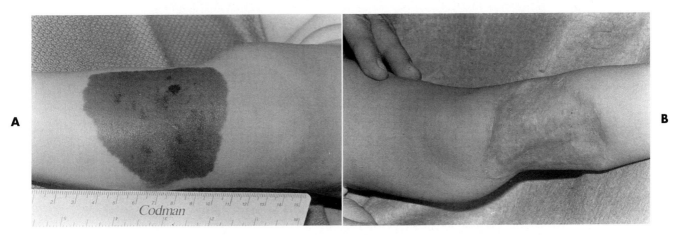

A   B

Figure 65-20.   The problem contour defect after excision of nevus to fascial level and graft (even full thickness) on the extremity. **A,** The nevus of the leg just distal to the knee is shown before excision. **B,** The result 1 year after coverage with an expanded full-thickness skin graft shows reasonable scar maturation and graft color but poor contour restoration.

the relatively poor aesthetics of split-thickness skin grafts in this area but still fall short of ideal, particularly when dealing with circumferential lesions (Figure 65-20). When planning skin graft reconstruction in these cases, it is recommended that the reconstruction be carried out in two procedures, addressing first the posterior and then the anterior aspect of the lesion. Scars are ideally placed along the mid-lateral and mid-medial lines of the extremity. With this sequence of procedures, an untoward flexion contracture after the posterior excision might

be addressed as the anterior half of the nevus is excised. With time and more experience, we would hope that the principles of reconstruction with free tissue transplantation and prefabricated flaps may provide for improved aesthetic and functional results in the lower and upper extremities. As with the hand, treatment of large and giant nevi of the feet are best addressed using skin grafts, with expanded or nonexpanded full-thickness grafts being of some benefit in terms of long-term durability (Figure 65-21).

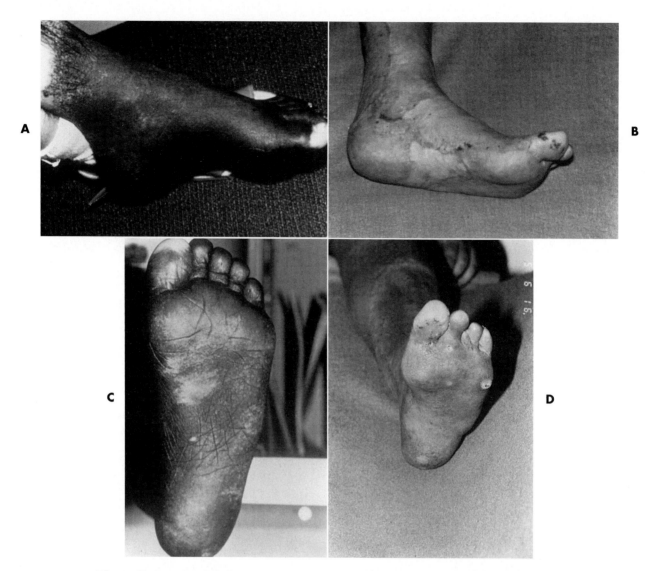

Figure 65-21. **A** and **B,** This stocking distribution giant nevus was treated initially with excision of the anterior aspect of the leg and foot and reconstruction with a split-thickness skin graft, then coverage of the plantar aspect of the foot and toes with an expanded full-thickness skin graft from bilateral lower abdomen and groin area. The result is shown 3 years after excision. **C,** A portion of the lesion of the plantar foot showed atypical cell changes before excision. **D,** Plantar view also shown at 3 years after reconstruction of the foot with some callous formation but stable, durable graft coverage.

OUTCOMES

The treatment of congenital nevi, whether pigmented or nonpigmented, follows similar principles based on size and location of the lesion, risk of malignant change, and age of the patient. Assessment of outcomes must consider issues of the effect of treatment on the risk of malignant change, the aesthetic appearance after reconstruction, and the potential functional consequences of the surgery. To a lesser extent, we also must look at the varied treatments in terms of how they affect hospital stay and how well they are tolerated by the patients.

In regard to the risk of malignant change, we would hope that continued evaluation of large series of patients with congenital pigmented nevi would one day answer the continued debate as to whether these lesions carry a risk of malignant degeneration or not. Although there are institutions that state that they have yet to see a case of malignancy in a giant congenital nevus, many series state otherwise and we ourselves have seen three patients develop malignancies in a giant nevus and go on to die from extensive metastases. With much variation in reporting, differing classifications of nevus by size, and variation in the age of the different populations followed, we may never have an answer. Certainly until we do have a more definitive answer, we must proceed on the premise that these lesions present both a risk of malignant change and a significant stigma because of their appearance. Treatment must be directed at both of these concerns. Outcome data at this time is limited to subjective assessment of different treatment options and assessment of how effectively these different options accomplish the removal of the lesion. However, it may be of some significance that, as of today, none of the patients who have undergone excision in our series has developed a malignancy, with follow-up of the earliest patients being greater than 15 years. One child who underwent excision of a borderline deviation melanoma in infancy is healthy without nevus or tumor at 14 years after surgical excision of her giant nevus.

Complications of the surgical procedures described within this chapter are primarily related to use of tissue expansion. Within our early group of patients undergoing excision and "large segment" split-thickness skin grafting, we had no graft losses. Although we have not reviewed our expander complications specifically in nevus cases only, our numbers give a general idea of the low risk of adverse outcomes from expansion. In fact, given the inclusion of complex wounds in the series, we would expect the complication rate to be somewhat lower in the current group. In our review of expansion in 1982-April 4, 1999, 622 expanders were used in 412 patients, with 69% for treatment of nevi. The patients ranged in age from 12 days to 19 years, averaging 4.7 years. The complications were similar to all series on expansion in respect to infection, exposure, and expander leakage. The complication rate by number of patients was 16% and by number of expanders was 12%, with failure rates (need to seek another reconstructive technique to address problem) of 3% and 2%, respectively. Of the expanded full-thickness skin grafts, 2 of 15 in this series had areas of minor loss. These results strongly support the safety of this treatment modality.

Although we have seen a reduction in inpatient stays even for children undergoing extensive skin grafting procedures, we also have noted that hospital stays of greater than 23 hours are rarities for patients undergoing nevus excision with tissue expansion. With increased experience, we have seen continued reduction in the complications of tissue expansion; this reduction in complications is occurring at the same time that we have observed continued increase in the effectiveness of the expanded tissue. With parental involvement in the expansion process, greater than two thirds of the expansion are performed at home, thereby reducing trips to the clinic and easing the anxiety of the children undergoing expansion. This shift of responsibility has not been at the expense of any increase in complications. Finally, in comparison of our patient population with similar-size lesions in similar locations treated with different treatment modalities, we have had the opportunity to compare outcomes of these procedures from both an aesthetic and a functional point of view.

Let us summarize these thoughts. In 1988, we presented a protocol for treatment of large and giant congenital pigmented nevi (greater than 2% TBS) based on a comparison of different treatment modalities in different body regions. Each area—head and neck, trunk, and extremity—seemed to lend itself to

different treatment options in accomplishing early nevus excision and reconstruction. To date, we have now treated 200 patients (from 1979 to 1997). Evaluation of this larger group has now demonstrated both the benefits of the previously described protocol and its weaknesses. Most of these are described above, but we should summarize them here.

We have seen little change in our approach to treatment of large congenital nevi of the head and neck. Tissue expansion is still the treatment modality of choice. However, as with other regions of the body, experience has demonstrated significantly better results in terms of hair direction, hairline restoration, and efficacy of coverage of larger surface areas (with reduced need for serial expansions) using expanded transposition flaps versus simple advancement of the expanded tissue. Although we have accepted the use of larger expanded full-thickness skin grafts for nevi of the combined periorbital area and medial cheek, we have confined the grafts as much as possible to the lids and have completed aesthetic unit reconstruction with expanded cheek flaps. Thoughtful integration of simple partial nevus excision and flap advancement or rotation before initial tissue expansion has seemed to reduce the need for serial expansion in the midfacial area and thereby has minimized some of the risks of expansion in this region. In addition, recent experience with prefabricated flaps, either carried on a transposed superficial temporal artery pedicle or transferred by microvascular technique from a more distant donor site, may further limit the need to use skin grafts in the reconstruction of some of these lesions (e.g., in the nasal region).

One of our greatest advancements has come in the treatment of giant nevi of the trunk, where improved flap design has allowed the excision of much larger nevi of the posterior trunk and buttocks. This is an area in which previously we believed there was little role for tissue expansion because of well-known problems with serial flap expansion and advancement on the back (i.e., increased likelihood of expander exposure and continuing decrease in the tissue gain). Previously, we recommended large segment grafting with nonmeshed split-thickness skin grafting. With continued experience in expansion and with a switch to the use of expanded transposition flaps, even the excision of giant nevi covering the entire buttocks, perineum, and perianal areas may be reconstructed without skin grafting.

The treatment of large and giant nevi of the extremities has been seen to improve as well, yet not to the extent seen in other regions. Although we accept the fact that large lesions, particularly those that are circumferential, are best treated with skin grafts, long-term follow-up of these patients has demonstrated a poor aesthetic result of many of these reconstructions and, on occasion, poor durability of the grafts, as well. We have just entered the era in which some of these problems are being addressed with use of pedicled flaps from the trunk and free tissue transfer from distant sites.

Although some surgeons might consider the innovations discussed in this chapter overkill for treatment of congenital nevi, we cannot diminish the psychologic impact of many of these large and very visible lesions without aiming for optimal aesthetic restoration, as well as treatment of a potentially premalignant lesion. It is through continued outcomes research that these latter "innovations" and others will prove their value.

REFERENCES

1. Alper JC, Holmes LB: The incidence and significance of birthmarks in a cohort of 4641 newborns, *Pediatr Dermatol* 1:58, 1983.
2. Alper J, Holmes LB, Mihm MC: Birthmarks with serious medical significance: nevocellular nevi, sebaceous nevi and multiple café-au-lait spots, *J Pediatr* 95:696-700, 1979.
3. Baader W, Kropp R, Tapper D: Congenital malignant melanoma, *Plast Reconstr Surg* 90:53-56, 1992.
4. Bauer BS, Vicari FA: An approach to excision of congenital gient pigmented nevi in infancy and early childhood, *Plast Reconstr Surg* 82:1012-1021, 1988.
5. Bauer BS, Vicari FA, Richard ME: Expanded full thickness skin grafts in children: case selection, planning and management, *Plast Reconstr Surg* 92:59-69, 1993.
6. Bauer BS, Vicari FA, Richard ME: The role of tissue expansion in pediatric plastic surgery, *Clin Plast Surg* 17:101-112, 1990.
7. Castilla EE, DaGraca-Dutra M, Orioli-Parreiras IM: Epidemiology of congenital pigmented nevi: I. Incidence rates and relative frequencies, *Br J Dermatol* 104:307-315, 1981.
8. Chretien-Marquet B, Bennaceur S, Fernandez R: Surgical treatment of large cutaneous lesions of the back in children by concentric cutaneous mobilization, *Plast Reconstr Surg* 100:926-936, 1997.
9. Cohen HJ, Minkin W, Frank SB: Nevus spilus, *Arch Dermatol* 102:433, 1970.
10. Constant E, Davis DG: The pre-malignant nature of the sebaceus nevus of Jadassohn, *Plast Reconstr Surg* 50:257-259, 1972.
11. Cordova A: The Mongolian spot, *Clin Pediatr* 20:714, 1981.
12. Cronin TD: Extensive pigmented nevi in hair-bearing areas, *Plast Reconstr Surg* 11:94, 1953.
13. Domingo J, Helwig EB: Malignant neoplasms associated with nevus sebaceous of Jadassohn, *J Am Acad Dermatol* 1:545, 1979.
14. Frieden IJ, Williams ML, Barkovich, AJ: Giant congenital melanocytic nevi: brain magnetic resonance findings in neurologically asymptomatic children, *J Am Acad Dermatol* 31:423-429, 1994.
15. Gexohemas RG: Q-switched ruby laser therapy of nevus of Ota, *Arch Dermatol* 128:1618, 1992.
16. Goldenhersh MA, Savin RC, Barnhill RL, et al: Malignant blue nevus: case report and literature review, *J Am Acad Dermatol* 19:712-722, 1988.
17. Horn MS, Sousker WF, Pierson DL: Basal cell epithelioma excising in a linear epidermal nevus, *Arch Dermatol* 117:247, 1981.
18. Hurwitz S: *Clinical pediatric dermatology*, ed 2, Philadelphia, 1993, WB Saunders.
19. Iconomore TG, Michelow BJ, Zuker RM: Tissue expansion in the pediatric patient, *Ann Plast Surg* 31:134-140, 1993.
20. Illig L, Weidner F, Hundeiken ME, et al: Congenital nevi <10 cm as precursors for melanoma, *Arch Dermatol* 121:1274-1281, 1985.
21. Johnson HA: Permanent removal of pigmentation from giant hairy nevi by dermabrasion in early life, *Plast Reconstr Surg* 30:321-323, 1977.
22. Kadonaga JN, Frieden IJ: Neurocutaneous melanosis: definition and review of the literature, *J Am Acad Dermatol* 24:747-755, 1991.
23. Kaplan E, Nicholoff BJ: Clinical and histologic features of nevi with emphasis on treatment approaches, *Clin Plast Surg* 14:277-300, 1987.
24. Kaplan EN: The risk of malignancy in large congenital nevi, *Plast Reconstr Surg* 53:421-428, 1974.
25. Keall J, McElwwain TJ, Wallace AF: Malignant melanomas in childhood, *Br J Plast Surg* 34:340-341, 1981.
26. Kopf AW, Bart RS, Hennesey P: Congenital nevocytic nevi and malignant melanomas, *J Am Acad Dermatol* 1:123-130, 1979.
27. Kopf AW, Levine LJ, Rigel DS, et al: Prevalence of congenital nevus like nevi, nevi spili and café-au-lait spots, *Arch Dermatol* 121:766, 1985.
28. Kopf AW, Weidman AS: Nevus of Ota, *Arch Dermatol* 85:195, 1962.
29. Leugh AK: Mongolian spots in Chinese children, *Int J Dermatol* 27:106, 1988.
30. Lorentzen M, Pers M, Bretleville-Jensen G: The incidence of malignant transformation in giant pigmented nevi, *Scand J Plast Reconstr Surg* 11:163-167, 1977.
31. Lovejoy FH, Boyle WE Jr: Linear nevus sebaceous syndrome: a report of two cases and a review of the literature, *Pediatrics* 52:382-387, 1973.
32. Mark GJ, Mihm MC, Liteplo MG, et al: Congenital melanocytic nevi of the small and garment type, *Human Pathol* 4:345-418, 1973.
33. Mehtegan A, Pinkas H: Life history of organoid nevi specia: reference to nevus sebaceous of Jadassohn, *Arch Dermatol* 91:574, 1965.
34. Moss ALH: Congenital "giant" nevus: a preliminary report of a new surgical approach, *Br J Plast Surg* 40:410-419, 1987.
35. Ozgur F, Akyurek M, Kayikcioglu A, et al: Metastatic malignant blue nevus: a case report, *Ann Plast Surg* 39:411-415, 1997.
36. Paller AS: Epidermal nevus syndrome, *Neurol Clin* 5:451-457, 1987.
37. Quaba AA, Wallace AF: The incidence of malignant melanoma (0 to 15 years of age) arising in "Large" congenital nevicellular nevi, *Plast Reconstr Surg* 78:174-179, 1986.
38. Reed WB, Becker SW Sr, Becker SW Jr: Giant pigmented nevi, melanoma, leptomeningeal melanocytosis: a clinical and histopathological study, *Arch Dermatol* 91:100-119, 1965.
39. Rhodes AR, Melsk JW: Small congenital nevocellular nevi and the risk of cutaneous melanoma, *J Pediatr* 100:219-224, 1982.
40. Rhodes AR, Silvermann RA, Harrist TJ, et al: A histologic comparison of congenital and acquired nevomelanocytic nevi, *Arch Dermatol* 121:1266-1273, 1985.

41. Rhodes AR, Wood WC, Sobr AJ, et al: Nonepidermal origin of malignant melanoma associated with giant congenital nevocellular nevus, *Plast Reconstr Surg* 67:782, 1981.

42. Rodriguez H, Ackerman LV: Cellular blue nevus: clinicopathologic study of forty-five cases, *Cancer* 21:393-405, 1968.

43. Rogers M: Epidermal nevi and the epidermal nevus syndromes: a review of 233 cases, *Pediatr Dermatol* 9:342, 1992.

44. Sandsmark M, Eskeland G, Ogaard AR, et al: Treatment of large congenital nevi, *Scand J Plast Reconstr Surg Hand Surg* 27:223-232, 1993.

45. Schachner L: *Pediatric dermatology,* New York, 1995, Churchill Livingstone.

46. Shaffer C, Walker K, Weiss GR: Malignant melanoma in a Hispanic male with nevus of Ota, *Dermatology* 1:146, 1992.

47. Solomon LM, Fretzin DF, Dewald RL: The epidermal nevus syndrome, *Arch Dermatol* 97:273-285, 1968.

48. Trozak DJ, Rowland WR, Hu F: Metastatic malignant melanoma in pre-pubertal children, *Pediatrics* 55:191, 1975.

49. Vergnes P, Taieb A, Maleville J, et al: Repeated skin expansion for excision of congenital nevi in infancy and childhood, *Plast Reconstr Surg* 91:450-455, 1993.

50. Wagner FR, Cottel WI: In situ malignant melanoma in a speckled lentiginous nevus, *J Am Acad Dermatol* 20:125, 1989.

51. Walton RG, Jacobs AH, Cox HJ: Pigmented lesions in newborn infants, *Br J Dermatol* 95:389-396, 1976.

52. Weidner N, Flanders DK, Jochmscur PR, et al: Neurosarcomatous malignant melanomas arising in neuroid giant congenital melanocytic nevus, *Arch Dermatol* 121:1302, 1985.

53. Weng C, Tsai YC, Chen TJ: Jadassohn's nevus sebaceous of the head and face, *Ann Plast Surg* 25:100, 1990.

54. Zhu N, Warr R, Cai R, et al: Cutaneous malignant melanoma in the young, *Br J Plast Surg* 50:10-14, 1997.

Microtia: Auricular Reconstruction

Satoru Nagata

Microtia (hypoplasia of the auricle) is known to result from incomplete embryonic development; thus the degree of severity of the deformity varies from case to case. Total auricular reconstruction for microtia is dependent on the degree of severity of hypoplasia in comparison with that of the normal auricle on which the specific auricular reconstruction is based. I have clinically classified microtia into three major types: (1) the lobule type, (2) the concha type, and (3) the small concha type. Regardless of which type, the ultimate goal is the reconstruction of an auricle with an appearance as close as possible to that of a normal auricle. The auricle constitutes only a small portion of the total body surface area, but it is probably one of the most sophisticated and complex morphologic structures of the body. Therefore it is necessary to fully comprehend the three-dimensional (3-D) morphologic properties of the auricle to attain more than satisfactory and favorable results in total and subtotal auricular reconstruction.

HISTORY OF AURICULAR RECONSTRUCTION

There have been numerous reports and publications concerned with auricular repair from as early as 1597, where Tagliacozzi[49] described the repair of upper and lower auricular deformities with retroauricular skin flaps. However, the first documented auricular reconstruction reference appeared in the Susruta Samhita,[3] in which the use of a cheek flap was suggested for repair of the missing lobule.

The actual milestone in modern auricular reconstruction came in 1959, when Tanzer[55] introduced the autogenous costal cartilage graft procedure. With his demonstrated excellence in results, this method has been used throughout the world.

On the other hand, use of inorganic and alloplastic auricular frameworks became common, and in 1966, Cronin[10] introduced the silicon ear framework, but because of complications and problems such as extrusion, this practice was discontinued.[9]

At present, the autogenous costal cartilage remains to the most ideal material source for fabrication of the 3-D auricular framework with the least number of complications.*

---

*References 4, 5, 16, 27-34, 54, 55.

ANATOMY AND EMBRYOLOGY

The subject of anatomy and embryology of the auricle is well documented in various publications and textbooks; therefore this subject will be excluded from this chapter.

ETIOLOGY

Incidence

An intensive study conducted by Grabb[17] and Kaseff[21] revealed that microtia occurs once in every 6000 births. The occurrence in Japan is estimated as 100 microtic births per year. An extremely high incidence rate of 0.1% has been reported among the Navajo tribe of Native Americans.[1] Microtia is twice as frequent among males as in females, and the estimated ratio of right-left-bilateral is 5:3:1.[13,42]

Hereditary Factors

Hereditary transmission of several types of auricular anomaly have been revealed: preauricular pits and sinuses, a combination of pits, preauricular appendages, cupping deformities, and deafness are all hereditary dominant transmissions.[26,58] Auricular abnormalities associated with deafness have revealed characteristics of both dominant and recessive hereditary transmissions,[23] cup ear deformity,[15,19,22,43] and mandibulofacial dysostosis.[41] Other associated relations were found among families with cleft and high palate[19] and first and second brachial arch syndromes.[52]

DIAGNOSIS

Classification

Numerous classifications for congenital deformities of the auricle have been suggested and reported, but none is completely satisfactory. Streeter[48] established his classification according to the pattern of embryologic development of the auricle, and Rogers[45] classified auricular hypoplasia according to a descending scale of severity. Tanzer[51] and Nagata[27-31] classified congenital auricular defects clinically according to the surgical approach. Present classification is clinically categorized as

(1) the lobule type: cases with the remnant ear and ear lobule but without the concha, acoustic meatus, and tragus[27-29]; (2) the concha type: cases with the remnant ear, ear lobule, concha, acoustic meatus, tragus, and incisura intertragica[27,28,30]; (3) the small concha type: cases with the existence of the remnant ear and lobule and a small indentation representing the concha[27,28,31]; (4) clinical anotia: cases with none or minute resemblance of a remnant ear; and (5) atypical microtia: cases that do not fall into any of the above classifications.

Associated Abnormalities

Microtia occurring as an isolated independent deformity is extremely unusual, and the most common associated defect involves the external auditory canal and the contents of the middle ear. The defect ranges from atresia of the canal combined with severely distorted, fused, and hypoplastic ossicles and failure of pneumatization of the mastoid cells and/or minor ossicular abnormalities to diminished external auditory canal diameter.

Other associated abnormalities include first and second brachial syndromes; defects of the external and middle ear; anomalies of the mandible, maxilla, malar, and temporal bones; macrostomia; lateral facial clefts; atrophy of the facial musculature; and occasional involvement of the lingual and palatal muscles and parotid gland.[7,17,24] There is also increased incidence of urogenital tract anomalies in the presence of microtia,[25,52] especially when accompanied by manifestations of first and second brachial arch syndromes.[56]

CLINICAL FEATURES

Microtia is a term describing severe types of hypoplasia of the auricle, from complete absence of auricular tissue (anotia) to a normal-appearing but small ear accompanied by a blind or absent external auditory canal. Microtia is characterized by the presence of a remnant lobule (usually a peanut-shaped or sausage-shaped vestige) along the vertical axis, surmounted by a vestige of skin containing remnant ear cartilage (lobule type). The location of the microtic lobule is variable, but usually it is displaced superiorly to the level of the lobule of the normal ear. The tomographic study conducted by Converse et al[7,8] revealed that skeletal deficiencies exist in all microtic cases.

ACOUSTIC FUNCTION AND PATHOLOGIC ABNORMALITIES

A significant correlation exists between the severity of auricular deformity and middle ear defects. Most common middle ear defects encountered are fusion or hypoplasia of the malleus and incus and/or isolated deformities of the ossicles, with increase in severity, complete atresia of the tympanic cavity, and the absence of the ossicles. Because of the middle ear's separate embryologic derivation, it has been assumed to be unaffected, but in recent polytomographic studies, dysplasia and hypoplasia have been reported.[41,44] Furthermore, uncertainty of the location and position of the facial nerve renders it susceptible to injury during surgery, especially in the absence of a pneumatized mastoid during middle ear surgery.

SURGICAL INDICATIONS

The topic of middle ear surgery in the presence of microtia still remains controversial, especially in unilateral cases. Even so, it is of major interest in improving acoustic function (hearing) among patients with bilateral microtia. It is necessary for the reconstructive plastic surgeon and the otologist to determine whether adequate auditory acuity is present in the patient for development of communication before 12 months of age. Insufficient restoration of impaired hearing with mechanical aids to acceptable levels is indicative of otologic surgical intervention for correction of impaired hearing. Technical surgical refinements for unilateral deafness have been reported,[20,50] even though this procedure is questioned for unilateral microtia patients with normal acoustic function on the opposite ear.[2,11-12,47]

Patients who have undergone middle ear surgery for correction of impaired hearing before auricular reconstruction are seldom observed with postsurgical complications, such as infection, chronic drainage, and gradual decrease in acoustic function. Thus numerous opinions on when the middle ear surgery should be performed have been reported. Nager[40] and Broadbent and Woolf[6] reported that auricular reconstruction can be performed after middle ear surgery in combination with lobular rotation in a transverse position. However, most reconstructive plastic surgeons would prefer to have the auricular reconstruction completed before middle ear surgery because valuable retroauricular skin is preserved and the surgical field for auricular reconstruction is free from scarring. Edgerton and Nager[14] proposed completing the auricular reconstruction and with an anteriorly based pedicle to flip the reconstructed auricle forward to provide the otologist ample space for middle ear surgery, although otologists object that the reconstructed auricle restricts the surgical field necessary for middle surgery.

AUTHOR'S METHOD OF AURICULAR RECONSTRUCTION

The method of total auricular reconstruction (microtia repair) is a two-stage operation in which the first stage involves fabrication and grafting of a three-dimensional costal cartilage framework (3-D frame) and the second stage is the projection of the constructed auricle.[27-32]

Initial Office Visit

During the initial office visit (usually within the first 12 months after birth), the surgical method and expectations (visual aids and illustrations are of great help for explaining surgical method and expectations), psychologic factors, hospitalization requirements, and limitations in postsurgical physical activities are to be thoroughly discussed with the patient and parents (guardian) and family. The patient is instructed to return annually until the patient reaches the proper age for surgery.

Follow-Up Annual Visits

The growth (development) of the patient, chest circumference (level of the xiphoid process), and acoustic analyses (if necessary) are determined and recorded. It is extremely important to establish a good patient-surgeon relationship with young children because they are most likely afraid of surgery.

Recommended Age of Surgery

The age of surgery may vary, but because a certain volume of costal cartilage is required for the fabrication of the 3-D frame and the growth of an auricle reaches adult size around the age of 10 years, the recommended age of surgery in Japan is 10 years. However, because of psychologic factors, surgeries in other countries are performed in the preschool years, around 5 years of age. In addition to the age factor, chest circumference (level of the xiphoid process) of 60 cm is recommended.

FIRST-STAGE OPERATION

The author's first-stage operation involves the harvesting of the costal cartilages, the fabrication of the 3-D frame, and the grafting of the 3-D frame.

Construction of the Paper Pattern (3-D Frame)

The average dimension of a normal adult ear in Japan is 32 mm × 60 mm, and the thickness of the skin covering the ear is about 2 mm.[27-31] Thus the dimension of the 3-D frame to be constructed should be 28 mm × 58 mm. For easier construction of the paper pattern, an 8-square outline is used, with the length of one side being 14 mm. Figure 66-1 shows how the paper pattern is made.

Fabrication of the 3-D Frame

The costal cartilages are harvested en bloc from the same side of microtia repair (Figure 66-2, A) with the anterior costal perichondrium and the anterior and posterior surfaces reversed (Figure 66-2, B). This is to utilize the natural configurations of the costal cartilages. A paper pattern of the 3-D frame is made (Figure 66-2, C), and each unit of the 3-D frame is outlined on the harvested costal cartilage (Figure 66-2, D). With a scalpel and special surgical sculpture knives (Hoshi Medical Co., Ltd., Tokyo), the base frame (Figure 66-2, E-F), crus helicis, and helical rim unit (Figure 66-2, G and I); superoinferior crus and anthelix unit (Figure 66-2, K); tragal unit (Figure 66-2, M-O); and incisura intertragica unit (Figure 66-2, P) are constructed. The constructed units are then fixed onto the base frame with specially made double-armed wire sutures (Figure 66-2, R; Hoshi Medical Co.) starting with the crus helicis and helical rim unit (Figure 66-2, G-J), followed by the superoinferior crus and anthelix unit (Figure 66-2, K-L), tragal unit (Figure 66-2, M-Q), and incisura intertragica unit (Figure 66-2, P-Q). The appearance of the fabricated 3-D frame is shown in Figure 66-2, Q. Special emphasis is placed on the construction of the inner surface of the crus helicis and helical rim unit (Figure 66-2, H) and the valvelike tragal unit (Figure 66-2, O).

For the fabrication of the 3-D frame for concha-type microtia, the inferior portion (lobule and tragal portion) is not fabricated (see Figure 66-7, H).

Skin Incision Outline

Because of insufficient skin surface area to cover the fabricated 3-D frame with the conventional methods available, through numerous modifications, refinements, and calculations, I selected the W-shaped skin incision as the ultimate type of skin incision for auricular reconstruction. The W-shaped skin incision eliminated the necessity of performing skin grafts to cover the insufficient exposed areas of the grafted 3-D frame.[35-39]

Lobule-Type Microtia

The schematic illustration of the first-stage surgical procedure for the lobule-type microtia is shown in Figures 66-3 and 66-4.

The skin incision for the anterior portion of the lobule forms three skin flaps, the anterior and posterior skin flaps of the lobule and the anterior skin flap of the tragus (see Figure 66-3, A and B). The inferior portion of the tragus is removed in a circular fashion with an estimated diameter of 2 mm to create a normal-appearing U-shaped configuration of the incisura intertragica (see Figure 66-3, B, arrow). The W-shaped skin incision outline is made on the posterior surface of the lobule to form the mastoid skin flap and the posterior skin flap of the lobule (see Figure 66-3, C and D). The remnant ear cartilage is removed completely with extreme care not to damage any of the subdermal layers (see Figure 66-3, F and G). The area outlined for the insertion and grafting of the 3-D frame is undermined to the point about 10 mm beyond the outline with the thickness of 1.5 to 2.0 mm (see Figure 66-3, H). It is of major importance that the area marker with the letter S is left attached to serve as the subcutaneous pedicle (see Figure 66-3, C, E, and H). Then the soft tissue located in the area corresponding to the external auditory meatus is removed to deepen the tragal cavity as if the external auditory canal were present (see Figure 66-3, I). The areas 1 cm in both directions from the center of the W-shaped skin flap (see Figure 66-3, D) are sutured together to construct the incisura intertragica (see Figure 66-4, A). Note that the lateral end of the W-shaped skin incision extends about 5 mm from the plotted outline of the auricle to be reconstructed (see Figures 66-3 and 66-4, A and B, arrow). The constructed 3-D frame is inserted from the tragal portion (Figure 66-5, A to C) and is centered with the subcutaneous pedicle (Figure 66-5, D). After anchor fixation of the 3-D frame, the skin flaps covering the 3-D frame are sutured (see Figures 66-4, C, and

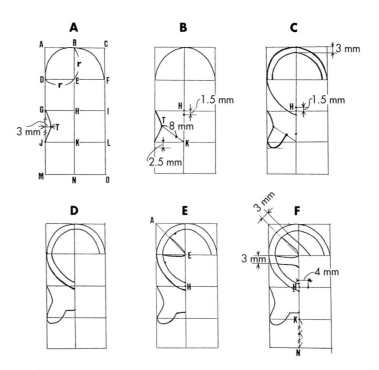

Figure 66-1. Construction of the paper pattern for the fabrication of the three-dimensional costal cartilage framework. **A,** Eight-square rectangular layout; length of *A-B* is 14 mm, *A-C* is 28 mm (width of 3-D frame), and *A-M* is 56 mm (length of 3-D frame). The superior margin of the helical rim is outlined from point *D* to point *F* as a semicircle with a radius of 14 mm (letter *R*). The tragus is constructed between point *G* and point *J* with the midpoint (letter *T*) being 3 mm from the *G-J* side of the square *G-K*. **B,** The area 1.5 mm from point *H* is marked, an imaginary line from point *K* to the midpoint of the tragus, letter *T*, is drawn, and 8 mm from letter *T* is marked along this line. A parallel line 2.5 mm inferior to side *J-K* of square *J-N* is drawn. **C,** A semicircle 3 mm (width of the helical rim) inferior and parallel to the superior margin of the helical rim is drawn. The anterior outer margin of the helical rim is extended in a smooth, circular fashion to the area 1.5 mm inferior to point *H* and the area 1.5 mm superior to point *H* is marked. A smooth, U-shaped intertragic notch is drawn with the opening of the U-shaped intertragic notch having the width of 8 mm and the area at the same height of the opening of the U-shaped intertragic notch on the antitragus side is marked along line *H-K*. **D,** The inferior margin of the helical rim is extended to the point 1.5 mm superior to point *H* (main body of the crus helicis is now constructed). A parallel line from the opening of the U-shaped intertragic notch to the point marked along line *H-K* is drawn. **E,** An imaginary line is drawn from point *A* to point *E*, and from the inferior border of the helical rim where this imaginary line traverses to point *E* is the inferior border of the superior crus and the line *D-E* under the same condition is the superior border of the inferior crus. **F,** The construction of the superior and inferior crus is done by constructing parallel lines at a distance of 3 mm (width of the superior and inferior crus), and the area 4 mm from point *H* along the line *H-I* is marked for the construction of the main body of the anthelix. The midpoint along line *K-N* is marked for the construction of the lobule. *Continued*

66-5, *E*). The excessive skin immediately superior to the tragal region (see Figure 66-4, *C*) is inverted to line the constructed pseudoexternal auditory meatus (see Figure 66-4, *D*). The skin covering the grafted 3-D frame is stretched evenly with aspiration (see Figure 66-4, *C*), and then rolled gauze with antibiotic ointment is placed in the indentations formed and fixed with bolster sutures (see Figures 66-4, *E*, and 66-5, *F* and *G*). The final procedure is to protect the grafted 3-D frame with a foam sponge (Reston Sponge, 3M Co., Minneapolis) and to dress the surgical site (see Figure 66-4, *F* and *G*). The bolster sutures are checked daily, and after removal of the rolled gauze and bolster sutures, cylindric cotton compresses

(White Cross Co., Japan) are placed in the indentations formed (see Figure 66-4, *J*). The diameter of the cylindric cotton compress can be easily adjusted by soaking it in antibiotic solution and stretching it with forceps to the desired diameter (see Figure 66-4, *H* and *I*).

Small Concha-Type Microtia

The schematic illustration for the first-stage surgical procedure for the small concha-type microtia is shown in Figure 66-6.

The skin incision for the small concha-type microtia is similar to that for the lobule-type microtia with the exception that the incision outline for the anterior portion of the lobule

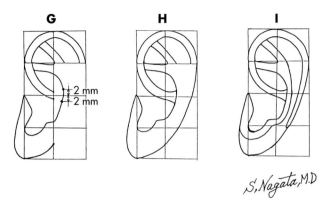

S. Nagata, M.D

Figure 66-1, cont'd. **G,** A line is drawn from the inferior margin of the inferior crus through the area marked 4 mm from point *H* to the line extending from the opening of the U-shaped intertragic notch. The area 2 mm superior and inferior to line *H-I* along the outer margin of the main body of the anthelix is marked (attachment of the crus helicis to the posterior surface of the 3-D frame). The outer border of the lobular region is drawn in an oblique manner from point *G* to point *M* exceeding the marginal line of *G-M* as shown and through point *M* to the marked midpoint of line *K-N*. **H,** The outer margin of the 3-D frame is completed by extending the line from the midpoint of line *K-N* to the superior margin of the helical rim terminating at point *F*. The crus helicis is completed by extending the lines of the crus helicis in a fan-shaped manner to the marked areas along the main body of the anthelix. **I,** The helical rim is completed as it tapers as it extends inferiorly and the anthelix is completed in a similar manner as shown.

must be modified (see Figure 66-6, *A*). The area directly posterior to the indentation is incised along the posterior border as illustrated. All other procedures are the same as for lobule-type microtia.

Concha-Type Microtia

The schematic illustration for the first-stage surgical procedure for the concha-type microtia is shown in Figure 66-7.

For the concha-type microtia, the modification in the W-shaped skin incision is necessary because the lobule and tragal portion of the 3-D frame is not constructed. Thus ample skin surface area is attained without using a large W-shaped skin incision (see Figure 66-7, *C*). In addition, the remnant ear cartilage is not completely removed. The inferior portion of the remnant ear cartilage corresponding to the lobule and tragal portion is left intact while the remaining superior portion of the remnant ear cartilage is removed (see Figure 66-7, *D* and *E*). All other steps of the procedure are the same as the lobule-type and small concha-type microtia, with the exception that the constructed 3-D frame must be fixed to the superior portion of the remnant ear cartilage left intact at the area corresponding to the superior border of the lobule.

SECOND-STAGE OPERATION

The second and final stage of auricular reconstruction is the projection of the constructed auricle. The second-stage surgery is usually performed 6 months after the first stage-operation.

The schematic illustration for the second-stage operation in primary auricular reconstruction cases is shown in Figures 66-8 and 66-9. The incision outlines for auricular projection (solid line posterior to the constructed auricle) and the harvesting of the ultradelicate split-thickness scalp skin (UDSTS; spindle-shaped outline) and for the elevation of the temporoparietal fascia flap (TPF; zig-zag outline) are shown in Figure 66-8, *A*. The surgical procedure is the harvesting of the UDSTS because a taut skin surface is required when harvesting with a scalpel (see Figure 66-8, *B* and *C*). The UDSTS is harvested so that the follicular buds are left at the donor site (see Figure 66-8, *E*) and harvested UDSTS is to be free of follicular buds (see Figure 66-8, *D* and *E*). If the harvested UDSTS is not free of follicular buds, postoperative hair growth at the recipient site and alopecia at the donor site will be unavoidable. Next the constructed auricle is elevated (see Figure 66-8, *F* and *G*), and the skin of the mastoid surface is undermined (about 1 cm from the outline for auricular projection) (see Figure 66-8, *H*) and advanced (see Figure 66-8, *I, arrows*). The excessive skin is excised in a triangular fashion (see Figure 66-8, *I*) to avoid dog-ear formation. The elevated TPF is passed through the skin tunnel constructed at the base of the TPF (see Figure 66-8, *J*). A costal cartilage block shaped to that of the eminentia concha is fabricated (see Figure 66-9, *B*) for the projection of the constructed auricle. The costal cartilage block is fixed to the posterior surface of the constructed auricle and the mastoid surface (see Figure 66-9, *A, arrow*). Then the TPF is used to cover the posterior surface of the projected auricle, costal cartilage block, and mastoid surface (see Figure 66-9, *C*). The harvested UDSTS is used to cover the posterior aspect of the projected auricle (see Figure 66-9, *A, D,* and *E*) and fixed with mattress sutures (see Figure 66-9, *D* and *F*). The donor site of the UDSTS is covered with porcine skin dressed with antibiotic ointment (see Figure 66-9, *G* and *H*). The cross-sectional view of the projected auricle is shown in Figure

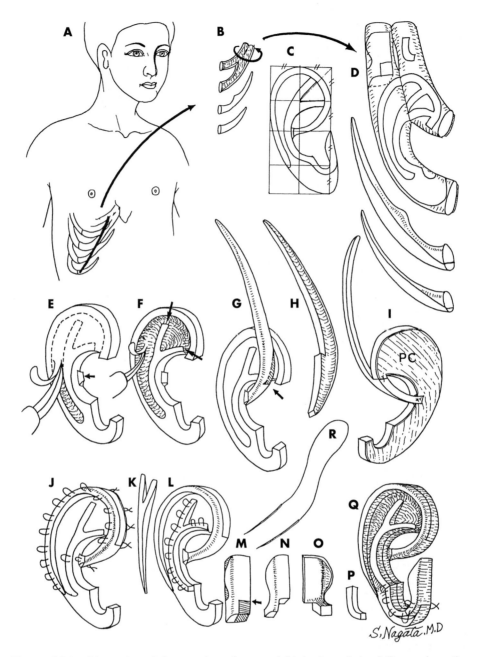

S. Nagata, M.D

Figure 66-2. Harvesting of the costal cartilages and fabrication of the 3-D costal cartilage framework. **A,** The costal cartilages are harvested en bloc from the same side of the auricle to be constructed, and the posterior perichondrium is left intact at the donor site. **B,** The anterior and posterior surfaces of the harvested costal cartilages are reversed to take advantage of their configurations. **C,** The paper pattern for the fabrication of the 3-D frame. **D,** The 3-D frame units outlined on the harvested costal cartilages. **E,** Rough sculpturing of the base frame. Note the presence of a notch *(arrow)* for the fixation of the crus helicis–helical rim unit to the base frame. **F,** Fine sculpturing of the base frame. Note that the superior and inferior crus terminates 3 mm from the helical rim. **G,** The fixation of the crus helicis–helical rim unit to the base frame with specially fabricated 38-gauge double-armed wire sutures. Note the presence of a steplike notch of the crus helicis–helical rim unit to strengthen the 3-D frame. **H,** The inner surface of the crus helicis–helical rim unit. **I,** The posterior surface of the base frame with the perichondrium and the fixation of the crus helicis portion of the crus helicis–helical rim unit to the base frame. **J,** The wire fixation of the crus helicis–helical rim unit to the base frame. **K,** The fabricated superior and inferior crus–anthelix unit. **L,** The wire fixation of the superior and inferior crus–anthelix unit to the base frame. **M** to **O,** Fabrication of the tragus unit. **P,** The intertragic notch rim unit. **Q,** The wire fixation of the tragus unit and the intertragic notch rim unit to the base-frame. The fabricated 3-D frame. **R,** Illustration of the specially fabricated 39-gauge double-armed wire suture.

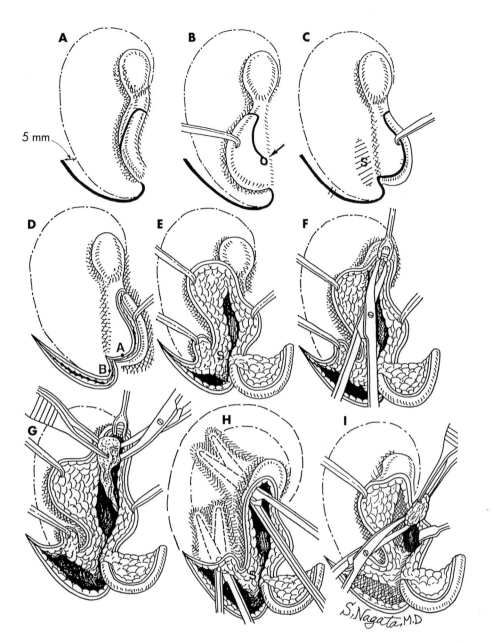

Figure 66-3. First-stage operation for noncomplicated lobule-type microtia (part 1). **A,** The outline area for auricular reconstruction for the lobule-type microtia *(dotted line).* **B,** The incision outline for the anterior surface of the auricle. Note that the inferior portion of the incision line (tragal portion) is removed in a circular fashion. **C,** The incision outline for the posterior surface of the auricle, known as the incision outline for the W-shaped skin flap. The shaded area, letter *S,* is the subcutaneous pedicle. **D,** The W-shaped skin flap formed and the areas 1 cm from the center of the W-shaped skin flaps are marked with letters *A* and *B.* **E,** The skin flaps formed and the subcutaneous pedicle (letter *S*). **F** and **G,** Complete excision of the remnant ear cartilage. **H,** Undermining procedure for the construction of the skin pocket for insertion of the 3-D frame. Note that the undermining procedure exceeds about 1 cm from the outline of the auricle to be constructed and extreme care must be exercised in the area of the subcutaneous pedicle. **I,** The soft tissue corresponding to the location of the external auditory canal is excised.

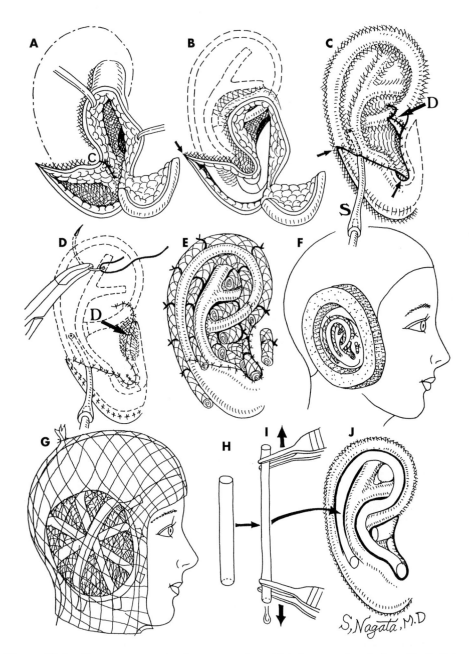

Figure 66-4. First-stage operation for noncomplicated lobule-type microtia (part 2). **A,** Points A and B are sutured together to form a smooth U-shaped configuration of the intertragic notch (letter C). **B,** After insertion of the 3-D frame, the W-shaped skin incision terminates about 5 mm from the outline of the auricle to be constructed *(arrow)*. **C,** Immediately after grafting of the 3-D frame. Note the presence of excessive skin (dog-eared, letter D) and that the terminal portion of the W-shaped skin ideally fits together after suturing *(arrow)* and aspiration (letter S). **D,** The excessive skin (Figure 66-4, C, letter D) inverted to construct the pseudoacoustic meatus *(arrow, letter D)* and bolster sutures for fixation of rolled gauze with antibiotic ointment. **E,** Appearance immediately after bolster suture fixation of rolled gauze with antibiotic ointment into the indentations formed and around the constructed auricle. **F,** Placement of Reston sponge for protective measure of the grafted 3-D frame after the first-stage operation for auricular reconstruction. **G,** Appearance after the first-stage operation. **H** and **I,** Cylindric cotton compress used after removal of bolster sutures and rolled gauze. Required diameter of the cylindric cotton compress can be obtained by soaking in antiseptic solution and by stretching with forceps. **J,** Appearance of how and where the cylindric compress are placed.

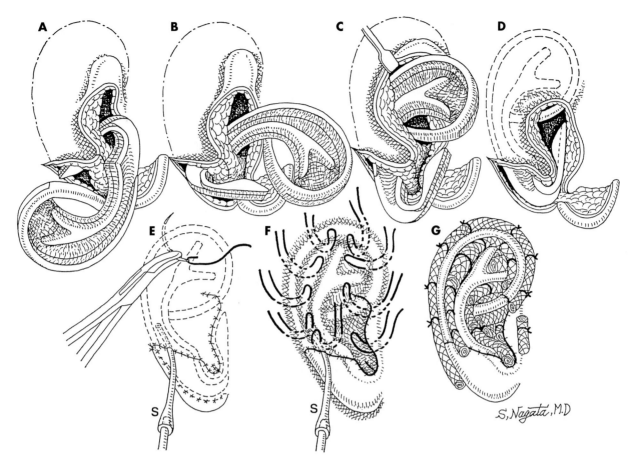

Figure 66-5. Insertion of the 3-D frame into the skin pocket. **A** to **D,** The fabricated 3-D frame is inserted from the tragus and centered with the subcutaneous pedicle. **E** to **G,** After suturing, the bolster sutures are placed for fixation of rolled gauze with antibiotic ointment in the indentations formed and around the constructed auricle.

66-9, *J.* Note the deep conchal cavity and the deep pseudo-acoustic meatus formed.

Representative Cases (Primary Typical Microtia Cases)

CASE 1 (Figure 66-10). The preoperative appearance revealed a left lobule-type microtia with a relatively small lobule and a large remnant (see Figure 66-10, *A*). The postoperative appearance after the second-stage operation revealed that the angle of projection of the constructed auricle is maintained and is practically identical to that of the opposite normal ear (see Figure 66-10, *C* to *E*). Furthermore, proportional and dimensional evaluation of the constructed auricle revealed that the proportion and dimension was within 1% to that of the normal ear, according to the study reported by Hale.[18]

CASE 2 (Figure 66-11). The preoperative appearance of a typical right lobule microtia is shown, and the postoperative results revealed that the proportional and dimensional evaluation of the constructed auricle was proportionally and dimensionally identical to that of a normal ear (see Figure 66-11, *E* and *F*).

CASE 3 (Figure 66-12). The preoperative appearance of a typical right small concha-type microtia is shown. Note that the constructed auricle is well projected and well maintained without any postoperative complications (see Figure 66-12, *C*).

CASE 4 (Figure 66-13). The preoperative appearance of a typical concha-type microtia is shown (see Figure 66-13, *A*). Note only the missing anatomic structures of the auricle are fabricated and the decrease in skin surface area required to cover the fabricated 3-D frame (see Figure 66-13, *B*). The postoperative appearances after the second-stage operation revealed that the constructed auricle is well projected and maintained (see Figure 66-13, *D* and *E*).

CASE 5 (Figure 66-14). The preoperative appearance of another concha-type microtia is shown (left) but with a proportionally large superior half of the remnant auricle (see Figure 66-14, *A*). The follow-up appointment after the second-stage operation revealed that the constructed auricle is well maintained and without complications (see Figure 66-14, *C*).

Text continued on p. 1036

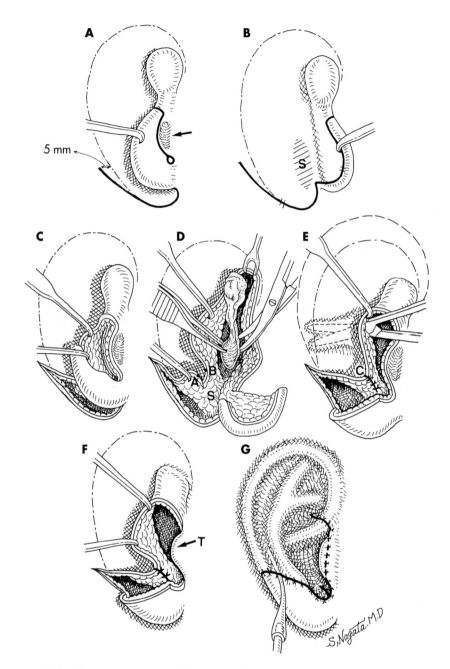

Figure 66-6. First-stage operation for noncomplicated small concha-type microtia. **A,** The surgical difference in the first-stage operation between the lobule-type microtia and the small concha-type microtia is in the incision line for the anterior surface of the auricle. The incision line *(solid line)* is located immediately posterior and along the indentation of the small concha *(shaded area, arrow)* to form the skin flap of the tragus. **B** to **G,** All other procedures are the same as for the lobule-type microtia with the exception that the indentation of the small concha is protruded and inverted (inverted cone of skin) to form the skin pocket to line the anterior and posterior surfaces of the tragus (**F,** letter *T*).

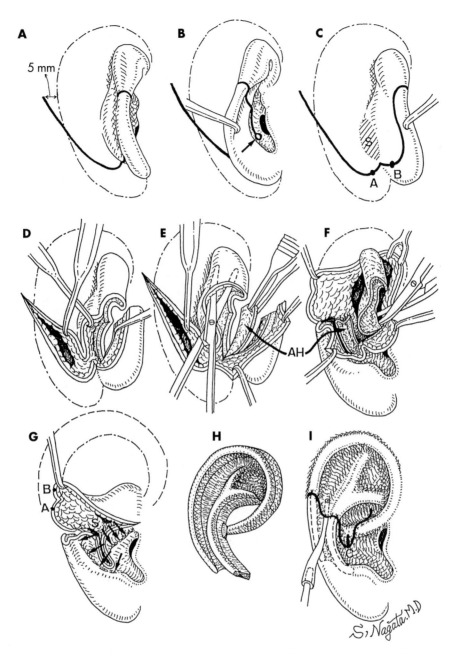

Figure 66-7.   First-stage operation for noncomplicated concha-type microtia. **A** to **C,** The line of incisions for the concha-type microtia are illustrated with the solid line. The incision for the anterior surface of the auricle extends from the helix to the anthelix and terminates at the posterior wall of the concha **(B).** The incision for the posterior surface of the auricle and mastoid surface uses a small W-shaped skin incision **(C). D** to **G,** The remnant cartilages of the superior portion of the auricle, the posterior wall of the concha, and the anthelix portion are excised **(E** and **F).** The excised area observed from the superior aspect of the skin flap corresponds to the area of the crus helicis, anthelix, and the area directly adjacent and anteriorly to the antitragus **(G,** *arrows*). **H,** The fabricated 3-D frame for the concha-type microtia. **I,** The appearance immediately after grafting of the 3-D frame.

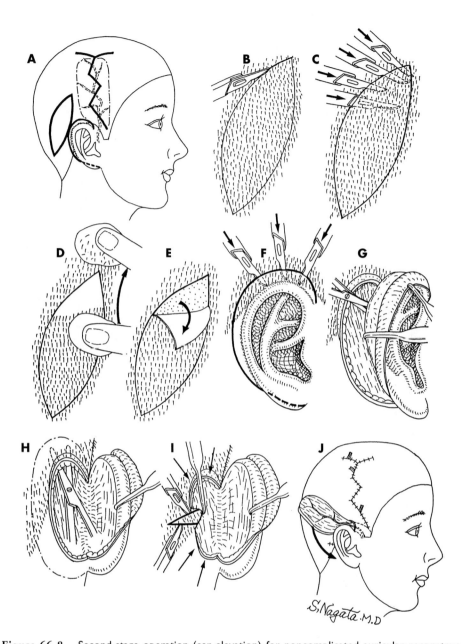

Figure 66-8. Second-stage operation (ear elevation) for noncomplicated auricular reconstruction (part 1). **A,** The incision outline for harvesting of the ultradelicate split-thickness scalp skin (UDSTS, *spindle-shaped*), harvesting of the temporoparietal fascia flap (TPF, *zig-zag line*) and for elevation of the constructed auricle *(solid and dotted line posterior to the constructed auricle)*. **B** to **E,** Schematic illustration on how the UDSTS is harvested. Extreme care is necessary in the harvesting of only the superficial layers of the scalp skin. **F** to **G,** Elevation of the constructed auricle for auricular projection. **H,** Undermining of the mastoid surface. **I,** The undermined skin of the mastoid surface is advanced *(arrows)* and the excessive skin is excised in a triangular shape in the hairline to avoid dog-ear formation *(triangle with scalpels)*. **J,** The elevated TPF is passed through the skin tunnel located at the base of the TPF.

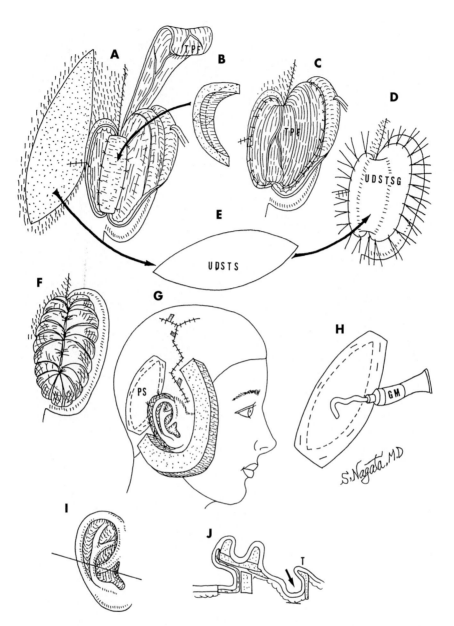

Figure 66-9. Second-stage operation (ear elevation) for noncomplicated auricular reconstruction (part 2). **A,** Appearance after fixation of the costal cartilage block for ear elevation. **B,** The fabricated costal cartilage block shaped to the morphologic configuration of the eminentia concha. **C,** Immediately after the posterior surface of the constructed auricle, costal cartilage block and the mastoid surface were covered with the TPF. **D** and **E,** The harvested UDSTS **(E)** is grafted to cover the raw surface area of the exposed TPF covering the posterior aspect of the elevated auricle. **F** and **G,** Mattress dressing and Reston sponge are used to protect the elevated auricle. **H,** Porcine skin with antibiotic ointment is used to cover the raw surface where the UDSTS was harvested (**G,** letters PS). **I** and **J,** Cross-sectional view of the elevated auricle. Note that the pseudoacoustic meatus (**J,** arrow) is located inferiorly to the protruding tragus (**J,** letter T).

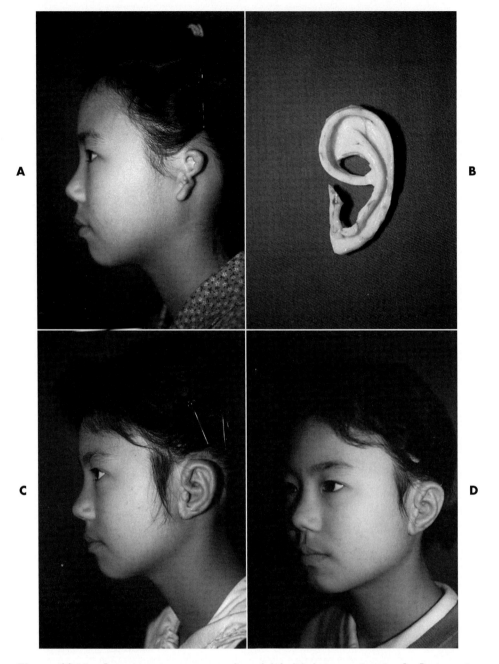

Figure 66-10. Representative case: complicated left lobule-type microtia. **A,** Preoperative appearance of a left lobule-type microtia. **B,** Fabricated 3-D frame. **C,** Lateral view after the second-stage operation. **D,** Anterior angle view after the second-stage operation.

Continued

The two-stage auricular reconstruction method introduced has been free of major complications, such as pneumothorax, during harvesting of the costal cartilage (posterior perichondrium is left intact at the donor site), extrusion of wire sutures and the 3-D frame (ample skin surface is attained with the W-shaped skin incision). Above all, total auricular reconstruction can be completed in two stages.

The follow-up results of the two-stage auricular reconstruction method revealed that more than satisfactory results are attained without postoperative complications and that the constructed auricle is well maintained.

NEW APPROACH FOR DIFFICULT AURICULAR RECONSTRUCTION

To a reconstructive plastic surgeon, there are numerous complicated auricular reconstruction cases that remain unsolved or extremely difficult to attain favorable results, whether the case is

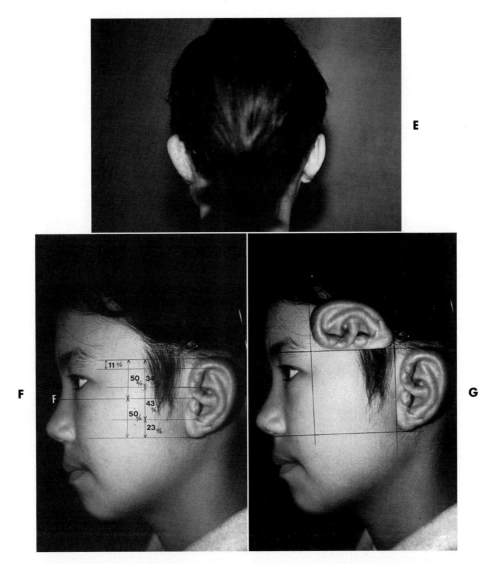

Figure 66-10, cont'd. E, Posterior view; note that the projected auricle is well maintained and without postoperative complications. **F** and **G,** The results of proportional and dimensional evaluation of the constructed auricle according to the study reported by Hale.[18]

total or subtotal auricular reconstruction, or congenital, acquired, or caused by unfavorable primary auricular reconstruction results.

Congenital Anotia, or Clinical Anotia

Congenital anotia, or clinical anotia, is an extremely rare case but can be encountered during practice, especially in Asian countries, because it is more common than in Western countries. The term *anotia* is self-explanatory: the anatomic ear is absent and/or only a minute amount of vestige is present, if any.

The major difficulty in auricular reconstruction is in the attainment of sufficient skin surface area to cover the fabricated 3-D frame without resorting to skin grafts; with anotia, it is even more difficult because the surgeon is dealing with a flat, taut skin surface area. Thus sacrifice in surgical procedures was inevitable and the results were unsatisfactory in view of the number of sacrifices. The anotia case taken up in this chapter is

further complicated with low hairline (see Figure 66-17, *A* and *B*). The topic of low hairline is discussed later as a separate entity.

Surgical Procedures

The schematic surgical procedures for the first-and second-stage operations are illustrated in Figures 66-15 and 66-16 for total auricular reconstruction for an anotia case further complicated with low hairline. Apart from the primary surgical method for auricular reconstruction, the TPF and UDSTS are used during the first-stage operation.

First-Stage Operation

The preoperative appearance is illustrated in Figure 66-15, *A,* and from the outline for auricular reconstruction (see Figure 66-15, *B* and *C*), over 70% of the surgical site for auricular reconstruction is covered with hair growth (low hairline). To secure ample skin surface area to cover the fabricated 3-D

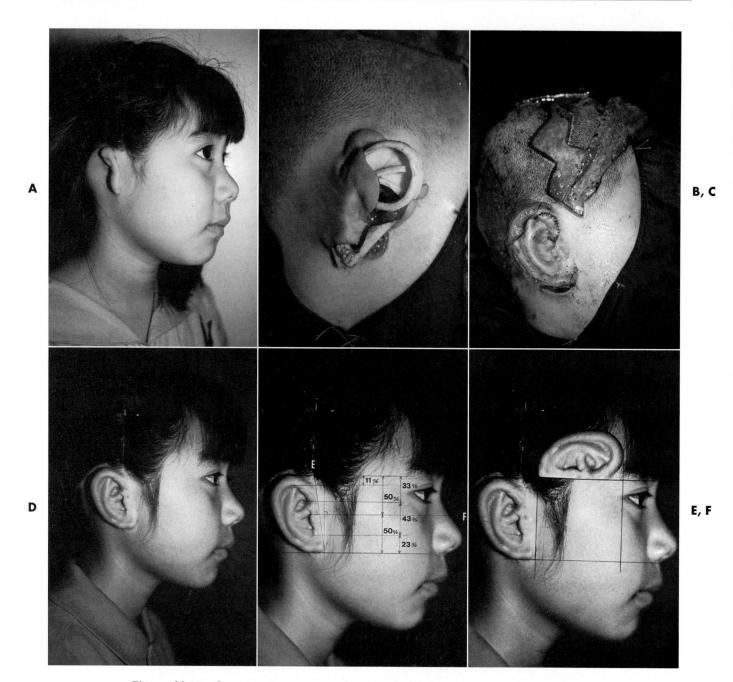

Figure 66-11. Representative case: complicated right lobule-type microtia. **A,** Preoperative appearance of a right lobule-type microtia. **B,** Intraoperative view showing how the 3-D frame is inserted into the skin pocket formed during the first-stage operation. **C,** Intraoperative view with the elevated TPF during the second-stage operation. **D,** Lateral view after the second-stage operation. **E** and **F,** The results of proportional and dimensional evaluation of the constructed auricle according to the study reported by Hale.[18]

frame, the area 15 to 20 mm from the anatomic outline of the auricle to be constructed is elevated as UDSTS (see Figure 66-15, *C* and *D*); note that the UDSTS is free of follicular buds. The subepidermal layer with the follicular buds is to be excised only in the area to which the 3-D frame is to be grafted (see Figure 66-15, *E* to *G*), or else postoperative hair growth is expected to occur from the constructed auricle. The TPF is

elevated to cover the anterior surface of the grafted 3-D frame (see Figure 66-15, *F* to *H*), and then the TPF is covered with UDSTS (see Figure 66-15, *H*).

Second-Stage Operation

The schematic illustration of the second-stage operation is shown in Figure 66-16. Because the TPF was used to cover the

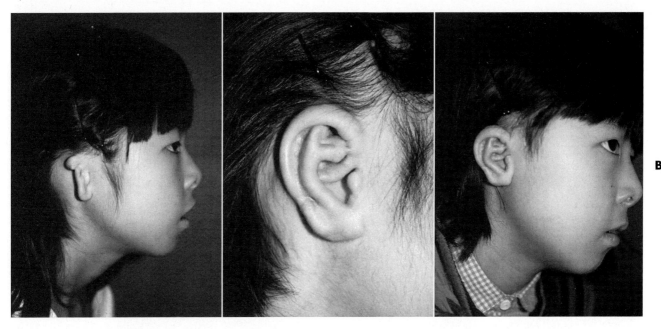

Figure 66-12. Representative case: complicated right small concha-type microtia. **A,** Preoperative appearance of a right small concha-type microtia. **B,** Postoperative appearance after the first-stage operation. **C,** Postoperative appearance after the second-stage operation.

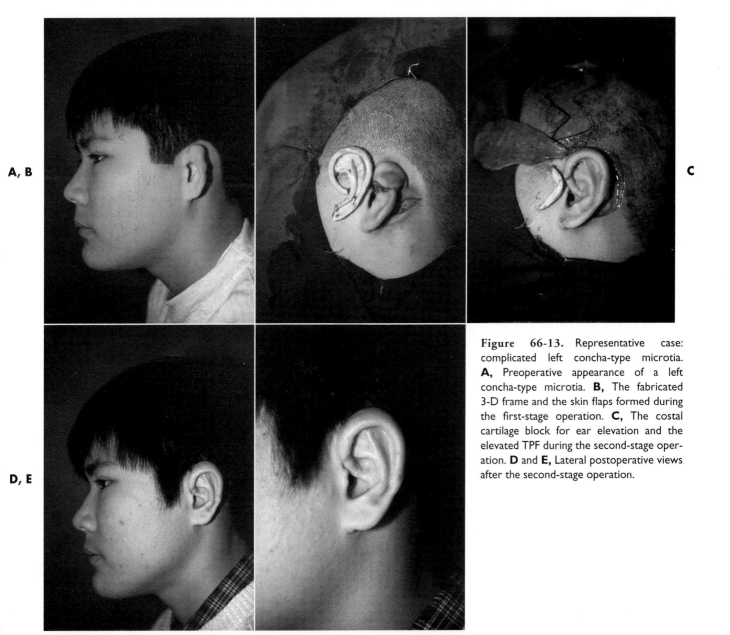

Figure 66-13. Representative case: complicated left concha-type microtia. **A,** Preoperative appearance of a left concha-type microtia. **B,** The fabricated 3-D frame and the skin flaps formed during the first-stage operation. **C,** The costal cartilage block for ear elevation and the elevated TPF during the second-stage operation. **D** and **E,** Lateral postoperative views after the second-stage operation.

Figure 66-14. Representative case: complicated left concha-type microtia with a proportionally large superior half of the remnant auricle. **A,** Preoperative appearance of a left concha-type microtia. **B,** The fabricated 3-D frame for the first-stage operation. **C,** Postoperative appearance after the second-stage operation.

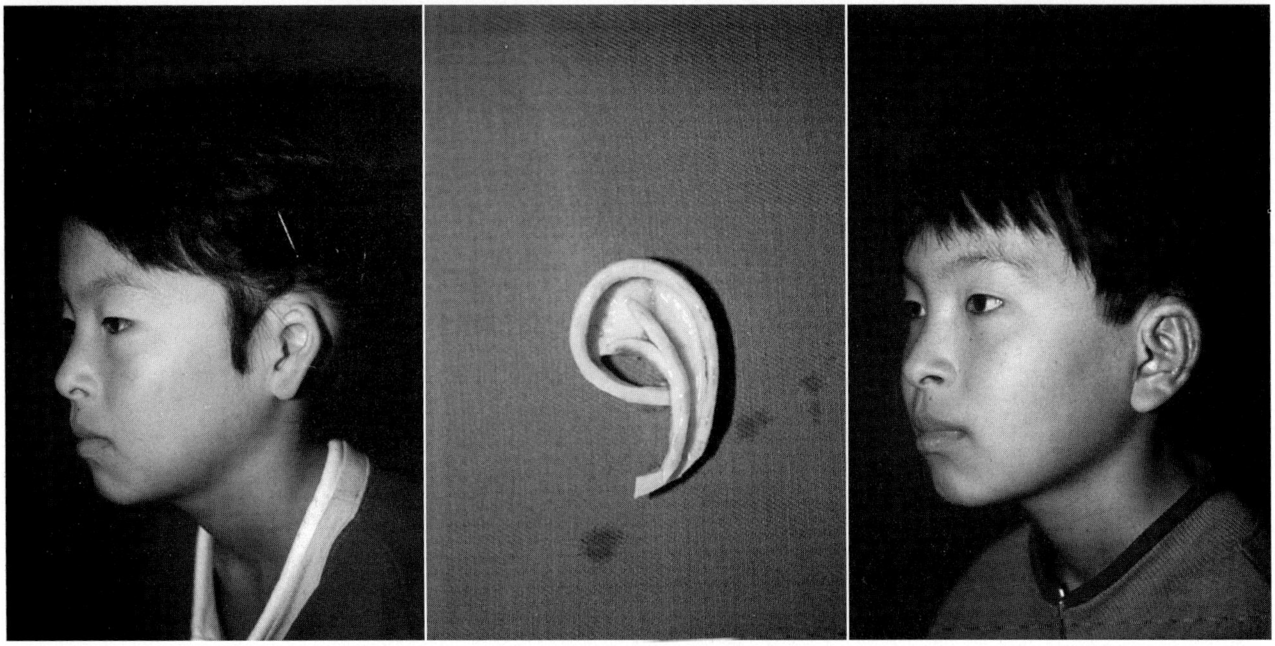

grafted 3-D frame in the first-stage operation, the deep temporoparietal fascia (DTF) and periosteum (PO) combined flap is used to cover the posterior surface of the project auricle, costal cartilage block, and mastoid surface. All other surgical procedures are the same as for the noncomplicated second-stage operation for auricular reconstruction.

REPRESENTATIVE ANOTIA CASE (Figure 66-17). The preoperative appearance of this anotia case revealed that a remnant lobulelike vestige was located posteriorly and distal to the normal anatomic location and that a pseudoexternal auditory canal was located below the hairline and anterior to the lobulelike vestige. This anotia case was further complicated with low hairline (see Figure 66-17, A and B). However, satisfactory results were attained with the two-stage auricular reconstruction method using the 3-D frame, UDSTS, TPF and DTF-OP combined flap (see Figure 66-17, E to G).

Secondary Auricular Reconstruction for Unfavorable Primary Auricular Reconstruction

Another extremely difficult auricular reconstruction is secondary auricular reconstruction for unfavorable primary auricular reconstruction results because of the abundance in scar tissue formation from the primary auricular reconstruction; the degree of difficulty in auricular reconstruction is directly proportional to the amount of scar tissue formed. However, with the application of the auricular reconstruction method for anotia, mentioned above, it is now possible to

treat these cases if and only if a 3-D frame can be fabricated or salvaged.

Representative Secondary Reconstruction Cases

CASE 1 (Figure 66-18). Because of diminished contour of the superior auricular structures and missing anatomic structures (see Figure 66-18, A), the patient strongly requested secondary reconstruction. Classification of scar tissue formation from primary reconstruction was moderate, and use of UDSTS was limited to the superior half of the anterior surface of the secondary reconstructed auricle during the first-stage operation (see Figure 66-18, C). Postoperative appearance revealed more than satisfactory results and a well-maintained and projected auricle.

CASE 2 (Figure 66-19). Because of unproportional dimensions and missing anatomic structures (see Figure 66-19, A), secondary reconstruction was performed. Note the difference in the 3-D frame fabricated, especially the anatomic features and the width of the superior portion of the 3-D frame (see Figure 66-19, B). With an increase in postoperative time, a well-defined contour of the auricular structures is attained (see Figure 66-19, E).

CASE 3 (Figure 66-20). Figure 66-20 shows an extremely difficult secondary reconstruction case with severe scar tissue formation from the primary auricular reconstruction. Preoperative examination revealed an extremely solidified

Text continued on p. 1046

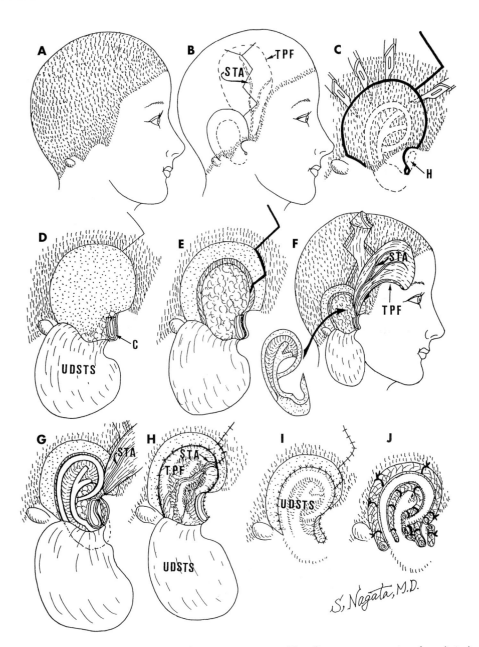

Figure 66-15. Complicated auricular reconstruction. The first-stage operation for clinical anotia with low hairline. **A,** Preoperative illustration of the clinical anotia case. **B,** The outline for the TPF to be harvested *(dotted line with arrow TPF),* the outline for the site for auricular reconstruction *(dotted line),* and the outer margin of the UDSTS to be elevated *(solid line).* **C** and **D,** Elevation of the UDSTS. Note the presence of a blind hole (**C,** *letter H*) and the remnant cartilage (**D,** *letter C*). **E,** The inferior layer with the presence of follicular buds is excised in the area where the 3-D frame is to be grafted. **F** and **G,** The TPF is elevated and the fabricated 3-D frame is grafted to the designated area free of follicular buds. **H,** The TPF is used to cover the grafted 3-D frame. **I,** Then the TPF-covered grafted 3-D frame is covered with the elevated UDSTS. **J,** The appearance immediately after rolled gauze with antibiotic ointments is fixed with bolster sutures.

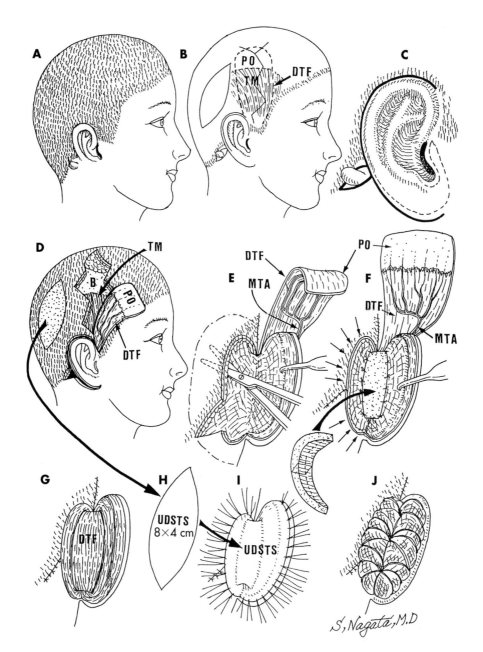

Figure 66-16. Complicated auricular reconstruction. The second-stage operation for clinical anotia with low hairline. **A,** The illustrated appearance of the patient immediately before the second-stage operation. **B,** The outline for the elevation of the combined deep temporal fascia (DTF) and the periosteum (PO) and for the harvesting of the UDSTS *(spindle-shaped)*. **C,** The incision outline for auricular projection and the excision of the polyplike vestige. **D,** The harvesting of the UDSTS and the elevation of the combined DTF-PO flap. Letters TM is the temporalis muscle, and letter B is exposed cranial bone. **E** to **J,** The remaining procedure is similar to the noncomplicated second-stage operation except that the combined DTF-PO flap is used instead of the TPF.

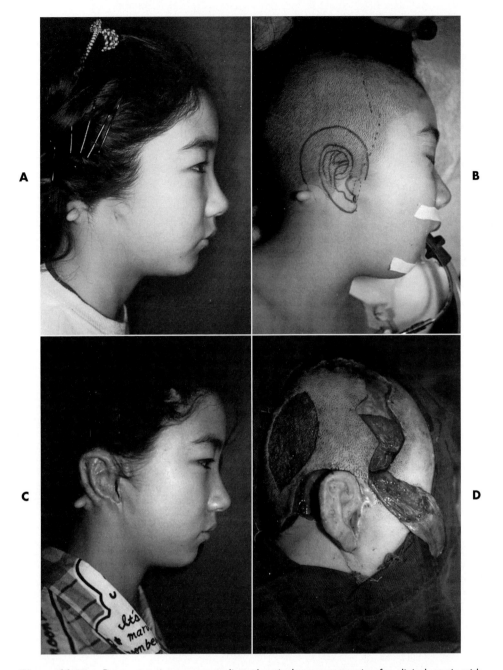

Figure 66-17. Representative case: complicated auricular reconstruction for clinical anotia with low hairline. **A,** Preoperative appearance of a clinical anotia case further complicated with low hairline. **B,** The incision outline and surgical layout for the first-stage operation. Note the polyplike vestige located posteriorly to the surgical site for auricular reconstruction. **C,** The postoperative appearance after the first-stage operation. **D,** The intraoperative view during the second-stage operation with the elevated combined DTF-PO flap. Note that the polyplike vestige has been excised. *Continued*

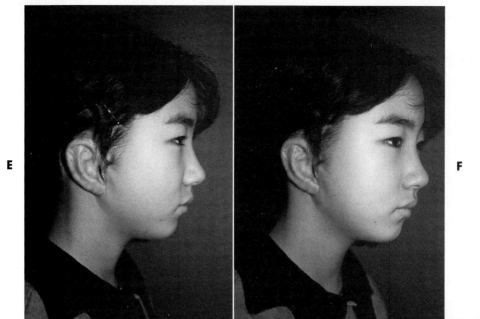

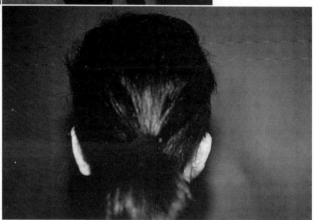

Figure 66-17, cont'd. **E** to **F,** Postoperative appearances after the second-stage operation. **G,** Postoperative posterior view after the second-stage operation. Note that the angle of projection of the constructed auricle is well maintained.

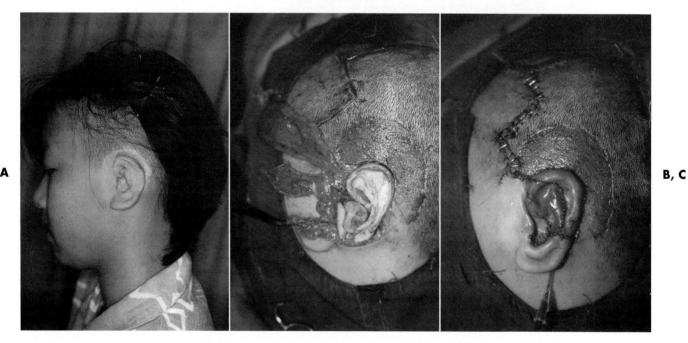

Figure 66-18. Representative case: complicated auricular reconstruction, secondary reconstruction of unfavorable primary auricular reconstruction. **A,** Preoperative appearance for secondary reconstruction. Note the diminished contour of the superior auricular structures and missing anatomic structures. **B,** Intraoperative appearance with the 3-D frame and skin flaps to cover the 3-D frame after grafting. **C,** Immediately after the grafting of the 3-D frame. Note that the majority of the superior portion of the constructed auricle is covered with UDSTS.

Continued

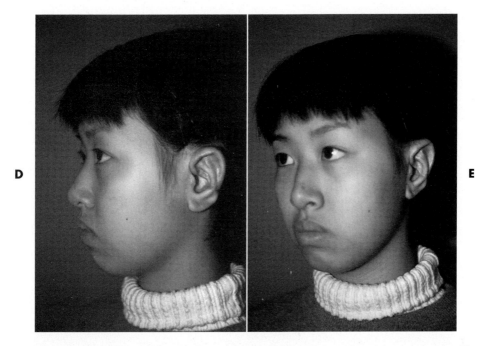

Figure 66-18, cont'd. **D** and **E,** The postoperative appearance after the second stage. The constructed auricle and the angle of projection of the constructed auricle are well maintained.

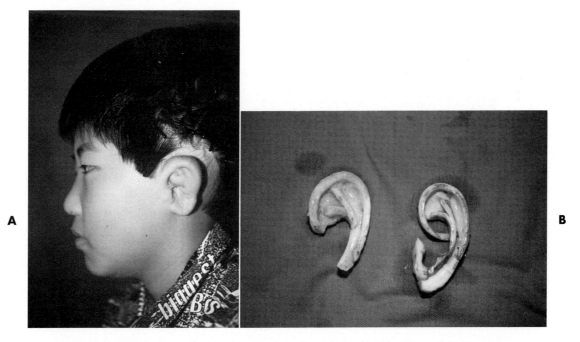

Figure 66-19. Representative case: complicated auricular reconstruction, secondary reconstruction for unfavorable primary auricular reconstruction. **A,** Preoperative appearance for secondary reconstruction. Note the unproportional dimensions and missing anatomic structures. **B,** The removed costal cartilage frame *(left)* and the fabricated 3-D frame *(right)*. Note the excessive width of the superior portion of the removed costal cartilage frame in comparison to the 3-D frame. *Continued*

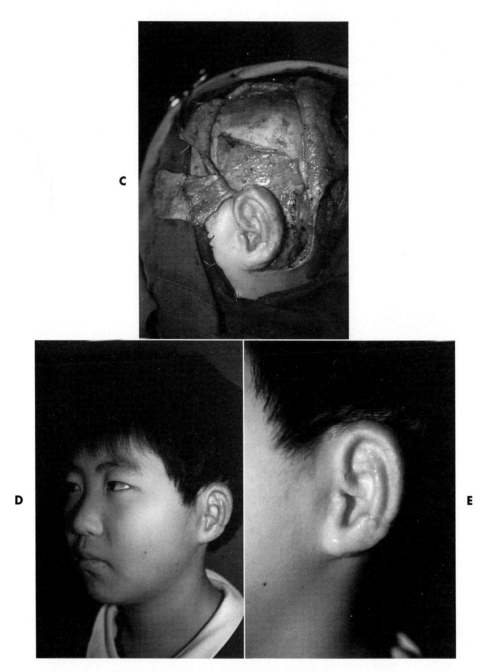

Figure 66-19, cont'd. C, Intraoperative appearance during the second-stage operation. The combined DTF-PO flap is used. **D** and **E,** Postoperative appearance after the second-stage operation.

scar tissue formation where the auricle was constructed during the primary auricular reconstruction (Figure 66-20, *A* and *B*). The preoperative condition of this case was identical to those classified as anotia or even more difficult becausedof insufficient skin surface area and abundant scar tissue formation. With application of the auricular reconstruction methods, satisfactory results were attained (Figure 66-20, *H* and *I*).

Low Hairline

As a separate entity in the category of complicated auricular reconstruction, low hairline has prompted numerous problems,

especially securing ample skin surface area free of hair growth to cover the grafted 3-D frame or an additional surgical procedure for epilation. An additional surgical procedure for epilation increases not only the risk of scarring but also hospitalization, financial costs, and, above all, discomfort and extra pain of surgery to the patient, especially if the patient is an infant.

With the use of the TPF and elevation of the UDSTS to cover the grafted 3-D frame during the first-stage operation, these problems were solved.

REPRESENTATIVE LOW HAIRLINE CASE (Figure 66-21). This low hairline case is represented by a concha-type

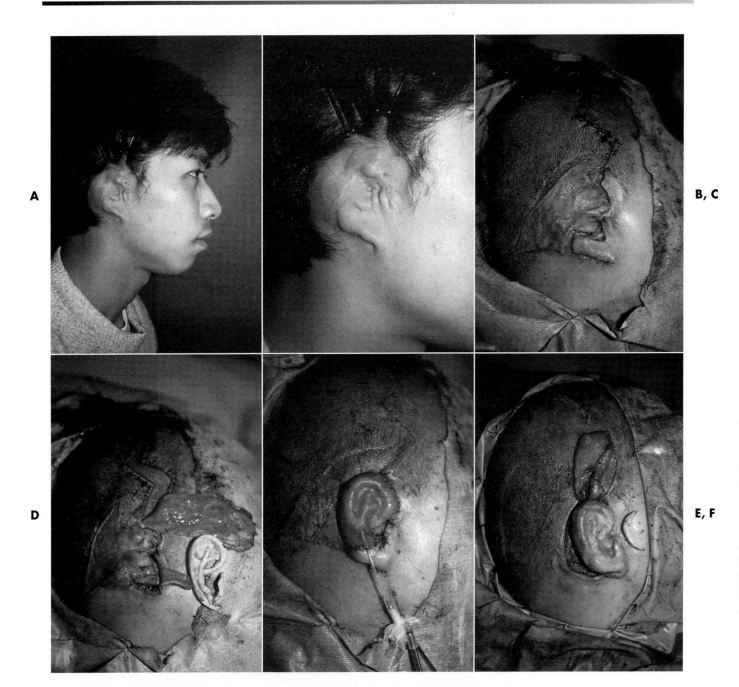

Figure 66-20. Representative case: an extremely complicated auricular reconstruction, secondary reconstruction of unfavorable primary auricular reconstruction; similar condition as for anotia. **A** and **B,** The preoperative appearance. Note the excessive scar tissue formed in the area of auricular reconstruction; extremely insufficient skin surface area to cover the 3-D frame is inevitable with the standard method of auricular reconstruction. **C** and **D,** Intraoperative view during the first-stage operation with the salvaged skin **(C)** and the fabricated 3-D frame **(D).** **E,** Immediately after covering the grafted 3-D frame with the TPF and UDSTS. **F,** Intraoperative view during the second-stage operation with the costal cartilage block shaped to that of the eminentia concha and the combined DTF-PO flap. *Continued*

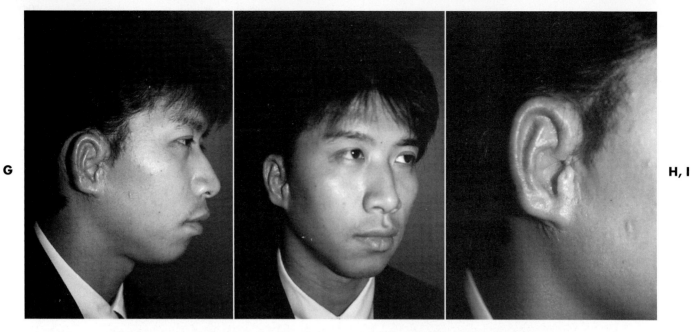

G
H, I

Figure 66-20, cont'd. **G** to **I,** Postoperative lateral, anterior angle, and close-up views after the second-stage operation. Note that the reconstructed auricle is well projected and maintained.

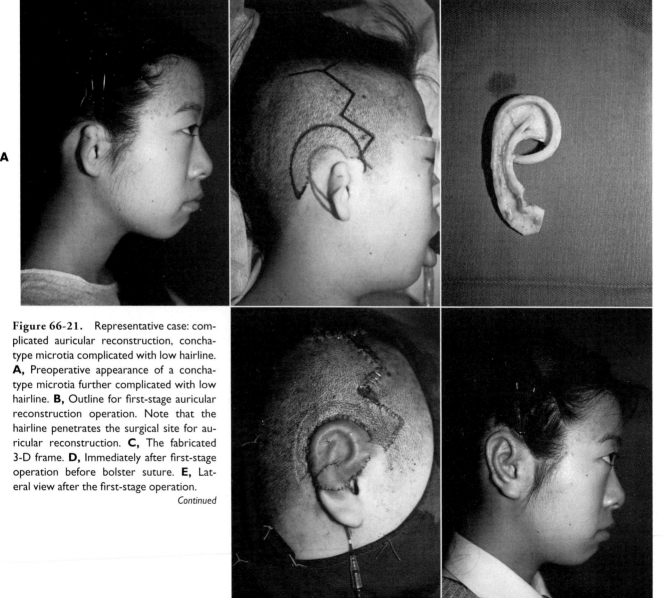

A
B, C
D, E

Figure 66-21. Representative case: complicated auricular reconstruction, concha-type microtia complicated with low hairline. **A,** Preoperative appearance of a concha-type microtia further complicated with low hairline. **B,** Outline for first-stage auricular reconstruction operation. Note that the hairline penetrates the surgical site for auricular reconstruction. **C,** The fabricated 3-D frame. **D,** Immediately after first-stage operation before bolster suture. **E,** Lateral view after the first-stage operation.

Continued

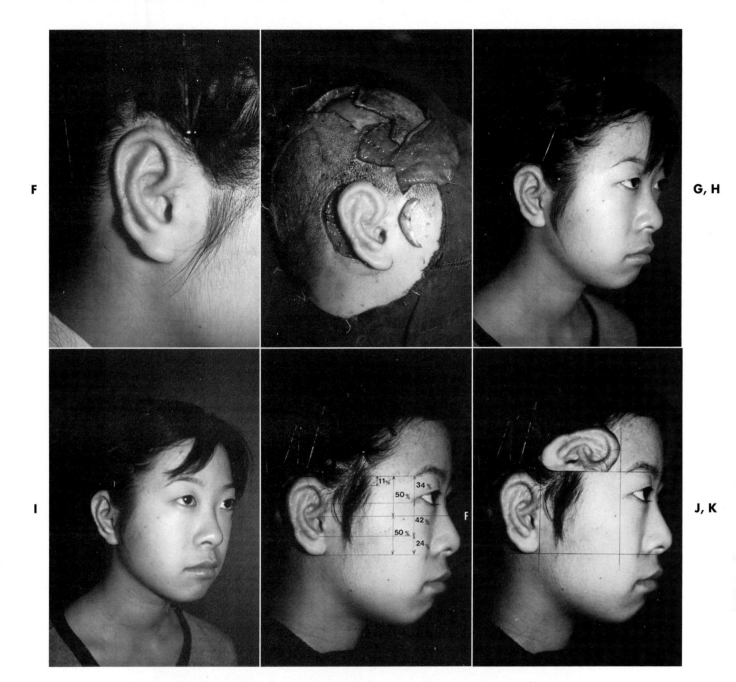

Figure 66-21, cont'd. F, Immediately before second-stage operation, close-up view. **G,** Intraoperative view during the second-stage operation with the costal cartilage block for auricular projection and the combined DTF-PO flap. **H,** Postoperative appearance after the second-stage operation. **I,** Anterior angle view. Note that the constructed auricle is well projected and maintained. **J** and **K,** Proportional and dimensional evaluation according the Hale.[18] Note that the constructed auricle is proportionally and dimensionally equivalent to that reported by Hale.

microtia, and from the plotted incision outline for auricular reconstruction during the first-stage operation, the low hairline or hair growth is identified to the superior region of the helical rim (see Figure 66-21, *A* and *B*). With use of the UDSTS, TPF, and DTF-OP combined flap, postoperative results revealed that the proportional and dimensional evaluation of the constructed auricle was proportionally and dimensionally within 1% deviation to that of a normal ear (see Figure 66-21, *I* and *J*).

Complications in Auricular Reconstruction in the Elderly

The most difficult problem in auricular reconstruction in elderly patients is in the fabrication of the 3-D frame. This is because the harvested costal cartilages are calcified and extremely brittle, and therefore modifications in the fabrication of the 3-D frame may be required. The crus helicis–helical rim unit may not be possible to fabricate as a one-piece unit as for younger patients because of limitations in elasticity and flexibility of the costal cartilages harvested. However, with extreme care in the fabrication of the 3-D frame, it is possible to perform auricular reconstruction in elderly patients.

REPRESENTATIVE ELDERLY AURICULAR RECONSTRUCTION (Figure 66-22). The representative case is a 65-year-old patient with left atypical-type microtia with

a pseudoexternal auditory canal located anteriorly to the normal anatomic location (see Figure 66-22, A and B). With extreme care, the fabrication of the 3-D frame was completed (see Figure 66-22, C) and the pseudoexternal auditory was transposed posteriorly during the first-stage operation. The postoperative results revealed more than satisfactory results and a well-maintained constructed auricle (see Figure 66-22, D).

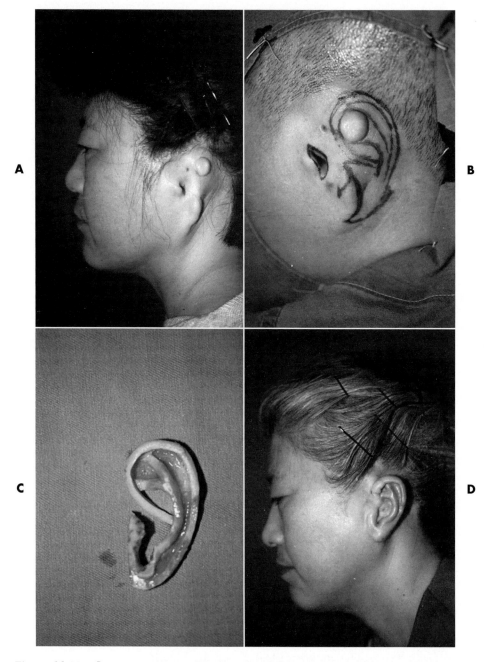

Figure 66-22. Representative case: complicated auricular reconstruction, atypical microtia in the elderly. A, Preoperative appearance of a left atypical-type microtia in a 65-year-old patient. Note a blind pseudoexternal auditory canal located anteriorly to the normal anatomic location. B, Outline for first-stage auricular reconstruction operation. The pseudoauditory canal was transposed posteriorly during the first-stage operation. C, The fabricated 3-D frame. Note that extreme care must be exercised in the fabrication of the 3-D frame because the costal cartilages harvested are usually calcified and brittle. D, The postoperative appearance after the second-stage operation. The constructed auricle is well projected and well maintained.

SUBTOTAL, OR PARTIAL, AURICULAR RECONSTRUCTION

The subtotal, or partial, auricular reconstruction method introduced in this chapter is a one-stage surgical method. Subtotal, or partial, auricular reconstruction is usually of acquired origin. The representative case for this category is of traumatic origin and is further complicated by low hairline.

One-Stage Surgical Method

The schematic illustration of the one-stage surgical method is shown in Figures 66-23 and 66-24. The importance of this method is in the construction and elevation of a combined full-thickness skin (FTS) and UDSTS skin (see Figure 66-23, *C* to *E*) to cover the grafted costal cartilage block fabricated to match the auricular defect (see Figure 66-24, *M* to *P*).

The subepidermal vascular circulation is lacking in the

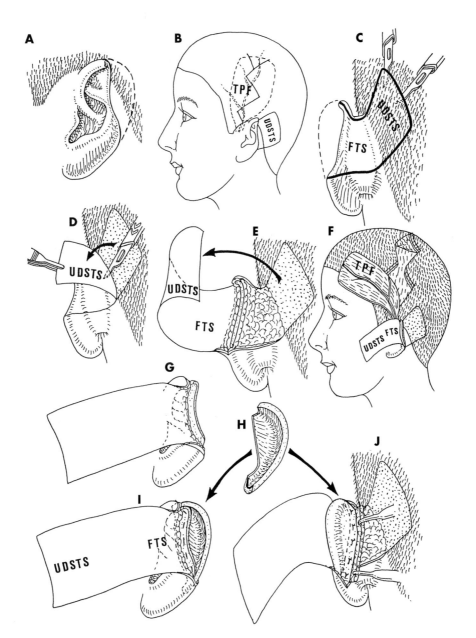

Figure 66-23. One stage subtotal, or partial, auricular reconstruction (part 1). **A,** Illustrated preoperative appearance of a traumatic auricular defect of traumatic origin further complicated with low hairline. **B,** Incision outline for then one-stage subtotal, or partial, auricular reconstruction. **C** to **E,** The elevation of the combined full-thickness skin (FTS) and UDSTS. Note that the skin elevated in the area of hair growth (low hairline) is the UDSTS portion. **F,** The TPF is elevated to cover the surface of the grafted costal cartilage block shaped to the auricular defect. **G,** The auricular cartilage is exposed. **H,** The fabricated costal cartilage block shaped to the auricular defect. **I** and **J,** The fabricated costal cartilage block is fixed to the auricular cartilage with specially fabricated 38-gauge double-armed wire sutures.

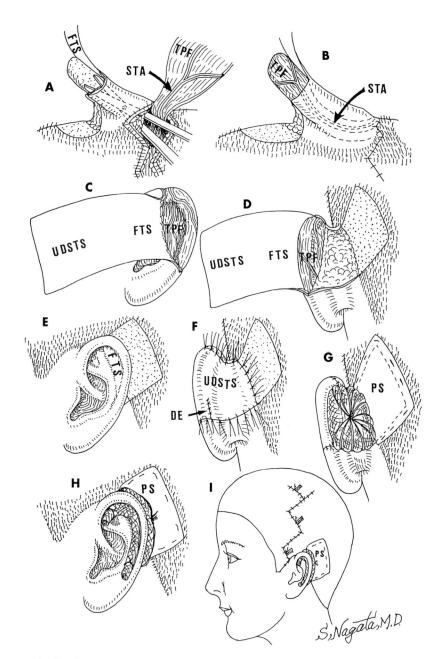

Figure 66-24. One-stage subtotal, or partial, auricular reconstruction (part 2). **A,** Superior view showing the skin tunnel being undermined for the passage of the TPF. **B** to **D,** The TPF completely covers the grafted costal cartilage block. **E,** The FTS portion of the combined FTS-UDSTS skin covers the anterior surface of the auricle. **F,** The UDSTS portion of the combined FTS-UDSTS skin covers the posterior surface of the auricle to the mastoid surface. Excessive skin of the combined FTS-UDSTS skin is excised to avoid dog ear formation *(letters DE, arrow).* **G** and **H,** Mattress sutures and bolster sutures are applied in the same manner as for total auricular reconstruction. Porcine skin with antibiotic ointment is used to cover the raw surface where the UDSTS was elevated. **I,** Illustrated appearance immediately after the one-stage subtotal auricular reconstruction further complicated with low hairline.

UDSTS section of the combined FTS-UDSTS skin, and therefore the TPF is elevated (see Figure 66-23, *F*) to cover the grafted costal cartilage block (see Figure 66-24, *K* to *N*) before being covered with the combined FTS-UDSTS skin.

REPRESENTATIVE CASE (Figure 66-25). A traumatic subtotal reconstruction of the auricle was performed on a patient who had lost part of her left ear resulting from laceration with broken glass. The initial office visit revealed that the partial acquired traumatic defect was further complicated with low hairline (see Figures 66-23, *A,* and 66-25, *A*); therefore the combined FTS-UDSTS skin (see Figure 66-25, *B*) and the TPF were elevated for auricular repair. The results of the one-stage subtotal reconstruction revealed more than satisfactory results and excellent color match with the UDSTS (see Figure 66-25, *C* and *D*).

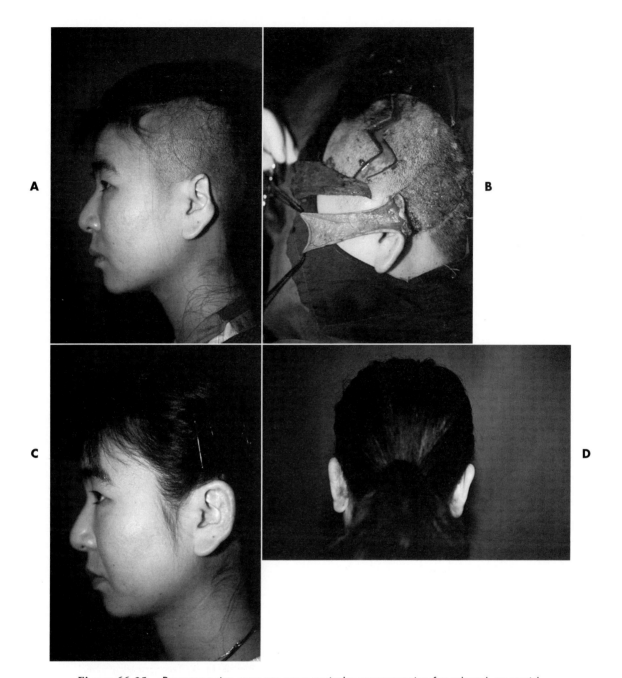

Figure 66-25. Representative case: one-stage auricular reconstruction for subtotal, or partial, auricular defect. **A,** Preoperative appearance of a traumatic subtotal, or partial, auricular defect (laceration caused by broken glass) further complicated with low hairline. **B,** Intraoperative view with the combined FTS-UDSTS. The proximal side portion is the FTS while the distal (forceps) is the UDSTS. **C,** Postoperative lateral view. **D,** Postoperative posterior appearance. The reconstructed auricle is well maintained.

CONCLUSION

It is conclusive that the results of auricular reconstruction are directly dependent on numerous factors, such as the fabrication of the 3-D frame; amount of skin surface area available to cover the fabricated 3-D frame; and the correct knowledge in the use of the UDSTS, TPF, and DPF.

PROPORTIONAL AND DIMENSIONAL EVALUATION OF THE AURICLE

A detailed proportional and dimensional evaluation study has been reported by Hale[18] in which the dimensions of the longitudinal axis were analyzed. The auricular length was 99%, and the width was 55% of the length of the auricle.

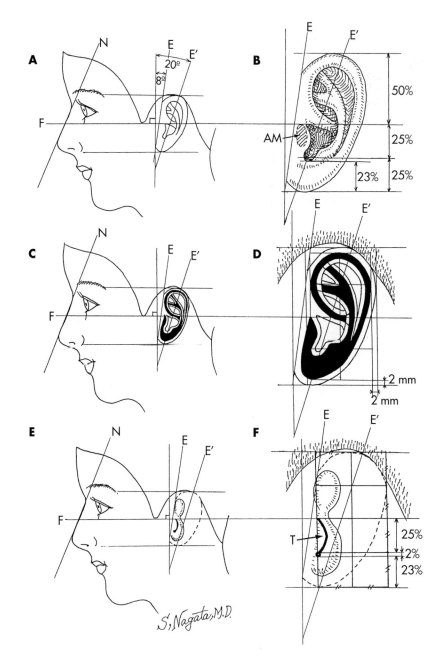

Figure 66-26. Anatomic positioning of the auricle to be constructed. **A,** The normal anatomic location of the auricle in reference to the Frankfurt Horizontal Line (FHL; letter F) is illustrated. **B,** The proportional evaluation of the normal auricle in reference to the FHL is illustrated. **C,** The anatomic position of the auricular cartilage is plotted in reference to the FHL. **D,** The proportional analyses is performed for the auricular cartilage (auricular cartilage + thickness of skin cover). **E,** The outline of the auricular reconstruction site plotted in respect to the FHL. **F,** The 8-square rectangle for the construction of the paper pattern is superimposed on the auricular reconstruction site in reference to the FHL. The tragus portion of the 3-D frame is the first structure of the outline and the remaining procedure for the construction of the paper pattern has been explained in Figure 66-1.

The average anatomic dimensions of an adult auricular cartilage (Japanese) are width of 28 mm and length of 56 mm. Therefore the paper pattern for the fabrication of the 3-D frame is constructed according to the specifications of the proportional and dimensional studies. To simplify the fabrication of the 3-D frame, I constructed 8 squares with the length of one side being 14 mm. The thickness of the skin covering the 3-D frame was calculated as being 1.5 to 2.0 mm[27-31]; therefore extreme care must be exercised during the undermining process for the construction of the skin pocket and the skin flaps to cover the 3-D frame. The total proportional length was analyzed as 99.9%, and the width was 54% of the length of the auricle.

Positioning of the Auricle to be Constructed

The anatomic location of the auricle is calculated by plotting a line through the inferior infraorbital margin and the center of the superior margin of the external auditory meatus; this line is called the Frankfurt horizontal line (FHL; Figure 66-26, *A, C,* and *E*). The FHL can also be considered the same line that connects the incisura anterior with the inferior infraorbital margin because the incisura anterior and the superior margin of the external auditory meatus are located at the same height. With a line drawn parallel to the FHL through the superior and inferior margin of the normal auricle, the distance between these lines is called the *auricular length.* The midpoint of the auricular length has been reported as the incisura anterior[18]; therefore the distance from the FHL to the superior and inferior margin parallel line must be equal in length. The distance from the inferior margin of the intertragic notch to the inferior margin of the ear lobule has been reported to be 23% of the auricular length. By adopting an acceptable degree of deviation of the constructed auricle of 2%, the distance from the incisura anterior to the intertragic notch will be 25% of the auricular length (see Figure 66-26, *B* and *F*). The line of incision and the tragal portion of the 3-D frame must therefore be designed to fit into this area (see Figure 66-26, *B, D,* and *F*), and the skin of the inferior portion of the tragus is removed in a circular fashion with a diameter of 2 mm for the construction of a smooth, U-shaped intertragic notch (see Figure 66-26, *F*).

With careful calculation and fabrication of the 3-D frame and positioning of the auricle to be constructed, it is now possible to reconstruct auricular defects with either total or subtotal (partial) auricular reconstruction.

REFERENCES

1. Aase JM, Tegtmeir RE: Microtia in New Mexico: evidence of multifactorial causation, *Birth Defects* 13:113, 1977.
2. Bellucci RJ, Converse JM: The problem of congenital auricular malformation. I. Construction of the external auditory canal. II. Construction of the auricle in congenital microtia, *Trans Am Acad Ophthalmol Otolaryngol* 64:840, 1980.
3. Bhishagratna KKL: *An English translation of the Susruta Samhita,* Calcutta, 1907, Wilkins Press.
4. Brent B: The correction of microtia with autogenous cartilage grafts. I. The classic deformity, *Plast Reconstr Surg* 66:1, 1980a.
5. Brent B: The correction of microtia with autogenous cartilage grafts. II. Atypical and complex deformities, *Plast Reconstr Surg* 66:13, 1980b.
6. Broadbent TR, Woolf RM: A bilateral approach to the middle ear. In Tanzer RC, Edgerton MT (eds): *Symposium on reconstruction of the auricle,* St Louis, 1974, Mosby.
7. Converse JM, Coccaro PJ, Becker M, et al: On hemifacial microsomia: the first and second branchial arch syndrome, *Plast Reconstr Surg* 51:268, 1973.
8. Converse JM, Wood-Smith D, McCarthy JG, et al: Bilateral facial microsomia: diagnosis, classification, treatment, *Plast Reconstr Surg* 54:413, 1974.
9. Cronin TD: Use of a Silastic frame for total and subtotal reconstruction of the auricle. In Tanzer RC, Edgerton MT (eds): *Symposium on reconstruction of the auricle,* St Louis, 1974, Mosby.
10. Cronin TD: Use of a Silastic frame for total and subtotal reconstruction of the external ear: preliminary report, *Plast Reconstr Surg* 37:399, 1966.
11. Derlacki EL: Pre-operative evaluation of congenital malformations of the conductive hearing mechanism. In Tanzer RC, Edgerton MT (eds): *Symposium on reconstruction of the auricle,* St Louis, 1974, Mosby.
12. Derlacki EL: The role of the otologist in the management of microtia and related malformation of the hearing apparatus, *Trans Am Acad Ophthalmol Otolaryngol* 72:980, 1968.
13. Dupertuis SM, Musgrave RM: Experiences with the reconstruction of the congenitally deformed ear, *Plast Reconstr Surg* 23:361, 1959.
14. Edgerton MT, Nager GT: Surgical reconstruction of the ear for congenital absence, *Transactions of the Fourth International Congress on Plastic Surgery,* Amsterdam, 1969, Excerpta Medica.
15. Erich JB, Abu-Jamra FN: Congenital cup-shaped deformity of the ears: transmitted through four generations, *Mayo Clin Proc* 40:597, 1965.
16. Fukuda O: The microtic ear: survey of 190 cases in 10 years, *Plast Reconstr Surg* 53:458, 1974.
17. Grabb WC: The first and second brachial syndrome, *Plast Reconstr Surg* 36:485, 1965.
18. Hale T: Artistic anatomy, dimensions and proportions of the external ear, *Clin Plast Surg* 5:337, 1978.
19. Hanhart E: Nachweis einer einfach-dominanten, unkomplizieren sowie einer nregelmassig-dominanten, mit Atresia auris, Palatoschisis und anderen Deformationen verbundenen Anlange zu Ohrmuschel-verkummerung (Mikrotie), *Arch der Julius Klaus Stift* 24:374, 1949.
20. Jahsdoerfer RA: Congenital ear atresia. In Tanzer RC, Edgerton MT (eds): *Symposium on reconstruction of the auricle,* St Louis, 1974, Mosby.
21. Kaseff LG: Investigations of congenital malformations of the ears with tomography, *Plast Reconstr Surg* 39:283, 1967.
22. Kessler I: Beobachtung einer uber 6 Generationen eindominant vererbten Mikrotie 1, *Grades HNO* 15:113, 1967.
23. Konigsmark BW: Hereditary deafness in man, *N Engl J Med* 281:713, 1969.
24. Longacre JJ, de Stefano GA, Holmstrand KE: The surgical management of the first and second brachial arch syndromes, *Plast Reconstr Surg* 31:507, 1963.
25. Longenecker CG, Ryan RF, Vincent RW: Malformations of the ear as a clue to urogenital anomalies: report of six additional cases, *Plast Reconstr Surg* 35:303, 1965.
26. Mikowitz S, Mikowitz F: Congenital aural sinuses, *Surg Gynecol Obstet* 118:4, 1964.
27. Nagata S: Total auricular reconstruction with a three-dimensional costal cartilage framework, *Ann Chir Plast Esthet* 40:371, 1995.
28. Nagata S: Secondary reconstruction for unfavorable microtia results: utilizing the temporoparietal and innominate fascia flaps, *Plast Reconstr Surg* 94:254, 1994.

29. Nagata S: A new method for total reconstruction of the auricle for microtia, *Plast Reconstr Surg* 92:187, 1993a.

30. Nagata S: Modification of the stages in total reconstruction of the auricle: Part I. Grafting of the three-dimensional costal cartilage framework for the lobule-type microtia, *Plast Reconstr Surg* 93:221, 1993b.

31. Nagata S: Modification of the stages in total reconstruction of the auricle: Part II. Grafting of the three-dimensional costal cartilage framework for the concha-type microtia, *Plast Reconstr Surg* 93:231, 1993c.

32. Nagata S: Modification of the stages in total reconstruction of the auricle: Part III. Grafting of the three-dimensional costal cartilage framework for the small concha-type microtia, *Plast Reconstr Surg* 93:243, 1993d.

33. Nagata S: Modification of the stages in total reconstruction of the auricle: Part IV. Ear elevation for the constructed auricle, *Plast Reconstr Surg* 93:254, 1993e.

34. Nagata S: A new reconstruction for microtia of the lobule, *Jpn Plast Reconstr Surg* 32:931, 1989.

35. Nagata S: Ear elevation with the use of a semilunar costal cartilage and the temporoparietal fascia flap: I. Lobule type microtia, *Jpn J Plast Reconstr Surg* 10:277, 1990.

36. Nagata S: A new reconstruction for lobule type microtia, *Jpn J Clin Exp Med (Igaku no Ayumi)* 150:540, 1989.

37. Nagata S: A new reconstruction for microtia of the lobule, *Jpn J Plast Reconstr Surg* 32:931, 1989.

38. Nagata S: New method of total reconstruction of the auricle for the lobule type microtia, *Jpn J Plast Reconstr Surg* 8:869, 1988.

39. Nagata S, Fukuda O: A new reconstruction for the lobule type microtia, *Jpn J Plast Reconstr Surg* 7:689, 1987.

40. Nager GT: Congenital aural atresia: anatomy and surgical management, *Birth Defects* 7, 1971.

41. Nauton R, Valvassori G: Inner ear anomalies: their association with atresia, *Laryngoscope* 78:1041, 1968.

42. Ogino Y, Yoshikawa T: Plastic surgery for the congenital anomaly of the ear, *Keisei Geka* 6:79, 1963.

43. Potter EL: A hereditary ear malformation transmitted through five generations, *J Hered* 28:255, 1937.

44. Reisner K: Tomography inner and middle ear malformations: value, limits, results, *Radiology* 92:11, 1969.

45. Rogers B: Microtia, lop, cup and protruding ears: Four directly inherited deformities? *Plast Reconstr Surg* 41:208, 1968.

46. Rogers B: Berry-Treacher Collins syndrome: a review of 200 cases, *Br J Plast Surg* 17:109, 1964.

47. Schuknecht H: Anatomical variants and anomalies of surgical significance (Gavin Livingstone Memorial Lecture), *J Laryngol Otol* 85:1238, 1971.

48. Streeter GL: Development of the auricle in the human embryo, *Carnegie Contrib Embryol* 14:111, 1922.

49. Tagliacozzi G: *De Curtorum Chirurgia per Instionem,* Venice, Italy, 1597, Bindoni.

50. Tanaka F, Ishimori Y, Sekiguchi J: An attempt to perform simultaneously plastic surgery for microtia and creation of the external auditory canal, *Transactions of the Sixth International Congress on Plastic Surgery,* Amsterdam, 1976, Excerpta Medica.

51. Tanzer RC: The constricted (cup and lop) ear, *Plast Reconstr Surg* 55:406, 1975.

52. Tanzer RC: Total reconstruction of the auricle. The evolution of a plan of treatment, *Plast Reconstr Surg* 47:523, 1971a.

53. Tanzer RC: Reconstruction of the auricle in four stages, *Transactions of the Fifth International Congress on Plastic Surgery,* Melbourne, 1971b, Butterworth.

54. Tanzer RC: An analysis of ear reconstruction, *Plast Reconstr Surg* 31:16, 1963.

55. Tanzer RC: Total reconstruction of the external ear, *Plast Reconstr Surg* 23:1, 1959.

56. Taylor WC: Deformity of ears and kidneys, *Can Med Assoc J* 93:107, 1965.

57. Vicent RW, Ryan RF, Longenecker CG: Malformations of ears associated with urogenital anomalies, *Plast Reconstr Surg* 28:214, 1961.

58. Wildervanck LS: Hereditary malformations of the ear in three generations: marginal pits, preauricular appendages, malformation of the auricle and conductive deafness, *Acta Otolaryngol* 54:533, 1962.

Prominent Ears

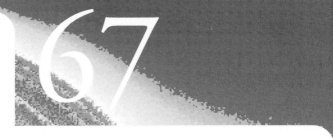

Stefan Preuss
Elof Eriksson

INTRODUCTION

Prominent ears have a normal chondrocutaneous component with an abnormal architecture that can be molded digitally to a normal shape.[29] It does not include the other types of deformed ears, such as lop ear, cup ear, or Stahl's ear. It also does not include the malformed ears in microtia, anotia, and cryptotia. The term *otoplasty* is commonly used for a surgical procedure that reduces the overprojection of an ear of normal size to 17 to 21 mm from the temporal scalp. This chapter describes the main principles of correction and details our preferred method. Incidence, embryology, anatomy, and nonsurgical treatment are discussed briefly.

INDICATIONS

INCIDENCE

It appears that various ear deformities vary in frequency in different parts of the world. For instance, in Japan, where the incidence of ear deformities has been studied carefully, prominent ears occur in 5.5% of infants at 1 year of age. According to Madzharov,[14] protruding ear constitutes the most common ear deformity (38.7%); it is usually bilateral and characterized by a cephaloauricular angle greater than 34 degrees. Appaix et al[2] reported an incidence of approximately 5% in Caucasians. Heredity seems to play a significant role.[9] Rogers[25] showed hereditary morphologic, anatomic, and genetic interrelationships among microtic, constricted, and protruding ears. Two thirds of the patients affected have a positive family history.[24]

EMBRYOLOGY

The auricle develops from the first (mandibular) and second (hyoid) branchial arches. During the sixth week of gestation,

six small tubercles appear on the mandibular and hyoid arches, demonstrating the first signs of development of the external ear. The tubercles develop into a protrusion that gradually increases and is quite prominent in the third month of gestation. During the sixth month, the helical margin curls, the antihelical fold forms, and the antihelical crura appear. According to Brent,[4] anything that interferes with the development of the intrinsic architecture of the ear will result in prominent ears. *Absence of an antihelical fold* is the most common deformity. The conchal scaphal angle can be increased from its normal size of 90 degrees to as much as 150 degrees or more. *Conchal hypertrophy* is the second most common deformity. The abnormalities are usually bilateral and are frequently noted in siblings and parents.[4] A practical way of subdividing the various deformities has been provided by Egloff[8]: (1) conchal hypertrophy, (2) no or insufficient antihelical folding, (3) both of these deformations, or (4) combinations of each of these three categories with lobular protrusion.

ANATOMY

The average height of the ear is 60 to 65 mm.[15,26,33] The width of the ear is usually 35 mm.[15,26,33] At age 3 the ear has achieved 85% of its total growth,[1] and at 5 to 6 years of age the growth is almost completed. Figure 67-1 shows the normal surface anatomy of the ear.

The structures of importance for this discussion are the helix, the antihelix, the concha, the superior and inferior crura, and the lobule. It is important to note that the lower portion of the helix continues in the cauda helicis. The protrusion of the ear from the temporal scalp is usually measured perpendicular to the temporal scalp, and the maximum protrusion is usually found in the upper half of the ear. The arterial supply of the ear comes from the posterior auricular, superficial temporal, and occipital arteries (Figure 67-2). The venous drainage will reach the posterior auricular, superficial temporal, and retromandibular veins. The innervation of the external ear is provided by the greater auricular nerve (C2-C3), the auriculotemporal nerve (V3), the lesser occipital nerve, and the auricular branch of the vagus (Figure 67-3). The lymphatic drainage of the external ear corresponds to its embryologic development. The concha and the meatus drain to the parotid and infraclavicular nodes, whereas the external ear canal and the cranial surface of the auricle drain to the retroauricular and mastoid lymph nodes.

TREATMENT

Nonsurgical Treatment

Nonsurgical correction of prominent ears with splinting has been reported by Japanese authors.[12,17,28] Tan et al[30] have reported on the use of the technique in England and the United States. Tan recommends that splinting be done in the neonatal period in any infant with an auricular deformity in which the ear can be brought into an acceptable shape and position by digital pressure. Several different materials have been used for molding of the deformed ears.[29,30] Most commonly, either a customized splint made of an alginate type of material or an insulated moldable wire is used. The splinting methods are very attractive because of their relative noninvasiveness, but the long-term outcome has yet to be determined.

Surgical Treatment

The goal of the surgical treatment is to create bilaterally symmetric ears that protrude 17 to 21 mm from the temporal scalp and that have a normal-appearing intrinsic anatomy. In principle, the surgical procedures should be uncomplicated, reliable, and adjustable and should allow for individualization to each patient.[9] Each of the three anatomic deformities of the prominent ear (underdevelopment of the antihelical fold, hypertrophy of the concha, and prominence of the lobule) should be evaluated and treated.

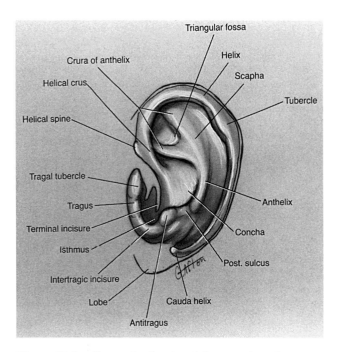

Figure 67-1. Composite drawing of the normal ear. Structures of importance in the surgical correction of prominent ears are helix, antihelix, concha, superior and inferior cruces, and lobule. (From McEvitt W: *Plast Reconstr Surg* 2:481-487, 1947.)

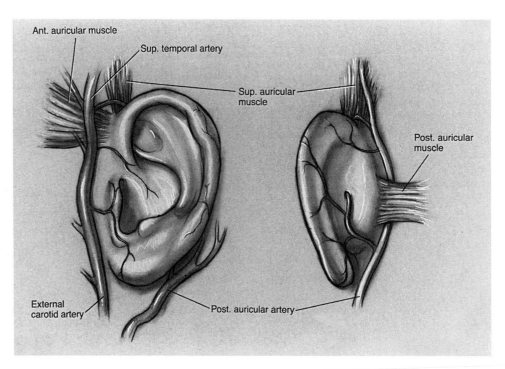

Figure 67-2. Arterial supply of the normal ear. (From Goycoolea MV, Paparella M, Nissen R: *Atlas of otologic surgery,* Philadelphia, 1989, WB Saunders.)

ANESTHESIA

We favor local anesthesia in all adults and most children. The local anesthesia starts with the application of EMLA cream, which is applied at least 1 hour before the procedure. Subsequently, at the beginning of the surgical procedure, the areas of incision are injected with 0.5% lidocaine with epinephrine to which bicarbonate has been added. The injection of the local anesthetic is started on the posterior side of the ear; the anterior surface of the ear is also infiltrated from the posterior side. We have not seen any problems related to the use of epinephrine.

OPERATIONS

POSTERIOR (MEDIAL) APPROACHES TO THE CARTILAGE

Dieffenbach (1845)[7] and later Ely (1881)[10] described how the prominence of the auricle could be reduced by excising skin and conchal cartilage in the cephaloauricular furrow. Their method was further developed by Luckett (1910),[13] who first conceptualized that prominent ears result from failure to form an antihelical fold. McEvitt (1947)[18] and several others

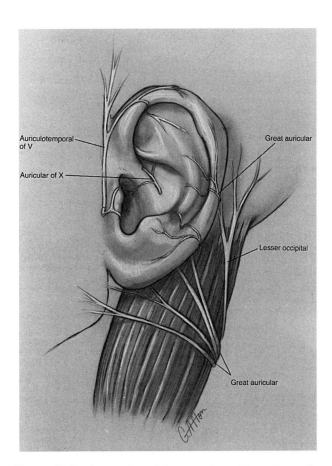

Figure 67-3. Innervation of the normal ear. (From Goycoolea MV, Paparella M, Nissen R: *Atlas of otologic surgery,* Philadelphia, 1989, WB Saunders.)

(Becker,[3] Converse,[6] and Tanzer [32]) created an antihelical fold by multiple parallel incisions from the posterior side of the cartilage (Figure 67-4).

Their goal was focused on creating a smoother antihelix than what Luckett[13] had been able to produce with his excisional technique. Converse (1955)[6] used abrasion from the posterior side of the cartilage to create a fold. Tanzer (1962)[32] suggested a technique in which a cartilage strip was created by two parallel incisions from posterior on either side of the antihelical fold. This partially isolated strip of cartilage was then tubed by the placement of sutures and could in this fashion create an antihelical fold. Morestin (1903)[19] had recommended permanent cartilage sutures in combination with excision in the area of the antihelical fold. Mustardè (1963)[20] described a technique in which a row of permanent mattress sutures was used to form an antihelical fold (Figure 67-5).

ANTERIOR (LATERAL) APPROACHES TO THE CARTILAGE

Gibson and Davis (1958)[11] studied the mechanical properties of ear cartilage. They found that the ear maintains its shape by a balance between the forces of the outer layers of the two sides of the cartilage. If only one layer is incised, the tension on that side is released and the cartilage will bend toward the opposite side. Chongchet (1963)[5] utilized this principle by superficially incising or scoring the anterior surface of the cartilage in the area of the antihelical fold. This method did create an antihelical fold and thus proved the utility of Gibson's findings,[27] but it was difficult to create a smooth fold with this technique. That same year, Stenstrøm (1963)[27] described how the anterior surface of the ear could be scratched with a specially designed rasp and in this way create an antihelical fold. Nordzell (1965)[21] took this principle one step further when he exposed the whole anterior or lateral framework of the ear through a posterior incision and used dermabrading equipment to create an antihelical fold. We prefer to call this an *open otoplasty.*

OPEN OTOPLASTY

We use a technique in which an incision is made through the posterior of the ear to enter the anterior surface of the cartilage. An antihelix is then created with the use of a motorized abrader in the area of the antihelical fold, as well as in the superior and inferior crura. Nordzell[21] originally described this technique in 1965, and in a recent report, he described the outcome of the procedure in 870 patients.[23] Manning et al[16] reported on the use of this technique in 1983.

The posterior incision is then made, and Nordzell described how this incision can be made through skin, cartilage, and anterior perichondrium at the same time (Figures 67-6, 67-7, and 67-8). The incision extends from the upper corner of the fossa triangularis to the antitragus. The anterior surface of the cartilage and perichondrium is then dissected free by elevating the skin. This can usually best be done with either a small

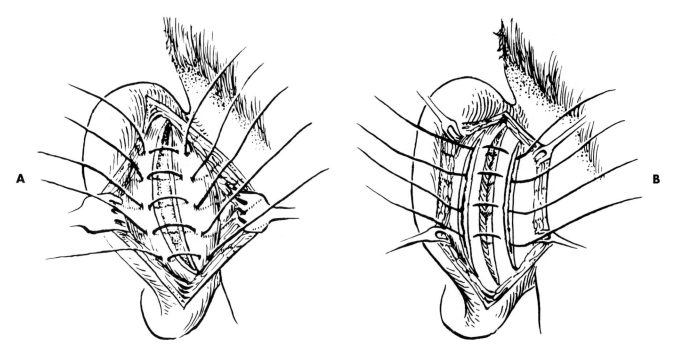

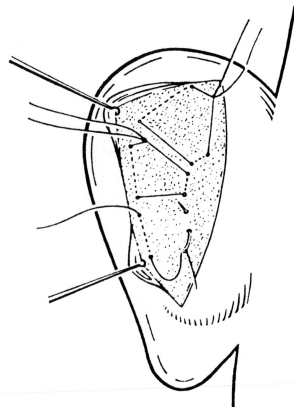

Figure 67-4. **A** to **C,** Evolution of the tubing principle for correction of prominent ears. (From Brent B: Reconstruction of the auricle. In McCarthy JG [ed]: *Plastic surgery,* vol 3, Philadelphia, 1990, WB Saunders.)

Figure 67-5. The Mustardè otoplasty technique. (From Mustardè J: *Br J Plast Surg* 16:172, 1963.)

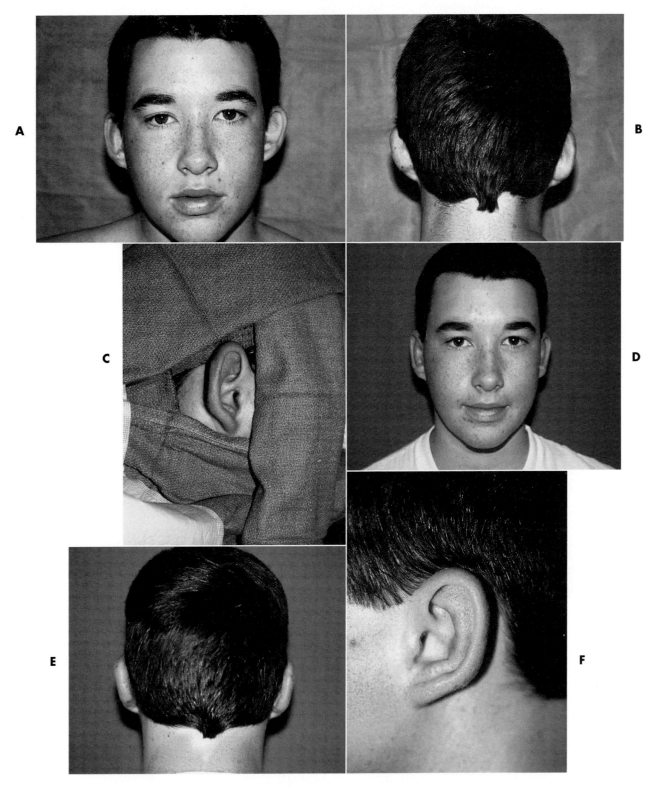

Figure 67-6. Case illustration: open otoplasty. **A** to **C,** Before otoplasty procedure. **D** to **F,** Results 8 weeks after otoplasty procedure.

periosteal elevator or a tenotomy scissors (Figure 67-9). It is very important not to injure the cartilage during this procedure because any break in the cartilage will impair the possibilities of folding in the desired fashion. Before becoming experienced with this technique, the surgeon may prefer to incise the skin first and the cartilage later. It is important to carry the incision anteriorly beyond the superior crux. At the lower end of the incision, the tail of the helix is left in place if it follows the contour of the helix. If it is rotated anteriorly, we prefer to resect it.

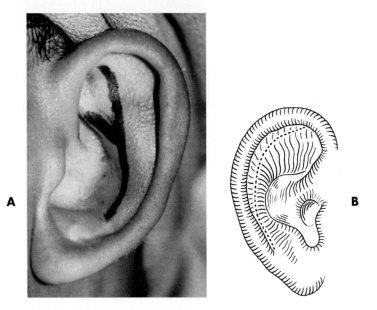

Figure 67-7. **A** and **B,** Planning of posterior auricular incision.

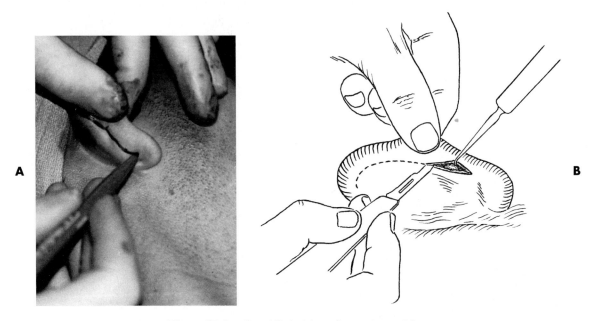

Figure 67-8. **A** and **B,** Incision of posterior auricle.

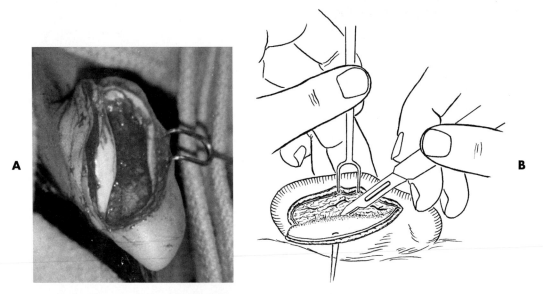

Figure 67-9. **A** and **B,** Dissection of the anterior surface of the cartilage and perichondrium with periosteal elevator and small tenotomy scissors.

The cartilage is then gently supported with a Brown-Adson forceps, and the areas of the antihelix and superior crus are abraded (it is not necessary to use saline irrigation) (Figure 67-10). We prefer a dermabrader with varying speed and an abrading stone with medium coarseness. The abrasion is continued until an antihelical fold has formed and the cartilage behind it is generally parallel to the temporal scalp. If the deformity consists of both a large concha and a missing antihelical fold, the abrasion of the cartilage can be combined with a wedge resection of the concha.

Abrasion of both the superior crus and particularly the inferior crus will allow the upper portion of the ear to fold toward the scalp along a horizontal axis, and this becomes a useful technique in setting back the upper pole of the ear.

If the lower concha and antitragus are very prominent, we prefer to reduce its height by removing a wedge of cartilage extending through the cavum conchae into the area just below the tragus. This not only reduces the height of the lower concha but also makes subsequent adjustments of the lobule much easier.

In general, no excision of skin is ever made in the middle third of the ear. A small excision of skin behind the upper pole and behind the lobule can facilitate the fine adjustment of the contour. It is very important that the ear does not have a "telephone ear" deformity at the end of the procedure. If this is the case, either the upper pole of the ear or the lobule or both needs to be moved closer to the temporal scalp. Tanzer[31] stated that it is desirable to be able to see the helix as the most lateral structure along the whole cartilaginous part of the ear. This is always the goal, but there are quite a few cases in which the helix is lacking its usual anterior curl in the midportion of the ear and one has to accept that the antihelix is slightly more prominent than the helix. This is also commonly seen in nonprominent, nonoperated ears.

When the desired correction of the cartilage framework has been achieved, the incision is closed. A chromic horizontal mattress suture is placed in the middle to upper portion of the ear to make certain that the lateral rim of cartilage becomes positioned behind the medial edge just posterior to the antihelix. Subsequently, the skin incision is usually closed with a running chromic suture. The procedure is quite expeditious and usually takes less than 30 minutes per ear. A dressing consisting of custom-cut strips of cotton moistened in mineral oil is used for packing into the various depressions of the ear. Practical cotton is also placed behind and in front of the ear, and a moderately compressive dressing is applied. This dressing is usually removed 3 days after the operation, and the patient is asked to wear an elastic headband over the ear for the next 2 weeks. The patient is also told not to participate in contact sports for 3 weeks postoperatively.

CONCHAL HYPERTROPHY

If the patient is also lacking an antihelical fold, a large concha can be significantly reduced by placing the antihelical fold more medially in the concha, thus reducing its height. If this is not sufficient, the concha can be further reduced by plicating it to the fascia with permanent sutures. If this still does not give a satisfactory correction, a posterior wedge can be taken out of the conchal cartilage (Figure 67-11). When possible, we prefer to use abrasion first, plication sutures second, and

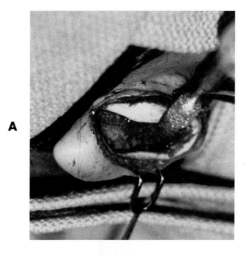

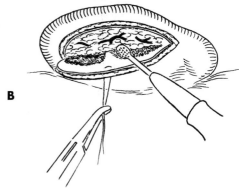

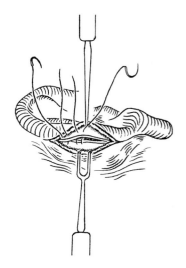

Figure 67-10. **A** and **B,** Abrasion of the antihelix and anterior crux until the formation of an antihelical fold.

Figure 67-11. Reduction of conchal hypertrophy. Excision of a posterior wedge of conchal cartilage and further conchal reduction by placement of plication sutures.

reserve cartilage excision for the most pronounced cases of conchal hypertrophy.

CORRECTION OF THE PROTRUDING LOBULE

There are several techniques for setback of the protruding lobule[13,18,19,20] that usually utilize a combination of skin resection and plicating sutures. If both the lower conchae with the antihelix and the lobule are protruding, we prefer to excise a transverse wedge of cartilage immediately above the antihelix.[9,21] This usually allows the inferior concha and the lobule to be rotated toward the mastoid process. If this is not sufficient, a plicating suture between the cartilage inferior to the antitragus and the fascia overlying the upper sternocleidomastoid muscle usually brings in the lobule. Additional adjustment can be achieved by a skin excision. Nordzell[22] recommends that the overprojecting lobule should be corrected by (1) an excision of the tail of the helix if this is rotated anteriorly and (2) a vertical excision of skin on the posterior side of the lobule.

OUTCOMES

Nordzell studied 80 consecutive patients in detail.[23] He found that five of these patients were *overcorrected by 2 to 3 mm,* and five were judged as slightly *undercorrected by 3 to 4 mm.* Four of the patients had minor cartilage irregularities, in the area of either the helix or the antihelix. Two patients had a significant asymmetry. Of the five undercorrected patients, three required an operation to correct one or both ears. In all three patients, the upper pole of the ear protruded too much. Most patients develop significant swelling and marked ecchymosis after the otoplasty procedure. In Nordzell's study, none of the patients required an operation for evacuation of hematoma, development of infection, or tissue necrosis.[23] The senior author used Mustardè's technique for many years before starting to use the open otoplasty. The technique of Mustardè was significantly more time consuming and also carried a greater risk of undercorrection or recurrence. With the open otoplasty, we have not seen any change in the position of the ear after the initial healing period of approximately 2 months. Similar to the open rhinoplasty, the open otoplasty allows for immediate evaluation of the antihelical fold, and we find it more powerful and versatile than closed techniques.

REFERENCES

1. Adamson P, McGraw B, Tropper G: Otoplasty: critical review of clinical results, *Laryngoscope* 101:883-888, 1991.
2. Appaix A, Pech A, Garcin M, et al: La chirurgie des oreilles decollées, *J Francais OtoRhinoLaryngologie Audiophonologie Chirurgie Maxillo-Faciale* 17:385-398, 1968.
3. Becker O: Correction of the protruding deformed ear, *Br J Plast Surg* 5:187, 1952.
4. Brent B: Acquired auricular deformity: a systemic approach to its analysis and reconstruction, *Plast Reconstr Surg* 59:475, 1977.
5. Chongchet V: A method of antihelix reconstruction, *Br J Plast Surg* 16:268-272, 1963.
6. Converse J, Nigro A, Wilson F, et al: A technique for surgical correction of lop ears, *Plast Reconstr Surg* 15:411-416, 1955.
7. Dieffenbach: *Die Operative Chirurgie,* Leipzig, Germany, 1845, FA Brockhaus.
8. Egloff D, Verdan C, Dupont C: L'oreille prominenté. Classificacion et techniques chirurgicales appropriées, *Ann Chir Plast* 24:291-295, 1979.
9. Elliot R Jr: Otoplasty: a combined approach, *Clin Plast Surg* 17:373-381, 1990.
10. Ely E: An operation for prominence of the auricles, *Arch Otolaryngol* 10:97-101, 1881.
11. Gibson T, Davis W: The distortion of autogenous cartilage grafts: its cause and prevention, *Br J Plast Surg* 10:257-274, 1958.
12. Kurozumi N, Ono S, Ishida H: Non-surgical correction of a congenital lop ear deformity by splinting with Reston foam, *Br J Plast Surg* 35:181-186, 1982.
13. Luckett W: A new operation for prominent ears based on the anatomy of the deformity, *Surg Gynecol Obstet* 10:635-637, 1910.
14. Madzharov M: A new method of auriculoplasty for protruding ears, *Br J Plastic Surg* 42:285-290, 1989.
15. Mallen R: Otoplasty, *Canadian Journal of Otolaryngology* 3:74-78, 1974.
16. Manning B, Finger R, Dibbell D: Diamond burr otoplasty, *Ann Plast Surg* 11:114-120, 1983.
17. Matsuo K, Hayashi R, Kiyono M, et al: *Clin Plast Surg* 17:383-395, 1990.
18. McEvitt W: The problem of the protruding ear, *Plast Reconstr Surg* 2:481-487, 1947.
19. Morestin H: De la reposition et du plissement cosmétiques du pavillon de l'oreille, *Rev Orthop* 14:289, 1903.
20. Mustardè J: Correction of prominent ears using buried mattress sutures, *Br J Plast Surg* 16:170-176, 1963.
21. Nordzell B: A new method for correction of protruding ears, *Acta Chir Scand* 129:317-324, 1965.
22. Nordzell B: Personal communication.
23. Nordzell B: Unpublished data.
24. Rhys Evans P: Prominent ears and their surgical correction, *J Laryngol Otol* 95:881-892, 1981.
25. Rogers B: Microtia, lop, cup and protruding ears: four directly inherited deformities? *Plast Reconstr Surg* 41:208-213, 1968.
26. Rubin L, Bromber B, Walden R, et al: An anatomic approach to the obtrusive ear, *Plast Reconstr Surg* 29:360-369, 1962.
27. Stenstrøm S: A "natural" technique for correction of congenitally prominent ears, *Plast Reconstr Surg* 32:509-518, 1963.
28. Takatoshi Y, Katsunori Y, Satoshi U, et al: Nonsurgical correction of congenital auricular deformities in children older than early neonates, *Plast Reconstr Surg* 4:907-914, 1998.

29. Tan S, Abramson D, MacDonald D, et al: Molding therapy for infants with deformational auricular anomalies, *Ann Plast Surg* 3:263-268, 1997.

30. Tan S, Shibu M, Gault D: A splint for correction of congenital ear deformities, *Br J Plast Surg* 47:575-578, 1994.

31. Tanzer R: An analysis of ear reconstruction, *Plast Reconstr Surg* 31:16, 1963.

32. Tanzer R: The correction of prominent ears, *Plast Reconstr Surg* 30:236-246, 1963.

33. Vuyk H: Cartilage-sparing otoplasty: a review with long term results, *J Laryngol Otol* 111:424-430, 1997.

Index